Lecture Notes in Artificial Intelligence 9238

Subseries of Lecture Notes in Computer Science

More information about this series at http://www.springer.com/series/1244

Willem-Paul Brinkman · Joost Broekens
Dirk Heylen (Eds.)

Intelligent
Virtual Agents

15th International Conference, IVA 2015
Delft, The Netherlands, August 26–28, 2015
Proceedings

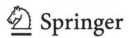 Springer

Editors
Willem-Paul Brinkman
Delft University of Technology
Delft
The Netherlands

Dirk Heylen
University of Twente
Enschede
The Netherlands

Joost Broekens
Delft University of Technology
Delft
The Netherlands

ISSN 0302-9743   ISSN 1611-3349   (electronic)
Lecture Notes in Artificial Intelligence
ISBN 978-3-319-21995-0   ISBN 978-3-319-21996-7   (eBook)
DOI 10.1007/978-3-319-21996-7

Library of Congress Control Number: 2015944453

LNCS Sublibrary: SL7 – Artificial Intelligence

Printed on acid-free paper

Springer International Publishing AG Switzerland is part of Springer Science+Business Media (www.springer.com)

Preface

Welcome to the proceedings of the 15th International Conference on Intelligent Virtual Agents (IVA). IVA is the interdisciplinary annual conference in which leading scientists from around the world present and discuss their latest work on intelligent virtual agents. These agents are interactive characters, which humans can interact with. They often have anthropomorphic elements to evoke responses that humans would exhibit when interacting with other humans. For this, agents could use natural human modalities such as facial expressions, speech, and gesture. Besides interaction modalities, these agents are capable of real-time perception, cognition, and actions in the social environment they operate in. Constructing and studying these IVAs requires knowledge, theories, methods, and tools from a wide range of fields such as computer science, psychology, cognitive sciences, communication, linguistics, interactive media, human–computer interaction, and artificial intelligence.

The IVA conference was started in 1998 as a workshop on Intelligent Virtual Environments at the European Conference on Artificial Intelligence in Brighton, UK, which was followed by a similar one in 1999 in Salford, Manchester, UK. Then dedicated stand-alone IVA conferences took place in Madrid, Spain, in 2001, Irsee, Germany, in 2003, and Kos, Greece, in 2005. Since 2006 IVA has become a full fledged annual international event, which was first held in Marina del Rey, California, then Paris, France, in 2007, Tokyo, Japan, in 2008, Amsterdam, The Netherlands, in 2009, Philadelphia, Pennsylvania, USA, in 2010, Reykjavik, Iceland, in 2011, Santa Cruz, USA, in 2012, Edinburgh, UK, in 2013, and Boston, USA, in 2014.

IVA 2015 was held in Delft, The Netherlands. The special topic of the conference was social training. Increasingly more research aims at utilizing the potential benefits of using intelligent virtual agents in automated training systems in domains with a strong emphasis on the social dimension of human–human interaction. Examples of such training domains are: negotiation, job interviewing, interrogation, aggression or conflict management, patient or customer conversation, but also social environments used for treatment of people with social anxiety or autism. The talks of the three keynote speakers each addressed social training from their own professional perspectives. Gerben van Kleef from the University of Amsterdam discussed emotions as social information, looking at implications for virtual interactions. Page Anderson from Georgia State University in Atlanta talked about how social training in virtual reality could be used to treat patients that suffer from social anxiety disorder. Michaël Bas as co-founder and CEO of Ranj serious games, looked at social training from a game perspective.

IVA 2015 received 70 submissions. Out of the 51 long paper submissions, only 11 papers were accepted as 14-page papers. Furthermore, there were 22 submissions accepted as 10-page papers, and 21 papers were included in the poster and demo track.

This year the conference also included two full-day workshops, one focusing on virtual health agents, and one focusing on engagement in social intelligent virtual agents. In addition four tutorials were given, respectively, on: using annotations for virtual human research; social signal interpretation for virtual agents; design and use of questionnaires in human–computer interaction; and introduction to the virtual human toolkit. A selected group of PhD students were also invited to participate in the doctoral consortium where they discussed their PhD project under the guidance of senior scholars in the field of intelligent virtual agents.

The conference was jointly organized by the University of Twente and Delft University of Technology. The Science Centre Delft was this year's conference venue. IVA conferences always depend on the contribution of a large number of people. For this year, we therefore would like to thank the senior Program Committee for their involvement in the review process, and the members of the Program Committee for their time and effort spent on reviewing all the submissions. Special thanks go to the three keynote speakers for reflection on the special topic. We would also like to thank Khiet Truong and Hannes Högni Vilhjálmsson for organizing the doctoral consortium, Tomoka Koda and Ronald Poppe for organizing the workshops, as well as Maaike Harbers and Marieke Peeters for chairing the poster and demonstration track. We thank the journal *Artificial Intelligence* for sponsoring the PhD students who attended the doctoral consortium. Finally, we would like to express our thanks to Anita Hoogmoed, the conference secretary, who managed the conference administration and logistics.

But all of this would of course not have been possible without all the authors of the various papers included in these proceedings. Their work, effort, and devotion in sharing their insights help the scientific community to move forward in this challenging field of intelligent virtual agents.

June 2015

Willem-Paul Brinkman
Joost Broekens
Dirk Heylen

Organization

Conference Co-chairs

Willem-Paul Brinkman   Delft University of Technology, The Netherlands
Joost Broekens   Delft University of Technology, The Netherlands
Dirk Heylen   Univeristy of Twente, The Netherlands

Doctoral Consortium Co-chairs

Khiet Truong   University of Twente, The Netherlands
Hannes Högni Vilhjálmsson   Reykjavík University, Iceland

Workshop Co-chairs

Tomoko Koda   Osaka Institute of Technology, Japan
Ronald Poppe   Utrecht University, The Netherlands

Poster and Demonstration Co-chairs

Maaike Harbers   Delft University of Technology, The Netherlands
Marieke Peeters   Delft University of Technology, The Netherlands

Conference Secretary

Anita Hoogmoed   Delft University of Technology, The Netherlands

Senior Program Committee

Elisabeth André   University of Augsburg, Germany
Ruth Aylett   Heriot-Watt University, UK
Norman Badler   University of Pennsylvania, USA
Timothy Bickmore   Northeastern University, USA
Jonathan Gratch   University of Southern California, USA
Stefan Kopp   University of Bielefeld, Germany
James Lester   North Carolina State University, USA
Stacy Marsella   Northeastern University, USA
Michael Neff   University of California, Davis, USA
Ana Paiva   Technical University of Lisbon, Portugal
Catherine Pelachaud   CNRS, TELECOM ParisTech, France

Candace Sidner	Worcester Polytechnic Institute, USA
David Traum	University of Southern California, USA
Hannes Högni Vilhjálmsson	Reykjavík University, Iceland
Michael Young	North Carolina State University, USA

Program Committee

Matthew Aylett	University of Edinburgh, UK
Tim Baarslag	University of Southampton, UK
Kirsten Bergmann	University of Bielefeld, Germany
Tibor Bosse	VU University Amsterdam, The Netherlands
Hendrik Buschmeier	University of Bielefeld, Germany
Angelo Cafaro	CNRS-LTCI, TELECOM ParisTech, France
Luísa Coheur	INESC-ID, Portugal
Celso De Melo	University of Southern California, USA
João Dias	Technical University of Lisbon, Portugal
Pedro Fialho	INESC-ID, Universidade de Évora, Portugal
Kerstin Fischer	University of Southern Denmark, Denmark
Mary Ellen Foster	Heriot-Watt University, UK
Patrick Gebhard	DFKI, Germany
Agneta Gulz	Linköping University, Sweden
Helen Hastie	Heriot-Watt University, UK
Koen Hindriks	Delft University of Technology, The Netherlands
Lewis Johnson	Alelo Inc., USA
Sophie Jörg	Clemson University, USA
Iwan de Kok	University of Bielefeld, Germany
Gert-Jan Lelieveld	Leiden University, The Netherlands
Bradford Mott	North Carolina State University, USA
Bilge Mutlu	University of Wisconsin–Madison, USA
Mark Neerincx	Delft University of Technology, TNO, The Netherlands
James Niehaus	Charles River Analytics, USA
Radoslaw Niewiadomski	University of Genoa, Italy
Aline Normoyle	University of Pennsylvania, USA
Elnaz Nouri	University of Southern California, USA
Magalie Ochs	LSIS, France
Rossana Queiroz	PUCRS, Brazil
Lazlo Ring	Northeastern University, USA
Justus Robertson	North Carolina State University, USA
Astrid Rosenthal-von der Pütten	University of Duisburg-Essen, Germany
Nicolas Sabouret	University of Paris-Sud, France
Daniel Schulman	VA Boston Healthcare System, USA
Mei Si	Rensselaer Polytechnic Institute, USA

Contents

Nonverbal Behavior and Gestures

Pedagogical Agents in Health and Training

Turn-Taking

Virtual Agent Perception Studies

Adaptive Dialogue and User Modeling

Towards a Socially Adaptive Virtual Agent

Atef Ben Youssef[1]([⊠]), Mathieu Chollet[2], Hazaël Jones[3], Nicolas Sabouret[1],
Catherine Pelachaud[2], and Magalie Ochs[4]

[1] LIMSI-CNRS UPR 3251, University Paris-Sud, Orsay, France
{atef.ben_youssef,nicolas.sabouret}@limsi.fr
[2] CNRS LTCI, Telecom-ParisTech, Paris, France
{mathieu.chollet,catherine.pelachaud}@telecom-paristech.fr
[3] SupAgro, UMR ITAP, Montpellier, France
hazael.jones@supagro.fr
[4] University Aix-Marseille, LSIS, DiMag, Marseille, France
magalie.ochs@lsis.org

Abstract. This paper presents a *socially adaptive virtual agent* that can adapt its behaviour according to social constructs (e.g. attitude, relationship) that are updated depending on the behaviour of its interlocutor. We consider the context of job interviews with the virtual agent playing the role of the recruiter. The evaluation of our approach is based on a comparison of the socially adaptive agent to a simple scripted agent and to an emotionally-reactive one. Videos of these three different agents in situation have been created and evaluated by 83 participants. This subjective evaluation shows that the simulation and expression of social attitude is perceived by the users and impacts on the evaluation of the agent's credibility. We also found that while the emotion expression of the virtual agent has an immediate impact on the user's experience, the impact of the virtual agent's attitude expression's impact is stronger after a few speaking turns.

Keywords: Social attitudes · Emotions · Affective computing · Virtual agent · Non-verbal behaviour · Adaptation

1 Introduction

Can you imagine a conversation where your interlocutors never change their behaviour, or do not react to your own behaviour? Intelligent virtual agents have the ability to simulate and express affects in dyadic interactions. However, the connection of these expressions with the interlocutor's verbal and non-verbal behaviour remains an open challenge. This results into what we can call "scripted" agents whose behaviour does not change in function of the human user's reactions. Our research motivation is that virtual agents should adapt their affective behaviour to the users' behaviour in order to be credible and to be able to build a relationship with them [32].

A first step in that direction is to build reactive agents that adapt their emotions according to their perceptions. A second step is to also consider long

© Springer International Publishing Switzerland 2015
W.-P. Brinkman et al. (Eds.): IVA 2015, LNAI 9238, pp. 3–16, 2015.
DOI: 10.1007/978-3-319-21996-7_1

term affects such as moods and attitudes. The expression of attitudes by the virtual character allows the human to build a social and affective relationship towards the character during the time of the interaction [32], because the character's behaviour does not only consist of emotional reactions, but also changes depending on the previous behaviours of the human and the previous reactions of the character towards the human's behaviours.

Social attitude can be defined as an affective style that spontaneously develops or is strategically employed in the interaction with a person or a group of persons, colouring the interpersonal exchange in that situation (e.g. being polite, distant, cold, warm, supportive, contemptuous). We propose in this paper an architecture for Socially Adaptive Agents, *i.e.* virtual agents that can adapt their behaviour according to social attitudes that they continuously update as the conversation progresses. More precisely, we propose to build agents that can perceive the non-verbal behaviour of their human interlocutor, build social constructs and adapt their non-verbal behaviour accordingly.

We apply this work to the domain of job interview simulation. We then evaluate our model to measure if this mode leads to more credible and natural agents.

2   Related Works and Theoretical Background

Our work refers to four different domains, as it involves the computation of agent's attitudes in real-time, with social adaptation, in the context of training.

Attitudes: A common representation for attitudes is Argyle's Interpersonal Circumplex [3], a bi-dimensional representation with a *Liking* dimension and *Dominance* dimension. Most modalities are involved in the expression of attitudes: gaze, head orientation, postures, facial expressions, gestures, head movements [6,9]. For instance, wider gestures are signs of a dominant attitude [9], while smiles are signs of friendliness [6]. Models of attitude expression for embodied conversational agents have been proposed in the recent years. Ballin *et al.* propose a model that adapts posture, gesture and gaze behaviour depending on the agents' social relations [4]. Cafaro *et al.* study how users perceive attitudes and personality in the first seconds of their encounter with an agent depending on the agent's behaviour [8]. Ravenet *et al.* propose a model for expressing an attitude as the same time as a communicative intention [27].

Social training background: The idea of using virtual characters for training has gained much attention in the recent years: an early example is the pedagogical agent Steve [18], which was limited to demonstrating skills to students and answering questions. Since then, virtual characters have also been used for training social skills such as public speaking training [12] or job interview training, for instance with the MACH system [15]. However, while the recruiter used in MACH can mimic behaviour and display back-channels, it does not reason on the user's affects and does not adapt to them.

Agents with real-time perception and reaction to affects: Several agent models have proposed to process users' behaviours to infer affects in real-time. Acosta and Ward proposed a spoken dialogue system capable of inferring the user's emotion from vocal features and to adapt its response according to this emotion, which leads to a better perceived *interaction* [1]. Prendinger and Ishizuka presented the Empathic Companion [26], which is capable to use users' physiological signals to interpret their affective state and to produce empathic feedback and reduce the stress of participants. The Semaine project [28] introduced Sensitive Artificial Listeners, *i.e.* virtual characters with different personalities that induce emotions in their interlocutors by producing emotionally coloured feedback. Audio and visual cues are used to infer users' emotions, which are then used to tailor the agent's non-verbal behaviour and next utterance. However the agents' behaviour is restricted to the face, and the agent mainly produces backchannels (*i.e.* listening behaviour). The SimSensei virtual human interviewer is designed to handle a conversation with users about psychological distress [13]. The agent can react to the user's behaviours as well as some higher level affective cues (*e.g.* arousal). However these cues only affect some of the dialogue choices of the agent and its reactive behaviour: no further adaptation is performed, such as long term adaptation of the expressed attitude. We try to overcome these limitations in our own work.

Social adaptation: The relational agent Laura introduced by Bickmore [5] is a fitness coach agent designed to interact with users over a long period of time. They use the amount of times the users interact with Laura as a measure of friendliness, and as the friendliness grows, Laura uses more and more friendly behaviours (*e.g.* smiles, nods, more gestures...). Buschmeier and Kopp [7] describe a model for adapting the dialogue model of an embodied conversational agent according to the common ground between a human and the agent. Their focus is on the dialogical aspect, while we consider the non-verbal dimensions in our work. The video game *Façade* uses unconstrained natural language and emotional gesture expression for all characters, including the player [22]. Its social games have several levels of abstraction separating atomic player interactions from changes in social "score". *Façade*'s discourse acts generate immediate reactions from the characters, it may take story-context-specific patterns of discourse acts to influence the social game score. The score is communicated to the player via enriched, theatrically dramatic performance. Yang et al. [36] analysed the adaptation of a participant body language behaviour to the multi-modal cues of the interlocutor, under two dyadic interaction stances: friendly and conflictive. They use statistical mapping to automatically predict body language behaviour from the multi-modal speech and gesture cues of the interlocutor. They show that people with friendly attitudes tend to adapt more their body language to the behaviour of their interlocutors. This work clearly shows a path to social adaptation, but the mechanism is not based on reasoning on the interlocutor's performance.

As a conclusion, progress has already been achieved in these different domains: from the computation of agent's affects in real-time, to social adaptation in the context of training. To our knowledge there is no system that combines all these aspects in a virtual agent.

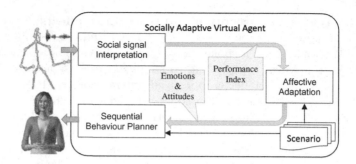

Fig. 1. Overview of our socially adaptative virtual agent architecture

3   Socially Adaptive Agents

Figure 1 presents the architecture of our socially adaptive agent. In our work, the context of the interaction is a one-to-one job interview in which the virtual agent is acting as a recruiter, and is leading the discussion by asking questions or proposing conversation topics to the human participant (interviewee), and reacts in real-time to his/her non-verbal behaviour. However, such a socially adaptive agent could be used in other contexts.

We follow a three-steps architecture. Firstly, a performance index (PI) of interviewee's non-verbal responses is computed using the Social Signal Interpretation (SSI) software [33]. Secondly, the performance index is passed to the affective module which computes the potentially expressed user's emotion and adapts the attitude of the virtual agent toward the interviewee. Lastly, the behaviour planner selects the appropriate social signals to express the emotion and the attitude of the agent. The rendering of this behaviour is based on the Greta/Semaine platform[1].

3.1   Social Signal Interpretation

The performance interpretation consists in evaluating the interviewee's non-verbal behaviour during his/her answer to the virtual agent's utterance. In this work, we only included cues from the interviewee's speech. We plan to include elements from the body language (head movement, crossing hand, etc.) in the computation of the performance index in the future.

We define $PI_d \in [0, 1]$ the detected Performance Index computed by the SSI system [33] as

$$PI_d = \sum_{i=1}^{N} \left(Param^i_{score} \times Param^i_{weight} \right) \tag{1}$$

where $Param^i$ is one the ($N = 5$) following parameters: speech duration, speech delay (hesitating before answering), speech rate, speech volume and pitch variation. The gender-dependency of the last three parameters was taken into account.

---

[1] http://semaine-project.eu/.

$Param^i_{weight}$ is the weight of the ith parameter fixed to $\frac{1}{N}$. The $Param^i_{score}$ is defined such that

$$Param^i_{score} = \left(\frac{Param^i_{detected} - Param^i_{reference}}{Param^i_{detected} + Param^i_{reference}} \right) \qquad (2)$$

where $Param^i_{detected}$ is the detected value using SSI while $Param^i_{reference}$ is the average value computed from a recorded data in preliminary study. This work is described in more details in [2].

3.2 Affective Adaptation

The detected performance index PI_d is compared to an expected one PI_e received from the scenario module that depends on the domain and the interaction situation. In our context of job interview simulation, experts (practitioners from a job centre) have anticipated possible non-verbal reactions from the interviewee to the questions defined in the job interview scenario, and defined values of PI_e accordingly.

Since we want to build a different reaction for good and low performances of the human interlocutor, we separate the affective state space of the virtual agent in two. Let PI^H and PI^L represent the good and low performances, which will lead to positive and negative affects for our virtual recruiter, respectively:

$$PI^H = \begin{cases} 2PI - 1 & if\ PI \geq 0.5 \\ 0 & otherwise \end{cases} \text{ and } PI^L = \begin{cases} 1 - 2PI & if\ PI < 0.5 \\ 0 & otherwise \end{cases} \qquad (3)$$

We compute the virtual agent's emotions by comparing detected PI_d and expected PI_e affect of the user, following the OCC theory of emotions [24]. In this study, we focus on 8 emotions: joy/distress, hope/fear, disappointment, admiration, relief and anger.

Joy follows from the occurrence of a desirable event: we simply assumed that youngster's detected positive index (PI^H_d) increase the joy of the agent. The intensity of joy felt by the agent is defined as:

$$E_f\,(Joy) = PI^H_d \qquad (4)$$

Similarly, *distress* is triggered by the occurrence of an undesirable event PI^L_d. Following the same approach, we define the intensity of *hope* and *fear* using the expected performance index PI^H_e and PI^L_e, respectively.

Disappointment is activated when the expected performance is positive and higher than the detected one: the youngster did not behave as good as the virtual agent expected it:

$$E_f\,(Disappointment) = \max\left(0, PI^H_e - PI^H_d\right) \qquad (5)$$

Similarly, we compute *admiration* (positive expectation with higher detected performance), *relief* (negative expectation with higher detected performance) and *anger* (negative expectation and even worse performance): $\max\left(0, PI_d^H - PI_e^H\right)$, $\max\left(0, PI_e^L - PI_d^L\right)$ and $\max\left(0, PI_d^L - PI_e^L\right)$, respectively.

Using these agent's emotions, we compute the mood of the agent, which represents its long-term affective state, from which we derive its attitude towards the interviewee. The computation of the mood relies on the ALMA model [14] and Mehrabian's theory [23], and is described in [19]. The outcome of this computation is a set of 7 categories of mood: *friendly, aggressive, dominant, supportive, inattentive, attentive* and *gossip*, with values in [0, 1]

Agent's moods are combined with the agent's personality to compute the attitude, following the work by [29] and [34]. The personality is defined, with values in [0, 1] of 5 traits: openness, conscientiousness, extroversion, agreeableness, neuroticism. Consequently, our virtual agent could have one of the 4 following personalities: provocative, demanding, understanding or helpful. For example, an agent with a non-aggressive personality may still show an aggressive attitude if its mood becomes very hostile. The exact combination, based on a logical-OR with fuzzy rules and transformation of categories into continuous values in Isbister's interpersonal circumplex [16], is given in [19]. In short, we obtain n attitude values $(val\,(a))$ positioned in the interpersonal circumplex which are used to compute values on the *friendliness* axis $(Axis_{Friendly})$ and the *dominance* axis $(Axis_{Dominance})$:

$$Friendly = \frac{1}{n}\sum\left(val\,(a_i) \times Axis_{Friendly}\,(a_i)\right) \tag{6}$$

$$Dominance = \frac{1}{n}\sum\left(val\,(a_i) \times Axis_{Dominance}\,(a_i)\right) \tag{7}$$

The levels of dominance and of friendliness represent the global attitude of the agent toward its interlocutor. The values of attitude are stored and their changes serve as inputs, together with the emotions and mood, to the *Sequential Behaviour Planner* for the selection of non-verbal behaviour.

3.3   Sequential Behaviour Planner

The *Sequential Behaviour Planner* module is in charge of planning the virtual agent's behaviour. It receives two inputs. The first input is the next utterance to be said by the virtual agent annotated with communicative intentions (*e.g. ask* a question, *propose* a conversation topic), defined in the scenario module. Communicative intentions are expressed by verbal and non-verbal behaviour, and the planning algorithm makes sure that appropriate signals are chosen to express the input intentions. The second input is the set of emotion values and attitude changes computed by the affective adaptation model presented in the Sect. 3.2.

In this paper, we do not present the emotion expression mechanism, as we merely reuse the existing emotion displays implemented in the Greta/Semaine platform [25]: the novelty of our agent is that we extended the Greta/Semaine platform with the capability for attitude expression. As shown in Sect. 2, attitudes can be displayed through multimodal cues (a smile, a frown, ...). However the context the cues appear in (*i.e.* the signals surrounding the cues) is crucial [20,35].

A smile may be a sign of friendliness, of dominance or even of submissiveness. Some models for attitude expression have already been proposed [4, 8, 27], but they only look at signals independently from each other, that is they do not consider the set of surrounding behaviours. This is the reason why we propose, in our model, to consider sequences of signals rather than signals independently of each other for expressing attitudes.

To choose an appropriate sequence of signals to express an attitude change, our algorithm relies on a dataset of signals sequences observed frequently before this type of attitude change.

Extraction of Sequences of Signals Characteristic of Attitude Changes. In order to obtain sequences of non-verbal signals characteristic of attitude changes, job interviews between human resources practitioners and youngsters performed in a job centre were recorded and annotated at two levels, the non-verbal behaviour of the recruiter and the expressed attitude of the recruiter. More details on the annotation process can be found in [11].

The attitude annotations are analysed to find the timestamps where the attitudes of the recruiters vary. The non-verbal signals annotation streams are then segmented using the attitude variations timestamps, and the resulting segments are regrouped in separate datasets depending on the type of attitude variation (we define 8 attitude variation types for: large or small rise or fall on the dominance or friendliness dimension). For instance, we obtain a dataset of 79 segments leading to a large drop in friendliness, and a dataset of 45 segments leading to a large increase in friendliness.

These datasets of sequences happening before a type of attitude variation are then mined by giving them as input to the Generalized Sequence Pattern (GSP) frequent sequence mining algorithm described in [30]. The GSP algorithm requires a parameter Sup_{min}, *i.e.* the minimum number of times a sequence happens in the dataset to be considered frequent. This algorithm follows an iterative approach: it begins by retrieving all the individual items (*i.e.* in our case, non-verbal signals) that happen at least Sup_{min} times in the dataset. These items can be considered as sequences of length 1: the next step of the algorithm consists in trying to extend these sequences by appending another item to them and checking if the resulting sequence occurs at least Sup_{min} times in the dataset. This step is then repeated until no new sequences are created. We run the GSP algorithm on each dataset and obtain frequent sequences for each kind of attitude variation. We also compute the *confidence* value for each of the extracted frequent sequences: confidence represents the ratio between the number of occurrences of a sequence before a particular attitude variation and the total number of occurrences of that sequence in the data [31].

Non-verbal Signals Sequences Planning. The Sequential Behaviour Planner takes as input an utterance to be said by the agent augmented with information on the communicative intentions it wants to convey. The planning algorithm starts by generating a set of *minimal non-verbal signals sequences* that express the communicative intentions. These *minimal sequences* are computed to make sure that the communicative intentions are expressed by the adequate signals.

Then, the algorithm creates *candidate sequences* from the *minimal sequences* by enriching them with additional non-verbal signals. We designed a Bayesian Network (BN) to model the relationship between pairs of adjacent signals and with the different attitude variations, and trained it on our corpus. Taking a *minimal sequence* as input, the algorithm looks for the available time intervals. It then tries to insert every kind of non-verbal signals considered in the network into this interval and computes the probability of the resulting sequence: if that probability exceeds a threshold , the sequence is considered as a viable *candidate sequence* and carries over to the next step.

Once the set of *candidate sequences* has been computed, the selected sequence is obtained using a majority-voting method derived from [17]. Full details on the Sequential Behaviour Planner can be found in [10].

4   Evaluation

The context of our study is job interview simulation. The developed virtual recruiter is capable of perceiving the participant's behaviour. It simulates emotions and attitudes dynamics and expresses them. We performed an experiment to evaluate whether our model of social adaptation improves the perception of the agent by users.

4.1   Experimental Setting

We used two different configurations for the socially adaptive virtual agent (and two different job seekers). Each configuration corresponds to a different set of values for the personality, the recruiter's questions and the corresponding expectations: one agent is considered as more demanding, while the other is supposed to have a more understanding personality.

We achieved the subjective evaluation through an online questionnaire. Each evaluator watched four scenes presenting the **agent-applicant dialogue**. The scenes were presented to the evaluators in a correct temporal order to evaluate the dynamic of the social model over time. Each scene was presented with three different conditions, followed by a set of questions to answer to. What changes from one condition to the other is the non-verbal behaviour of the agent, which correspond to three different versions of the virtual agent. Each condition was presented in a different video clip, where the evaluators could concentrate on the observation of the agent's non-verbal behaviour and compare the three conditions. The first condition of the agent is a scripted agent with predefined behaviour. During the answer phase, the agent occasionally shows affective behaviours (*i.e.* predefined emotions and attitude), regardless of the input. Note that the agent's behaviour is not exaggerated in our model. The second condition of the agent expresses emotions computed by our affective model, during the question phase. The role of

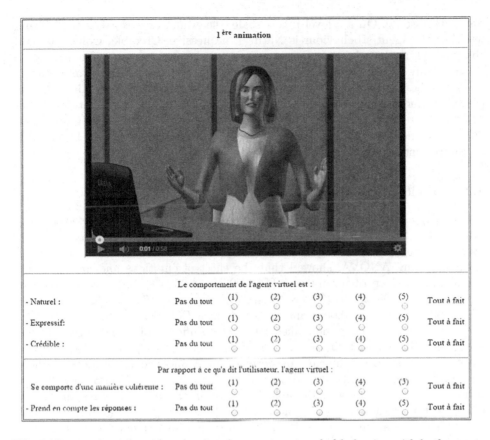

Fig. 2. Screen-shot of a video showing the agent non-verbal behavior with both agent and applicant speech

this condition is to verify that the computation of affects does not have a negative impact on the perception of the agent's behaviour (actually, our hypothesis is that it should improve the quality of the agent). The third virtual agent condition is the socially adaptive agent that displays both emotion and attitude computed from the applicant's behaviour. It is also the configuration that was used to collect the data.

With the two variants for the personality of the agent (demanding or understanding), we have a total of 24 videos (2 variants × 4 scenes × 3 agent versions). Evaluators could assess either the demanding or understanding agent, but each evaluator had to evaluate the three animations for each four scenes.

The subjective tests were performed by 83 evaluators (29 with the understanding variant and 54 with the challenging one), aged between 22 and 79 years old. 33 evaluators were males and 50 were females. 45 were already familiar with subjective evaluation tests while the remaining 38 were not. 51 of the participants were native speakers.

Our subjective evaluation is based on a questionnaire that was presented after each one of the 4 animations corresponding to 3 different versions of agent for a given scene. On a 5-level Likert scale, the evaluator was asked to indicate whether the agent's behaviour is Natural, Expressive, Credible, Coherent with the job seeker's speech, and takes into account what the human participant said (Consideration). In addition, the evaluator was asked to rank the 3 animations, from the best (*i.e.* 1) to the worst (*i.e.* 3). The goal of this ranking was to perform a forced A/B/C test: comparison of the 3 versions in order to obtain a "global impression". Figure 2 presents an example of a video of a random and anonym version of agent displaying agent's non-verbal behavior with both agent and applicant speech.

4.2   Results and Discussion

Figure 3a presents the results of evaluators' perception of the different agent versions. On all five criteria, the emotion-only agent outperforms the scripted agent and the socially adaptive agent outperforms the two other ones. An analysis of variance, using ANOVA, showed that the effect of emotions and attitude was significant on term of naturalness ($F(2, 993) = 4.93, p < 0.01$), expressiveness ($F(2, 993) = 11.69, p < 10^{-5}$), credibility ($F(2, 993) = 3.15, p < 0.05$), coherence ($F(2, 993) = 5.27, p < 0.005$) and consideration ($F(2, 993) = 10.16, p < 10^{-4}$). Post hoc analyses using the Tukey's honest significant difference criterion for significance indicated that the differences between the scripted version and the emotion version are significant on term of naturalness, expressiveness, coherence and consideration ($p < 0.05$) and are significant for all criteria between the scripted agent and the socially adaptive agent ($p < 0.05$). The first important result in this evaluation is that an emotional agent is judged as more natural and coherent than an agent using predefined emotions (independent from the participant's reaction). This validates our cognitive model for computing affects, presented in Sect. 3.2. Moreover, it shows that the expression of affects, as we have achieved it (see Sect. 3.3), has a positive impact on the user's perception of

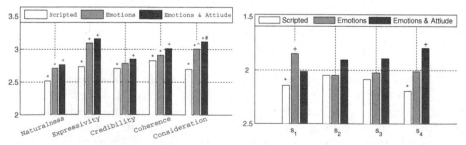

(a) Average evaluators' perception of the different agent versions

(b) Average rank of the agent during each scene

Fig. 3. Results of the evaluation of the virtual agent's behaviour over 83 participants.* denotes significant differences ($p < 0.05$) found from $^+$. Similarly, ^denotes a quasi-significant difference ($p < 0.08$) from $^\#$, using ANOVA.

the agent's behaviour. The second important result is that expressing emotions and attitude improves the performance of the agent on all criteria: the participants did notice the difference in the non-verbal behaviour when the attitude is implemented. This validates the attitude expression model in the behaviour planner presented in Sect. 3.3.

Figure 3b presents the evolution of the evaluation over the 4 scenes. For the first scene s_1, people rank the scripted agent between 2nd and 3rd on average, and the agent with emotions, on the contrary, is the 1st. It shows that towards the end (last scenes s_3 and s_4), the agent expressing and adapting its attitude is ranked better than the agent with only emotions, itself ranked better than the scripted agent, while this is not the case in the first scene. In the ranking result, the difference between the different agents version is not significant in the beginning of the interaction ($F(2, 249) = 2.83, p < 0.07$). Post hoc analyses using the Tukey's honest significant difference criterion show a significant difference between the emotional agent and the scripted agent ($p < 0.02$), in the first scene s_1. The difference with the adaptive agent becomes visible only after a few speaking turns and is significant at the end of the interview s_4 ($F(2, 243) = 5.14, p < 0.01$). Note that these results are derived form both understanding and demanding agents. There is a slight difference between these 2 variants. However, we have the same tendency with the same conclusion.

This confirms the hypothesis that our social and affective adaptation model makes the agent behaviour evolve during the interview, which impacts the perception that the user has of the agent over time. This corresponds to the idea that social attitude is a long-term mechanism, that may not have immediate effects on the interlocutor. In our affective model, the attitude value is only changing slowly (while the emotional reaction is immediate) : the adaptation process becomes visible after a few minutes of conversation.

5   Conclusion and Future Work

In this paper, we propose an architecture for a socially adaptive agent in the context of dyadic interactions. Our virtual agent is able to analyse the behaviour of the human participant, to update a cognitive model with social constructs (*e.g.* attitude, relationship) depending on the behaviour of their interlocutor, and to show coherent social attitude expression. This approach has been evaluated in the context of job-interview simulation, by comparing the behaviour of our agent with a scripted and a reactive approach. Results show that our socially adaptive agent performs significantly better in term of naturalness, expressiveness, credibility, coherence and user's consideration. It also shows that, while the emotion expression has an immediate impact on the user's experience, the attitude expression's impact is stronger after a longer period of time. The impact on the evaluation of the agent's credibility increases as the interview progresses. While most evaluations in the literature rely on immediate reactions, we show that adaptation takes time and is visible after few minutes of interaction.

Our model strongly relies on the computation of the performance index. We intend to consider additional signals to compute this performance index such as body language (head movements, crossing hands, postures, ...) and facial expressions (smile, surprise, ...). Yet, this performance index is currently seen as an exact value, while it is computed from social cues detected with perception software that can produce errors. The next version of our socially adaptive agent should rely on an extended model with uncertainty values. A second extension would be to consider the social cues as possible inputs to the non-verbal behaviour planner, to better control the coherence and credibility of the agent's behaviour. Indeed, several research works show that the agent's reaction should not only be based on internal mental state, but also on adaptation mechanisms to the interlocutor's expressed emotions [21, 36]. Lastly, we believe that allowing the agent to reason about the actual and potential behaviour of the interlocutor, following a Theory of Mind paradigm, will lead to a more credible decision process both for the dialogue model and for the appraisal mechanism.

References

1. Acosta, J.C., Ward, N.G.: Achieving rapport with turn-by-turn, user-responsive emotional coloring. Speech Commun. **53**(9–10), 1137–1148 (2011)
2. Anderson, K., André, E., Baur, T., Bernardini, S., Chollet, M., Chryssafidou, E., Damian, I., Ennis, C., Egges, A., Gebhard, P., Jones, H., Ochs, M., Pelachaud, C., Porayska-Pomsta, K., Rizzo, P., Sabouret, N.: The TARDIS framework: intelligent virtual agents for social coaching in job interviews. In: Reidsma, D., Katayose, H., Nijholt, A. (eds.) ACE 2013. LNCS, vol. 8253, pp. 476–491. Springer, Heidelberg (2013)
3. Argyle, M.: Bodily Communication. University paperbacks, Methuen (1988)
4. Ballin, D., Gillies, M., Crabtree, B.: A framework for interpersonal attitude and non-verbal communication in improvisational visual media production. In: First European Conference on Visual Media Production, pp. 203–210 (2004)
5. Bickmore, T.W., Picard, R.W.: Establishing and maintaining long-term human-computer relationships. ACM Trans. Comput. Hum. Interact. (TOCHI) **12**(2), 293–327 (2005)
6. Burgoon, J.K., Buller, D.B., Hale, J.L., Turck, M.A.: Relational messages associated with nonverbal behaviors. Hum. Commun. Res. **10**(3), 351–378 (1984)
7. Buschmeier, H., Baumann, T., Dosch, B., Kopp, S., Schlangen, D.: Combining incremental language generation and incremental speech synthesis for adaptive information presentation. In: Proceedings of the 13th Annual Meeting of the Special Interest Group on Discourse and Dialogue, pp. 295–303 (2012)
8. Cafaro, A., Vilhjálmsson, H.H., Bickmore, T., Heylen, D., Jóhannsdóttir, K.R., Valgarsson, G.S.: First impressions: users' judgments of virtual agents' personality and interpersonal attitude in first encounters. In: Nakano, Y., Neff, M., Paiva, A., Walker, M. (eds.) IVA 2012. LNCS, vol. 7502, pp. 67–80. Springer, Heidelberg (2012)
9. Carney, D.R., Hall, J.A., LeBeau, L.S.: Beliefs about the nonverbal expression of social power. J. Nonverbal Behav. **29**(2), 105–123 (2005)

10. Chollet, M., Ochs, M., Pelachaud, C.: From non-verbal signals sequence mining to bayesian networks for interpersonal attitudes expression. In: Bickmore, T., Marsella, S., Sidner, C. (eds.) IVA 2014. LNCS, vol. 8637, pp. 120–133. Springer, Heidelberg (2014)
11. Chollet, M., Ochs, M., Pelachaud, C.: Mining a multimodal corpus for non-verbal signals sequences conveying attitudes. In: International Conference on Language Resources and Evaluation, Reykjavik, Iceland, May 2014
12. Chollet, M., Sratou, G., Shapiro, A., Morency, L.-P., Scherer, S.: An interactive virtual audience platform for public speaking training. In: Proceedings of the 2014 International Conference on Autonomous Agents and Multi-agent Systems, AAMAS 2014, pp. 1657–1658. Richland, SC (2014)
13. Artstein, R., Benn, G., Dey, T., Fast, E., Gainer, A., Georgila, K., Gratch, J., Hartholt, A., Lhommet, M., et al.: Simsensei kiosk: a virtual human interviewer for healthcare decision support. In: Proceedings of the 2014 International Conference on Autonomous agents and Multi-Agent Systems, pp. 1061–1068 (2014)
14. Gebhard, P.: ALMA - A layered model of affect. Artificial Intelligence, pp. 0–7 (2005)
15. Hoque, M.E., Courgeon, M., Martin, J.-C., Mutlu, B., Picard, R.W.: Mach: my automated conversation coach. In: Proceedings of the 2013 ACM International Joint Conference on Pervasive and Ubiquitous Computing, pp. 697–706. ACM (2013)
16. Isbister, K.: Better Game Characters by Design: A Psychological Approach (The Morgan Kaufmann Series in Interactive 3D Technology). Morgan Kaufmann Publishers Inc., San Francisco (2006)
17. Jaillet, S., Laurent, A., Teisseire, M.: Sequential patterns for text categorization. Intell. Data Anal. 10(3), 199–214 (2006)
18. Johnson, W.L., Rickel, J.: Steve: an animated pedagogical agent for procedural training in virtual environments. ACM SIGART Bull. 8(1–4), 16–21 (1997)
19. Jones, H., Sabouret, N.: TARDIS - A simulation platform with an affective virtual recruiter for job interviews. In: IDGEI (2013)
20. Keltner, D.: Signs of appeasement: evidence for the distinct displays of embarrassment, amusement, and shame. J. Pers. Soc. Psychol. 68, 441–454 (1995)
21. Kendon, A.: Movement coordination in social interaction: some examples described. Acta Psychol. 32, 101–125 (1970)
22. Mateas, M., Stern, A.: Structuring content in the façade interactive drama architecture. In: Proceedings of Artificial Intelligence and Interactive Digital Entertainment (AIIDE), pp. 93–98 (2005)
23. Mehrabian, A.: Pleasure-arousal-dominance: a general framework for describing and measuring individual differences in temperament. Curr. Psychol. 14(4), 261 (1996)
24. Ortony, A., Clore, G.L., Collins, A.: The Cognitive Structure of Emotions. Cambridge University Press, Cambridge (1988)
25. Poggi, I., Pelachaud, C., de Rosis, F., Carofiglio, V., De Carolis, B.: Greta. a believable embodied conversational agent. In: Stock, O., Zancanaro, M. (eds.) Multimodal Intelligent Information Presentation, pp. 3–25. Springer, The Netherlands (2005)
26. Prendinger, H., Ishizuka, M.: The empathic companion: a character-based interface that addresses users' affective states. Appl. Artif. Intell. 19(3–4), 267–285 (2005)

27. Ravenet, B., Ochs, M., Pelachaud, C.: From a user-created corpus of virtual agent's non-verbal behavior to a computational model of interpersonal attitudes. In: Aylett, R., Krenn, B., Pelachaud, C., Shimodaira, H. (eds.) IVA 2013. LNCS, vol. 8108, pp. 263–274. Springer, Heidelberg (2013)
28. Schroder, M., Bevacqua, E., Cowie, R., Eyben, F., Gunes, H., Heylen, D., Ter Maat, M., McKeown, G., Pammi, S., Pantic, M., et al.: Building autonomous sensitive artificial listeners. IEEE Trans. Affect. Comput. 3(2), 165–183 (2012)
29. Snyder, M.: The influence of individuals on situations: implications for understanding the links between personality and social behavior. J. Pers. 51(3), 497–516 (1983)
30. Srikant, R., Agrawal, R.: Mining sequential patterns: generalizations and performance improvements. Adv. Database Technol. 1–17, 1996 (1057)
31. Tan, P.-N., Steinbach, M., Kumar, V.: Introduction to Data Mining, 1st edn. Addison-Wesley Longman Publishing Co. Inc., Boston (2005)
32. Vardoulakis, L.P., Ring, L., Barry, B., Sidner, C.L., Bickmore, T.: Designing relational agents as long term social companions for older adults. In: Nakano, Y., Neff, M., Paiva, A., Walker, M. (eds.) IVA 2012. LNCS, vol. 7502, pp. 289–302. Springer, Heidelberg (2012)
33. Wagner, J., Lingenfelser, F., Baur, T., Damian, I., Kistler, F., André, E.: The social signal interpretation (ssi) framework-multimodal signal processing and recognition in real-time. In: Proceedings of the 21st ACM International Conference on Multimedia, Barcelona, Spain (2013)
34. Wegener, D.T., Petty, R.E., Klein, D.J.: Effects of mood on high elaboration attitude change: the mediating role of likelihood judgments. Eur. J. Soc. Psychol. 24(1), 25–43 (1994)
35. With, S., Kaiser, W.S.: Sequential patterning of facial actions in the production and perception of emotional expressions. Swiss J. Psychol. 70(4), 241–252 (2011)
36. Yang, Z., Metallinou, A., Narayanan, S.: Analysis and predictive modeling of body language behavior in dyadic interactions from multimodal interlocutor cues. IEEE Trans. Multimedia 16(6), 1766–1778 (2014)

An Ontology-Based Question System for a Virtual Coach Assisting in Trauma Recollection

Myrthe Tielman[1]([✉]), Marieke van Meggelen[3], Mark A. Neerincx[1,2], and Willem-Paul Brinkman[1]

[1] Delft University of Technology, Delft, The Netherlands
{m.l.tielman,w.p.brinkman,m.a.neerincx}@tudelft.nl
[2] TNO Human Factors, Soesterberg, The Netherlands
[3] Erasmus University Rotterdam, Rotterdam, The Netherlands
m.vanmeggelen@fsw.eur.nl

Abstract. Internet-based guided self-therapy systems provide a novel method for Post-Traumatic Stress Disorder patients to follow therapy at home with the assistance of a virtual coach. One of the main challenges for such a coach is assisting patients with recollecting their traumatic memories, a vital part of therapy. In this paper, an ontology-based question system capable of posing appropriate and personalized questions is presented. This method was tested in an experiment with non-patients ($n = 24$), where it was compared with a non-ontology-based system which did not provide personalization. Results show that people take more time answering questions with the ontology-based system and use more words describing properties, such as adjectives. This indicates that the ontology-based system facilitates more thoughtful and detailed memory-recollection.

Keywords: Virtual coach · PTSD · Dialogue system · Ontology · Memories

1 Introduction

Post-Traumatic Stress Disorder (PTSD) is a mental disorder caused by one or more traumatic experiences [1]. Several treatments for PTSD are available, with the most common element being exposure, which is the process of exposing patients to their traumatic memories [8]. One problem for PTSD treatment is that there is often a barrier to talk about problems and a stigma on seeking help from the mental health-care system. One new method for exposure treatment for PTSD which addresses this issue is, a self-therapy system with a virtual coach [7,16]. With such a system, patients follow their therapy at home behind their computer with the assistance of a virtual coach and a human therapist is only remotely involved. One of the main challenges for a virtual coach in such a self-therapy system is providing the assistance PTSD patients need for exposure sessions. PTSD patients often have fragmented memories of their trauma

© Springer International Publishing Switzerland 2015
W.-P. Brinkman et al. (Eds.): IVA 2015, LNAI 9238, pp. 17–27, 2015.
DOI: 10.1007/978-3-319-21996-7_2

and are very reluctant to recall them, requiring detailed questions to stimulate memory retrieval. For a virtual coach to know which questions to ask, it needs some understanding of the traumatic experience and the personal story of the patient. Aside from needing detailed and personalized questions, it is also important to get it right, because of the sensitivity of the topic. To solve this problem, we propose an ontology-based conversational system with minimal natural-language processing with which a virtual coach can pose relevant and personalized questions to assist individuals with memory recollection.

For our system we envision that our virtual coach can apply similar techniques for motivation and behavioral change as human coaches would, and can achieve the same effect, even though patients know they are interacting with a digital agent. Blanson-Henkemans et al. [6] already showed that a virtual coach with emotional facial expressions can motivate people to live a healthier life, and Bickmore et al. [4] showed the effectiveness of an application with virtual character to elicit healthier behavior in older adults. For mental health-care, virtual characters have been employed for complex user groups such as people suffering from depression [11]. For PTSD, Rizzo et al. [14] developed the SimCoach, a virtual coach guiding veterans who potentially have PTSD towards treatment. Even though virtual avatars have some limitations compared to human coaches, such as the lack of full language abilities, they also have their own advantages, like full-time availability. Moreover, the anonymous nature of a virtual character can increase self-disclosure by patients [10].

Despite a lack of full natural language capabilities, virtual agents which can communicate with humans in a meaningful way have been developed. Schulman et al. [15] developed a conversational agent using Motivational Interviewing (MI, [12]) for health-behavior change. Their method relied on multiple-choice and free text input based on which specific dialogue acts for MI were selected. Also considering MI, Friedrichs et al. [9] developed a system which repeats back utterances of the user and employs multiple-choice input to personalize the content. Both these systems have been evaluated with users, showing that even without natural language understanding a system can hold a personalized and meaningful dialogue with a user and elicit behavior change.

Ontologies are often used in dialogue systems to add additional meaning and world knowledge. For example, Bickmore et al. [5] developed an ontology-based counseling framework which described a patient's mental states and therapist's actions affecting these states. Another possible use of ontologies is to add meaning to the speech of the agent itself, something often used for chatbots [2,3]. This shows that ontologies can be used in dialogue systems to add knowledge and meaning. In this paper, we propose to use ontologies in such a way that they assist in interpreting the user input, to steer the conversation towards its goal, and giving meaning to the dialogue of the virtual agent.

2   Ontology

Several definitions of the term *ontology* have been proposed. In this paper we use the working definition as formulated by Noy & McGuiness [13], where an ontology is *a formal explicit description of concepts in a domain of discourse (classes) properties of each concept describing various features and attributes of the concepts (slots), and restrictions on properties.* Ontologies enable a structured knowledge base of a domain. For trauma, this means that the ontology allows a system to have an understanding of traumatic events. It could understand, for instance, that whenever an abuse victim never mentions a perpetrator, something is missing from the discourse and the system should ask an appropriate question.

The first thing to consider when designing an ontology for a question system is the type of the expected answers. For this paper, we consider the possibilities of the self-therapy Multi-Modal Memory Restructuring system (3MR) [7]. This system allows users to employ different types of media, namely text, images, music, video, google maps, websites, and emotion labels. For a user, all these are available to expose them to their memory and a question system can employ these as possible answers. An example would be the question *Where did this happen?*, which might be answered in the form of text, but also through adding a map. For this reason, our ontology is based around these types of media.

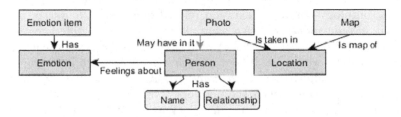

Fig. 1. Section of an ontology based on diary items in the 3MR system, showing the types Emotion, Photo and Map and its relations and properties.

Figure 1 shows an example of an ontology based on types of answers. In this way, every answer type has properties, which can again be instances of other classes again having their own properties. Which classes and properties these are, is determined by the type of memory one wants to retrieve. For a war veteran, the location of the trauma in a foreign country is very relevant, while for abuse victims this might be the type of room they were in.

3   Question System

Together with the ontology, a question dialogue based on this ontology needs to be in place. The ontology led the design of the natural language questions, whenever a specific item was entered, such as a photo, the resulting questions could be derived from the ontology. Whenever the ontology was not specific enough to decide on the order of the questions (for instance what to start with), a basic *when, where, who, what,* paradigm was used. We asked for both memories relating to a general time period and those relating to a specific moment.

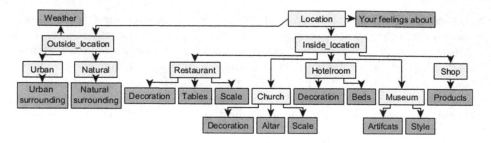

Fig. 2. Ontology of holiday moment locations. The light boxes are the classes, the darker ones their properties.

Both types are an important aspect of exposure therapy for PTSD and with the 3MR system, the therapy follows a gradual exposure paradigm where people first confront their general memories before working on the trauma itself. Two similar ontologies were in place, both asking for the when, where, who and what of the memory. The main deviation was that only the general ontology contained photo and movie questions (*Add a photo taken in that general period*) and only the specific ontology contained emotion related questions (*How were you feeling in that specific moment?*). An example of the general difference between those conversations for war veterans would be that in the general conversation the *where* question would be *Where was your mission?*, while in the specific conversation this would be *At which exact spot were you in that moment?*.

Personalization begins when the ontology is filled in and specific questions are asked. This could happen for instance, by knowing if a photo was taken in an inside or outside location. These have different properties and only those appropriate would be asked after. While a system not knowing this could still ask for properties of the location, it could only ask for those applying to all locations and give examples. To illustrate this concept, Fig. 2 shows a section of an ontology of a location of a holiday memory. The classes, or light boxes would correspond to multiple-choice questions and possible answers. The darker boxes, or properties would correspond to open questions asking after these properties. For example, once one has indicated that the location was inside in a shop, the questions would be *What kind of items were they selling in the shop?* corresponding to *products* and *How did you feel being in this place?* corresponding to *Your feelings about* (which is inherited from being a *location*). In contrast, in a naive system where a patients' answers are not taken into account, there would only be the following questions in all situations: *Can you describe your location? If you were outside, think of what your surroundings looked like and what the weather was like, and if you were inside, what type of place you were in and what it looked like?* followed by *If google streetview is available for this spot, could you find it and add it to the diary?* In this example it is clear that the naive conversation will consist of more general and longer questions. Moreover, with an ontology is that one has a clear overview of all the topics of the questions. If the ontology contains classes and properties for every concept in a certain memory, one knows the question dialogue will also be complete. Another expected advantage is that with an ontology one can draw new conclusions. Knowing the 2 facts that 1, a shop is a type of location, and 2, that one can have feelings about a location, one can infer that one can have feelings about being in a shop. This reasoning quality is what separates the ontology from a tree-based dialogue. It can be expected, that an ontology based system can assist people better at recollecting memories than a naive system where answers are not taken into account (from this point referred to as non-ontology based). To test this hypothesis, an experiment was set up comparing an ontology-based to a non-ontology based question dialogue.

4 Experiment

A within-subject experiment with two conditions was conducted. We wished to know if an ontology-based system would allow people to recollect their memories better than a system where answers were not taken into account (non-ontology based). Our ontology-based system was compared with such a non-ontology-based question system which had the same topics and order of questions, but without any of the personalization. The effect this difference had on people's opinions and experiences with the system was tested, as well as the effect it had on the level of detail in the answers.

4.1 Participants

Giving exposure sessions to PTSD patients without providing full treatment was not considered ethically appropriate. For this reason 24 healthy participants (10 female, mean age 28.4, SD 3.1) were recruited from the University staff and student population. Eight Participants performed the experiment in their native language (English or Dutch), all others in their second language (English). Because the participants did not have traumatic experiences, the memories they had to recollect were of holidays. This topic was chosen because it was universal for this sample and could be modelled with an ontology quite well. Furthermore, in exposure treatment PTSD patients would also start with a positive memory to get familiar with the system.

4.2 Question System

The question system was based on two ontologies, one for a general holiday memory and one focusing on a specific moment within that same holiday. For the non-ontology based system, the questions followed the exact same order and topics as the ontology-based system, such as destination and travelling companions. An example of the ontology and the difference between the systems can be found in Sect. 3. Multiple-choice options were used to ensure that the ontology-based system could react to answers appropriately. The non-ontology based system did not include any multiple-choice options. Finally, in the ontology-based system it was possible to pose a constraint on the type of answers possible, in this case the length of the answers. For the questions asking for descriptions, the answer needed to be at least six words long. Whenever this was not the case, a follow-up question would ask the participant to tell more. All open questions were answered through adding items to the diary, be it in form of media or typed text in a text item to answer the question.

4.3   Wizard of Oz and Procedure

A Wizard of Oz procedure was followed. The full dialogue was written in advance and the procedure was fully specified to avoid any influence from the wizard. The order of the questions was set and participants could signal they were finished answering through a button. The wizard was in the same room as the participants, but they could not see the wizard controlling the system. All questions appeared on the screen of the participant as typed text. The whole question would appear at once, along with multiple-choice options if applicable.

Prior to the experiment, all participants were asked to bring media (photos, video & music) from four holidays. The two memories which were used in the experiment were randomly chosen. All participants started with an introductory exercise to get to know the system. After this, the agent posing the questions gave a short introduction explaining its function and that it could communicate through text. After this, two dialogue sessions followed in which participants were asked to describe two holiday memories, one with the ontology-based and one with the non-ontology based question system. Each dialogue session consisted of 10 min of questions on the general experience and 10 min of questions on a specific moment, the order of sessions was counter-balanced. Participants had the option to take a short break between the two dialogue sessions. The experiment was approved by the University ethics committee.

4.4   Measures

Both subjective experience and the amount of detail in participant's answers were studied. The subjective experience was examined in three ways. The first was the emotion experienced when thinking back to the memory. In particular, if the subjective feeling changed when the memory was recollected. Pre and post-measures were taken with the 5-point Self-Assessment Manikin scale (SAM) scale (Lang, 1980) of Arousal and Valence for both memories recollected. The second subjective measure was how well people felt the system helped them in recollecting their memory. The third way was how people experienced the conversation with the system. These two measures were examined with 6 questions each in a questionnaire answered on a 7-point Likert scale. Examples of these questions are *The questions assisted me well in recollecting my memory* for the memory recollection and *The conversation did not run smoothly* for the conversational experience. This questionnaire was presented directly after each dialogue session. Finally, each participant answered four questions on their overall preference of one system over the other. The first was on which system helped recollect the memory best, the second which system was most pleasant to work with, the

Table 1. Annotations and definition

Annotation	Consists of
Objects	All nouns, except those referring to a person (or multiple, such as *people*), and those referring to a period of time (e.g. *day* or *moment*).
People	All nouns referring to people (e.g. *girl, tourists*) and names of people.
Descriptives	Adjectives (including terms as *very* and *three*), as well as words describing aspects of something (e.g. *cold*, in *the room is cold*). Excluding adjectives of feelings. Double adjectives were counted apart (*a very cold room*, and *a large cold room* both counting 2 descriptives)
Feelings	All words referring to feelings (e.g. *excited*), including *looking forward to* and *tired*, as well as all adjectives of feelings (*very excited* counting both words).
Time	All nouns referring to time, such as *month* or *period*.

third on which asked the best questions to trigger the memory and the fourth on which system they would use again. The objective measure considered was the amount of detail in the answers of the patients. On a general level, the number of words typed and the number of question topics posed were checked. The number of question topics could differ per participant because the dialogue sessions had a fixed time, i.e. some participants would answer only questions about location and travel, while others were quicker and would also answer questions on travel companions. To consider the amount of detail present in the texts, all answers were annotated and the number of objects, people, descriptives, feelings and time references were counted. The description of the categories in this annotation can be found in Table 1. A second annotator annotated 1235 words to ascertain reliability of the rating. Interrater reliability was assessed with Cohen's Kappa and showed a good agreement between annotators $\kappa = 0.86$, $p<0.0001$.

4.5   Data Preparation and Analysis

Two questionnaires were designed for this experiment, one measuring how well people felt the system helped them in memory recollection, and one measuring how people experienced the conversation with the system. The validity of these was tested with Cronbach's alpha, after which one question was removed from the recollection questionnaire and two from the conversation questionnaire to improve internal validity. Internal validity after this was acceptable to good (α 0.72 to 0.81 for the recollection and α 0.54 to 0.63 for the conversation questionnaire). For objective measures we considered the answers given to the questions. For one of the participants, the answers to the questions were lost due to a technical error, so the answers of only 23 participants were taken into account. When considering the amount of detail in the answers, we only considered the comparable answers. Here *comparable*, means the answers to question topics which were actually posed and answered in both conditions. This gives a measure where we can compare, as if per question, how detailed the actual answers were. As it is possible that more questions were posed in one condition than the other, comparing all texts could result in comparing answers of, for instance, answers to five questions to answers to three questions. This would give a distorted image of how detailed the response to each question actually was.

5   Results

5.1   Questionnaires

The first questionnaire measured if recollecting a memory changed peoples arousal and/or valence regarding the memory. A doubly multivariate repeated measures was done for both arousal and valence, with moment of measurement (pre/post) and system (ontology/non-ontology based) as within-subject factors. No significant results were found ($p >.05$). For both the recollection and the conversation questionnaire, a paired samples t-test was done to compare scores between conditions. Neither of these two questionnaires yielded any significant results between conditions (Recollection: $t(23) = -.38$, $p = .71$, Conversation: $t(23) = -.27$, $p = .79$). On the overall preference, a single-sample t-test showed no significant difference between the result of any of the 4 questions and the middle position on the scale (50), signifying that there was no significant preference for one system over the other (Recollection: $t(23) = 1.26$, $p = .22$, Pleasant: $t(23) = 1.82$, $p = .81$ Questions: $t(23) = 1.17$, $p = .25$ Use again: $t(23) = .1.57$, $p = .13$).

5.2   Answers

A paired t-test was performed on the amount of words typed in answers and the number of question topics answered in both conditions, the results of which are presented in Table 2. The table shows that there is a significantly higher number of total words in the answers with non-ontology based system compared to the answers with the ontology-based system. The result for the number of topics is similar, a significantly higher number of topics was covered with the non-ontology-based system compared to the ontology-based system.

Table 2. Comparison between the number of words and number of topics for the ontology-based and non-ontology-based system.

Measurement	Mean(SD)		t	df	p	Cohen's d
	Ontology	Non-Ontology				
Nr. of words	237 (114)	285 (11)	-2.37	22	0.027	0.33
Nr. of topics	8 (3)	10 (4)	-3.98	22	0.001	-0.54

Table 3. Comparison between the ontology-based and non-ontology-based system based on the total number of objects, people, descriptives, feelings and time references in the participants comparable texts.

Category	Mean(SD)		$F(1,22)$	p	η^2
	Ontology	Non-Ontology			
Objects	21 (14)	20 (13)	1.00	0.328	0.044
People	7 (7)	6 (4)	0.66	0.425	0.029
Descriptive	22 (13)	16 (9)	8.91	**0.007**	0.288
Feeling	5 (3)	6 (4)	0.34	0.567	0.015
Time	4 (3)	3 (3)	0.32	0.263	0.057

Finally, the amount of detail in comparable texts in the two conditions was considered. An omnibus test was done on the annotations of the total number of comparable texts, showing a trend of a higher number of words in the ontology-based system, but no significant result $F(5, 18) = 23.63$, $p = .084$, $\eta^2 = .87$. Table 3 shows the univariate analysis for the individual annotation categories. Here we see that there was a significantly higher number of descriptive words used in the ontology-based system even after a Bonferroni correction which sets the α level at 0.01. None of the other categories showed significant results.

6   Discussion and Conclusion

The first conclusion we can draw based on the results is that no subjective difference between the ontology-based and the non-ontology-based system was found. The second conclusion is that people answered the questions more quickly with the non-ontology based system, as shown by a higher number of topics answered with the non-ontology-based system, while both conditions lasted equally long. This result might indicate that people put more effort into answering the questions from the ontology-based system. When making statements about effort in memory recollection it is, however, also important to consider the amount of detail in the answers and not just the time taken. Concerning this, we see that there is a significantly higher number of descriptive terms for the ontology-based system. From this we can conclude that people describe memories in more detail with this system. Taken together with the result that people take more time, this suggest that people recollect their memories in more detail with an ontology-based system. This study also has some limitations, the main drawback being that the participants tested were healthy individuals, and not PTSD patients. We believe, however, that our results do provide a valid insight in memory recollection with an ontology-based system as it shows that such a system can assist in detailed memory recollection. Future work will have to study the effect of an ontology-based system on the recollection of memories which people would rather forget. One contribution of this study has been to show that aside from high-level planning [5], and adding domain knowledge [2], ontologies can also be used to store specific knowledge of the user and steer the conversation based on this. It has also shown that the use of multiple-choice options to personalize the conversation [9,15] can be combined with such an ontology. Finally, we have shown that an ontology-based question system is effective in assisting users with detailed memory recollection, as necessary in PTSD exposure therapy [8].

Acknowledgements. *This work is part of the programme Virtual E-Coaching and Storytelling Technology for PTSD, which is financed by the Netherlands Organization for Scientific Research (pr. nr. 314-99-104).*

References

1. Diagnostic and statistical manual of mental disorders: American Psychiatric Association, 5th edn. Washington DC (2013)
2. Al-Zubaide, H., Issa, A.A.: Ontbot : ontology based chatbot. In: Innovation in Information and Communication Technology (2011)
3. Augello, A., Pilato, G., Vassallo, G., Gaglio, S.: Chatbots as interface to ontologies. In: Gaglio, S., Lo Re, G. (eds.) Advances in Intelligent Systems and Computing, pp. 285–299. Springer, Switzerland (2014)
4. Bickmore, T.W., Nelson, R.A.S.K., Cheng, D.M., Winter, M., Henault, L., Paasche-Orlow, M.K.: A randomized controlled trial of an automated exercise coach for older adults. J. Am. Geriatr. Soc. **61**(10), 1676–1683 (2013)
5. Bickmore, T., Schulman, D., Sidner, C.: A reusable framework for health counseling dialogue systems based on a behavioral medicine ontology. J. Biomed. Inform. **44**, 183–197 (2011)
6. Blanson-Henkemans, O., van der Mast, C., van der Boog, P., Neerincx, M., Lindenberg, J., Zwetsloot-Schonk, B.: An online lifestyle diary with a persuasiv computer assistant providing feedback on self-management. Tech. Health Care **17**, 253–267 (2009)
7. Brinkman, W.P., Vermetten, E., van der Steen, M., Neerincx, M.A.: Cognitive engineering of a military multi-modal memory restructuring system. J. Cyber Ther. Rehabil. **4**(1), 83–99 (2011)
8. Foa, E., Hembree, E., Rothbaum, B.O.: Prolonged Exposure Therapy for PTSD: Emotional Processing of Traumatic Experiences Therapist Guide (Treatments That Work). Oxford University Press, New York (2007)
9. Friederichs, S., Bolman, C., Oenema, A., Guyaux, J., Lechner, L.: Motivational interviewing in a web-based physical activity intervention with an avatar: randomized controlled trial. J. Med. Internet Res. **16**(2), e48 (2014)
10. Lucas, G., Gratch, J., King, A., Morency, L.P.: Its only a computer: virtual humans increase willingness to disclose. Comput. Hum. Behav. **37**, 94–100 (2014)
11. Martínez-Miranda, J., Bresó, A., García-Gómez, J.M.: Look on the bright side: a model of cognitive change in virtual agents. In: Bickmore, T., Marsella, S., Sidner, C. (eds.) IVA 2014. LNCS, vol. 8637, pp. 285–294. Springer, Heidelberg (2014)
12. Miller, W.R., Rollnick, S.: Motivational Interviewing: Preparing People to Change Addictive Behavior. Guilford Press, New York (1991)
13. Noy, N.F., McGuinness, D.L.: Ontology development 101: a guide to creating your first ontology. Stanford Knowledge Systems Laboratory Technical Report (2001)

14. Rizzo, A., Lange, B., Buckwalter, J.G., Forbell, E., Kim, J., Sagae, K., Williams, J., Rothbaum, B.O., Difede, J., Reger, G., Parsons, T., Kenny, P.: An intelligent virtual human system for providing healthcare information and support. Med. Meets Virtual Reality **18**, 503–509 (2011)
15. Schulman, D., Bickmore, T., Sidner, C.: An intelligent conversational agent for promoting long-term health behavior change using motivational interviewing. In: AAAI Spring Symposium Series (2011)
16. Tielman, M., Brinkman, W.-P., Neerincx, M.A.: Design guidelines for a virtual coach for post-traumatic stress disorder patients. In: Bickmore, T., Marsella, S., Sidner, C. (eds.) IVA 2014. LNCS, vol. 8637, pp. 434–437. Springer, Heidelberg (2014)

Adaptive Grounding and Dialogue Management for Autonomous Conversational Assistants for Elderly Users

Ramin Yaghoubzadeh[1]($\boxtimes$), Karola Pitsch[2], and Stefan Kopp[1]

[1] Social Cognitive Systems Group, CITEC, Bielefeld University,
P.O. Box 10 01 31, 33501 Bielefeld, Germany
ryaghoubzadeh@uni-bielefeld.de
[2] Institute for Communication Studies, University of Duisburg-Essen,
Universitätsstraße 12, 45141 Essen, Germany

Abstract. People with age-related or congenital cognitive impairments require assistance in daily tasks to enable them to maintain a self-determined lifestyle in their own home. We developed and evaluated a prototype of an autonomous spoken dialogue assistant to support these user groups in the domain of week planning. Based on insights from previous work with a WOz study, we designed a dialogue system which caters to the interactional needs of these user groups. Subjects were able to interact successfully with the system and rated it as equivalent in terms of robustness and usability compared to the WOz prototype.

Keywords: Assistive technology · Cognitive impairment · Conversational agents

1 Introduction

Many older adults, when impacted by the aging processes, are able to continue living in their accustomed home environment if they receive support for their gradually declining capacities. The same holds true for people with congenital or acquired cognitive impairments[1] who, thanks to improved social integration and better-suited healthcare, nowadays can also enjoy the boon of independence, if given support. The factors that most often lead to an end of independent living, besides fall events, are cognitive problems in both user groups that lead to an erratic or completely lost day structure. This can range from forgetfulness to a total lack of the sense of time, hindering their management of activities like meals, medication, appointments or social events.

We present work towards an assistive conversational agent for self-determined daily schedule management and maintenance, a cooperation with one of Europe's largest health and social care providers for elderly people and people with various disabilities. We previously explored the principal suitability and acceptability of

---

[1] In this paper, we adopt the terminology recommended by ACM SIGACCESS [4].

© Springer International Publishing Switzerland 2015
W.-P. Brinkman et al. (Eds.): IVA 2015, LNAI 9238, pp. 28–38, 2015.
DOI: 10.1007/978-3-319-21996-7_3

spoken-language virtual assistants for these users, identifying constraints for successful interaction [16]. In the present work we explored how interaction between an *autonomous* system and people from those groups could be made robust and effective, ensuring both mutual understanding and assessment as an acceptable interactant. After highlighting existing work in our field and the foundations from our previous work, we will describe our dialogue management framework `flexdiam` designed with these requirements in mind, and results of an initial evaluation of the autonomous system with older adults.

2   Related Work

Dialogue management has received much attention, and a number of established approaches exist; see McTear [10] for an overview. Of particular relevance here are flexible grounding mechanisms with error and repair handling. Larsson [9] proposed an issue-based dialogue management capable of ellipsis resolution and accomodating unaddressed questions; Skantze dealt with errors and repair in spoken dialogue and tracked the grounding status of concepts and confidence scores in the Galatea discourse modeller [14]. Roque & Traum [11] proposed a model to track the extent to which material has reached mutual belief in a dialogue by distinguishing between several discrete degrees of groundedness, demonstrating an improved appraisal of an agent's dialogue skills. Crook et al. [5] presented an approach for dealing with user barge-ins in a dialogue system, discerning between continue, abort and replan actions. Buschmeier & Kopp [3] proposed a Bayesian model incorporating evidence from back-channel feedback to infer continuous degrees of understanding or acceptance. These systems have generally not been confronted with the special interactional needs of elderly or cognitively impaired users. Interaction in that domain has mostly been text-based or multiple-choice, e.g. the Always-On Companion for isolated older adults [13].

There is a substantial body of work on the requirements and potentials of interactive assistive systems especially for elderly people. The GUIDE project [7] identified dimensions of user models for different impairments, and potential domains of support, remarking that spoken language is the preferred modality for older users without technical experience. The use of speech input by older adults has been explored systematically [17], taking into account the detrimental effect of dysarthria and articulation disorders on recognition quality, although even then limited speech interaction, e.g. for environmental control, can be realized [6,8]. Beskow et al. [2] evaluated a prototype multimodal reminder agent for people with cognitive problems that combined handwriting recognition and spoken dialogue. Studies for people with general cognitive impairments are still few; a first study showed that parallels to older adults exist in interactions with spoken dialogue systems, such as a diminished awareness of system errors [16].

3   Background and Requirements

Lessons from Previous Work. Previously [16], we engaged in a participatory design process with two user groups – older adults (n=6) living autonomously in apartments attached to a nursing home, and people with cognitive impairments (n=11) from an institution offering technological experience and training. The design process comprised interviews, focus groups, interaction experiments and concluding focus groups or interviews (depending on specific impairments, in accord with care personnel). In the interaction experiments, we used a WOz version of a spoken dialogue virtual assistant with a graphical calendar. Subjects were asked to enter fictional appointments using natural speech. They were able to use image cue cards depicting the day of the week, time, and topic of an activity. Subjects could at least read the days of the week and times, but images were required for topics. Crucially, we manipulated the "agent's" understanding of entered appointments by introducing systematic errors in the summaries at predefined times. In a between-subject design with two conditions, we contrasted two methods for grounding and confirming information provided by the user: asking for confirmation for each "slot", or summarizing the whole appointment in one utterance. We found a noticeable difference in error detection rates, most pronounced for the group with at least mild mental retardation (APA-DSM-IV F70 [1]). We used a simplified process of usability rating involving nine interview questions and a graphical scale on which subjects with numerical or abstraction problems could visually point out ratings. There were no differences in rating between the conditions for any user group.

The central insight from the experiments is that the information grounding process in a multimodal spoken dialogue system for people with cognitive impairments must be highly adaptive, to avoid situations in which the users are overwhelmed by large chunks of information and fail to spot system errors. Grounding must thereby extend to very fine-grained and explicit strategies, in which each piece of information is best negotiated individually. This did not lead to negative usability assessment, in contrast to our inital assumptions. Anecdotally, we found in informal focus groups and meetings that participants looked forward to further studies, primarily stating their positive impression of the agent. This was especially pronounced in the group of people with cognitive impairments, but also with the older adults. One older participant hung a picture of the agent on her mirror and chatted about the agent, showing images to her grandchildren.

Requirements for an Autonomous Assistant. The analysis of our initial interaction studies, related work, and interviews with subjects and care personnel, led to the following central requirements and design principles for robustness and interaction quality in a spoken-dialogue assistant for our user groups: **(1)** The system must satisfy critical requirements for fluid dialogue: it has to present and process information in an *incremental* fashionr to facilitate the reception of the other party by maximizing both the duration of presentation and the *timeliness* of its feedback. Feedback and corrections must be flexibly processed *at any time*, in the form of barge-ins, but also as later revisions. The system must therefore be able to reason about changes in assumptions and evidence between *arbitrary points* in the past and the present and also to refer to past discourse units. **(2)** The system has to be prepared for uncertainty in the interaction in two ways: firstly, input variables can be *uncertain,* e.g. due to inaccuracies in speech recognition, exacerbated by articulation disorders. Wherever possible, the system must maintain parallel *alternative hypotheses* and resolve them in a controlled manner. Secondly, even explicit feedback signals from the user cannot always be presumed to accurately reflect the result of a comprehensive assessment of the common ground by them. The system must hence be able to employ optimal strategies for information presentation that maximize the *incidence of meaningful feedback* but are not perceived as intrusive. **(3)** Information should be structured in a way suited to the user groups in terms of its simplicity. When a hierarchical task structure is required (such as asking clarification questions or solving sub-tasks to contribute to a more complex task), the system must offer *transparency.* It should be able to summarize the current state of the hierarchical task, and to *inquire about the user's understanding* of it. Thus, when communication problems arise, such as a lack of contributions or evidence that the user is confused, it should attempt to successively *request explicit feedback* from the user by descending the task hierarchy, or back-track to a previously grounded point.

4   The `flexdiam` Dialogue Manager

In order to realize the aforementioned requirements, we developed and evaluated a dialogue management framework called `flexdiam`, written in Python and first presented here. The design of this framework was inspired by the analysis of the requirements and possible interaction problems of our variously impaired user groups, to allow for robust, flexible, and acceptable, mostly task-related, spoken-language interactions.

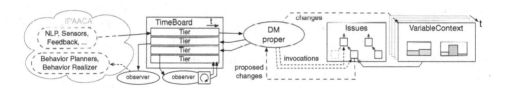

Fig. 1. Architecture overview of `flexdiam`

Information in the system is spread over three complementary data structures with specific capabilities contributing to this end (see Fig. 1 for an architecture overview). The **temporal structure** of dialogue is represented in a central data structure, termed `TimeBoard`, which stores all events, past, ongoing, or future (projected), in thematically grouped *tiers* (Fig. 3). It serves as the interface for communication between input processing, dialogue management proper, and behavior planning and realization. It is a globally modifiable blackboard, and it is by convention that strict governance of the flexible temporal aspects of dialogue is guaranteed. Entries on the board have a payload content (usually an *incremental unit* in our middleware IPAACA [12]) as well a as start and end time, possibly undefined to reflect open intervals. The board provides a set of interval relations enabling predicates over a set of tiers, describing their structure for any requested interval of time. The board receives any changes as write operations on the start, end, or content of events, storable with timestamps for full rollback capability. Any set of tiers can have attached *observers* to which all changes of event parameters on those tiers are relayed, and which can act as pipelines or concurrent processors. Data other than events with temporal extent, i.e. **knowledge and propositional information** are represented via a structure termed `VariableContext`, (Fig. 4, left), a blackboard satisfying two requirements: firstly, all information may reside there in the form of distributions with attached entropy values. Modules may analyze the distributions or entropies or instantiate maximum-likelihood versions. Secondly, the `VariableContext` has full temporal independence. All changes are stored as time-stamped deltas, providing the means both for rollbacks and for analysis between two points in time, e.g. changes in distributions. In order to represent **task and discourse states**, the system follows a hybrid approach that centers around a forest of structures called `Issues`, terminology adapted from Larsson [9], that represent (attributed) common current topics or current questions that have to be resolved cooperatively. In `flexdiam`, they are independent agents that encapsulate the structure of the task addressed so far, localized planning, as well as situated interpretative capability and situated capability for action, encompassing both dialogue contributions and other side effects. Moreover, they contain a local success and failure test which the dialogue manager proper uses to decide on finalizing an Issue to defer processing back to the parent. The dialogue manager proper can invoke six operations on an Issue object: `interpret`, which is used to interpret an NLU result (Fig. 4, center), `can_interpret`, which performs a shallower check of whether a NLU result can be (partially) used by the issue object, `introduce`, which must be called and completed exactly once for any system-introduced issue opening a new sequence before the issue is considered a valid acceptor for user contributions (preemptive user contributions inside a sequence are however acceptable and expected), `reintroduce`, which is used to pick up the previously introduced issue when the system takes the floor from idle state, `child_closed`, which is invoked whenever a child issue has been finalized by the DM proper due to a flagged local success or failure condition, and `make_certain`, which is the meta-dialogue operation to summarize the current state of the issue object and explicitly ask for confirmation. Issues can themselves mark local progress using the `progressed` function. This invalidates all children (see below) and invokes `child_progressed` on the parent. Whenever an **Issue object is invoked**, it processes the respective input and proposes a comprehensive change set, termed `IssueReturn` (Fig. 4, right), composed of (1) a change set to merge into the VariableContext, (2) a set of *transmits*, which are objects that the DM proper should insert on the TimeBoard, publishing them to external components, (3) a flag indicating whether the issue object deems the invocation to have been an exhaustive operation on the input, and (4) optionally, a child issue that the DM

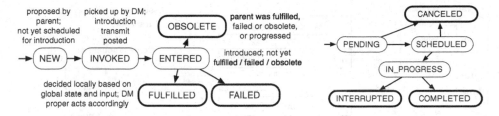

Fig. 2. Left: State machine for `Issue` objects. Terminal states (=issue inactive) in bold. **Right:** State machine for `Transmit` objects. State transitions closely correspond to planners/realizers.

proper should in the future pick as the preferential entry point for invocation in lieu of the presently invoked issue. In line with the general notion of temporal variability and uncertainty, all operations that do not have immediate effect are treated as **asynchronously performed operations**. New issue or transmit objects are not guaranteed to fully come to pass in the dialogue, nor assumed to be successfully completed a-priori. Both traverse state machines dependent upon external events, starting as incomplete and unreliable entities (cf. Fig. 2). The invocation of the **DM proper** is realized by observers on the input and structure tiers that call corresponding functions in the DM when new parses are received or a change in structure is detected (such as a prolonged silence after a user utterance).

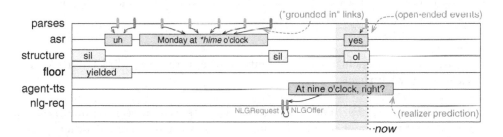

Fig. 3. The `TimeBoard` encapsulates the temporal structure and dependency of events. The typical setup encompasses input tiers (*asr* and dependent incremental *parses*), information derived by helper agents (*structure*: sil=silence, ols=overlap; *floor* is explicitly yielded by system after questions), and output tiers (*nlg-req* contains posted requests and offers received from NLG program, *agent-tts* contains agent utterances as reported by realizer feedback). **Example situation:** The user barges in with a reply after the agent asked a clarification question since the preceding user utterance was misarticulated. In the setup of the present work, the agent would interrupt himself.

5 Evaluation

After the basic functionality tests accompanying the design of `flexdiam`, we carried out an early evaluation with our user groups, in line with the approach

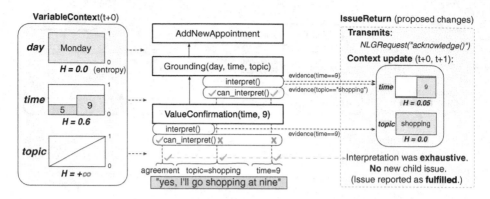

Fig. 4. Uncertain information in `VariableContext` and unfolded discourse in `Issue` forest. **Left:** Relevant subset of prior context: *day* has been established, *time* is uncertain, *topic* is unknown. The Grounding issue chose to propose a ValueConfirmation for *time*, primed for a yes/no answer, because the entropy was less than 1 bit (state from Fig. 3). **Center:** Hierarchical situated interpretation, moments after Fig. 3; the confirmation part of the utterance is understood as a reply to the most recent (bottom-most) issue, while the remainder is captured here by the immediate parent. **Right:** IssueReturn contains proposed updates from interpret(). Context is to be updated with new distributions. An *acknowledge()* will be requested from the NLG as contingent feedback. No new children are proposed and since the issue deems its success condition (processing a yes/no reply) fulfilled, it will henceforth report its fulfilled() predicate as True. **N.B.** Had the user omitted the "yes", the remaining evidence might, depending on configuration, have been sufficient for the parent to *progress*, silently deactivating the child to *OBSOLETE* state (cf. Fig. 2).

of an user-centered, inclusive design, with a system resulting directly from our previous work with them.

Study Design and Setup. The task for participants was entering appointments into a calendar using spoken conversation with the virtual assistant "Billie". The setup comprised a dedicated ASR machine running Windows ASR and DragonNaturallySpeaking Client edition, with a desk microphone, and a touch-screen PC running `flexdiam`, parser, NLU, behavior planner, a 3D environment with a character driven by ASAPrealizer [15], and CereVoice TTS. During interactions, participants met the virtual agent as their conversation partner, next to a calendar with real-time visualization of intermediate results of the incremental interpretation of user input. The scene on the touch screen included a red button with a back arrow, introduced as an 'emergency button' should the agent constantly fail to understand the participant. The button was "wired" to reset the system to the top-most dialogue state (clarifying whether the participants wanted to enter anything else). We set up the system to cope with various expected verbalizations for the topic of calendar management, to be able to handle all types of repair patterns that we previously found, and set up the Issue structure accordingly. For all participants, we chose the slow-paced, explicit grounding strategy of asking for confirmation for every slot, which had been identified as the most reliable one for impaired participants. In contrast to a previous WOz experiment [16], we did not provide cue cards with completely predefined fictional appointments. Rather, participants were free to enter whatever they wished – but we provided a single cue sheet with textual and iconic representations of possible activities (Fig. 6, left). We prepared the NLU to preferentially spot those topics and respective synonyms. Yet, all other inputs were also valid; they were subjected to a simple heuristic extraction to reduce them to short entries.

Participants and Procedure. After an initial test run with three people from the group with cognitive impairments, in which additional failure modes were detected and addressed, we conducted a controlled small-scale experiment with the group of older adults (n = 6, 4f, 2m, ages 77–86). The same group had already participated in the previous experiment, so they had cursory acquaintance with the task and the agent Billie from about 14 months earlier. After initial written consent, participants were asked to participate in a short speech recognizer training process by calmly reciting excerpts from a recipe book in three episodes of about 30 s each. While the training program operated in the background, they were instructed about their task for the experiment proper. We split the interaction into two parts, an initial phase where participants should attempt to make up to three entries without further instruction as to the format, followed by an intermission in which we would be able to intervene should the system be totally overwhelmed by the user's interactional style. The primary hints provided where to avoid excessive verbosity and to use verbal instead of paraverbal feedback. A second interaction phase followed, for which participants were asked to make at least five entries. After this final phase, participants were asked to participate in a structured interview including the following usability questions (the same as in previous work; translated): (1) How did you like to plan your week with Billie (B)? (2) Did B always do what you wanted? (3) Did B provide sufficient help? (4) Could you understand B's language well? (5) Did B express himself in an easy way? (6) Did B understand you correctly? (7) How did you like the image-based calendar? (8) Do you think B could be of help to you? (9) Do you think B could be a good appointment assistant?

Results. All participants were generally able to enter appointments successfully. Concessions were made by participants in accepting entries that were altered by the system based on topic extraction heuristics (for topics not on the cue sheet). In total, 46 entries were negotiated, of which 7 (15.2 %) did not correspond to the user's original wishes. All errors occurred in the first phase (Fig. 5). Topic negotiation was counted as successful if a suitable paraphrase was settled on (e.g. VP05 tried to enter "hairdresser", initially not recognized; she then elaborated "shampoo and cut", which she later ratified – we counted that as a success). Communication problems mainly resulted from the inability of the system to process long, convoluted utterances properly. In particular, one participant (VP04) used a very verbose style with back stories and indirect replies. He produced noticeably more utterances compared to the average of the other

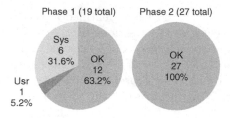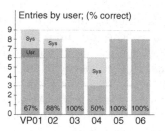

Fig. 5. Left: Completed topic negotiations in the two interaction phases. *OK*: entered verbatim as dictated or with acceptable paraphrase; *Sys*: ratified, but system failed to offer acceptable topic; *Usr*: false entry due to the user not detecting a system error (cf. previous work). **Right:** Total, correct and erroneous negotiations, by participant, with proportion of correct entries.

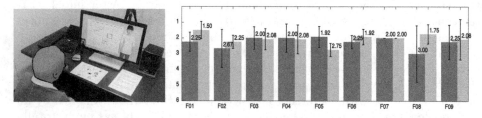

Fig. 6. Left: Interaction with autonomous system (older participant, anonymized). **Right:** Comparison of usability ratings (see text) between previous WOz experiment [16] (pale) and the present autonomous system (dark), for elderly users. German school grades (1–6, 1 is best).

participants (170 vs. 104), used more than twice the utterances per negotiation (28.33 vs. 13.16), while 50.6 % were three words or longer (the maximum for the others was 27 %). Several times, the ASR computer was causing lag due to processing of several conjoint utterances. The explanatory intervention in the intermission did not make the participant alter his interactional style in a lasting way. Further, as the study was conducted in the field (a care facility), there were fluctuations in noise due to simultaneous events in neighboring rooms, affecting portions of two other interactions. However, no participant made use of the "fallback" touch-screen reset button, which was the only supported non-speech interaction mode. Remarkably, the ratings of the usability questions differed only slightly from the WOz experiment conducted in our previous work [16] (overlaid in Fig. 6, right). That is, the *autonomous* assistant based on `flexdiam` achieved ratings similar to a WOz system in which the entire input processing and system response selection tasks were performed by a human wizard. The least favorable ratings came from VP04, for whom the system failed to provide a pleasant and effective interaction. Consequently, his intention-to-use (question F08) was minimal (grade 6).

6   Discussion and Conclusion

The general goal of the present work is to develop conversational assistants that can work autonomously and robustly with user groups like older adults or cognitively impaired people. Such groups often bring about special interactional challenges. Based on the results from previous WOz studies with these user groups, we have developed the dialogue manager `flexdiam` that specifically aims to enable flexible and adaptive grounding mechanisms, including barge-ins, repairs and interactively negotiated content. The evaluation study we have conducted with older adults showed that the general design of the system, along with the explicit grounding and ratification strategy selected for allowing users to detect system errors, is suitable to almost match the results obtained with the WOz version of the assistant – only one error was never detected. Participants with a relatively brief interaction style could effectively enter information error-free. This results lends support to the notion that autonomous conversational assistants in domains as confined as calendar management (although including relatively open sub-tasks like entering activities) are in principle possible.

In general, the challenge for such assistants is to maximize robustness of spoken dialogue, while at the same time ensuring acceptable interactions. This holds especially with elderly users who sometimes exhibit excessive verbosity, even when explicitly instructed to adhere to a brief interaction style. Consequently, the system must take initiative where it cannot cope, to actively "make life easier" for itself and preserve operability. Here, a virtual agent, by virtue of its ability to convey subtle interactional information, can be a socially acceptable "pace controller" by emitting successively more explicit turn management behavior instead of just barging in to grab the floor. Extending the assistant in this direction will be one of the areas for our future work. Moreover, we plan to extend the evaluation study to the other user group of people with congenital or acquired cognitive impairments.

Acknowledgements. This research was partially supported by the German Federal Ministry of Education and Research (BMBF) in the project 'VERSTANDEN', by the Deutsche Forschungsgemeinschaft (DFG) in the Center of Excellence 'Cognitive Interaction Technology' (CITEC), and by the Volkswagen Foundation.

References

1. American Psychiatric Association: Diagnostic and Statistical Manual of Mental Disorders DSM-IV-TR, 4th edn. American Psychiatric Publication, Arlington (2000)
2. Beskow, J., Edlund, J., Granström, B., Gustafson, J., Skantze, G., Tobiasson, H.: The MonAMI reminder : a spoken dialogue system for face-to-face interaction. In: 10th Annual Conference of the International Speech Communication Association INTERSPEECH 2009, pp. 300–303 (2009)
3. Buschmeier, H., Kopp, S.: Using a Bayesian model of the listener to unveil the dialogue information state. In: SemDial 2012: Proceedings of the 16th Workshop on the Semantics and Pragmatics of Dialogue, pp. 12–20, Paris, France (2012)

4. Cavender, A., Trewin, S., Hanson, V.: ACM SIGACCESS Accessible Writing Guide. www.sigaccess.org/resources/accessible-writing-guide. (Accessed 10–March-2015)
5. Crook, N., Smith, C., Cavazza, M., Pulman, S., Moore, R., Boye, J.: Handling user interruptions in an embodied conversational agent. In: Proceedings of the AAMAS International Workshop on Interacting with ECAs as Virtual Characters, pp. 27–33 (2010)
6. Fager, S.K., Beukelman, D.R., Jakobs, T., Hosom, J.-P.: Evaluation of a speech recognition prototype for speakers with moderate and severe dysarthria: a preliminary report. Augment. Altern. Comm. **26**(4), 267–277 (2010)
7. GUIDE Consortium: User Interaction & Application Requirements - Deliverable D2.1. (2011)
8. Hawley, M.S., Enderby, P., Green, P., Cunningham, S., Brownsell, S., Carmichael, J., Parker, M., Hatzis, A., ONeill, P., Palmer, R.: A speech-controlled environmental control system for people with severe dysarthria. Med. Eng. Phys. **29**(5), 586–593 (2007)
9. Larsson, S.: Issue-Based Dialogue Management. University of Gothenburg, Gothenburg (2002)
10. McTear, M.: Spoken Dialogue Technology: Towards the Conversational User Interface. Springer, London (2004)
11. Roque, A., Traum, D.: Improving a Virtual Human Using a Model of Degrees of Grounding. In: Proceedings of International Joint Conference on Artificial Intelligence IJCAI 2009, Pasadena, CA (2009)
12. Schlangen, D., Baumann, T., Buschmeier, H., Buß, O., Kopp, S., Skantze, G., Yaghoubzadeh, R.: Middleware for incremental processing in conversational agents. In: Special Interest Group on Discourse and Dialogue, pp. 51–54 (2010)
13. Sidner, C., Bickmore, T., Rich, C., Barry, B., Ring, L., Behrooz, M., Shayganfar, M.: An Always-On Companion for Isolated Older Adults. In: SIGdial 2013, Metz, France (2013)
14. Skantze, G.: Galatea: a discourse modeller supporting concept-level error handling in spoken dialogue systems. Recent Trends in Discourse and Dialogue. Text, Speech and Language Technology, vol. 39, pp. 155–189. Springer, Netherlands (2008)
15. van Welbergen, Herwin, Reidsma, Dennis, Kopp, Stefan: An incremental multimodal realizer for behavior co-articulation and coordination. In: Nakano, Yukiko, Neff, Michael, Paiva, Ana, Walker, Marilyn (eds.) IVA 2012. LNCS, vol. 7502, pp. 175–188. Springer, Heidelberg (2012)
16. Yaghoubzadeh, Ramin, Kramer, Marcel, Pitsch, Karola, Kopp, Stefan: Virtual agents as daily assistants for elderly or cognitively impaired people. In: Aylett, Ruth, Krenn, Brigitte, Pelachaud, Catherine, Shimodaira, Hiroshi (eds.) IVA 2013. LNCS, vol. 8108, pp. 79–91. Springer, Heidelberg (2013)
17. Young, V., Mihailidis, A.: Difficulties in automatic speech recognition of dysarthric speakers and implications for speech-based applications used by the elderly: a literature review. Assist. Technol. **22**(2), 99–112 (2010)

Opponent Modeling for Virtual Human Negotiators

Zahra Nazari[(⊠)], Gale M. Lucas, and Jonathan Gratch

Institute for Creative Technologies, University of Southern California,
Los Angeles, USA
{zahra, lucas, gratch}@ict.usc.edu

Abstract. Negotiation is a challenging domain for virtual human research. One aspect of this problem, known as *opponent modeling,* is discovering what the other party wants from the negotiation. Research in automated negotiation has yielded a number opponent modeling techniques but we show that these methods do not easily transfer to human-agent settings. We propose a more effective heuristic for inferring preferences both from a negotiator's pattern of offers and verbal statements about their preferences. This method has the added advantage that it can detect negotiators that lie about their preferences. We discuss several ways the method can enhance the capabilities of a virtual human negotiator.

1 Introduction

Negotiation is an important and challenging domain for virtual human research. Several efforts have advanced the design of conversational agents that negotiate with human users, both as a means for teaching negotiation skills [1] and as a means to advance the social intelligence of virtual agents [2, 3]. Negotiation engages a wide range of individual and interpersonal skills that are not only crucial for people, but essential for machines that socially engage with humans. In this paper, we present a novel algorithm for advancing one of these skills – opponent modeling.

Understanding what the other party wants is key to successful negotiation [4]. Unfortunately, these must often be inferred from words and actions, and many negotiation contexts, parties may feel they should withhold or misrepresent their true preferences. Opponent modeling is a focus of research in the multi-agent community and various models are proposed. However, models developed in the context of agent-agent negotiations may be inappropriate in human negotiations. In this paper, we illustrate that standard opponent modeling approaches do not perform well on human data and we introduce a heuristic that performs far better.

Opponent modeling is part of a larger effort of ours to create a virtual human platform that teaches negotiation skills (see Fig. 1). The agent allows students to engage with different virtual human role-players across a variety of negotiation problems via natural language and nonverbal expressions of emotion. Opponent modeling plays a crucial role for this agent to (a) understand what the student wants, (b) understand how the agent's own behavior is influencing the student's beliefs, and (c) a metric for quantifying the information being exchanged between parties. For example,

W.-P. Brinkman et al. (Eds.): IVA 2015, LNAI 9238, pp. 39–49, 2015.
DOI: 10.1007/978-3-319-21996-7_4

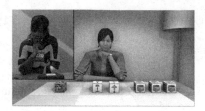

Fig. 1. The conflict resolution agent and a human user [5].

a student might think they are accurately communicating their preferences but their actual words and deeds might communicate something quite different to the other party, and the difference between the true and inferred models can serve to quantify this discrepancy.

The rest of this paper is organized as follows. Section 2, explains the negotiation setting considered for this paper and an overview of the currently existing models. In Sect. 3, we use a large corpus of human negotiations to address the differences between human-involved and multi-agent settings, and propose alternative models that address these differences. In Sect. 4, results from the existing and proposed models are shown. Finally, Sect. 5 provides a summary and discusses the future work.

2   Preliminaries/Background

We adopt a standard formulation of a bilateral negotiation. Parties must find agreement over set of independent issues. Each issue consists of a set of discrete levels (levels might correspond to attributes of an agreement, such as salary and benefits of a job offer). A negotiation succeeds if both players agree on a level for each issue, at which point each party receives a utility (unknown to the other party). Here, we adopt the conventional assumption of a linear additive utility function in the range of [0, 1]. The value of ω, is the weighted (w_i) sum of assigned levels for each issue (l_i):

$$u(\omega) = \sum_{i=1}^{n} w_i \cdot l_i \tag{1}$$

The weight w_i represents the preference the opponent holds for issue i. The set of all possible deals are known as outcome space (Ω) that is known for both parties and negotiators try to reach an outcome that maximizes their own utility.

An important concept in negotiation is *Pareto efficiency* which is a measure of the quality of a negotiated agreement. A deal is inefficient if it is possible to improve the other party's position without harming one's own. Rational agents should only offer Pareto efficient deals as this maximizes joint gains and increases the chance of a beneficial agreement for oneself. Unfortunately, one needs perfect information about both parties' preference to calculate the efficiency of a deal. Having a good estimate of the opponent's preferences helps the negotiators to make offers that are closer to Pareto optimal and are more likely to be accepted by their opponent.

Several algorithms have been proposed to estimate the opponent' utility function (see [4] for a recent review). These models only use the pattern of offers for their estimations and fall into two main types: Bayesian models and frequency models. Bayesian models generate a set of candidate preference profiles first, and then use certain assumptions about the opponent concessions to update their models. One of the main assumptions in this set of models is that the opponent starts with asking for maximum possible utility and then gradually concedes towards lower utilities. Among Frequency models, N.A.S.H Frequency [4] learns the issue weights based on how often the best value for each issue is offered. Hardheaded [6] learns the issue weights based on how often the level of an issue changes, assuming when a party changes an asked level for an issue frequently, they must assign lower utility for that issue.

Various metrics have been proposed to assess the quality of an opponent modeling approach. In this paper, we use a standard accuracy measure in negotiation contexts called rank distance of the deals [7]. This metric compares the utility of all possible deals in the outcome space (Ω), given the estimated (u'_{op}) and the actual weights (u_{op}), and calculates the average number of conflicts in how deals are ranked using the estimated vs. actual utility function:

$$d_r\left(u_{op}, u'_{op}\right) = \frac{1}{|\Omega|^2} \sum_{\omega \in \Omega, \omega' \in \Omega} c_{<u, <u'}(\omega, \omega') \tag{2}$$

The function c, the *conflict indicator*, takes any pair of deals (ω and ω') and returns 1 if the ranking between the deals changes when calculated by the actual vs. estimated weights; otherwise it returns 0. An opponent modeling approach is considered to be more accurate if it produces a *smaller* rank distance than another approach.

One limitation of rank distance is that it minimized the average number of errors that can arise from the estimated weights but not the severity of these errors. An alternative strategy, known as *minmax regret,* is to minimize the worst-case negative consequences that arise from using the estimated weights. Minmax regret is considered a more conservative and robust procedure for selecting amongst models. To capture this intuition in the opponent modeling context, we propose the following measure.

Max-regret finds the maximum absolute difference between the utility of a deal given actual weights $\left(u_{op}(\omega)\right)$ and its utility given estimated weights $\left(u'_{op}(\omega)\right)$ over all possible deals (Ω):

$$d_M\left(u_{op}, u'_{op}\right) = \max_{\omega \in \Omega} \left|u_{op}(\omega) - u'_{op}(\omega)\right| \tag{3}$$

As we assume utility has been normalized to the range [0...1], a max-regret of 0.5 indicates that the estimate may be off by half of its maximum possible value. For example, if our opponent could receive $1000 for his best deal, with a max-regret of 0.5 we estimate his payout at only $500, leading us to think we're getting a great deal when we could have extracted greater concessions. We will use both rank distance and max-regret to assess the value of different opponent modeling techniques.

3 Challenges with Modeling Human Negotiation Preferences

Opponent modeling techniques do a reasonable job of inferring the preferences of automated negotiation agents [4], but they may fail to capture the true preferences of human negotiators. A review of the literature on human negotiations emphasizes several differences between how people and automated negotiation agents behave:

1. Automated agents tend to start with the offer that is best to them, and concede monotonically from that point. Human negotiators (especially novice negotiators) tend to start much closer to what they perceive to be a fair offer [8, 9]. As fairness depends on an estimate of the Pareto frontier, which may be incorrect, a 'fair' offer may differ considerably from what is truly fair, adding noise into any algorithm that focuses strictly on offers.
2. Automated agents impose strict mechanisms to structure the negotiation process. Most algorithms assume that parties take turns exchanging complete offers. In contrast, humans are more flexible and usually make partial offers (i.e., offers that specify levels on only a subset of the issues [8].
3. Automated agents can be tediously patient and often exchange thousands of offers before reaching a deal, whereas humans may only exchange a few offers before concluding a negotiation [10].
4. Most importantly, people communicate via language whereas most agents only communicate via a pattern of offers. Language allows people to distinguish between preferences and deals (e.g., I'd prefer the best stereo possible for this car but can only afford $10,000). Of course, people often lie in negotiations, so there may be differences between what people say and do.

In this section, we describe a large corpus of face-to-face negotiation data, illustrate that humans indeed violate the assumptions of current opponent modeling techniques, and propose some simple heuristics to infer the preferences of human negotiators.

3.1 Corpus

Participants: 113 same-sex dyads (38 female dyads, 75 male dyads) were recruited from craigslist for participation in this study. Participants were paid for completing the study, and based on the outcome they achieved in the negotiation, were given additional entries into a lottery for a cash prize. They reported a mean age of 26.83 (SD = 12.77), and 41.6 % racially identified as African-American, 32.3 % as Caucasian, 8.8 % as Hispanic, 8.0 % as other, 6.2 % as Asian, 3.1 % as Native American/Hawaiian.

Design: Each dyad engaged in a negotiation task, in which they role-played characters who are negotiating over six antique items (three crates of LP records, two art deco lamps, and one art deco painting), which have varied levels of value to them. They are told that their task is to decide how to divide up these six items with another participant, and if they fail to reach agreement, that they will receive the number of lottery tickets that they would have received for one of their highest value items.

Table 1. Participant's preferences for different issues across task and side.

Task	Side	Records	Lamps	Painting
Distributive	A	High (30)	Moderate (15)	Low (5)
	B	High (30)	Moderate (15)	None (0)
Integrative	A	High (20)	Moderate (10)	Low (5)
	B	Moderate (10)	High (30)	None (0)

Dyads were randomly assigned to either a distributive or integrative task: the items either have the same level of value to each participant, or different levels of value to each partner (Table 1). Specifically, in the distributive task, for both participants, the records are the highest value items, and the lamps have moderate value to them, whereas in the integrative task, for participant A, the records are the highest value items and the lamps have moderate value, but for participant B, the lamps have the highest value and the records have moderate value. In both conditions, the painting is of little value to participant A, and of no value at all to participant B.

Of the original 226 participants, 8 were removed for non-compliance with procedures (e.g., obvious intoxication, beginning the negotiation before reading all instructions), 5 dyads were excluded for failing to reach agreement in the negotiation, and an additional 28 participants were excluded from analyses because, after the study, they failed to accurately report the preferences to which they had been assigned.

All dialogues were manually transcribed and annotated with several different dialog acts. Two dialog acts are relevant for the current paper (the complete annotation scheme is described here [11]). *Offers* correspond to statements about a division of items. For example, the statement "How about if I take two records and you take both lamps?" is a partial offer. It is also partial in two distinct senses as (a) fails to mention the painting, and (b) it requests two records while leaving the third record unspecified.

Preference-assertions correspond to statements about an individual issue such as "I like records" or "I don't like paintings." The full annotation scheme makes several distinctions in preferences (e.g., I-like-best, i-like, i-might like, etc.), however, for the purpose of this paper, we collapse these into two broad classes (I-like-ITEM, and I-don't-like-ITEM) as more subtle distinctions would be problematic for automatic language recognition. Thus, to summarize, preference-assertions indicate an issue (e.g., records) and a sentiment (positive or negative) expressed toward that issue. If multiple issues are stated in a single utterance ("I like the records and the lamps"), these are represented as two preference assertions.

· Preference-assertions are annotated for their veracity. False statements do not necessarily mean the participant is lying (they could have misspoken), however it was clear that many participants attempted to misrepresent their true preferences.

3.2 Testing the Assumptions of Standard Opponent Models

In this section, we report some statistics from the corpus explained above as empirical evidence illustrating the differences between human and agent negotiators.

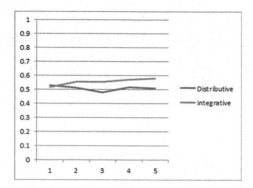

Fig. 2. Concession rates: y-axis is relative amount of total value claimed by each offer by round.

1. Participants did not start high and concede over time, as assumed by many opponent modeling methods. Figure 2 shows the average strength of offers by round and by the type of negotiation. A value of 1.0 would indicate that the participant made the high-utility offer they could obtain. Instead, they only asked for about half of this on the first round. Rather than conceding over time, participants, if anything, show the opposite trend. This can be explained as participants in the integrative condition discover a win-win solution is possible (i.e., they revise their demands upward as they form a more accurate model of their opponent).
2. The complete offer protocol adopted in automated agent frameworks was indeed violated. Of the 522 offered in the dataset, 370 (70 %) were partial.
3. In contrast to the thousands of offers exchanged by automated agents, human participants exchanged only 5.8 offers on average per negotiation.
4. People talked extensively about their preferences. People made 9.9 statements about their preferences on average in each negotiation (as compared to 5.8 explicit offers). Therefore, about twice as much as the information relevant for preference standard opponent modeling methods discards modeling. Most of this information was truthful, although 18 % of participants misstated their preferences, which emphasizes a challenging in using human data.

The observed differences between agent and human negotiators clearly emphasize the need for models that are better suited to the characteristics of human negotiators. We approached this problem by proposing three straightforward heuristic models: the *Issue-ratio heuristic* uses the sequence of offers to estimate the preference profile, the *Issue-sentiment heuristic* derives an estimate from explicit preference assertions, and the *Offer/Sentiment heuristic* simply uses the mean of these two models to integrate information in both offers and language. Note these are the simplest models we could imagine and future work could improve on these using machine-learning methods.

Issue-Ratio Heuristic: Rather than looking at concession rates, this heuristic examines each issue separately and assumes (1) if an issue is important, the participant will offer a greater percentage of the possible value to themselves, and (2) if an issue is important, they will include it more often in their partial offers. We realize these two intuitions in the following metric. If an issue (i) is discussed in an offer (k), it is assumed to have two parts: which level of that issue was claimed for self (l_k) and which level was assigned to the opponent (l'_k). The heuristic estimates each issue weight (w_i) for a participant by comparing the average level claimed for self ($\bar{l}_k$) to the average level offered to the opponent ($\bar{l}'_k$) across all offers made by that participant:

$$w_i = \frac{\bar{l}_k}{\bar{l}'_k} \tag{4}$$

Issue-Sentiment Heuristic: Participants made a large number of explicit statements about their preferences (e.g., "I like the records the most"). Although the trustworthiness of these expressions remains unknown, they could be considered as a valuable source of information for our preference models. We propose a very simple heuristic based merely on counting the number of times a preference is expressed towards an issue. More precisely, every time a positive preference is asserted towards an item ("I like the painting"), we add one to a weight associated with the issue. Every time a negative preference is expressed ("I don't really care for the painting"), we subtract one to the weight associated with the issue. All weights are normalized to compute a set of weights that are comparable to the weights derived from offers:

$$w_i = |P_i| - |N_i| \tag{5}$$

P_i is the set of all positive statements a participant asserted about issue i, and N_i is the list of all negative statements that participant made about issue i.

Offer/Sentiment Heuristic: As negotiators reveal preferences both through their offers and through explicit preference statements, a heuristic that incorporates both sources of information might perform best. A simple way to combine these two factors is to average the weights that arise from these two estimates. Our Offer/Like heuristic accomplishes just this. If no information is given by one source (e.g., the participant makes offers but does not make any preference assertions), we use just one estimator. If both estimators produce valid weights, we simply take the mean of the two estimates.

Offer/Sentiment Discrepancy: Finally, the fact that we have two sources of preference information (through offers and through explicit preference statements) it becomes possible to examine the discrepancy between these two estimates. This might have potential for lie detection. For example, if a negotiator implies one thing through his words but makes offers inconsistent with these preferences; we would have reason to be suspicious. Alternatively, this might suggest the negotiator is confused. Either way, such discrepancies are important to note and could be valuable to a pedagogical negation agent. We define Offer/Like discrepancy as the rank distance between the weights estimated via offers and the weights estimated via preference statements.

4 Evaluation

Here, we contrast the performance of our heuristics against the state-of-the art in opponent modeling techniques. We compare the performance of all heuristics on the dataset discussed above and report their accuracy in terms of rank-distance and max-regret. We also considered if Offer/Like discrepancy could be used for lie detection.

4.1 Heuristic Accuracy

We chose HardHeaded and N.A.S.H. Frequency as representatives of the state-of-the-art in opponent modeling. Hardheaded won the 2011 automated negotiation agents' competition and had one of the highest accuracies in modeling opponents (see [4]). N.A.S.H. Frequency did not perform as well in practice but represents the standard Bayesian view on how to model opponents.

Hardheaded is designed to solve a more general problem than was faced by our human participants, so we also created a *HardHeaded_Modified* to allow a more direct comparison. In the human negotiation task, participants were given knowledge about the ranking of levels within an issue (i.e., 2 lamps had more value than 1 lamp which had more value than no lamps). HardHeaded estimates this ranking from the pattern of offers. Thus, to create a fair comparison, we created a version of the algorithm with these parameters were fixed to their true values. In this way, both humans and the algorithms started the negotiation with the same knowledge about the task.

Each model was given the sequence of offers and preference assertions that were produced by each participant in the corpus (preference assertions were only used by the Issue-Sentiment model and the hybrid Offer/Sentiment model). For each participant, we calculate the rank distance of the deals, and Max-regret between the estimated weights produced by the model and the true weights provided to the participant. We also include a model that produces random weights as a point of comparison. Results are shown in Fig. 3. There were significant differences between models (Rank distance: $F (4, 176) = 85.242$, $p < .001$), Max-regret: $F (4, 176) = 44.148$, $p < .001$). As predicted, the existing models did not fare well on human data and their performance was close to random. Issue-sentiment and issue-ratio heuristics, however, made significantly better estimations in terms of both rank distance of the deals, and Max-regret measures. The composite Offer/Sentiment heuristic made the best estimation for the participants' preferences. These differences are significant ((Offer/Sentiment)/issue-ratio, Rank distance: $t(1, 179) = 5.006$, $p < .001$), Max-regret: $t(1, 179) = 3.195$, $p = .002$) ((Offer/Sentiment)/Issue-sentiment, Rank distance: $t(1, 179) = 7.656$, $p < .001$), Max-regret: $t(1, 179) = 7.21$, $p < .001$).

4.2 Lie Detection

We next tested if the Offer/Sentiment heuristic could serve as the basis of a lie detector. We compared the discrepancy of the weights estimated by the Issue-Ratio heuristics

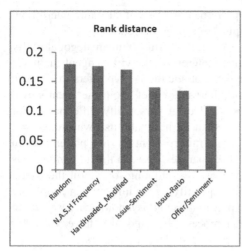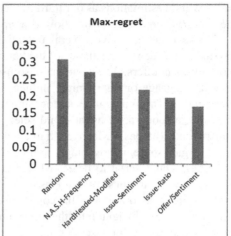

Fig. 3. Performance of various models based on two measures, rank distance of the deals, and max-regret [Note that the smaller our measures are the better that prediction is]

with the weights estimated by the Offer-Sentiment heuristic. This discrepancy was significantly positively correlated with the number of false preference assertions made by each participant ($r = 0.174$, $p = 0.03$), which confirms our hypothesis that agents can use the discrepancy between language channel and the pattern of offers to detect suspicious information. This is especially promising as both heuristics are quite simplistic and we expect even stronger correlations with more improved estimators.

5 Conclusion

Opponent preference modeling is an important skill for a virtual agent who intends to have efficient negotiations with humans or engage with them as a trainer. Despite the wide attention this area of research has received in agent-agent frameworks, negligible work was done for human involved settings. Using a corpus of human-human negotiations, we addressed the main differences between human and agent negotiators. Human negotiators violate many of the assumptions of automated negotiation agents, rendering these existing models useless for our purpose. Human participants made frequent use of partial offers, whereas agents typically assume complete offers; humans started with fair offers, whereas agents assume initial offers will be tough. Most importantly, humans use language to communicate their preferences whereas agents only focus on the pattern of offers. As a result of these differences, state-of-the-art opponent modeling methods perform close to chance on human data.

We proposed a new set of simple methods to estimate opponent preferences in human negotiations. Our first heuristic used this pattern of behavior to capture people's preferences and showed a significantly better performance than other existing models. Our second heuristic only used participants' preference assertions and performed as good as the offer heuristic. We used the average between offer based and the assertion based weight estimations as our third model performed the best of all. More interesting, the Offer/Sentiment heuristic allowed a simple form of lie detection.

These heuristics have several potential uses for a virtual human negotiator. By having a more accurate estimate of the human's preferences, the virtual agent can make more efficient offers. The agent can also use the heuristic on its own offers to estimate how its language or offers might influence the human's belief about the agent's own preferences. This can guide dialog strategies and even personality differences. For example, a cooperative agent could select speech acts that make its own preferences transparent, whereas a Machiavellian agent might misrepresent its own preferences in order to gain strategic advantage. Similarly, discrepancies between the human's words and offers could serve to detect when the human is attempting to exploit the agent. Finally, these heuristics can serve as metrics for quantifying the information people are exchanging in negotiations. This could have potential use in psychological research on emotion to give insight into the negotiation process. It could also have value for pedagogical agents for assessing the performance of student negotiators.

Future work will proceed on several fronts. First, we hope to improve upon these heuristics using machine-learning approaches. The current heuristics are very simple and we expect substantial improvements are possible, both in how to estimate weights from issues and language separately, but also how to best combine these two sources of information. Second, we plan to use active probing to improve our estimates. In the current paper, we passively observed a sequence of assertions and offers, but in a real negotiation, negotiators can select offers or ask about preferences in order to reduce uncertainty about the opponent's preferences [12]. Finally, we will incorporate these methods into a virtual human negotiator being developed at our lab [5].

Acknowledgement. This research was supported by the US Army. The content does not necessarily reflect the position or the policy of any Government, and no official endorsement should be inferred.

References

1. Kim, J.M., Hill, R.W., Technologies, C., Lane, H.C., Forbell, E., Core, M., Marsella, S., Pynadath, D., Hill Jr, R.W., Durlach, P.J., Hart, J.: BiLAT: A game-based environment for practicing negotiation in a cultural context. Int. J. Artif. Intell. Educ. **19**, 289–308 (2009)
2. Traum, D.R., Marsella, S.C., Gratch, J., Lee, J., Hartholt, A.: Multi-party, multi-issue, multi-strategy negotiation for multi-modal virtual agents. In: Prendinger, H., Lester, J.C., Ishizuka, M. (eds.) IVA 2008. LNCS (LNAI), vol. 5208, pp. 117–130. Springer, Heidelberg (2008)
3. Rosenfeld, A., Segal-halevi, E., Drein, O., Kraus, S., Zuckerman, I.: NegoChat: a chat-based negotiation agent. In: Proceedings of the 2014 International Conference on Autonomous Agents and Multi-agent Systems, International Foundation of Autonomous Agents and Multi-agent Systems (2014)
4. Baarslag, T., Hendrikx, M., Hindriks, K., Jonker, C.: Predicting the performance of opponent models in automated negotiation, vol. 2, pp. 59–66. In: Proceedings of 2013 IEEE/WIC/ACM International Conferences on Intelligent Agent Technologies (IAT 2013) (2013)

5. Gratch, J., Devault, D., Lucas, G., Marsella, S.: Negotiation as a challenge problem for virtual humans. Paper presented at the 15th international conference on intelligent virtual agents, Delft (2015)
6. van Krimpen, T., Looije, D., Hajizadeh, S.: HardHeaded. In: Ito, T., Zhang, M., Robu, V., Matsuo, T. (eds.) Complex Automated Negotiations: Theories, Models, and Software Competitions. SCI, vol. 435, pp. 225–230. Springer, Heidelberg (2012)
7. Hindriks, K.V., Tykhonov, D.: Towards a quality assessment method for learning preference profiles in negotiation. In: Ketter, W., La Poutré, H., Sadeh, N., Shehory, O., Walsh, W. (eds.) AMEC 2008. LNBIP, vol. 44, pp. 46–59. Springer, Heidelberg (2010)
8. Kelley, H.: A classroom study of dilemmas in interpersonal negotiations. Strategic Interaction and Conflict, pp. 49–73. Institute of International Studies, University of California, Berkeley (1966)
9. Fehr, E., Schmidt, K.M.: The economics of fairness, reciprocity and altruism - experimental evidence and new theories. Handb. Econ. Giving Altruism Reciprocity 1(6), 615–691 (2006)
10. Lin, R., Kraus, S.: Can automated agents proficiently negotiate with humans? Commun. ACM 53, 78 (2010)
11. Devault, D., Mell, J., Gratch, J.: Toward natural turn-taking in a virtual human negotiation agent. In: Paper Presented at the AAAI Spring Symposium on Turn-taking and Coordination in Human-Machine Interaction. Stanford (2015)
12. Boutilier, C., Sandholm, T., Shields, R.: Eliciting bid taker non-price preferences in (combinatorial) auctions, pp. 204–211. In: Proceedings of Nineteenth National Conference on Artificial Intelligence (2004)

Adapting Virtual Patient Interviews for Interviewing Skills Training of Novice Healthcare Students

Stephanie Carnell[✉], Shivashankar Halan, Michael Crary,
Aarthi Madhavan, and Benjamin Lok

University of Florida, Gainesville, FL 32611, USA
scarnell@ufl.edu

Abstract. The purpose of this paper is to explore the potential of using a selection-based interaction method to adapt virtual patient interviews for training novice healthcare students in interviewing skills. We outline a method for identifying topics about which novices are likely to ask by reviewing previous transcripts of novice interactions, and results indicate that the method was successful in such identification. Additionally, we examine the possibility of using a selection-based virtual patient as a modeling tool for learning interviewing skills. Our initial results support the possibility of such question modeling and reveal that healthcare students already view selection-based virtual patient interactions as modeling opportunities.

Keywords: Virtual patients · Healthcare education · Interview skills training · Interaction methods

1 Introduction

Of the available virtual patient (VP) technology, the potential of designing VPs to accommodate the experience level of different learners, particularly novices, is relatively unexplored [1]. Usually, a VP creator's aims are to make all aspects of a VP as realistic, or high fidelity, as possible. The decision to use high fidelity design is usually supported by findings from high-fidelity simulations, but the decision does not examine whether such a design has particular advantages for the given educational context [1]. Further study may reveal low fidelity designs may be more useful to novices, as low fidelity designs may better fit their educational needs.

One potential design choice that could be explored for novice users is the type of interaction method. Typically, the goal for the interaction method is a chat-based virtual patient that responds to user-generated questions. However, there are two important limitations to chat-based VPs: these designs rely on existing interview experience to progress the interview, which may frustrate novices who lack the requisite interviewing skills, and such frustrations may be further aggravated by a chat-based interaction method's varying performance. Chat-based interactions must have high accuracy rates and controlled performance degradation [2], both of which are limited by current natural language processing technology. With these limitations, a chat-based interaction is likely to inhibit a novice's ability to complete an interview.

© Springer International Publishing Switzerland 2015
W.-P. Brinkman et al. (Eds.): IVA 2015, LNAI 9238, pp. 50–59, 2015.
DOI: 10.1007/978-3-319-21996-7_5

However, a selection-based interaction method, the lower fidelity implementation, will not experience the challenges of a chat-based interface. Selection-based interactions have the advantage of displaying the available, answerable questions [3]. Additionally, a selection-based interaction could further ease novices' interview experiences by utilizing questions on topics novices are likely to consider. Finally, a further benefit of a selection-based interaction method for novices is the potential of the selection questions to act as models for appropriate interview questions.

This study explores the potential of using a selection-based interaction method to design a novice-oriented VP. Previous work shows that novice and expert interviewers focus on different topics during VP interviews [4], making the best source for novice-oriented content other novices. Thus, our first objective was to determine whether using previous novice interactions with an existing VP was an effective method of identifying novice-oriented topics. In Sect. 3, we outline our method of creating a novice-oriented, selection VP. Another one of our goals was to discover if healthcare students viewed selection-based interactions as opportunities for question modeling and whether such modeling effects may occur after using a selection-based VP.

2 Related Work

In this section, we outline the existing need for interview modeling in the medical field, based on the current methods of interview skills training. We also point out existing uses of a selection-based interaction and their application areas.

2.1 Patient-Centered Interviewing

Using a patient-centered approach in a medical interview has been shown to lead to improved patient satisfaction and cooperation [5], and this conclusion is the basis of the paradigm in medical education to emphasize a "holistic, patient-centered" approach [6]. However, this approach is at odds with clinicians' tendencies to reach focused biomedical questions early in the interview [7], which can cause the clinician to overlook the patient's perspective and thus leave the patient unsatisfied.

Several sources, however, indicate that a patient-centered approach can be taught [5, 7]. Teaching methods for such skills were evaluated by Smith et al. when they evaluated biopsychosocial training programs [8]. Several of the evaluated successful programs provided demonstrations of appropriate interviewing [9], which indicates that good interview skills can be acquired through modeling, an established learning method [10], and shows the usefulness of a system that provides demonstrations.

2.2 Selection-Based Interactions

Several interactive experiences with virtual agents have been designed using selection interactions. SIDNIE, an nursing interview system, allows users to conduct a pediatric interview using a selection-based interface [11]. The designers of SIDNIE found that, after using the system, nurses' interview skills improved from the baseline and that a selection interface rated highly among participants in usability.

Another use of a selection-based interaction is Operation ARIES!, a game designed to teach scientific, critical thinking [12]. In Operation ARIES!, players develop interviewing skills while playing the interrogation module. Early levels of interviews provide examples from a character that, when a topic is clicked, asks questions related to the clicked topic. The player is meant to interpret the examples as models for good critical thinking questions. Though testing of Operation ARIES! is ongoing, the use of a selection-based interaction as a modeling method in scientific inquiry provides basis for the use of such an interaction in other fields.

3   Selection Generator

In this section, we outline a method for creating a selection-based VP. This method was based on another system that generated virtual medical students to train standardized patients [13]. Using this method, a selection-based VP is created from an existing chat-based VP and novice interviews. Given such data, the selection generator calculates the most frequently asked questions and the average locations of the patient responses in interviews. Using this information, the selection generator then creates a set of questions for a selection-based VP. The selection generator is designed on top of our current system, Virtual People Factory 2.0 (VPF2).

VPF2 is a web application that allows users to create, edit, and interact with a VP. A VPF2 virtual patient can include many components, but of particular interest are the *question-answer pairs*. These question-answer pairs define the statements the VP can make and the corresponding questions. In addition to the question-answer pairs, the system also saves transcripts from previous interactions. The transcript is similar to a list that stores the statements made by both the interviewer and the patient.

This brief overview of VPF2 defines the two primary objects on which the selection generator operates: the question-answer pairs and the transcripts. The selection generator process begins by creating a list of all of the patient responses pulled from a given set of transcripts. For each patient response, the selection generator also saves the "location" of the answer in the transcript. The location is calculated by dividing an answer's index location in the transcript by the length of the overall transcript.

Because each of the transcripts represent independent interviews, some of the patient responses will be duplicates. The duplicate answers are counted to give the frequency of a response. Also calculated at this time are the average location values. This stage of the process ends with a list of non-duplicate patient responses and their associated frequency and location values. This list is then sorted by descending frequencies and ascending average locations, based on the assumptions that the most significant questions will be asked most often and earliest in the transcripts.

At this stage, the patient's question-answer pairs are retrieved to get the selection questions. A most popular question list is created from the questions with answers that match the first fifty patient responses in the response list. Next, the entirety of the patient response list is used to create another question list that features questions organized by topic. The *topic* refers to the domain area to which a patient's response relates and is stored with the question-answer pair. The selection generator organizes the questions within topics based on increasing average location values stored in the patient response list. The most popular question list and the topic-sorted question list are then sent to the interaction page and are displayed as collapsible lists (see Fig. 1).

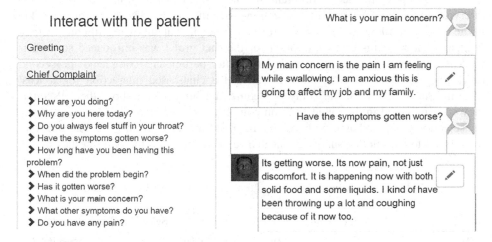

Fig. 1. A sample selection list with a user's interaction

4 Experimental Study

To explore the validity of using a selection-based interaction for interview skills training, we conducted a user study in which healthcare students interviewed VPs using chat-based and selection-based interfaces. University of Florida healthcare students enrolled in a course on dysphagia in spring 2015 were the participants. Participation was voluntary and was compensated with five extra-credit points on a participant's final exam score. 22 out of the 27 students (81.5 %) enrolled in the class volunteered, and the majority of 22 students were graduate students completing a Master's degree in speech-language pathology. 19 of the 22 participants were female (86.4 %). The average age of the participants was 24.36 (SD = 3.59). This participant population was well suited for our investigation because the students would later have to interview real patients suffering from dysphagia, a medical condition in which patients experience difficulty swallowing, as part of their profession. According to the course's instructor, the participants have had minimal exposure to real dysphagia patients. All 22 participants self-reported no prior interview skills training. This led us to categorize this population as a novice population with regards to patient interviewing.

As part of the extra-credit exercise, students completed five VP-based tasks related to dysphagia during the semester. In this paper, we examine the first three tasks. During the first class meeting, the investigators demonstrated an interview using the chat-based interaction method and described the requirements for the extra-credit exercise. Students were given a week to sign up. During the second week of classes, all 22 students completed the first task of the study, a minimum fifteen-minute interview with a dysphagia VP using the chat-based interface. After all the students completed this interview, their performance—specifically, the number of discoveries made—was analyzed in order to divide the students pseudo-randomly into two groups. This division was done to make both groups equivalent in discoveries found during task one.

Each group completed a different second task. The selection group ($n = 11$) interviewed a second VP using the selection-based interaction. The chat group ($n = 11$) wrote a 650-word case description for a dysphagia patient who suffered from a brainstem stroke. This case description for the chat group was introduced so participants spent equal time working with VPs. After participants completed the second tasks, they all interviewed a third VP using the chat-based interaction for at least 15 min. An overview of the study procedure and information about the VPs interviewed is provided in the Table 1. Upon completion of task two, the participants from the selection group had used both the chat interface and the selection interface and were then asked to complete a survey about their experiences with the two interfaces.

Table 1. Study procedure and information about the VPs interviewed

	Chat Group		Selection Group	
Task 1		**Interview Vinny Devito**		
	Interaction Method	**: Chat-based interaction**		
	Diagnosis	: Brainstem Stroke		
	Available Questions	: 1360		
	Number of Discoveries	: 11		
Task 2	**Create new patient description**		**Interview Marty Graw**	
	Interaction Method: **None**		Interaction Method:	
	Participants typed out a 650-word		**Selection-based interaction**	
	case description for dysphagia VP		Diagnosis: Stricture	
			Available Questions: 150	
			Number of Discoveries: 17	
Task 3		**Interview Lilly Smith**		
	Interaction Method	**: Chat-based interaction**		
	Diagnosis	: Brainstem Stroke		
	Available Questions	: 1360		
	Number of Discoveries	: 11		

4.1   Interaction Methods

Chat-Based Interaction. VPF2 VPs typically utilize a chat-based interaction method. Users chat with a patient by typing a question in the area labeled "Type Here" (see Fig. 2a). After the typed question is received, the chat log on the right of the screen is updated with the patient's response; a recording of a human reading the response is also played and lip-synced with a three-dimensional representation of the virtual human on the left of the screen.

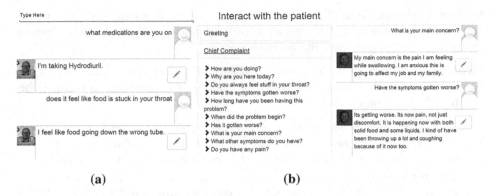

Fig. 2. (a) A sample chat log from the first chat-based VP versus (b) a sample chat from the selection-based VP

Selection-Based Interaction. The interface for the selection-based interaction was built on the chat-based interface, so the two pages share many features. The selection page also incorporates human audio and a 3D representation of the patient. The main difference between the two interfaces is the selection interface's reduction of the chat log's screen space. This reduction allows for the placement of the selection questions.

4.2   Metrics

We outline the metrics used in this study below. Each of these values is calculated per participant, per VP.

Total Time. The total time is a measure of how long the participant spent interacting with the VP. This time is the sum of all transcript times and is measured in seconds.

Percentage of Discoveries Found. A *discovery* is an important piece of information that a user should extract from the patient in the course of the interview. The total discoveries made is the sum of discoveries made in each transcript with duplicates removed. The percentage of discoveries found is the total discoveries made divided by the number of discoveries associated with the VP.

Number of Questions Asked. The number of questions asked is the sum of all questions asked across all transcripts. This sum includes answers that elicited a response and those that did not.

Response Accuracy. The response accuracy refers to the total number of questions that elicited a response divided by the number of questions asked. This accuracy can vary per user for the chat-based interaction method but should theoretically be 100 % for the selection-based interaction method. However, the response accuracy can fall below 100 % if the user clicks questions quickly and does not wait for the patient to respond. For the analysis reported in this paper, we have assumed that the response elicited from the patient is correct. We did not account for false positives where a response was elicited but was not relevant to the question asked, due to limitations of the matching algorithm that fetches the response for each question.

Average Response Time. The average response time is the average of all response times across all transcripts. A response time is the difference between when the current question was asked and when the previous question was asked.

Feedback from the Survey. The survey consisted of twelve questions about the user's experience using the interaction methods. Half of the questions concerned the chat-based interaction method:

1. *I became frustrated while using the chat-based interaction method.*
2. *I was able to ask the questions I wanted to using the chat-based interaction method.*
3. *Using the chat-based interaction method helped me learn dysphagia interviewing skills significantly.*
4. *Did the interview with the chat-based interaction method feel like a real-world interview? Please explain why or why not.*
5. *For what types of learning tasks do you think the chat-based interaction method is appropriate? For which tasks would it be inappropriate?*
6. *What did you like or dislike about the chat-based interaction method?*

The same six questions were repeated with "chat-based" replaced by "selection-based." Questions one through three allowed responses on a seven-point Likert scale, and the remaining questions were free response.

5   Results

Of the 22 students in the study, all 22 completed both chat-based interactions. The survey was sent to the 11 students who also completed the selection-based interaction, and all 11 completed the survey.

5.1   Transcript Analysis

Analysis of the transcript data was performed using independent t-tests and Mann-Whitney tests (see Table 2; t-tests indicated by asterisk and significance indicated in bold). There were no significant differences in any metric between the selection and creation groups for task one. For task three, there were no significant differences except the response accuracy $t(22) = -2.40$, $p = 0.029$. On average, the selection group's response accuracy (M = 85.05, SE = 1.48) was greater than the chat group's response accuracy (M = 78.71, SE = 2.24) for task three.

5.2   Survey Feedback

The numerical survey data was analyzed using Wilcoxon Signed Rank tests. There were no significant differences in any of these questions. The frustration item was low for both selection (M = 2.91) and chat (M = 3.55), and the ability to ask questions item was high for selection (M = 5.55) and chat (M = 5.45). The impact on learning item indicated a positive response for both selection (M = 4.09) and chat (M = 4.00).

Table 2. Means, standard deviations, and p-values per metric for tasks 1 and 3

	Task 1			Task 3		
	Chat	Selection	p	Chat	Selection	p
Total time (s)	4298.3 ± 2729.8	3831.7 ± 1819.4	0.642*	2921.9 ± 1812.8	2169.4 ±1222.0	0.606
Percent discoveries	89.3 ± 10.6	86.8 ± 11.0	0.606	81.8 ± 9.73	81.1 ± 13.5	0.898
No. questions asked	106.1 ± 67.7	82.9 ± 29.4	0.748	93.5 ± 59.6	72.1 ± 21.9	0.797
Response accuracy (%)	84.1 ± 7.08	86.5 ± 6.50	0.42*	78.7 ± 7.42	85.0 ± 4.90	**0.029***
Avg. response time (s)	30.2 ± 8.97	27.5 ± 7.06	0.478	24.7 ± 7.67	23.6 ± 7.84	0.562

Table 3. Free response data gathered from the eleven participants who completed the survey

Free response feedback	
Felt chat was like a real-world interview	9 (81.8 %)
Felt selection was like a real-world interview	4 (36.4 %)
Suggested chat be completed after some instruction was provided	5 (45.5 %)
Found selection appropriate for novice users	9 (81.8 %)

Responses for the free response questions are represented in Table 3. 9 out of 11 participants described the chat-based interaction method as similar to a real-world interview, while 4 out of 11 said the selection-based interview was similar to a real-world interview. 5 out of 11 participants described the chat-based interaction as a suitable exercise for learning interviewing skills only after some training or instruction has been provided. 9 out of 11 participants described the selection-based interaction as appropriate for novice users.

6 Discussion

Our hypothesis on using a selection-based interaction as a modeling tool received possible support in the difference in response accuracy. A larger response accuracy indicates that the selection group asked more questions answerable by the chat-based VP; this ability to ask the correct types of questions could be because of modeling from the selection-based interaction. Additionally, because the two groups used the same amount of time and of questions, greater response accuracy also indicates that the selection group gained more patient information than the chat group did.

The modeling potential was also supported by the participants' free response survey answers. The majority of the participants, when asked for which tasks the selection-based interaction is appropriate, responded with answers similar to the following:

> "It [selection-based interaction] would be appropriate for the very first interview because then we get an idea of what types of questions we should be asking." — Participant 3

Even though participants felt the chat-based interaction was more like a real-world interview, such statements were qualified, as below:

"Chat-based interaction is appropriate once the students are aware of what types of questions to ask; otherwise it's inappropriate. For example, I thought having the chat-based interaction as our first interview was a little difficult since I had no clue what to ask." – **Participant 7**

Such feedback indicates that the many participants already view the selection-based interaction as a modeling tool and as an appropriate training exercise for novices.

That 81.8 % of the participants described the selection interaction as appropriate for novices also supports Cook and Triola's claim that low-fidelity interaction methods may be more appropriate for certain educational contexts [1]. Further, the high mean value for "I was able to ask the questions I wanted to using the selection-based interaction method" could indicate that the selection generator's method of choosing content from novice transcripts seems appropriate for creating a novice-oriented VP.

However, the greater response accuracy for the selection group could originate from more experience with VPF2 rather than a modeling effect, as the chat group did not interact directly with the system while writing their case descriptions. However, we feel that the two activities are comparable enough in time and in dysphagia content that such learning of the system is probably not the cause of the significance.

7 Conclusion and Future Work

This study explored the creation of a selection-based VP for novice users. Our method used novice transcripts and an existing chat-based VP to produce a new selection-based VP. After creating the VP, we had actual healthcare students interview the patient, as well as two chat-based VPs. Our initial findings indicate that the selection generator can be used to design novice-oriented VPs.

Other contributions include support for the potential modeling benefits of a selection-based VP, as it appears that interacting with a selection-based VP can impact interview questions several weeks later. Relatedly, several participants suggested that interviewing practice should begin with a selection VP in order to learn what questions should be asked. Such a suggestion could mean that healthcare students already view selection VPs as opportunities for modeling.

In future work, novice-oriented VP creation should draw content from novice interviews, as we did in this study, and add expert validation for question phrasing. This step should provide the appropriate models of questions to be asked, while still maintaining the novice-oriented content. Other potential research could explore whether the organization of the selection questions has an effect on interview question order.

References

1. Cook, D.A., Triola, M.M.: Virtual patients: a critical literature review and proposed next steps. Med. Educ. **43**, 303–311 (2009)

2. Lester, J., Branting, K., Mott, B.: Conversational agents. In: Munindar, P.S. (ed.) The Practical Handbook of Internet Computing, pp. 220–240. Chapman & Hall, London (2004)
3. Pence, T.B., Dukes, L.C., Hodges, L.F., Meehan, N.K., Johnson, A.: The effects of interaction and visual fidelity on learning outcomes for a virtual paediatric patient system, pp. 209–218. In: Proceedings of 2013 IEEE International Conference Healthcare Informatics, ICHI 2013 (2013)
4. Kenny, P.G., Parsons, T.D., Rizzo, A.: A comparative analysis between experts and novices interacting with a virtual patient with PTSD. Annu. Rev. CyberTherapy Telemed. 7, 122–124 (2009)
5. Smith, R.C., Lyles, J.S., Mettler, J.A., Marshall, A.A., Van Egeren, L.F., Stoffelmayr, B.E., Osborn, G.G., Shebroe, V.: A strategy for improving patient satisfaction by the intensive training of residents in psychosocial medicine: a controlled, randomized study. Acad. Med. 70, 729–732 (1995)
6. Coulehan, J.L., Block, M.R., NetLibrary, I.: The Medical Interview Mastering Skills for Clinical Practice. F.A. Davis Co, Philadelphia (2006)
7. Haidet, P., Paterniti, D.A.: "Building" a history rather than "taking" one. Arch. Intern. Med. 163, 1134–1140 (2010)
8. Smith, R.C., Marshall, A.A., Cohen-Cole, S.A.: The efficacy of intensive biopsychosocial teaching programs for residents - a review of the literature and guidelines for teaching. J. Gen. Intern. Med. 9, 390–396 (1994)
9. Smith, R.C., Osborn, G., Hoppe, R.B., Lyles, J.S., Van Egeren, L., Henry, R., Sego, D., Alguire, P., Stoffelmayr, B.: Efficacy of a one-month training block in psychosocial medicine for residents - a controlled study. J. Gen. Intern. Med. 6, 535–543 (1991)
10. Cox, R., McKendree, J., Tobin, R., Lee, J., Mayes, T.: Vicarious learning from dialogue and discourse: a controlled comparison. Instr. Sci. 27, 431–458 (1999)
11. Dukes, L.C., Pence, T.B., Hodges, L.F., Meehan, N., Johnson, A.: SIDNIE: scaffolded interviews developed by nurses in education, pp. 395–405. In: Proceedings IUI International Conference on Intelligent User Interfaces (2013)
12. De, Freitas S., Liarokapis, F.: Serious Games and Edutainment Applications, pp. 9–23. Springer, London (2011)
13. Rossen, B., Cendan, J., Lok, B.: Using virtual humans to bootstrap the creation of other virtual humans. In: Allbeck, J., Badler, N., Bickmore, T., Pelachaud, C., Safonova, A. (eds.) Intelligent Virtual Agents. Lecture Notes in Computer Science, vol. 6356, pp. 392–398. Springer, Berlin, Heidelberg (2010)

On Conversational Agents with Mental States

Tibor Bosse[1,2(✉)] and Simon Provoost[1]

[1] Department of Computer Science, VU University Amsterdam,
De Boelelaan 1081, 1081 HV Amsterdam, The Netherlands
{t.bosse,s.j.provoost}@vu.nl
[2] Department of Training and Performance Innovations, TNO, Kampweg 5,
3769 DE Soesterberg, The Netherlands

Abstract. Embodied conversational agents (ECAs) have been put forward as a promising means for the training of social skills. The traditional approach to drive the behaviour of ECAs during human-agent dialogues is to use conversation trees. Although this approach is easy to use and very transparent, an important limitation of conversation trees is that the resulting behaviour of the ECAs is often perceived as predictable. To provide ECAs with more sophisticated behaviour, the current paper proposes an approach to endow them with mental states. The approach is illustrated by a motivational example in the domain of aggression de-escalation training.

Keywords: Virtual training · Aggression de-escalation · Cognitive modelling

1 Introduction

Embodied conversational agents (ECAs) are computer-generated characters 'that demonstrate many of the same properties as humans in face-to-face conversation, including the ability to produce and respond to verbal and nonverbal communication' [5]. ECAs have been put forward as a promising means for the training of social skills [8]. Recent applications can be found in domains varying from negotiation [9] to sales conversations [3].

To effectively train users in developing such social skills, an important requirement for ECAs is *believability*, as believable agents permit their conversation partners to 'suspend their disbelief', which is an important condition for learning [2]. Although much progress has been made with respect to the physical appearance of ECAs, it still remains difficult to develop agents with believable behaviour. The traditional approach to drive the behaviour of ECAs during a human-agent dialogue is to use *conversation trees*, i.e. tree structures representing all possible developments of the dialogue, where users can decide between different branches using multiple choice. Although this approach can be quite successful due to its transparency, an important limitation of conversation trees is that they are quite rigid. Consequently, the resulting behaviour of the ECAs is often perceived as stereotypical and predictable. This can be overcome by constructing very large conversation trees (with many branches), but this approach is highly labour-intensive and difficult to re-use.

© Springer International Publishing Switzerland 2015
W.-P. Brinkman et al. (Eds.): IVA 2015, LNAI 9238, pp. 60–64, 2015.
DOI: 10.1007/978-3-319-21996-7_6

As an alternative, several authors have proposed the use of cognitive models to endow ECAs with more sophisticated behaviour (e.g., [3, 7]). Using such models, agents base their behaviour not only on their current observations (or input), but also on internal mental states, for example an emotional state that resulted from previous interactions. The abstract nature of cognitive models however, makes it difficult to unify them with conversation trees.

Elaborating upon similar approaches (like [3, 7]), the current paper makes a step towards building a bridge between the traditional conversation tree approach (transparent, but rigid) and cognitive models (dynamic, but abstract). The approach is illustrated by an example in the domain of simulation-based training for aggression de-escalation.

2 Aggression De-escalation Training

Aggressive behaviour against employees in the public sector, such as tram drivers, police officers, and ambulance personnel, is an ongoing concern worldwide. The current paper is part of a project that explores to what extent simulation-based training using ECAs can be an effective method for employees to develop these types of social skills[1]. In the envisioned training environment, a trainee will be placed in a virtual scenario involving verbal aggression, with the goal of handling it as adequately as possible. The scenarios emphasise dyadic (one-on-one) interactions. For instance, the trainee plays the role of a tram driver, and is confronted with a virtual passenger who starts intimidating him in an attempt to get a free ride. The trainee observes the behaviour of the ECA, and has to respond to it by selecting the most appropriate responses from a multiple choice menu.

The main learning goal of the training system is to help trainees develop their *emotional intelligence*: they should be able to recognise the emotional state of the (virtual) conversation partner, and choose the right communication style. Here, an important factor is the distinction between *reactive* and *proactive* aggression made within psychological literature: reactive aggression is characterised as an emotional reaction to a negative event that frustrates a person's desires, whereas proactive aggression is the instrumental use of aggression to achieve a certain goal [6]. Based on the type of aggressive behaviour that is observed, the trainee should select the most appropriate communication style. More specifically, when dealing with a reactive aggressor, empathic, *supportive* behaviour is required to de-escalate a situation, for example by showing understanding for the situation. Instead, when dealing with a proactive aggressor, a more dominant, *directive* type of intervention is assumed to be most effective, e.g. by making it clear that aggressive behaviour is not acceptable [1, 4, 10]. By ensuring that the ECAs respond in an appropriate manner to the chosen responses, the system provides implicit feedback on the chosen communication style.

---

[1] More information on this project, called 'Simulation-based Training of Resilience in Emergencies and Stressful Situations', can be found at http://stress.few.vu.nl.

3 Conversational Agents with Mental States

The proposed training system is based on the InterACT software[2], developed by the company IC3D Media[3]. InterACT is a software platform that has been specifically designed for simulation-based training. The system assumes that a dialogue consists of a sequence of spoken sentences that follow a turn-taking protocol. That is, first the ECA says something (e.g. "I forgot my public transport card. You probably don't mind if I ride for free?"). After that, the user can respond, followed by a response from the ECA, and so on. In InterACT, these dialogues are represented by conversation trees, where vertices are either atomic ECA behaviours or decision nodes (enabling the user to determine a response), and the edges are transitions between nodes. The atomic ECA behaviours consist of pre-generated fragments of speech, synchronised with facial expressions and possibly extended with gestures.

Each decision node is implemented as a multiple choice menu. Via such a menu, the user has the ability to choose between multiple sentences. In the current version, for every decision node, four options are used, which can be classified, respectively, as *letting go*, *supportive*, *directive*, and *call for support*. Here, the supportive and directive option relate to the communication styles that were explained above. The other two options are more 'extreme' interventions, which should be applied, respectively, in case the aggressor has calmed down or in case the aggression is about to escalate, for example when personal threats are being made [10]. Additionally, the choice of the user determines how the scenario continues (or whether it ends immediately) by triggering a corresponding branch in the tree. Because a correct or wrong user choice is always followed by, respectively, a positive or negative ECA response, this approach is potentially predictable and repetitive.

We therefore propose to endow the ECA with an internal *state of aggression* that is represented numerically. Additionally, each ECA has a personality, which specifies whether it is a reactive or a pro-active aggressor. Based on this, the dynamics of the ECA's state of aggression are influenced by the observed communication style of the user in the following way: if a reactive aggressor is approached in a supportive manner, he calms down, but if he is approached in a directive manner, he becomes more aggressive. For the proactive aggressor, this works exactly the other way around.

This approach allows us to create a large variation in scenarios with relatively limited effort, because the ECA's internal states keep track of the *history* of the conversation. To start with, threshold values determine which ECA verbal response matches which level of aggression. By designing additional verbal statements that contain language of an increasingly aggressive nature, but otherwise carry the same message, *every* user choice can now be followed by a wider variety of ECA responses. Because we no longer require a new user choice leading to the new ECA response, we can actually create more different scenarios with half the work (see Fig. 1).

Lastly, under the proposed approach, the precise path that is taken through the conversation tree no longer solely depends on what the user does, but also on the

---

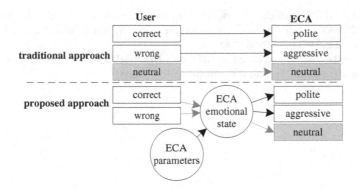

Fig. 1. The benefits of the proposed approach. The red verbal behaviours entail the extra work involved when adding a new ECA response, the green arrows the resulting new scenarios.

ECA's personality, i.e. the nature of the ECA's aggression and the parameter configuration that determines the rate at which its internal states change.

Acknowledgements. This research was supported by funding from the National Initiative Brain and Cognition, coordinated by the Netherlands Organisation for Scientific Research (NWO), under grant agreement No. 056-25-013. The authors would like to thank Karel van den Bosch for a number of fruitful discussions.

References

1. Anderson, L.N., Clarke, J.T.: De-escalating verbal aggression in primary care settings. Nurse Pract. **21**(10), 95–102 (1996)
2. Bates, J.: The role of emotions in believable agents. Commun. ACM **37**(7), 122–125 (1994)
3. Van den Bosch, K., Brandenburgh, A., Muller, T.J., Heuvelink, A.: Characters with personality! In: Nakano, Y., Neff, M., Paiva, A., Walker, M. (eds.) IVA 2012. LNCS, vol. 7502, pp. 426–439. Springer, Heidelberg (2012)
4. Bosse, T., Provoost, S.: Towards aggression de-escalation training with virtual agents: a computational model. In: Zaphiris, P., Ioannou, A. (eds.) LCT. LNCS, vol. 8524, pp. 375–387. Springer, Heidelberg (2014)
5. Cassell, J., Sullivan, J., Prevost, S., Churchill, E.: Embodied Conversational Agents. MIT Press, Cambridge (2000)
6. Dodge, K.A.: The structure and function of reactive and proactive aggression. In: Pepler, D., Rubin, H. (eds.) The Development and Treatment of Childhood Aggression, pp. 201–218. Erlbaum, Hillsdale (1990)
7. Gebhard, P., Kipp, M., Klesen, M., Rist, T.: Adding the emotional dimension to scripting character dialogues. In: Rist, T., Aylett, R.S., Ballin, D., Rickel, J. (eds.) IVA 2003. LNCS (LNAI), vol. 2792, pp. 48–56. Springer, Heidelberg (2003)
8. Kenny, P., Hartholt, A., Gratch, J., Swartout, W., Traum, D., Marsella, S., Piepol, D.: Building interactive virtual humans for training environments. In: Proceedings of 2007 Interservice/Industry Training, Simulation and Education Conference, Orlando (2007)

 9. Kim, J., Hill, R.W., Durlach, P., Lane, H.C., Forbell, E., Core, C., Marsella, S., Pynadath, D., Hart, J.: BiLAT: a game-based environment for practicing negotiation in a cultural context. Int. J. AI Educ. **19**(3), 289–308 (2009)
10. Ministry of the Interior and Kingdom Relations: Handboek agressie en geweld - voorkomen, beperken, afhandelen. Technical report (in Dutch) (2008)

Cognitive, Affective and Social Models

Virtual Suspect William

Merijn Bruijnes[1]([✉]), Rieks op den Akker[1],
Arno Hartholt[2], and Dirk Heylen[1]

[1] Human Media Interaction, University of Twente,
PO Box 217, 7500 AE Enschede, The Netherlands
m.bruijnes@utwente.nl
[2] Institute for Creative Technology, University of Southern California,
12015 Waterfront Drive, Playa Vista, CA 90094, USA

Abstract. We evaluate an algorithm which computes the responses of
an agent that plays the role of a suspect in simulations of police interrogations. The algorithm is based on a cognitive model - the response
model - that is centred around keeping track of interpersonal relations.
The model is parametrized in such a way that different personalities of
the virtual suspect can be defined. In the evaluation we defined three different personalities and had participants guess the personality based on
the responses the model provided in an interaction with the participant.
We investigate what factors contributed to the ability of a virtual agent
to show behaviour that was recognized by participants as belonging to
a persona.

Keywords: Social interaction · Police interview · Response model ·
Data analysis · Mental models · Virtual agents · Tutoring application

1 Introduction

We aim to build embodied conversational agents that can play the role of a suspect in a tutoring system by means of which police trainees learn to interrogate
suspects. Trainees are taught how the behaviour of a suspect is related to their
own behaviour, for instance to the interpersonal stance they adopt. Interpersonal
stance (e.g. [7]) is a core construct in the theory used to understand and explain
how a suspect behaves in a police interview. Adopting the right stance may be
instrumental in arriving at a confession. Currently, actors play the role of a suspect in training sessions in trainings offered by the Dutch Police Academy. They
play a suspect persona from a specific scenario based on historical material. If we
want to use an artificial actor that plays a suspect we need to know how to relate
the behaviour of our virtual suspect to the behaviour of the trainee in a way that
is consistent with the persona the virtual suspect is playing. The agent needs to
model the dynamics of such interpersonal relations. Ideally, the agent can analyse
the speech and non-verbal messages of the trainee to determine the level of friendliness or aggression and use these interpretations to update the interpersonal values. The response of the virtual suspect is based on the interpersonal status of the
suspect (e.g. if you make him angry, he will respond angrily). Virtual humans in

© Springer International Publishing Switzerland 2015
W.-P. Brinkman et al. (Eds.): IVA 2015, LNAI 9238, pp. 67–76, 2015.
DOI: 10.1007/978-3-319-21996-7_7

social skill learning offer learning by experience; the student can experience a social interaction. Using virtual humans to train students in social skills is not a new idea. There are many examples of virtual humans used in social skill training and some in the interrogation domain. For example in [10] a virtual Arabic civilian is questioned by US military personnel to hone their interrogation skills. Afterwards reflecting on the interaction can provide reflective learning of the trainee, particularly when this is a reflection on his or her own interaction [1]. A virtual suspect which can provide experiential and reflective learning has to be able to provide information on the interaction it had using terms the students understands. The real actor describes, using terms of psychological, social, and interpersonal theories, how the personality of the suspect influenced the effects of the actions by the student had on the suspect. Bruijnes et al. [4,5] created a response model (RM) based on observations of (practice) police interrogations ([3]). In this paper we evaluate how well this RM can portray a suspect persona in an interaction. Participants played the role of police interviewer and used natural language to interact with the virtual suspect.

2   Response Model

In [3] we analysed videos of police officers practising interrogations and defined several interpersonal, psychological, and linguistic concepts which are necessary to understand what goes on during an interview, including the concepts of *interpersonal stance* [7], *face* [2], and *rapport* [9] and the concepts *information* and *strategy*. The RM by Bruijnes et al. [4], which we evaluate in this paper, is rule-based and the rules are based on these psychological theories and concepts. The implementation consists of four components: the *personality* of the suspect persona; a *question frame* that describes the question of the interviewer; the *interpersonal state* as 'felt' by the suspect; and an *answer frame* that holds a description of the answer of the suspect (see Fig. 1 top). The *question frame* influences the interpersonal state of the RM, taking into account the personality of the persona, and the 'current' interpersonal state. The answer frame depends on this (updated) interpersonal state, the question frame, and the personality, see Fig. 1. For example, a persona with a friendly personality does not immediately become aggressive when confronted with an unfriendly question but if it is repeatedly confronted with unfriendly behaviour it can become aggressive.

2.1   Personas

The personality of the suspect in the RM can be set to reflect different personas. In [5] three personas were used to evaluate the RM. Participants interacted with one of three personas or a random generator that provided random *answer frame* output. The question was whether people can distinguish with which persona they interact; a 'Guess who you were talking to'-task. We follow the approach in [5] and use the same personas to allow a comparison between this study and the work in [5]. The personas are defined as follows, see for example interactions Table 1:

Huls: Mr. Huls is a friendly and mild family-man. Recently he got into debt as he has no work. He takes this as a personal failure towards his family, he feels guilty for failing them. He is emotional and considers the feelings of others important.
RM summary: Dependent personality. High affiliation, sensitivity to rapport, and sensitivity to internal and external pressure. Low attitude to opposed.

Remerink: Mr. Remerink married a wealthy woman and hold his high social status in high regard. He is helpful when treated with respect, but gets very upset when disrespected. He perceived his arrest as an insult.
RM summary: Friendly personality. High dominance. Other variables moderate.

vanBron: Mr. vanBron has a criminal record of drugs related crimes, assault, nuisance, and failure to comply with police requests. Has a history of abuse, neglect, and was raised in different foster care homes and boarding schools. He prefers to resolve situations with a large mouth and is prone to violence.
RM summary: Aggressive personality. High dominance, attitude to being opposed, and sensitivity to internal pressure. Low affiliation, sensitivity to rapport, and sensitivity to external pressure.

2.2 Behaviour Realisation

We used components from the Virtual Human Toolkit [6] to build the virtual suspect. Specifically, we used the NPCEditor [8], a statistical text classifier that provides question-answer matching. It uses information retrieval techniques to match the user's input with a 'known' question and return the answers that are paired with this question. The questions and answers were authored by the authors and based on observations of many (practice and real) police interviews. All answers in the NPCEditor were annotated in terms of the *answer frame* of the RM. The NPCEditor provided several appropriate answers to a question of the user. A wizard interpreted the user's questions in the terms of the *question frame* of the RM. This triggered an update of the RM state. From the answers provided by the NPCEditor, the answer which annotation matched *interpersonal state* and *answer frame* state of the RM best was selected (see Fig. 1). For example, if the RM was in a 'good mood' it selected a 'friendly' instead of an 'unfriendly' answer. The selected answer was send to the VHToolkit Renderer that realised the behaviour. For all personas we used model 'Brad' from the VHToolkit, the voice of one of the authors, and the same NPCEditor script. The only difference between the personas was the setting of the personality in the RM.

The question is whether the RM can accurately portray a suspect in an interaction. Can users differentiate between different personalities and can they agree on a description of the suspect. Problematic with evaluating a virtual human is that it often remains unclear what each component contributes to the evaluation. For example, the cause of inappropriate behaviour might be in the virtual human's speech recognition, interpersonal or emotional interpretation,

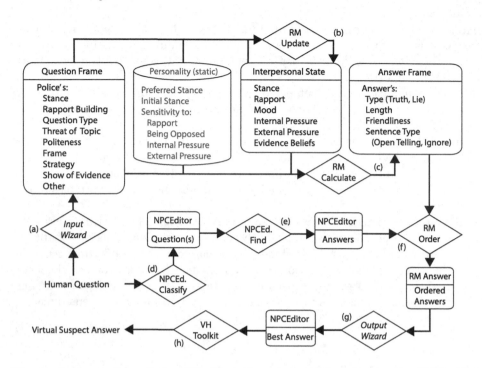

Fig. 1. A description of the RM (Sect. 2) and its integration in the VHToolkit (Sect. 2.2). The user asks a question. A wizard provides values of the question frame (describing the question of the user) to the RM (a). The RM has a static personality (the persona representation). It has an interpersonal state (holds values describing how the suspect 'feels') that updates when a question frame is presented (b). The output of the RM is the answer frame (describing the answer the suspect will give) and it is calculated based on the question frame, personality, and (new) interpersonal state (c). Please refer to [3–5] for details on the terms in the RM. The NPCEditor finds appropriate answers to the human's question (d, e) and the RM orders those answers based on the answer frame (f). The answer that the RM selected to be most appropriate is executed by the VHToolkit (h). A wizard had the option to deviate from the RM suggestion and select a different answer if the NPCEditor selected answers that are inappropriate for the scenario (g), for example by misclassifying the question asked.

reasoning, or the authoring of the response behaviours available to the system. By means of a 'Guess who you were talking to'-test, Bruijnes et al. [5] presented an evaluation of the RM, in which participants interacted with the RM using the terms from the *question frame* and the *answer frame* without having to formulate their question. They found the personality of the suspect was classified correctly 81.25 % of the time by the participants, showing the 'error' of the RM alone being 18.75 %. In this paper we investigate how the virtual suspect fares when participants have to use natural language in the interaction with the suspect. We expect the accuracy with which participants can 'Guess who they were talking to' will decrease as there are more potential sources for confusion.

Table 1. Example Q&As for the three personas in different phases of interaction. The officer's question is in italic and the virtual suspect's answer is shown below it for each of the personas. Q1 and Q2a are asked at the beginning of the interaction, showing the effect of the initial RM status of the persona on the answers A1 and A2a. Q2b is asked after a pleasant conversation in which the police officer managed to build rapport etc. A2b shows the answers for each of the personas after this pleasant interaction. Q2c is asked after an unpleasant conversation where the officer was unfriendly and intimidating. A2c shows the effect this has on the answers of the suspect personas.

Q&A	Huls	Remerink	vanBron
Q1		*Where do you live?*	
A1	I'm living at Mainstreet 12 in Venice.	Why should I tell you where I live, didn't you guys just arrest me at my place? Go figure it out you dumbass!	I live on the moon, I'm actually from Mars.
Q2a		*Do others use your desk?*	
A2a	Well, sometimes when I have guests they sleep in the office. I guess they might use the desk when they are in there.	Access smackes! It's my desk. No one got any business there. No one gets access... get it? Smackses!	Access smackes! It's my desk. No one got any business there. No one gets access... get it? Smackses!
	Interaction where the officer is building rapport, being friendly, etc. ↓		
Q2b		*Do others use your desk?*	
A2b	Well, sometimes when I have guests they sleep in the office. I guess they might use the desk when they are in there.	Well, sometimes when I have guests they sleep in the office. I guess they might use the desk when they are in there.	I guess when I have guests they could use the desk.
	Interaction where the officer is intimidating, unfriendly, face threatening etc. ↓		
Q2c		*Do others use your desk?*	
A2c	What ever. It's like the public library in my office. The whole neighbourhood uses my desk.	Access smackes! It's my desk. No one got any business there. No one gets access... get it? Smackses!	Access smackes! It's my desk. No one got any business there. No one gets access... get it? Smackses!

3   Experiment

We asked 42 participants (age $M = 28.3$, $SD = 9.4$, 12 female) to interact with William, our virtual suspect. There were four conditions, the RM personality of William was set to the personality of one of the three personas or the RM was a random answer frame generator. The session started with an explanation on how to interact with the virtual suspect (see Sect. 3.2). Participants interviewed the suspect until they completed their task: get him to say the name of an accomplice (see Sect. 3.1). Afterwards, they had to 'Guess who they were talking to'.

3.1   Case

The following case description, which resembles a police report, was provided to the participants:

> *William* is a suspect in a drug smuggling case. He was observed by a team of detectives delivering a suitcase filled with 20.000 XTC pills to the airport. He left the suitcase with suspected accomplice Shannon. Shannon was arrested with the drugs in her possession. This is proven and the suspect does not need to make statements about this. The house of the suspect was searched by detectives. In an office at the second floor a desk was found. This desk had a locked top drawer. A photo of Shannon was found in this drawer. It is not proven that this photo belongs to the suspect. It is not proven that Shannon and William know each other.

The police create an interview plan when they prepare for an interview. They determine the topics they want to address during the interview based on the tactical clues they have and they prepare questions for each of these topics. We prepared an interview plan and participants were told to follow it during their interview of the virtual suspect. The interview was over when William admitted to knowing Shannon, which was the inevitable eventual outcome of the interview.

3.2   Interacting with the Virtual Suspect

Participants had to follow the interview plan, but we explicitly encouraged them to add 'social padding' to the questions in the interview plan and make their contributions as natural as possible. The participants had to type their contribution to the conversation, when satisfied with the contribution press *ENTER*, and then pronounce their contribution in the way it was meant. The virtual suspect would respond based on *what* the participant typed and *how* they said it. The written contribution (the 'what') was processed automatically by the NPCEditor and the social spoken contribution (the 'how') was interpreted by a wizard (see Fig. 1). The contribution participants typed had to be what we called a 'complete contribution'. This meant that it should include something for the suspect to respond to like a question or a statement. For example, *'OK.'* is not a complete contribution but *'OK, but what else can you tell me about your office?'* is. The virtual suspect responded when the participant finished pronouncing his or her sentence. Alternatively, it could occur that the virtual suspect was unable to understand the participant's sentence. In this case the suspect would interrupt after they pressed *ENTER* and said 'What do you mean?'. This meant the participant had to change the written contribution and try again. We gave written and oral explanations and gave ample opportunity for questions. During the start of the interview we provided a reminder of the interaction procedure if necessary. All participants understood the procedure and had a meaningful interaction with the virtual suspect. After the interaction, participants received a description of the personas and had to choose which of the three personas they thought was most similar to William and report the confidence in their choice.

4   Results

In total there were 42 participants of which 53.1 % or 17 guessed correctly whom they were talking with resulting in $\kappa = 0.295$. This is better than chance (33.3 %), but worse than [5]'s result of 81.25 % correct. There is no correct answer for the 10 participants that interacted with a random generator. Overall, vanBron is recognized best: 60 % of the RM acts of vanBron were perceived as vanBron (*recall*) and 66.7 % of the people who thought they were interacting with vanBron were correct (*precision*). Remerink has a recall of 54.5 % and precision of 46.2 %, and Huls has a recall of 45.5 % and precision of 50 %, see Table 2.

Table 2. Table showing the relation between the RM personality setting (the persona it *acted*) and what persona the participants *perceived* most similar to the virtual suspect. It includes the totals for the RM settings and the totals for the perceived personas. For each persona it includes the accuracy of the perception (recall) and the accuracy of the RM (precision). Finally, the perceptions of the random interactions are presented.

Perceived \	Acted (RM setting) Huls	Remerink	vanBron	Total Perc.	Precision	*random*
Huls	5	2	3	10	50%	*0*
Remerink	6	6	1	13	46.2%	*8*
vanBron	0	3	6	9	66.7%	*2*
Total RM Setting	11	11	10	32		*10*
Recall	45.5%	54.5%	60%			

Table 3. The confidence the participants had in their choice for a persona.

	Huls	Remerink	vanBron	random
Mean	5,45	5,91	4,80	5,20
SD	0,82	1,22	0,92	0,79

The confusion personas tells us something about the possible reason for the mistakes and thus how serious these mistakes are. From the descriptions of the personas Huls, Remerink, and vanBron we could argue that they increase in offensiveness and decrease in friendliness. Following this rationale we argue that Remerink is more similar to Huls and vanBron than Huls is to vanBron. This is also reflected in the data. Huls is mistaken for Remerink 6 times but never for vanBron. Remerink is mistaken for Huls 2 times and 3 times for vanBron. Finally, vanBron is perceived as Huls 3 times and as Remerink 1 time. If we consider the differences between personas as a step (e.g. the difference between Huls and Remerink is one step, but Huls and vanBron is two steps) we see that 12 out of 15 misclassifications are one step from the intended persona and only three are 2 steps. This tells us that the confusion is not random. Rather, the system is able to answer extremely unfriendly (which is necessary to act as vanBron) but can do this even when it acts as Huls when the user is very unfriendly and gets Huls angry (or when the system has no friendly answers available).

The random setting for the RM provided random *Answer frame* output. There is no correct answer for the 10 participants that interacted with the random generator. In this condition, the content of the answer was appropriate but the interpersonal form was random. We might expect a uniform distribution of choices of personas. However, Remerink was chosen 8 times, vanBron 2 times, and Huls never, see Table 2. Possibly people were confused by the inconsistency of the behaviour as the suspect could for example go from friendly to unfriendly and back every turn. Remerink might be the persona that fits such behaviour best. From the Remerink description: 'He is *helpful* when treated with respect, but gets very *upset* when disrespected'. This makes explicit that he is capable of a wide range of interpersonal behaviours, perhaps wider than the other two personas. The random responses are very likely to include at least some unfriendly or aggressive responses which might explain why Huls was never chosen. Also, the random responses are unlikely to be only unfriendly and aggressive which is what participants might have expected from vanBron. This might explain the lower number of choices for vanBron.

The confidence observers have in their 'Guess who you were talking to'-choice tells us something about the clarity of the persona acts of the response model. If the virtual suspect displays confusing behaviour it is likely that participants are less certain about their choice. Participants answered on a 7-point scale how confident (lowest (1) or highest (7)) they felt about their choice. We expect the confidence to be lower when the responses of the virtual human lack clarity as they do in the random condition. Indeed, we find that the confidence in choice for each of the RM settings (the three personas and the random) differs close to significance level, (Kruskal-Wallis) $\chi^2 = 7.532, p = 0.057$. However, people who interacted with vanBron were less certain about their choice than people in other RM settings, where participants who interacted with Remerink were most confident in their choice, see Table 3. Moreover, the difference in confidence was only significant (or approaching significance) for Remerink-random (Mann-Whitney $U = 30.0, p = 0.066$) and Remerink-vanBron ($U = 22.5, p = 0.018$), all other RM settings did not produce significant differences on confidence. So, our hypothesis that the random condition would result in lower confidence ratings holds true only when comparing random to persona Remerink. This is interesting because we earlier expected that the random condition was interpreted as Remerink often because Remerink was most likely to show a wide variety of behaviours. However, people that interacted with random were less certain about their choice than when they were interacting with Remerink. Note that this is regardless of whether participants were correct. When we look at the confidence of those that were correct the difference between RM persona-settings again differs almost significantly, $\chi^2 = 5.349, p = 0.069$. However, the confidence of participants that were incorrect does not differ significantly, $\chi^2 = 0.387, p > 0.5$. For the participants that were correct only the confidence between RM setting vanBron and Remerink differed significantly

($U = 7, p = 0.044$). It seems that vanBron showed behaviour that made participants doubt their choice for him. This might be due to the volatile nature of his personality: he can be easily swain from friendly to aggressive. Also, most participants were doing their best to be friendly and build rapport. This made even the nasty persona vanBron friendly if they persisted and participants might have been confused by their 'success' in turning him friendly towards the end of the interrogation.

5   Discussion

Getting the behaviour of a virtual character right is not easy. Getting the persona right is an important step towards a believable virtual suspect that can be used to train police officers to interrogate suspects. The RM from [4] calculates an answer frame; interpersonal features of responses of a virtual suspect, based on a persona and the question asked. In [5] an attempt was made to isolate the performance of that RM; how well its responses could be interpreted as belonging to one of three personas. Their participants interacted using question frame values as input and received answer frame values as output. In this work we expanded on their results and investigated what effect using a virtual agent that can understand and use natural language in the interaction has. In [5], participants were able to guess correctly with which persona-setting in the RM they were interacting in about 80 % of the time. This would indicate that the RM leads to confusion about who the RM is trying to enact in about 20 % of the participants. In our study we found the accuracy of the 'Guess who you were talking to'-test decreased to about 53 %, showing the influence of natural language in the interaction and the importance of good authoring of responses for a virtual human. Other possible reasons for the decrease in performance include the appearance and voice of the virtual suspect.

We found that the personas that differed most were less likely to be confused. This means the RM was indeed able to select different behaviour for different personas and that the behaviour differed more when the personas were more different. So, it appears that confusion was not random. In fact, we argue that some participants managed to change a persona's initial mood and overcome its personality so that it showed behaviour not characteristic for the persona. The ability of the RM to do this is what caused the confusion. In police trainings this is exactly what the (virtual) suspect actor must do: respond to the behaviour of the trainee. The virtual suspect William is not yet able to provide a reflection after the interaction that tells the participant how (un)successful they were at changing the 'mood' of the suspect. We feel participants would have been more accurate at the 'Guess who you were talking to'-test if they had such information.

To create a virtual suspect that requires no wizard and that is capable of having a more natural interaction, we need to include automatic recognition of speech and the interpersonal features of speech. Also, the system will have to be able to give feedback on the interaction in terms of the RM to facilitate reflective learning. These issues are future work.

Acknowledgements. This publication was supported by the Dutch national program COMMIT.

References

1. Boud, D., Keogh, R., Walker, D.: Reflection: Turning Experience into Learning. Nichols Publishing Company, New York (1985)
2. Brown, P., Levinson, S.C.: Politeness: Some Universals in Language Usage. Cambridge University Press, Cambridge (1987)
3. Bruijnes, M., Linssen, J., op den Akker, R., Theune, M., Wapperom, S., Broekema, C., Heylen, D.: Social behaviour in police interviews: relating data to theories. In: D'Errico, F., Poggi, I., Vinciarelli, A., Vincze, L. (eds.) Conflict and Multimodal Communication, pp. 317–347. Springer International Publishing, Switzerland (2015)
4. Bruijnes, M., Wapperom, S., op den Akker, H., Heylen, D.: A virtual suspect agents response model. In: Ring, L., Leite, Y., Dias, J. (eds.) Fourteenth International-Conference on Intelligent Virtual Agents (IVA 2014); Proceedings of the Workshop on Affective Agents, pp. 17–24 (2014)
5. Bruijnes, M., Wapperom, S., op den Akker, R., Heylen, D.: A method to evaluate response models. In: Bickmore, T., Marsella, S., Sidner, C. (eds.) IVA 2014. LNCS, vol. 8637, pp. 67–70. Springer, Heidelberg (2014)
6. Hartholt, A., Traum, D., Marsella, S.C., Shapiro, A., Stratou, G., Leuski, A., Morency, L.-P., Gratch, J.: All together now. In: Aylett, R., Krenn, B., Pelachaud, C., Shimodaira, H. (eds.) IVA 2013. LNCS, vol. 8108, pp. 368–381. Springer, Heidelberg (2013)
7. Leary, T.: Interpersonal Diagnosis of Personality: Functional Theory and Methodology for Personality Evaluation. Ronald Press, New York (1957)
8. Leuski, A., Traum, D.: NPCEditor: creating virtual human dialogue using information retrieval techniques. AI Mag. **32**(2), 42–56 (2011)
9. Tickle-Degnen, L., Rosenthal, R.: The nature of rapport and its nonverbal correlates. Psychol. Inquiry **1**(4), 285–293 (1990)
10. Traum, D., Roque, A., Leuski, A., Georgiou, P., Gerten, J., Martinovski, B., Narayanan, S., Robinson, S., Vaswani, A.: Hassan: a virtual human for tactical questioning. In: Proceedings of the 8th SIGdial Workshop on Discourse and Dialogue, pp. 71–74 (2007)

Modeling a Social Brain for Interactive Agents: Integrating Mirroring and Mentalizing

Sebastian Kahl$^{(\boxtimes)}$ and Stefan Kopp

Social Cognitive Systems Group, Faculty of Technology, Bielefeld University,
Inspiration 1, 33619 Bielefeld, Germany
{skahl,skopp}@uni-bielefeld.de

Abstract. Human interaction has a distinct collaborative quality based on the attribution of communicative intentionality. Two networks in the human brain are often described as part of the "social brain": the mirror system for recognizing intentional behavior and the mentalizing (theory of mind) system for processing it. We equip virtual agents with both systems and model their interaction during embodied communication. Results of simulation experiments demonstrate how higher orders of theory of mind lead to more robustness of communication by enabling interactive grounding processes.

Keywords: Embodied virtual agents · Social cognition · Mentalizing · Mirroring · Coordination · Gesture

1 Introduction

Building artificial agents for natural interaction with humans eventually requires a deep understanding of the mechanisms underlying human social behavior. We are particularly interested in the perceptual and cognitive mechanisms that shape human behavior in social interaction. Those mechanisms have been receiving growing interest in fields such as Cognitive Science and Cognitive Neuroscience in the last decade. Two partially overlapping networks have been identified in the "social brain" [17]: an *action observation system* for perceiving and recognizing others' behaviors, and a *mentalizing system* for understanding others in terms of attributed mental states or theory of mind (ToM). Action observation is widely assumed to rest upon principles of prediction-based processing [2], where predictions about expected sensory stimuli are continuously formed and evaluated against incoming sensory input to inform further processing. A core mechanism to derive such predictions are sensorimotor simulations of the observed behavior, also referred to as *mirroring*. Prediction-based processing has also been argued to underlie language production and comprehension [9] or the social brain more generally [5].

We argue that learning from these mechanisms may help to substantially improve the interactive capabilities of virtual agents. Furthermore, developing models and

© Springer International Publishing Switzerland 2015
W.-P. Brinkman et al. (Eds.): IVA 2015, LNAI 9238, pp. 77–86, 2015.
DOI: 10.1007/978-3-319-21996-7_8

testing them in human-agent interaction contributes to a more detailed understanding of how the social brain works. For example, it is not clear so far how the mentalizing system and the mirroring system work together: How does perception change when a behavior is assumed to be "for me"? How are pathways between perception and action modulated by mentalizing in social interaction? And how do these mechanisms participate in coordination processes like feedback, joint attention, or grounding? Indeed, interacting with agents assumed to be "intentional" is fundamentally different from interacting with non-intentional objects [6]. For example, it has been shown that intentionality-attribution and underlying mentalizing influence sensory processing to become "social perception", an altered understanding of each other's actions [14,19], which is also known as an "intentional stance" [4]. Clearly, these processes play an important role not only in solitary observation events, in which they have been studied mostly so far, but even more so in continuous online interaction [8,13].

In this paper, we present work towards virtual agents with social brain-like functions by realizing and integrating mirroring and mentalizing abilities in a cognitively inspired fashion. In the following sections, we first review related modeling attempts and then present a model that formalizes the two systems in terms of computational processes, as well as their roles and dynamic interplay in inter-agent communication. Finally, we report results from simulations of embodied communication between two virtual agents, each of which equipped with its own model. We analyze how different abilities for mentalizing enable increasingly complex social coordination, from mere mimicry to eventually shared understanding.

2   Related Work

Researchers interested in embodied conversational agents (ECAs) have explored many ways that enable agents to respond in interactive settings of verbal and non-verbal communication. The Smart Body animation system [15] enables responsive combination of behavior animations and has been integrated with an improved text and speech analysis system, called Cerebella, to better react by mapping appropriate behavioral responses to derived mental states [7]. The Thalamus framework [10] employs a perceptual loop for continuous interaction with the environment mediated through the agent's body. It has been extended to a generation process shared between "mind" and "body", modeled as a network of behavior models that interface with a body representation [11]. Contradicting with (though referring to) tenets of embodied cognition, this model separates mind and body dualistically. We do not follow this modularized approach but strive for a more consequently embodied and situated account, in which cognitive processes ground in or even arise from sensorimotor layers and bodily shaped interaction with the environment, mediated through perception-action couplings.

As one of the few modeling attempts to combine mentalizing, perception and action control in dynamic social interaction, Wolpert et al. [18] underline in their MOSAIC model that a true communicative model needs to close the communicative loop and must be perceptive to the observer's responses and ultimately her understanding. They hypothesize a hierarchy of paired forward and inverse models as a basic mechanism for processing movement as well as beliefs or intentions. Sadeghipour and Kopp [12] proposed an Empirical Bayesian Belief Update model (EBBU), a probabilistic model that implements a mirroring-based account of the perception and production of gestural behavior. They use a hierarchically organized representation of motor knowledge for action perception through forward models that formulate probabilistic expectations about possible continuations of observed gestures. The same representation is used for action generation, with probabilistic interactions between both processes to explain priming and resonance effects. Representations are dynamically augmented by way of inverse models when an unknown action is encountered.

Few attempts have been made to clarify the interaction between mentalizing and mirroring. A meta-analysis of studies on mentalizing found that mirror areas are not recruited unless the task involves inferencing intentionality from action stimuli [17]. Teufel et al. [14] present the "Perceptual Mentalizing Model" which focuses on the influence of the mentalizing system on the mirror system via perceptual processing. They differentiate between explicit and implicit ToM (what we call here mentalizing and mirroring, respectively). Importantly, both kinds of ToM are assumed to be influenced by social sensory processing. Explicit ToM processes are associated with processing of intentionality of a movement and strongly influence perception-action coupling in implicit ToM processing. Wykowska et al. [19] present a model of social attention, the "Intentional Stance Model", in which the mentalizing system either exhibits an intentional stance towards agents (attributing intentionality) or a design stance towards objects. The mentalizing system is assumed to influence sensory processing in a top-down fashion, but also to affect sensory gain control in attention mechanisms. They report the sensory gain manipulation for attentional reorienting mechanisms to be stronger in the intentional stance than in the design stance. A key aspect in triggering this intentional stance seems to be social gaze, which has been found to lead to the attribution of communicative intent [1], which in turn differentially recruits the mirroring and mentalizing system networks in processing the behavior of the interlocutor.

3   Towards an Integrated Model of the Social Brain

In this paper we present first steps towards a model of how a predictive sensorimotor subsystem and a mentalizing subsystem for attributing mental states interact during situated communication. We thereby not only devise the model but also implement and test it in simulation of social (nonverbal) interactions between two virtual agents, to explore how communicative coordination emerges from the dynamic interplay between the two systems.

We base our modeling approach on a number of assumptions (see Fig. 1): First, we define successful communication to be a process that requires *shared* communicative intentionality and establishes perceptual or conceptual common ground between the participants [16]. This state is achieved in a dynamic grounding process [3], in which communicating agents reciprocally reveal and coordinate

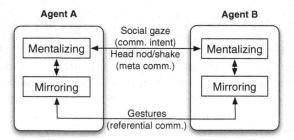

Fig. 1. The simulated nonverbal communication between our two virtual agents.

their beliefs about each other as well as the state of their interaction. Second, mentalizing plays a pivotal role by facilitating information integration and self-other distinction for coordinated action. It affects and receives information from the mirroring system, which itself processes perceived action in an immediate fashion. Third, we assume that coordinated action in communication highly depends on the degree of ToM realized by the mentalizing system: 2nd order reasoning, i.e. beliefs about other-beliefs, is minimally necessary for any cooperative behavior that goes beyond accidental coordination. Finally, gaze plays a special role in signaling and regulating social attention and is an indicator of communicative intent [1]. Mirror areas were found to be recruited especially when intentional action is expected [17]. We hence assume that gaze triggers mentalizing and thus also mirroring activity. Staying within the confines of the nonverbal domain, we also include head-nods and head-shakes as meta-communicative feedback for signalling agreement or disagreement.

3.1   Mentalizing Subsystem

The mentalizing subsystem is a model of an agent's subjective ToM, which processes definite information about itself and infers others' mental states from perceptual input. A detailed depiction of the mentalizing subsystem is given in Fig. 2, which we will refer to and describe in more detail in Sect. 3.3. In its current version, the system utilizes a simple set of inference heuristics to model how mental state attributions arise and change in social interaction. In detail, this model consists of three sets of mental state attributes for different orders of ToM reasoning: Beliefs held about mental states of myself (me) or the interlocutor (you) constitute what we call '1st order ToM'. Further, in pursuit of a minimal cognitive model of mentalizing, we assume that only one order of ToM higher is needed for what we want to model. In contrast to the classical recursively nested beliefs, however, we stipulate these beliefs to be held about mental states that both interlocutors have in common (we). This is what we call '2nd order ToM'. The functional role that we ascribe to 2nd order ToM is to keep track of common ground, the desire to agree, and the collaborative state of communication more generally. Generally, mental states consist of beliefs, desires, and intentions.

3.2   Mirroring Subsystem

The mirroring subsystem employs the abovementioned EBBU model [12] for action observation and production. It implements a probabilistic hierarchical representation of sensorimotor knowledge about hand gestures, along with basic prediction, evaluation and activation processes that are used in both perception and generation of gestures. On the lowest level, *motor commands* are stored that represent segmented movements in time and space. Hand trajectories are given as directed graphs with edges representing motor commands. On the intermediate level, *motor programs* represent paths in the motor command graph and thus stand for meaningful movements. The highest level of abstraction stores *motor schemas* that cluster and represent similar motor programs. When observing a hand trajectory the hierarchical motor knowledge structure is activated and "resonates" to the observed gesture. In each time step the model predicts possible continuations of the observed gesture and compares them to the actual perception. Results lead to updated posterior probability distributions and hence activation of the corresponding motor commands, programs, or schemas. We equipped the mirroring subsystem with knowledge of different trajectories for three iconic ('circle', 'square', 'surface') and one emblematic gesture ('waving'). Those were learned from real human motion data. Single motor programs for a schema can take up to five seconds to produce, with motor commands being activated every tenth of a second. For every new observation of a hand trajectory entering the system the top-most level posterior distributions over motor schemas are taken as a proxy for a gesture's meaning, and are linked to first order mental state attributes in the mentalizig system.

3.3   Integration and Interplay

Our goal is to integrate mentalizing with mirroring-based action perception to account for how behavior and mental states arise and interact dynamically in a communicative interaction. As a working hypothesis, we consider both systems to be separate but with continuous interactions and projections between each other. In the mentalizing subsystem, any observation of actions can have a direct influence on the mental states held about *you*, where desires, beliefs and intentions are heuristically inferred. For any observed gesture processed by the mirroring subsystem, the most likely motor schema hypothesis is immediately projected into the mentalizing subsystem where it forms a mental state attributed as a *you*-belief, as long as the intention to communicate can be inferred. Correspondingly, a *me*-belief would cause the mirroring subsystem to recruit the intended motor schema for production. The current version of the mirroring subsystem is only capable of processing hand gestures; gaze and head movements are thus directly asserted to the mentalizing subsystem.

Depending on the degree of ToM processed in the agent's mentalizing module, communicative intent can trigger an inferred desire to reach mutual agreement about the understanding of the produced gesture. This is assessed applying a threshold for *good-enough* understanding to the likelihood of beliefs about mental states of *me* and *you* (1st order ToM). Note, however, when this threshold is exceeded the producer agent still cannot be certain about the correct understanding in the recipient unless sufficient feedback is provided. Here we require at least one correct reproduction of the gesture. Further, head-shake and head-nod signals are employed for meta-communication and can either increase or decrease confidence in the respective *you*-belief.

4   Simulation Results

In order to test the model in online interactions we implemented the model and ran simulations with two virtual agents, each of which equipped with its own integrated model. At the start of the simulation, both agents only have a predefined set of mental states about themselves. They can communicate using four gestures ('circle', 'square', 'surface', and 'waving') that are perceived and generated as 3D hand trajectories, as well as head nods/shakes that are transferred as simple timed key-value pairs. Gestures are produced with a configured amount of white noise, normalized to the maximum movement vectors in the motor schema, so that 10 % noise reflect only a small amount of deviation during gesturing. The amount of noise, the ability for 2nd order ToM, and the good-enough threshold for minimal confidence in observing a gesture are the independent variables to parametrize the simulation. We ran six simulation setups: 10 %/20 %/30 %

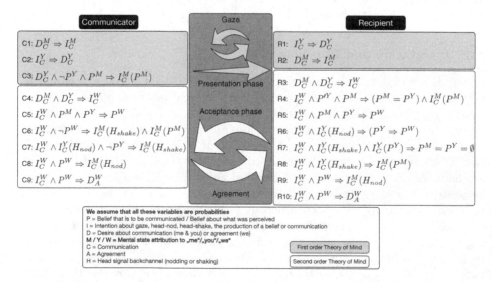

Fig. 2. Attributes and inference heuristics in the mentalizing subsystem applied during different phases of the interaction. The basis for complex inference is "Communicative Intention", inferred from social gaze. The "Communicator" agent enters the "Presentation Phase", followed by an "Acceptance Phase" of interactive grounding, where higher order mental attributions are needed for both agents to reach "Agreement".

noise with enabled or disabled 2nd order ToM capacity, and a static confidence threshold of 0.8. Each of the setups was run 100 times, always with identically configured agents. Simulations ended either when both agents believed to have reached agreement, or without 2nd order ToM, as soon as the *Communicator* finished its gesture production. As dependent variables we collected the probability distribution of the attributed *you*-belief about a gesture's meaning after every processing of a hand trajectory. We were particularly interested in the effects that different degrees of mentalizing have on the inter-agent coordination dynamics. The complexity of the communication depends on inferred communicative intent, signaled via social gaze. As soon as mutual communicative intent is established, the simulation follows a typical grounding process with presentation and acceptance phases [3], where the *Communicator* always starts with producing a 'circle' gesture.

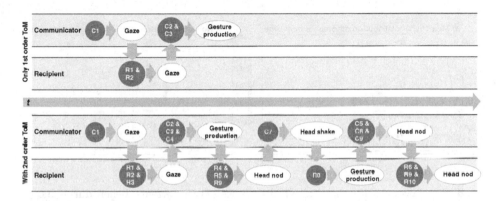

Fig. 3. Example interactions from our simulation when both agents have 1st order ToM (top) or 2nd order ToM (bottom). Overt behavior is shown along with the triggered mentalizing inferences (gray circles; indices referring to Fig. 2).

To examplify the effect of the mental attributions and inferences possible in 1st and 2nd order ToM, Fig. 3 illustrates two typical interaction patterns from our simulation study. The overt behavior of two agents, a *Communicator* and a *Recipient*, are shown along with the inferences drawn after perceiving or producing a certain behavior, with indices referring to the inference rules as shown in Fig. 2. The interaction at the top shows a sequence of behavior and inferences typical for 1st order ToM mentalizing. The configured desire to communicate triggers *rule C1*, hence gaze behavior is perceived by the *Recipient* (*rule R1*). Since the *Recipient* is equally configured, its reciprocal gaze behavior (*rule R2*) triggers an inference about the *Recipient's* desire to communicate in the *Communicator* (*rule C2*), and consequently a gesture is produced(*rule C3*). The interaction at the bottom shows behavior and inferences enabled through 2nd order ToM. While in the beginning there is a similarity to the 1st order ToM interaction, additionally *rules R3 and C4* are triggered and establish the agents' common communicative intent and thus the foundation for meaningful coordination behavior. After the initial gesture production the *Recipient's* mirroring subsystem provides the mentalizing subsystem with the most likely interpretation for the *Communicator's* behavior. That novel behavior triggers *rule R4*, by which the *Recipient* would ideally produce the understood gesture back to the *Communicator*, but in this interaction the gesture was understood with a likelihood above the good-enough threshold. This triggers *rule R5 and R9* as well, leading to a head-nod. Since the *Communicator* has no idea what the *Recipient* has understood the head-nod behavior is answered by a head-shake (*rule C7*), which triggers the *Recipient* to produce its understood gesture back to the *Communicator* (*rule R8*). The *Communicator* understands the gesture, which triggers rules equivalent to those in the *Recipient* (*rule C5, C8, and C9*), leading to a head-nod, which is equivalently answered by the *Recipient* (*rule R6, and R9*) and finalizes the interaction through mutually believed agreement (*rule R10*).

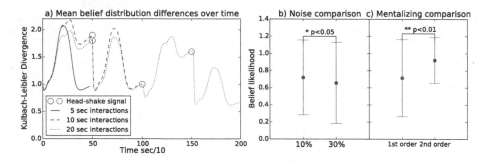

Fig. 4. Simulation results show (a) KL-divergence between agents' beliefs during interactions of different extend, averaged over noise and ToM conditions, (b) mean differences between noise conditions, and (c) total mean differences between achieved likelihood about another's belief between ToM conditions.

To test the agents' ability to coordinate with and without 2nd order ToM enabled, we analyzed the Kulbach-Leibler Divergence between the probability distributions of the *Recipient's you*-belief and the *Communicator's me*-belief, i.e. the "target belief". Figure 4(a) shows the divergence over interaction time. Without 2nd order ToM only one gesture was produced within 5 s. With 2nd order ToM the duration was strongly dependend on the correct understanding of observed gestures. The more mistakes, likely due to noise, the more correction effort emerged and hence longer interactions. Analyzed were interactions with length of at least 10 s and 20 s, respectively. These plots show the average success of coordination, especially in longer interactions. To test the effect of noise we compared the success of both agents reaching the target belief after 5 s, averaged over ToM conditions (Fig. 4(b)). The comparison shows a significant difference ($t = 2.4$, $p < 0.05$) between 10 % ($M = 0.6$, $SD = 0.4$) and 30 % ($M = 0.7$, $SD = 0.5$) noise conditions on gesture understanding. Subsequently, we tested the influence of 2nd order ToM, also by analyzing the success of reaching the target belief (Fig. 4(c)). A comparison of the final beliefs averaged over all noise conditions with 2nd order ToM ($M = 0.9$, $SD = 0.27$) and without ($M = 0.7$, $SD = 0.45$) showed that 2nd order ToM leads to significantly more likely success in coordination ($t = 6.8$, $p < 0.01$).

5   Conclusions

In this paper we have presented work towards equipping virtual agents with a cognitively inspired model of a "social brain". Our approach is based on the notion that in social interaction, abilities for higher order mentalizing come to interact with predictive action observations in particular ways, and it is this interplay that accounts for the dynamic coordination mechanisms responsible for successful communication. The present step was to implement a 'minimal' mentalizing model that enables distinct mental perspectives, corresponding to beliefs about *me*, *you*, and *we*, and to let it interact with a mirroring-based EBBU model. Actual simulations of dynamically unfolding interaction were run to investigate whether higher order mental state attributions can give virtual agents a distinct advantage in inferring information necessary to successfully act towards a communicative goal. The results we obtained so far demonstrate that endowing IVAs with mechanisms found in the "social brain" enables interactive grounding without scripting it, and thus makes communication significantly more robust and efficient. However, even with higher order mentalizing capacities, a too large perturbation of the communicative signals led to long interaction times due to the inefficient error correcting mechanism emerging from both agents' goal for successful communication. Still, our first prototypical modeling attempt established that mentalizing is crucial for meaningful coordination behavior and success in communication could not be guaranteed without 2nd order ToM. We see the present framework as a good basis for further investigations how an understanding of social cognitive processes can help in the endeavour towards more natural and robust embodied agents, just as the analysis of interactions of humans with agents equipped with our framework will contribute to testing our understanding of how the social brain works. As next steps we will include an account for strategic noise compensation through altered signaling behavior, and want to pursue the question how self-other distinctions can manifest in the sensorimotor system during action observations to help in that attempt.

Acknowledgements. This research/work was supported by the Cluster of Excellence Cognitive Interaction Technology 'CITEC' (EXC 277) at Bielefeld University, which is funded by the German Research Foundation (DFG).

References

1. Ciaramidaro, A., Becchio, C., Colle, L., Bara, B.G., Walter, H.: Do you mean me? communicative intentions recruit the mirror and the mentalizing system. Soc. Cogn. Affect. Neurosci. **9**(7), 909–916 (2014)

2. Clark, A.: Whatever next? predictive brains, situated agents, and the future of cognitive science. Behav. Brain Sci. **36**(03), 181–204 (2013)
3. Clark, H.H., Brennan, S.E.: Grounding in communication. In: Perspectives on socially shared cognition, vol. 13, pp. 127–149. American Psychological Association, Washington, DC, US (1991)
4. Dennett, D.C.: The Intentional Stance. The MIT Press, Cambridge (1987)
5. Frith, U., Frith, C.: The social brain: allowing humans to boldly go where no other species has been. Philos. Trans. R. Soc. Lond. B Biol. Sci. **365**(1537), 165–176 (2010)
6. Gangopadhyay, N., Schilbach, L.: Seeing minds: a neurophilosophical investigation of the role of perception-action coupling in social perception. Soc. Neurosci. **7**(4), 410–423 (2012)
7. Lhommet, M., Marsella, S.C.: Gesture with meaning. In: Aylett, R., Krenn, B., Pelachaud, C., Shimodaira, H. (eds.) IVA 2013. LNCS, vol. 8108, pp. 303–312. Springer, Heidelberg (2013)
8. Myllyneva, A., Hietanen, J.K.: There is more to eye contact than meets the eye. Cognition **134**, 100–109 (2015)
9. Pickering, M.J., Garrod, S.: An integrated theory of language production and comprehension. Behav. Brain Sci. **36**(4), 329–347 (2013)
10. Ribeiro, T., Vala, M., Paiva, A.: Thalamus: closing the mind-body loop in interactive embodied characters. In: Nakano, Y., Neff, M., Paiva, A., Walker, M. (eds.) IVA 2012. LNCS, vol. 7502, pp. 189–195. Springer, Heidelberg (2012)
11. Ribeiro, T., Vala, M., Paiva, A.: Censys: a model for distributed embodied cognition. In: Aylett, R., Krenn, B., Pelachaud, C., Shimodaira, H. (eds.) IVA 2013. LNCS, vol. 8108, pp. 58–67. Springer, Heidelberg (2013)
12. Sadeghipour, A., Kopp, S.: Embodied gesture processing: motor-based integration of perception and action in social artificial agents. Cogn. Comput. **3**(3), 419–435 (2011)
13. Schilbach, L., Timmermans, B., Reddy, V., Costall, A., Bente, G., Schlicht, T., Vogeley, K.: Toward a second-person neuroscience. Behav. Brain Sci. **36**(4), 393–414 (2013)
14. Teufel, C., Fletcher, P.C., Davis, G.: Seeing other minds: attributed mental states influence perception. Trends Cogn. Sci. **14**(8), 376–382 (2010)
15. Thiebaux, M., Marsella, S., Marshall, A.N., Kallmann, M.: SmartBody: behavior realization for embodied conversational agents. In: Proceedings of the 7th International Joint Conference on Autonomous Agents and Multiagent Systems, vol. 1, pp. 151–158 (2008)
16. Tomasello, M.: Origins of Human Communication. The MIT Press, Cambridge (2008)
17. Van Overwalle, F.: Social cognition and the brain: a meta-analysis. Hum. Brain Mapp. **30**(3), 829–858 (2009)
18. Wolpert, D.M., Doya, K., Kawato, M.: A unifying computational framework for motor control and social interaction. Philos. Trans. R. Soc. of Lond. B Biol. Sci. **358**(1431), 593–602 (2003)
19. Wykowska, A., Wiese, E., Prosser, A., Müller, H.J.: Beliefs about the minds of others influence how we process sensory information. PLoS ONE **9**(4), e94339 (2014)

Modeling Sensation for an Intelligent Virtual Agent's Perception Process

Tobias Haubrich[1], Sven Seele[1(✉)], Rainer Herpers[1,2,3], Christian Bauckhage[4], and Peter Becker[1]

[1] Institute of Visual Computing, Bonn-Rhein-Sieg University of Applied Sciences, Grantham-Allee 20, 53757 Sankt Augustin, Germany
[2] University of New Brunswick, Fredericton E3B 5A3, Canada
[3] York University, Toronto M3J 1P3, Canada
[4] University of Bonn, 53115 Bonn, Germany
sven.seele@h-brs.de

Abstract. Perception is an important aspect of cognition since it forms the basis for further decision-making processes. In this contribution, the overall architecture of our synthetic perception for agents framework (SynPeA) for simulating a virtual entities perception is presented. We discuss aspects of modeling visual sensation and propose mechanisms for virtual sensors and memory. Different visual sensing approaches are compared by applying them to an artificial evaluation scenario. The evaluations show promising results with respect to performance and quality.

Keywords: Intelligent virtual agents · Perception · Virtual environments

1 Introduction

In virtual environments (VEs), intelligent virtual agents (IVAs) play an important role in bringing the virtual world they inhabit to life. The problem of simulating plausible behaviors for virtual agents is increasingly attracting researchers. Believable simulations of virtual humans or animals are used to predict behavior in real-life scenarios (e.g., evacuation, traffic, military campaigns, etc.), to create virtual tutors, or to realize engaging non-player characters in video games.

While perception processes are mentioned in most of the existing work on IVAs, they are rarely the focus. Yet, some researchers emphasize that every decision an entity makes, and thus its behavior, depends on its perception of its environment (e.g., [1,17]). We argue that simulating believable perception is indeed an integral part of simulating believable IVAs.

This contribution focuses on the "starting point" of the perception-action cycle: sensation. Sensation is the process of receiving stimuli from the environment through sensory organs before any signal is transferred to the brain. To solve the general problem of implementing believable behavior for IVAs, we present the *synthetic perception for agents* framework (SynPeA). We focus on

© Springer International Publishing Switzerland 2015
W.-P. Brinkman et al. (Eds.): IVA 2015, LNAI 9238, pp. 87–97, 2015.
DOI: 10.1007/978-3-319-21996-7_9

the problem of modeling visual sensation and propose mechanisms for virtual sensors and memory. Different approaches for virtual visual sensing were evaluated and showed promising results with respect to performance and accuracy.

2   Related Work

In the literature, perception processes for virtual entities are frequently mentioned but seldom focused on. In the simplified model by Russel and Norvig, the term percept refers to an agent's perceptual inputs at any given instant [18, p.34]. In our model, we differentiate between stimuli – collected from the environment – and percepts of which the IVAs themselves are *aware* (cf. [14]).

The challenge of modeling perception processes is the *"god's eye"* described by Luck and Aylett [9]. IVAs do not need to distinguish between their virtual world and models of the world. However, to show believable behavior, IVAs should have approximately the same limitations as their real counterparts [9].

For VEs artificial and synthetic perception processes have to be distinguished. We define artificial perception as processes that take signals from the environment and try to deduce an internal representation of this environment (cf. [20]). Integrating artificial processes into VEs is possible, but might entail problems that are still not sufficiently solved. In contrast, synthetic perception processes do not have to address problems such as object recognition and interpretation [10]. Instead they exploit existing semantical descriptions when a signal (possibly from an object) is sensed; making them more appropriate for use in VEs.

Semantics facilitate efficient perception processes by avoiding recognition and interpretation. In [21] three forms of semantics for games and simulation are distinguished: object semantics, object relationships, and world semantics.

IVAs generally possess a set of virtual sensors that represent the sensory organs of their real counterparts. Most research deals with simulating visual sensation. This emphasis is due to the fact that the visual channel is the most important for humans. Thus, simulating the visual channel is considered a convenient way to make the behavior of simulated entities more authentic. In a simplified manner, synthetic vision is about solving the visibility problem known from computer graphics. If an object is determined as visible, all geometric and all semantic information about the object is considered as sensed. Consequently, approaches to visual sensation are generally object-based. Many problems arise because virtual objects are clearly defined, whereas the definition of a visual object in the real world is anything but clear (cf. [4]). Advanced synthetic vision systems could include clarity or saliency calculations for certain objects.

We divide the process of visual sensation into a set of subprocesses and arrange them in a *visual sensing pipeline*. The process starts with preselection followed by physical filtering, e.g., field of view (FOV) filters and occlusion filters.

There are two common approaches to implementing visual sensors. Peters et al. differentiate geometric approaches, which do not render the scene at all, and pure synthetic approaches, where the scene is rendered from an agent's point of view [12]. However, we categorize the approaches by the way they solve the above-mentioned visibility problem. The approaches considered in this contribution are ray cast-based synthetic vision and depth buffer-based synthetic vision.

The basic approach for FOV tests in ray cast-based synthetic vision is to use a view cone. Since conic FOVs have some disadvantages, building a FOV from multiple view cones was proposed in [8]. Rabin and Michael describe an approach where FOVs are modeled as ellipses [15]. One advantage is that it can be efficiently calculated whether a point lies within the elliptic area. Occlusion tests are realized using ray casts (cf. [20]). Generally, a single ray is cast to one point of each object. If this point can be hit, the entire object is declared visible.

Depth buffer-based synthetic vision approaches reuse existing graphics pipeline processes. The primary idea is to render a low-resolution image from an agent's point of view. Information is obtained from the fact that it is known to which virtual object a fragment belongs and how distant the fragment is [16]. The FOV test is covered by culling processes, whereas the occlusion test is performed by constructing the depth buffer. Over the years, several ideas have been proposed to enhance this approach. One important idea, called *false coloring*, was presented by Noser et al. [10], who simplified the image analysis by rendering objects with a unique color while omitting textures and shadows in the rendering process. Thus, an object can be declared visible if the rendered image contains at least one pixel of the object's unique color. Several other researchers applied and extended this approach (cf. [2,3,6,13]), such as coloring objects by type or group [19] or simplifying the rendered 3D models [11].

Virtual sensors are often attached to a unified sensor interface that aggregates data acquired by different sensors in a common (sensory) memory (cf. [3,7]). An example of a memory concept is provided by Peters [13]. His concept is based on a theory proposed by the psychologists Atkinson and Shiffrin. It includes three memory stages: a short-term sensory storage (STSS), a short-term memory (STM), and a long-term memory (LTM). Entries are moved between the different layers of the memory hierarchy depending on how much attention they receive. In this contribution we only consider the STSS as part of our sensation process (see Fig. 1). Its content represents the *environmental stimulus*.

3 Sensation for IVAs

The overall architecture of our perception process is decomposed into two cycles (s. Fig. 1). The *environmental stimulus cycle (ESC)* extracts stimuli from the virtual environment via virtual sensors. The sensors determine *sensible* objects from the VE and store appropriate stimuli inside the sensory storage. In the real world, sensors need to receive signals (stimuli) provided by the environment. In a virtual world, the process is often inverted. Sensors send signals to the objects to determine whether they emit stimuli that affect the sensor. The *information attention cycle (IAC)* acquires information from the environmental stimulus that the agent is (possibly) interested in. Further details can be found in [5].

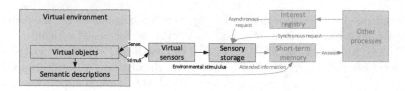

Fig. 1. Architecture of the SynPeA (synthetic perception for agents) framework. The parts on the left represent the environmental stimulus cycle (ESC) detailed in this contribution, while the grayed-out parts represent the information attention cycle (IAC).

3.1   Semantic Modeling

In our system, every virtual object that should be perceivable is enhanced with semantic information (in the form of a *perceivable* object), which provides the perceivable data. Each *perceivable* consists of a list of properties ($\mathcal{P}$). Every property in $\mathcal{P}$ contains a name, a sensory modality, a generic value, and a value describing the minimum clarity needed to perceive the property.

3.2   Virtual Sensors

Virtual sensors need to determine which signals or objects could be perceived by an agent. Generally, it is sufficient to determine whether an object can be sensed to grant access to its semantic information. In future iterations, clarity and saliency of the sensation could be used to inhibit access to specific parts of the semantic information. According to Enns, a visual signal needs at least $200\,ms$ to reach the brain and cause an according action under optimal circumstances [4]. Thus, it is possible to process the sensors, e.g., every $100\,ms$ without becoming unrealistic. We investigated the two following approaches to solving the visibility problem by implementing them as virtual sensors. A comparison of accuracy and performance of the prototypical implementations is provided in Sect. 4.

Ray Cast-Based Approach. The ray cast-based sensor complies with the visual sensing pipeline mentioned in Sect. 2. First, one or more *preselectors* should identify subsets of interesting objects out of the set of all objects. The union of these subsets is reduced to the set that represents the sensor's part of the *environmental stimulus*. The reduction is executed by applying *physical filters*. We apply an elliptic FOV filter (cf. [15]) parameterized by view range and view angle. Afterwards, a ray cast-based line-of-sight filter is applied. It implements an occlusion check that is realized using ray cast operations in combination with multiple mass points for each virtual object (cf. [20]). To avoid increasing the required computations, one mass point of each object is randomly chosen in each sensing step. The non-determinism of this approach is counteracted by keeping objects in the sensory storage for more than one sensing step (see Sect. 3.3).

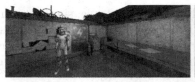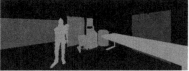

Fig. 2. A scene from an NPC's view (left) rendered using the false coloring-based vision sensor (right). The scene is based on Unity's Project: Stealth (Color online figure).

Depth Buffer-Based Approach. The depth buffer-based sensor uses the false coloring approach (cf. [10]). The parts of the visual sensing pipeline are mapped to different stages of the graphics pipeline. The FOV test is performed by culling processes and the occlusion test is performed by analyzing the pixels of an image calculated by the depth buffer algorithm. Every virtual object is assigned a unique color defining its appearance in the rendered image. The pixels of the image are perused, and the associated objects are added to the sensor's set of sensed objects. Two approaches for evaluating the images were integrated.

In a serial approach pixels are evaluated sequentially, which means runtime mainly depends on texture resolution. The second approach runs in parallel by transferring the pixel array back to the GPU. A result buffer includes an integer value for every sensible object. For every pixel a thread is executed which uses its pixel's value as an index for incrementing the color value in the result buffer. Finally, the returned result buffer is perused. Every object whose value is bigger than 0 is considered as sensed. One advantage of this approach is that it also determines how many pixels are covered by an object, which could be used for determining saliency values. Due to the parallel evaluation the runtime depends less on the texture size but mainly on the number of sensible objects.

Especially in the serial case, the dimensions of a rendered image should be small to save computational resources. Due to this low resolution, parts of more than one object could be visible in the area of one pixel, but the pixel will only be filled with one color. As a result, objects may not be sensed by the sensor although they are visible. To improve the results of the approach a tremor is added that changes the sensor's viewport such that the rendering camera's FOV differs slightly in every sensing step. Thus, the color of different objects is written to the pixels. In conjunction with the persistence in the sensory storage, this alteration improves the accuracy of sensors that use low resolution images. Figure 2 demonstrates our implementation of the false coloring approach.

3.3 Sensor Interface and Memory

To enable the integration of sensors of different approaches, we integrate a uniform interface into our model, which is similar to that of Kuiper et al. and Conde and Thalmann [3,7]. To fulfill the interface requirements, each sensor has to implement a sense function that returns a set of generic stimuli objects.

A basic visual stimulus is comprised of the following 6-tuple, similar to the definition used by Kuffner et al. [6]: ID of the perceived object (id), point in time when the sensation took place (t), properties of the perceived signal/object ($\mathcal{P}$), clarity of the sensation ($\mathcal{C}$), saliency of the sensation ($\mathcal{S}$), transformation of the perceived object (T), velocity of the perceived object (v).

The clarity ($\mathcal{C}$) and saliency ($\mathcal{S}$) parameters were added for future iterations. Clarity describes how clearly an object or signal was sensed (e.g., based on distance, fog, or darkness). Saliency describes how outstanding a sensed object or signal was (e.g., based on conspicuous colors or fast movement).

The chosen memory model is an adaptation of the one introduced in [13]. As of now, our concept considers two of the original model's three stages: a short-term sensory storage (STSS), which is the focus of this contribution, and a short-term memory (STM), which is important as soon as attention processes are examined. Entries in each stage are affected by memory decay, which is the time an entry sustains without being utilized. As suggested in [6] the STSS is implemented as a list avoiding the administration of complex data structures.

The STSS gathers all stimuli received by the virtual sensors. By storing the stimuli's information over a short period of time, a sensory persistence is provided. Thus, briefly sensed signals or objects are not forgotten too quickly. Since entries in the STSS have a rapid decay, there does not need to be a difference between entries referring to static or dynamic objects in the STSS. If memory entries sustain over a longer time period (e.g., entries in the STM), dynamic information must be copied to allow information to become obsolete. For example, if an object vanishes behind a wall, its last perceived state must be preserved.

4   Evaluation

Two evaluations of the implementation were performed using a consumer-level PC (Intel Core i7-2600 K, 8 GB RAM and NVIDIA GeForce GTX560). The first evaluation investigated sensor accuracy based on what the sensors sensed and what they were expected to sense. The second evaluation considered sensor performance which is critical if real-time capability is to be achieved.

To perform the evaluations an artificial evaluation scenario was defined. The scenario includes a scene with several visually sensible cubes that are distributed on a fixed 3D grid. During the evaluations, the scene was sensed by an agent using alternating sensors. The applied sensor configurations are listed in Table 1. Configurations A and B utilized the ray cast-based vision sensor. In A only the cube origin (midpoint) and in B one random mass point was checked. Each cube included 9 mass points of which 8 were near the corners and the 9th was at the origin. In C to K the false coloring-based vision sensor was applied. Four configuration pairs used the same texture size; one without camera tremor and one with a tremor of 0.3°. From pair to pair the texture size was quadrupled. Additionally, the configurations were applied to a serial and a parallel version of the sensor. In configuration K a texture of 256 × 256 pixels was used. This

Table 1. Evaluated sensor configurations (view angle: $120°$, view range: $100\,m$).

Type	ID	Configuration	ID	Configuration
Ray cast-based	A	Without mass points		
Ray cast-based	B	With mass points		
False coloring-based	C	$16^2 = 256\,px$, no tremor	D	$16^2 = 256\,px$, tremor $0.3°$
False coloring-based	E	$32^2 = 1024\,px$, no tremor	F	$32^2 = 1024\,px$, tremor $0.3°$
False coloring-based	G	$64^2 = 4096\,px$, no tremor	H	$64^2 = 4096\,px$, tremor $0.3°$
False coloring-based	I	$128^2 = 16384\,px$, no tremor	J	$128^2 = 16384\,px$, tremor $0.3°$
False coloring-based	K	$256^2 = 65536\,px$, no tremor		

configuration was only applied to the parallel version because a serial analysis of the texture was no longer feasible.

In the sensor accuracy evaluation the same static scene of randomly distributed cubes was used for all configurations to achieve comparable results (see Fig. 3 (a)). The visible cubes were counted manually in a high resolution rendering of the scene to obtain the ground truth: 121 of 137 cubes were not fully occluded, i.e. sensible. Every sensor configuration was executed for $60\,s$ to obtain stable results. The STSS's decay was $0.5\,ms$ and the number of its entries was logged after every sensing step ($0.1\,s$). Since false positives are not possible, the values determined how many of the de facto sensible cubes were actually sensed.

In the sensor performance evaluation the number of cubes in the scene was increased over time to examine how the number of sensible objects correlates with the sensor execution times. All cubes were placed at the same depth level since occlusion has no influence on sensor run times. The STSS's decay was set to $0.5\,ms$. The sensor execution times and the number of entries in the STSS were logged after every sensing step.

Results and Analysis. The results of the different approaches are individually analyzed before a comparison is provided in the next subsection. The accuracy of the ray cast-based sensors (A and B) depends on the number and distribution of the objects' mass points. While in A 91 of 121 visible cubes were sensed, between 108 and 119 cubes were sensed in B. Results in B were not constant because the mass point checked in each sensing step was chosen randomly. At no time were all 121 cubes sensed because the tested object origins or mass points were not visible, even when other parts of the cube were.

The sensor execution times depend mainly on how much rays need to be cast. Since we restricted the ray casts to one per object and sensing step, the execution time depends only on the number of objects to be checked. Figure 4 indicates a linear increase of the execution time for more then 100 objects.

As expected, the false coloring-based sensors (C-K) show varying results. Figure 3 (b) shows that the accuracies of the serial and the parallel sensors do

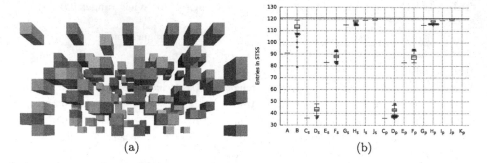

(a)   (b)

Fig. 3. Setup (a) and results (b) of the sensor accuracy evaluation. 121 of 137 cubes were not fully occluded (horizontal line). The sensor configurations from Table 1 including a serial (subscript s) and a parallel (subscript p) version of the false coloring-based sensor were applied. (b) shows the number of entries in the STSS for each configuration.

not differ. Furthermore, the number of memory entries converges to the true number of visible objects with an increasing number of pixels. Configurations I_s and I_p already nearly sensed the correct value of 121. In the other configurations (C–H) the image was not detailed enough to include all cubes. Unrecognized cubes result from the rasterization performed as a part of the camera's rendering. In this case, non-occluded objects can be missed, as in configurations C and D. Configurations utilizing tremor show a general increase of accuracy. The slightly altered raster of the camera causes other objects to occupy the image's pixels. J_s and J_p show that sometimes less cubes are sensed because the tremor can cause slightly visible cubes to become occluded. Similarly, slightly occluded cubes could become visible. However, in the case of a small tremor, both effects are negligible. If the image is sufficiently dimensioned, the tremor becomes unnecessary.

The execution times are mainly affected by two steps. First, for both approaches (linear and parallel) the time is increased due to the number of objects to be rendered. As Fig. 4 shows, this increase is insignificant. Second, the time increases with texture size. In the linear case the pixel array is converted into a hash set structure to remove duplicate entries. The remaining increase is due to the reduction operation, which has $\mathcal{O}(n)$ complexity. In the parallel case the rendered images' pixels are concurrently analyzed on the GPU. The main increase results from the data transfer between the working memory and the GPU. This explains why the serial approach is (slightly) faster for low resolution images (C, E). For higher resolutions the parallel sensor outperforms the serial allowing dimensions that are not feasible with the serial sensor, e.g., $256 \times 256\text{px}$ (K) .

Comparison. In conclusion, both approaches provide any desired accuracy depending on the configuration. In the ray cast-based approach, the number and distribution of mass points influence the results, whereas the dimensions of the texture are the decisive factor in the depth buffer-based approach.

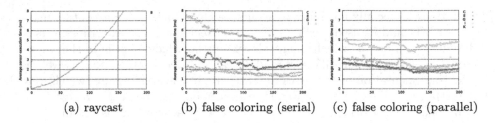

(a) raycast   (b) false coloring (serial)   (c) false coloring (parallel)

Fig. 4. Average sensor execution times in relation to the number of perceivable cubes. Cubes were added every 5 s from 0 to 200. All cubes were always visible.

The performance of the sensors depends on the number of perceivable objects (cf. Fig. 3). If only a small number of objects (≤ 100) needs to be checked, the ray cast-based sensors provide better execution times because each object is checked separately, instead of rendering the entire scene. However, with an increasing number of objects the false coloring-based approach becomes more efficient, because it profits from the usage of highly optimized graphics hardware.

An appropriate approach for a small number of sensible objects would be to use the ray cast-based sensor as default and to swap to a false coloring-based sensor when high quality results are required. In cases where many objects are to be sensed, we recommend using the false coloring approach.

5   Conclusions

Although numerous authors consider perception for virtual agents, the area has seldom been the focus of their work. We defined an independent architecture based on selected existing concepts and divided the process into sensation, memory and retrieval, with sensation being the main focus of this contribution.

Our visual sensation approach is object-based. A set of virtual sensors are attached to a unified sensor interface. The sensors return references to sensed virtual objects (and their semantic information) in the form of stimuli. The stimuli are stored in a sensory storage that provides short persistence.

In the visual case, the sensors have to solve the visibility problem known from computer graphics. A ray cast-based approach and a depth buffer-based approach were examined, which provide arbitrary accuracy dependent on their configuration. While the ray cast-based approach provides good run times for a small number of objects, the false coloring-based approach provides better results for large object sets. Based on the results, the applied sensing approach should be selected based on the use case that is considered. A dynamic swapping of different sensors to fit certain situations might also be beneficial.

Future challenges lie in the calculation of clarity and saliency values to guide subsequent attention processes. Additionally, it would be interesting to investigate how sensing of partial objects or object features might be possible. A big challenge is to improve the applicability of more complex perception processes, which is mainly related to their performance. To restrict the amount of required calculations (especially for multiple agents), a global perception execution manager (PEM) could be used. Such a PEM could decide when to execute sensors of different agents and at which quality level. Further challenges lie in the implementation of sensors for different modalities (auditive, tactile, etc.) as well as in the implementation of processes for the parts of the architecture, which were not further described here (see Fig. 1), e.g., memory and retrieval processes.

In conclusion, a plausible or even realistic virtual sensation is the first step towards a comprehensible information base, which could drastically improve the realism of the behavior of simulated entities.

Acknowledgments. The presented work was partially funded by the FHprofUnt program of the BMBF (project AVeSi, grant 17028X11).

References

1. Blumberg, B.M.: Old Tricks, New Dogs: Ethology and Interactive Creatures. PhD thesis, Massachusetts Institute of Technology (1996)
2. Bordeux, C., Boulic, R., Thalmann, D.: An efficient and flexible perception pipeline for autonomous agents. Comput. Graph. Forum. **18**, 23–30 (1999)
3. Conde, T., Thalmann, D.: An integrated perception for autonomous virtual agents: active and predictive perception. Comput. Anim. Virtual Worlds **17**, 457–468 (2006)
4. Enns, J.T.: The Thinking Eye, the Seeing Brain: Explorations in Visual Cognition. W. W. Norton and Company, New York (2004)
5. Haubrich, T., Seele, S., Herpers, R., Bauckhage, C., Becker, P.: Synthetic Perception for Intelligent Virtual Agents. In: Proceedings of the 1st ACM SIGCHI Annual Symposium on Computer-Human Interaction in Play (CHI PLAY) (2014)
6. Kuffner, Jr., J., Latombe, J.-C.: Fast synthetic vision, memory, and learning models for virtual humans. In: Proceedings of Computer Animation (1999)
7. Kuiper, D.M., Wenkstern, R.Z.: Virtual agent perception combination in multi agent based systems. In: Proceedings of the 2013 International Conference on Autonomous Agents and Multi-agent Systems (2013)
8. Leonard, T.: Building an AI Sensory System: Examining the Design of Thief: The Dark Project (2003). http://www.gamasutra.com/view/feature/131297
9. Luck, M., Aylett, R.: Applying artificial intelligence to virtual reality: intelligent virtual environments. Appl. Artif. Intell. **14**, 3–32 (2000)
10. Noser, H., Renault, O., Thalmann, D., Magnenat-Thalmann, N.: Navigation for digital actors based on synthetic vision, memory, and learning. Comput. Graph. **19**, 7–19 (1995)
11. Ondřej, J., Pettré, J., Olivier, A.-H., Donikian, S.: A synthetic-vision based steering approach for crowd simulation. ACM TOG **29**(4), 123:1–123:9 (2010)
12. Peters, C., Castellano, G., Rehm, M., Andre, E., Raouzaiou, A., Rapantzikos, K., Karpouzis, K., Volpe, G., Camurri, A., Vasalou, A.: Fundamentals of agent perception and attention modelling. In: Cowie, R., Pelachaud, C., Petta, P. (eds.) Emotion-Oriented Systems. Cognitive Technologies, pp. 293–319. Springer, Heidelberg (2011)
13. Peters, C., O'Sullivan, C.: Synthetic vision and memory for autonomous virtual humans. Comput. Graph. Forum **21**, 743–752 (2002)

14. Peters, C., O'Sullivan, C.: Bottom-up visual attention for virtual human animation. In: Proceedings of the 16th International Conference on Computer Animation and Social Agents (2003)
15. Rabin, S., Michael, D.: Game programming gems 7, chapter designing a realistic and unified agent-sensing model. Course Technology, Boston (2008)
16. Renault, O., Magnenat-Thalmann, N., Thalmann, D.: A vision-based approach to behavioural animation. Vis. Comput. Animation 1, 18–21 (1990)
17. Reynolds, C.W.: Flocks, herds and schools: a distributed behavioral model. SIGGRAPH Comput. Graph. 21, 25–34 (1987)
18. Russell, S.J., Norvig, P., Canny, J.F., Malik, J.M., Edwards, D.D.: Artificial intelligence: a modern approach. Prentice hall, Englewood Cliffs (1995)
19. Strassner, J., Langer, M.: Virtual humans with personalized perception and dynamic levels of knowledge. Comput. Animation Virtual Worlds 16, 331–342 (2005)
20. Terzopoulos, D., Rabie, T.: Animat vision: active vision in artificial animals. In: Proceedings of the 5th International Conference on Computer Vision (1995)
21. Tutenel, T., Bidarra, R., Smelik, R.M., Kraker, K.J.D.: The role of semantics in games and simulations. Comput. Entertainment 6(4), 57:1–57:35 (2008)

Towards Adaptive, Interactive Virtual Humans in Sigma

Volkan Ustun[1](✉) and Paul S. Rosenbloom[1,2]

[1] Institute for Creative Technologies, University of Southern California,
Los Angeles, CA, USA
ustun@ict.usc.edu
[2] Department of Computer Science, University of Southern California,
Los Angeles, CA, USA

Abstract. Sigma is a nascent cognitive architecture/system that combines concepts from graphical models with traditional symbolic architectures. Here an initial Sigma-based virtual human (VH) is introduced that combines probabilistic reasoning, rule-based decision-making, Theory of Mind, Simultaneous Localization and Mapping and reinforcement learning in a unified manner. This non-modular unification of diverse cognitive, robotic and VH capabilities provides an important first step towards fully adaptive and interactive VHs in Sigma.

1 Introduction

Virtual humans (VHs) are synthetic characters that can take the part of humans in a variety of contexts. The main goal for VHs is to look and behave as real people to the extent possible [17], including: (1) using their perceptual capabilities to observe their environment and other virtual/real humans in it; (2) acting autonomously in their environment based on what they know and perceive, e.g. reacting and appropriately responding to external events; (3) interacting in a natural way with both real people and other VHs using verbal and non-verbal communication; (4) possessing a *Theory of Mind* (*ToM*) to model their own mind and the minds of others; (5) understanding and exhibiting appropriate emotions and associated behaviors; and (6) adapting their behavior through experience. Most critically, this broad range of capabilities must be integrated together and work coherently. This integration can be quite hard, but if it can yield more than the sum of its parts, it can simplify a variety of other aspects.

Sigma [13] is being built as a computational model of general intelligence that is based on combining what has been learned from over three decades worth of independent work in cognitive architectures [7] and graphical models [3]. The long-term goal is to understand and replicate the *architecture of the mind*; i.e., the fixed structure underlying intelligent behavior in both natural and artificial systems. This ambitious goal strives for the complete control of VHs (and robots in the future) that behave as closely as possible to humans, primarily by achieving and integrating the list above in a manner that should ultimately yield *plug compatibility* between humans and artificial systems. Such compatibility potentially creates very flexible VHs and simulation environments.

© Springer International Publishing Switzerland 2015
W.-P. Brinkman et al. (Eds.): IVA 2015, LNAI 9238, pp. 98–108, 2015.
DOI: 10.1007/978-3-319-21996-7_10

Sigma's development is guided by a trio of desiderata: (1) *grand unification*, uniting the requisite cognitive and non-cognitive aspects of embodied intelligent behavior in complex real worlds; (2) *functional elegance*, yielding broad cognitive (and sub-cognitive) functionality from the interactions among a small general set of mechanisms; and (3) *sufficient efficiency*, executing rapidly enough for anticipated applications. The first and last desiderata are directly relevant to the construction of broadly capable, real-time, VHs, while the middle one implies a rather unique path towards them, where instead of a disparate assembly of modules, all of the required capabilities are constructed and integrated together on a simple elegant base. Most of the work to date on Sigma has individually explored particular capabilities for learning, memory and knowledge, decision making and problem solving, perception, speech, Theory of Mind, and emotions. These individual capabilities are important in building human-like intelligence but getting them to work together is also quite challenging [17]. *Sigma's* non-modular, *hybrid* (discrete + continuous) *mixed* (symbolic + probabilistic) character supports attempting a deep integration across these required VH capabilities, straddling the traditional boundary between symbolic cognitive processing and numeric sub-cognitive processing.

The work here combines a subset of these capabilities within Sigma to construct an adaptive, interactive VH in a virtual environment. The VH is adaptive not only in terms of dynamically deciding what to do, but also in terms of embodying two distinct forms of relevant learning: (1) the automated acquisition of maps of the environment from experience with it, in the context of the classic robotic capability of Simultaneous Localization and Mapping (SLAM); and (2) reinforcement learning (RL), to improve decision making based on experience with the outcomes of earlier decisions. The VH is interactive both in terms of its (virtual) physical environment – through high-level perception and action – and other participants, although the latter is still quite limited. Although speech and language are being investigated in Sigma, neither is deployed in this VH, so social interaction is limited to constructing – actually, learning, with the help of RL – models of the self and others.[1] These forms of adaptivity and interaction are combined together within Sigma and, for this initial VH, with a basic rule-based decision framework.

Sigma provides the ability to exhibit this combination of capabilities in a unified manner because of its grounding in a *graphical architecture* that is built from graphical models [3] (in particular, factor graphs and the summary product algorithm [5]), n-dimensional piecewise linear functions [10], and gradient descent learning [14]. The required VH capabilities emerge in a functionally elegant manner from the interactions among this small but general set of mechanisms, plus knowledge. For example, RL arises from the interactions between gradient descent learning and particular forms of both domain-specific and domain-independent knowledge [11].

Chen et al. [1] discussed the fusion of symbolic and probabilistic reasoning at an earlier stage of the development of Sigma. In that study initial steps towards grand unification were demonstrated when perception, localization and decision-making were implemented within a single graphical model, with interaction among these capabilities

---

[1] As explained later, what the VH actually does is to model itself as if it were a different VH.

modulated through shared variables. The work here greatly expands on this approach to yield a more significant combination of capabilities, plus a deployment in a VH that is embodied in the SmartBody character animation system [15] and that operates within a 3D virtual environment rather than a toy one-dimensional space. In the work here, SmartBody's internal movement, path-finding and collision detection algorithms are used in animating the VH's actions, although eventually much of this is to be moved within Sigma. Sigma has no direct access to the virtual environment, but can perceive and act on it through a (deliberately) noisy interface.

In addition to the contributions of this work to the creation of adaptive, interactive VHs, it is also thus an important step in the maturation of Sigma. The hope is that this will serve as a foundation towards developing even more complete and functional VHs. It also should help better understand how to handle the interactions between VHs and their environments in a robust manner that is similar to, but still somewhat simpler than, interactions between robots and the real world.

The conceptual model(s) for the VHs, and their interactions with the virtual environment, are described in Sect. 2. A basic introduction to Sigma is provided in Sect. 3. Section 4 provides a discussion of the Sigma models that control the VH(s). Conclusions and possible extensions to this work are discussed in Sect. 5.

2   Conceptual Model and Environment

Physical security systems are comprised of structures, sensors, protocols, and policies that aim to protect fixed-site facilities against intrusions by external threats, as well as unauthorized acts by insiders. Physical security systems are generally easy to understand but they also allow complex interactions to emerge among the agents. These properties make physical-security-systems simulation a natural candidate as a testbed for developing cognitive models of synthetic characters [18]. Similar to the discussion in [18], a physical-security-system scenario in a retail store has been selected as a platform to develop and test Sigma VH models.

In a typical retail-store shoplifting plot, offenders first pick up merchandise in a retail store and then try to leave without getting caught by any of the store's security measures. A simple grab-and-run scenario is considered in this paper, but a large number of different scenarios are possible. In this scenario, the intruder needs to locate the desired item in the store, grab it, and then leave the store. The role of security is to detain the intruder before s/he leaves the store. A basic assumption is that it is not possible to tell what the intruder will do until s/he picks up an item and starts running. The security can immediately detect the activity and start pursuing the intruder once the item is picked up (assuming CCTV). If the intruder makes it to the door, it is considered a success for the intruder.

For the basic setup, it is assumed that the intruder does not know the layout of the store and hence it has to learn a map and be able to use it to localize itself in the store. When the intruder locates the item of interest, it grabs the item and leaves the store via one of the exits. In the hypothetical retail store used here (Fig. 1), there are shelves (gray rectangles), the item of interest (the blue circle) and two entry/exit doors (red rectangles). The intruder leaves the store via either (1) the door it used to enter or

(2) the door closest to the item of interest. The main task for security is to learn about the exit strategies of intruders and use this to effectively detain them.

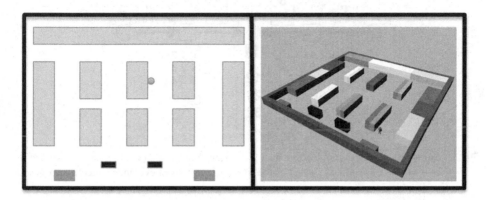

Fig. 1. Layout of the store and its SmartBody representation (Color figure online)

SmartBody [15], a Behavior Markup Language (BML) [4] realization engine, is used as the character animation platform for this study, with communication between the Sigma VH model and SmartBody handled via BML messages. In the current setup, locomotion and path finding are delegated to the SmartBody engine. Sigma sends commands and queries to SmartBody to perform these tasks and to return perceptual information. Two basic types of perception are utilized by the Sigma VH model: (1) information about the current location of the agent, mimicking the combination of direction, speed and odometry measurements for a robot; and (2) objects that are in the visual field of the agent and their relative distances, mimicking the perception of the environment for a robot (currently the agents have x-ray vision, but a more realistic visual system is in the works). Location information is conveyed to the Sigma VH model with noise added; perfect location information is not available to the model.

3 Sigma

The Sigma cognitive architecture is built on *factor graphs* [5] – undirected graphical models [3] with variable and factor nodes, and functions that are stored in the factor nodes. Graphical models provide a general computational technique for efficient computation with complex multivariate functions – implemented via hybrid mixed *piecewise-linear functions* [10] in Sigma – by leveraging forms of independence to: decompose them into products of simpler functions; map these products onto graphs; and solve the graphs via message passing or sampling methods. The *summary product algorithm* [5] is the general inference algorithm in Sigma (Fig. 2). Graphical models are particularly attractive as a basis for broadly functional, yet simple and theoretically elegant, cognitive architectures because they provide a single general representation and inference algorithm for processing symbols, probabilities and signals.

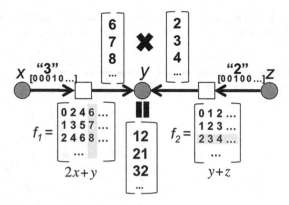

Fig. 2. Summary product computation over the factor graph for $f(x, y, z) = y^2 + yz + 2yx + 2xz = (2x + y)(y + z) = f_1(x, y)f_2(y, z)$ of the marginal on y given evidence concerning x and z.

The Sigma architecture defines a high-level language of *predicates* and *conditionals* that compiles down into factor graphs. Predicates specify relations over continuous, discrete and/or symbolic arguments. They are defined via a name and a set of typed arguments, with *working memory* (WM) containing predicate instantiations as functions within a WM subgraph. Predicates may also have perception and/or long-term memory (LTM) functions. For perceptual predicates, factor nodes for *perceptual buffers* are connected to the corresponding WM subgraphs. For example, Observed (object:object visible:boolean) is a perceptual predicate with two arguments: (1) object of type object; and (2) visible of type boolean. This predicate specifies which objects are visible to the agent at any particular time. For memorial predicates, *function factor nodes* (FFNs) are likewise connected to the corresponding WM subgraphs. Messages into FFNs provide the gradient for learning the nodes' functions.

Conditionals structure LTM and basic reasoning, compiling into more extended subgraphs that also connect to the appropriate WM subgraphs. Conditionals are defined via a set of *predicate patterns* – in which type specifications are replaced by constants and variables – and an optional *function* over pattern variables. *Conditions* and *actions* are predicate patterns that behave like the respective parts of rules, pushing information in one direction from the conditions to the actions. The example conditional in Fig. 3 updates the information about which objects have been seen so far, based on the information in the Observed predicate. *Contacts* are predicate patterns that support the bidirectional processing that is key to probabilistic reasoning, partial matching, constraint satisfaction and signal processing. Overall, conditionals provide a deep combination of rule systems and probabilistic networks.

```
CONDITIONAL Seen
        Conditions: Observed(object:o visible:true)
        Actions: Seen-Objects(object:o)
```

Fig. 3. Conditional for context information.

Processing in Sigma is driven by a *cognitive cycle* that comprises input, graph solution, decisions (selection of best elements from distributions), learning, and output. Graph solution occurs via the summary product algorithm. Most of perception and action is to occur within graph solution in Sigma, rather than within external modules [3]. Decisions in Sigma, in the classical sense of choosing one among the best operators to execute next, are based on an architecturally distinguished selection predicate: `Selected(state:state operator:operator)`. Typically the operator associated with the highest value, or utility, in the distribution is selected. Once an operator is selected, it can be applied by conditionals with actions that modify the state in working memory. As in Soar [6], a single cognitive cycle yields *reactive* processing; a sequence of cognitive cycles yields *deliberative* processing; and if no operator can be selected, or a selected operator can't be applied, a Soar-like impasse [6] occurs, leading to *reflective* processing.

4 The Sigma Virtual Human (VH) Model

In a typical physical security system setting there are intruders (shoplifters) and security personnel. There may also be neutrals, but they are not modeled in this work. In this initial implementation, only an intruder is modeled as a VH, although part of the capability of a security agent – of learning a model of the intruder based on witnessing the intruder's actions – has been grafted onto the implementation of the intruder, as if it were observing itself from the outside (although the intent is eventually to move this into a distinct VH). In the current scenario, the intruder does not know the layout of the store in advance, and so it must learn a map of the store while simultaneously localizing itself in the learned map (Sect. 4.1). The intruder also needs a decision framework to dynamically decide what to do based on its immediate circumstances (Sect. 4.2). Learning the strategy of the intruder – i.e., whether it exits through the entry door or the closest door – occurs by learning a policy for the agent via RL and then using this policy and the agent's actions to determine on each trial the relative likelihoods of the two strategies being used (Sect. 4.3).

4.1 Simultaneous Localization and Mapping (SLAM)

The intruder has no a priori knowledge about the layout of the retail store (which is as shown in Fig. 1). Therefore, it has to learn a map of the store while simultaneously using the map to localize itself within the store. A 31×31 grid is imposed on the store for map learning. A VH only occupies a single grid cell, whereas objects in the environment – such as shelves – may span multiple cells.

The Sigma VH model defines two perceptual predicates – `Location-X(x:location)` and `Location-Z(z:location)` – to represent the location of the VH on the grid (the `location` type is discrete numeric, with a span of 31). Together these two predicates span the space of 2D cells in the grid, with perception of x and z involving a noise model that assumes any neighboring cell of the correct cell may be perceived as the agent's current location. The objects in the visual field are also perceived, along with the relative distances of the center of these objects to the agent's location.

To perform SLAM, a Dynamic Bayesian Network (DBN) [2] is defined via two almost identical conditionals, one for x (Fig. 4) and a similar one for z. These conditionals convert relative locations of objects given the agent to absolute locations in the map, using the affine transform *translation* to offset the agent's current location by the distance to the object. In Fig. 4, `Object-Location-X` is a memorial predicate that has a function that represents the map that is learned via gradient descent. Since both the `Location-X` and `Object-Location-X` patterns are contacts, processing is bidirectional between them; both perception of the VH's location and perception of the objects' locations have an impact on the posterior for the VH's location. This bidirectional processing forms the basis for SLAM, where the map is learned while it is simultaneously used for localization.

```
CONDITIONAL SLAM-X
      Conditions:   Observed(object:o visible:true)
                    Object-Distance-X(dist-x:dx object:o)
      Condacts:     Location-X(x:lx)
                    Object-Location-X(object:o x:(lx-dx))
```

Fig. 4. SLAM conditional for the x coordinate

4.2   Behavior Rules

The objective of the intruder is to grab the item of interest (Fig. 1) and then to leave the store through one of the exits without being detained. In the current implementation, four basic behaviors, with corresponding Sigma operators, are available to the intruder: (1) *walk towards target object*; (2) *run towards target object*; (3) *pick up target object*; and (4) *walk towards random object*. Target objects play a role in the intruder achieving its goals, while random objects drive exploration of the store.

The intruder is initialized with a sequence of target objects that it needs either to walk towards or to pick-up. Given that the intruder does not have a priori knowledge of the store, it may need to explore the store, mapping it in the process, to locate the target objects. The basic operator used for exploration is *walk towards random object*. The intent is that doing this will help the agent eventually discover the target object.

This exploratory operator is always available; however, if other more task-relevant behaviors are available, they take precedence. For example, Fig. 5 shows a conditional in which the operator *walk towards target object* is suggested for selection with a utility of 0.5 when the VH has seen the target object (and hence, there is an estimate of its location). Exploration has a lower utility, so walking to a target object takes precedence if both operators are available. When the VH is within a threshold distance of the target object, a new operator – *pick up target object* – is then selected. The model terminates when the intruder reaches its preferred exit door, which acts as the target object for the *run towards target object* operator.

```
CONDITIONAL WALK-TOWARDS-TARGET
    Conditions:        Target-Object(object:o)
                       Seen-Objects(object:o visible:true)
    Actions:    Selected(operator:walk-target)
    Function:   0.5
```

Fig. 5. Conditional suggesting the *walk towards target object* operator

4.3   Leveraging Reinforcement Learning (RL) to Model Others

One basic assumption made in this paper is that it is easy to recognize that a grab-and-go scenario has been initiated, by observing the pick-up behavior of the intruder.[2] However, even though security can easily recognize when such a scenario has been initiated, it still needs to intercept the intruder before it leaves the retail store. As there are two exit doors, early anticipation of the intruder's choice increases the chances of a successful detention.

Theory of Mind (ToM) involves formation of models of others and generation of expectations about their behavior based on these models to enable effective decisions in social settings [19]. In decision-theoretic approaches to ToM, such models can be represented as reward functions. For the intruder in our scenario there are two possible models, distinguished by whether a reward is received when the agent returns to its door of entry or when it reaches the nearest door from the item of interest. This corresponds to Bayesian approaches to multi-agent modeling that use a distribution over a set of policies to specify the beliefs that one agent has about another [8].

In general, RL enables agents to learn effective policies for task performance based on rewards received over a sequence of trials [16]. In Sigma, RL is not a separate architectural learning algorithm, but occurs through a combination of gradient-descent learning and the appropriate knowledge expressed in predicates and conditionals. Here, as in [9], RL is leveraged in selecting among models of other agents; in particular it is used to emulate the process by which a separate security agent would learn a model of the intruder. First a form of multiagent RL is used to learn a distinct *policy*, or *Q function*, for the intruder under each possible model, and then these policies are used in combination with the perception of the intruder's actions to yield a gradient over the two models that is proportional to the models' Q values for the performed actions. In particular, the model for which the observed action has higher Q values will have an increased likelihood in the posterior distribution.

The conditional that compares the Q values and generates a posterior distribution for the models is shown in Fig. 6. It multiplies the Q values for the observed action – specified by the location of the intruder and the direction of movement from that location – in each policy by 0.1, to scale down utilities in [0, 10] to values for selection

---

[2] The details of this recognition process are beyond the scope of this paper but there are a variety of behavioral cues (e.g. posture changes while concealing an item, gait changes under stress etc.) that could be revealing. Exhibiting and detecting such cues is one of a number of intriguing future directions for this work.

in [0, 1], and then projects these values onto the model predicate to generate a posterior distribution on the model of the intruder.

```
CONDITIONAL PREDICT-MODEL
      Conditions:    Previous-RL-Loc(location:loc)
                     RL-Direction(direction:d)
                     Q(model:m location:loc direction:d
                       value:[0.1*q])
      Actions:       Model(model:m)
```

Fig. 6. Model prediction conditional

Ultimately, this approach to model learning needs to be evaluated in terms of how well it helps security catch the intruder, but for now we will only consider how quickly it helps determine through which door the intruder is attempting to escape. Here the VH was first run for 20 trials for each exit-door scenario to learn the policies on a low fidelity 4×4 grid, which was reduced for efficiency purposes, but with the VH still actually moving on the full 31×31 grid. Then each model was run for 5 trials for testing. The average number of cognitive cycles required to complete the scenario after picking up the item of interest is 31.2 for door 1 and 17.2 for door 2. The Sigma model correctly selects the exit strategy – P (Correct Exit Strategy) > 0.65 – after 12.4 cognitive cycles for door 1 (39.7 % of the time to needed to reach the door) and 11.8 cognitive cycles for door 2 (68.6 % of the time needed to reach the door). Thus, at least in a preliminary form, this demonstrates how model learning can help identify the correct door considerably before it is reached.

5   Conclusion

A first adaptive, interactive VH based on Sigma has been created that combines short-term rule-based adaptivity in decision making with two forms of long-term adaptivity (i.e., learning) – *mapping* in the context of SLAM, and *modeling* of others via RL – plus both interaction with a virtual environment and social interaction (in terms of ToM reasoning and learning). This VH, even as initial and limited as it is, provides an initial indicator of the potential for grand unification. To expand further on this potential, we are prioritizing the development of multiple VHs, plus the ability for them to interact via speech and language.

There are different types of participants – intruders, security, and neutrals – in a typical physical security system. Such variety makes the physical-security-system setting very flexible for the generation of scenarios that encompass many different interactions among VHs, and between VHs and humans. Consequently, an extended version of the current retail store security setting should yield a useful testbed for further exploration of this potential. As the scenarios get more complex, we expect the forms of cognition exhibited to become comparably sophisticated, going beyond simple rule-based reasoning to more involved combinations of reactive, deliberative and reflective processing.

In addition to grand unification, the VH here leverages Sigma's functionally elegant approach to providing and combining capabilities such as rule-based reasoning, SLAM, ToM, and RL. It also stretches, but does not quite break the desideratum of sufficient efficiency. Although the decision cycles were longer than the desired 50 ms [12] – around 250 ms – the impact on the performance of the VH was minimal because those activities requiring faster decisions were delegated to SmartBody's inner algorithms. Further analysis and optimizations are clearly required, but this should not detract significantly from how the VH here exhibits simple interactive, adaptive behavior by combining different types of reasoning and learning mechanisms under a unified model in a functionally elegant manner.

Acknowledgments. This effort has been sponsored by the Office of Naval Research and the U. S. Army. Statements and opinions expressed do not necessarily reflect the position or the policy of the United States Government, and no official endorsement should be inferred. We would also like to thank Ari Shapiro for his overall support with SmartBody.

References

1. Chen, J., Demski, A., Han, T., Morency, L.P., Pynadath, D.V., Rafidi, N., Rosenbloom, P.S.: Fusing symbolic and decision-theoretic problem solving + perception in a graphical cognitive architecture. In: Biologically Inspired Cognitive Architectures (2011)
2. Grisetti, G., Kummerle, R., Stachniss, C., Burgard, W.: A tutorial on graph-based SLAM. Intell. Transp. Syst. Mag. IEEE **2**(4), 31–43 (2010)
3. Koller, D., Friedman, N.: Principles and Techniques: Probabilistic Graphical Models. MIT Press, Cambridge (2009)
4. Kopp, S., Krenn, B., Marsella, S.C., Marshall, A.N., Pelachaud, C., Pirker, H., Thórisson, K.R., Vilhjálmsson, H.H.: Towards a common framework for multimodal generation: the behavior markup language. In: Gratch, J., Young, M., Aylett, R.S., Ballin, D., Olivier, P. (eds.) IVA 2006. LNCS (LNAI), vol. 4133, pp. 205–217. Springer, Heidelberg (2006)
5. Kschischang, F.R., Frey, B.J., Loeliger, H.A.: Factor graphs and the sum-product algorithm. IEEE Trans. Inf. Theor. **47**(2), 498–519 (2001)
6. Laird, J.E.: The Soar Cognitive Architecture. MIT Press, Cambridge (2012)
7. Langley, P., Laird, J.E., Rogers, S.: Cognitive architectures: research issues and challenges. Cogn. Syst. Res. **10**, 141–160 (2009)
8. Pynadath, D.V., Marsella, S.C.: PsychSim: modeling theory of mind with decision-theoretic agents. In: IJCAI (2005)
9. Pynadath, D.V., Rosenbloom, P.S., Marsella, S.C.: Reinforcement learning for adaptive theory of mind in the sigma cognitive architecture. In: Goertzel, B., Orseau, L., Snaider, J. (eds.) AGI 2014. LNCS, vol. 8598, pp. 143–154. Springer, Heidelberg (2014)
10. Rosenbloom, P.S.: Bridging dichotomies in cognitive architectures for virtual humans. In: Proceedings of the AAAI Fall Symposium on Advances in Cognitive Systems (2011)
11. Rosenbloom, P.S.: Deconstructing reinforcement learning in sigma. In: Bach, J., Goertzel, B., Iklé, M. (eds.) AGI 2012. LNCS, vol. 7716, pp. 262–271. Springer, Heidelberg (2012)
12. Rosenbloom, P.S.: Towards a 50 ms cognitive cycle in a graphical architecture. In: Proceedings of the 11th International Conference on Cognitive Modeling (2012)
13. Rosenbloom, P.S.: The sigma cognitive architecture and system. AISB Q. **136**, 4–13 (2013)

14. Rosenbloom, P.S., Demski, A., Han, T., Ustun, V.: Learning via gradient descent in Sigma. In: Proceedings of the 12th International Conference on Cognitive Modeling (2013)
15. Shapiro, A.: Building a character animation system. In: Allbeck, J.M., Faloutsos, P. (eds.) MIG 2011. LNCS, vol. 7060, pp. 98–109. Springer, Heidelberg (2011)
16. Sutton, R.S., Barto, A.G.: Reinforcement Learning: An Introduction. MIT Press, Cambridge (1998)
17. Swartout, W.: Lessons learned from virtual humans. AI Mag. **31**(1), 9–20 (2010)
18. Ustun, V., Yilmaz, L., Smith, J.S.: A conceptual model for agent-based simulation of physical security systems. In: Proceedings of the 44th Annual Southeast Regional Conference. ACM (2006)
19. Whiten, A. (ed.): Natural Theories of Mind. Basil Blackwell, Oxford (1991)

Beyond Believability: Quantifying the Differences Between Real and Virtual Humans

Celso M. de Melo[1($\boxtimes$)] and Jonathan Gratch[2]

[1] USC Marshall School of Business, Los Angeles, CA 90089-0808, USA
demelo@usc.edu
[2] Institute for Creative Technologies, University of Southern California,
12015 Waterfront Drive, Building #4, Playa Vista, Logs Angeles,
CA 90094-2536, USA
gratch@ict.usc.edu

Abstract. "Believable" agents are supposed to "suspend the audience's disbelief" and provide the "illusion of life". However, beyond such high-level definitions, which are prone to subjective interpretation, there is not much more to help researchers systematically create or assess whether their agents are believable. In this paper we propose a more pragmatic and useful benchmark than believability for designing virtual agents. This benchmark requires people, *in a specific social situation, to act with the virtual agent in the same manner as they would with a real human.* We propose that perceptions of mind in virtual agents, especially pertaining to *agency* – the ability to act and plan – and *experience* – the ability to sense and feel emotion – are critical for achieving this new benchmark. We also review current computational systems that fail, pass, and even surpass this benchmark and show how a theoretical framework based on perceptions of mind can shed light into these systems. We also discuss a few important cases where it is better if virtual humans do *not* pass the benchmark. We discuss implications for the design of virtual agents that can be as natural and efficient to interact with as real humans.

Keywords: Believability · Mind perception · Emotion · Virtual vs. real humans

1 Introduction

The intelligent virtual agents community has always been fascinated with building "believable" agents. These agents are meant to provide the "illusion of life" and support the audience's "suspension of disbelief" [1–4]. The notion emerged from the arts and was a natural reaction to the focus, at the time, artificial intelligence researchers placed on simulating proper reasoning, problem solving, and logical-analytical skill. This fresh new perspective led researchers to, among others, develop agents that were driven by personality and expressed emotion.

Believability was, nevertheless, left mostly underspecified. As researchers attempted to determine the requirements for achieving believable agents, it became

© Springer International Publishing Switzerland 2015
W.-P. Brinkman et al. (Eds.): IVA 2015, LNAI 9238, pp. 109–118, 2015.
DOI: 10.1007/978-3-319-21996-7_11

clear that believability was hard to measure with any precision or reliability. Some researchers did attempt to refine the notion of believability [5, 6] but, ultimately, the concept remained prone to subjective interpretation and, consequently, hard to study from a scientific point of view.

In this paper we propose a more pragmatic, clearly defined, and useful benchmark than believability. The benchmark is that: *in a specific social setting, people behave with the virtual agent in the same manner as they would with a real human*. In social decision making, this benchmark is achieved when, for instance, people are as fair, generous, or cooperative with virtual as with real humans. In a learning task, the benchmark is achieved when people learn as much and as efficiently with virtual as with real humans. In a therapy session, the benchmark is achieved when, for instance, people self-disclose as much with the virtual as with the real doctor. The benchmark is, thus, really a point in a continuum, where there are virtual agents that fall below it (probably the majority) and others that actually surpass it. Finally, in contrast to believability which originally came from the arts, achieving our benchmark can be informed by rigorous communication and psychological theories. Section 2 overviews these theories. Section 3 reviews critical work that demonstrates how these theories and benchmark can guide the design of virtual agents in various domains. Section 4 will, then, present our conclusions.

2   Theoretical Framework

Clifford Nass and colleagues were among the first to advance a general theory of how humans interact with machines [7–9]. The theory's main tenet is that to the extent that machines display social cues (e.g., interactivity, verbal and nonverbal behavior, filling of typically human roles), people will treat them in a fundamentally social manner. The argument is that people "mindlessly" treat computers that exhibit social traits like other people as a way to conserve cognitive effort and maximize response efficiency [8]. These automatic cognitive heuristics lead people to use the easily accessible social rules from human-human interaction and apply them in human-machine settings. To support their theory, they replicated in a human-computer context various findings from the human-human interaction literature. For instance, they demonstrated that people were polite to computers [10], treated computers that were perceived to be teammates better [11], and even applied gender and race stereotypes to computers [12].

These initial findings were so promising that they actually proposed that it was possible to replicate any finding in human-human interaction with computers:

"Findings and experimental methods from the social sciences can be applied directly to human-media interaction. It is possible to take a psychology research paper about how people respond to other people, replace the word 'human' with the word 'computer' and get the same results" ([7], p. 28).

Thus, a strict interpretation of the theory suggests that, in social settings, people will treat machines – virtual agents included – just like real humans and, thus, immediately meet our proposed benchmark.

Subsequent studies, however, showed that, even though people treat machines in a social manner, people still make important distinctions between humans and machines. For instance, these studies showed that, in certain social settings, people experienced higher social presence [13, 14], inhibition [15], learning [16], flow [17], arousal [18, 19] and engagement [14] with humans than machines. These kind of findings led Blascovich and colleagues [20, 21] to propose that social influence would be greater in machines, the higher the perceived mindfulness[1]. According to this view, thus, the higher the attributions of mind people make, the more likely machines are to pass our benchmark.

Research shows that people are, in fact, quite adept at anthropomorphizing – i.e., attributing human-like qualities, including mental states – to non-human entities [22, 23]. Perceiving mind in (human or non-human) others matters because, when we see mind in others, we attribute more responsibility, moral rights, and respect to others [24]. On the other hand, when we deny mind to others, we dehumanize, and consequently, discriminate others [25].

Recent research, furthermore, suggests that we perceive mind in others according to two core dimensions [26]: *agency*, the ability to act and plan; and, *experience*, the ability to sense and feel emotion. When we deny agency to others [25, 27], we treat others like "animals" that possess primitive feelings, but no higher reasoning skills. When we deny experience to others, we treat others like "cold emotionless automata" ("business people"). Accordingly, in a survey involving thousands of participants, Gray et al. [26] showed that: (a) adult humans were rated high in perceived agency and in perceived experience; (b) animals and babies rated high in experience, but low in agency; finally, (c) machines rated high in agency but very low in experience. According to this view, therefore, machines are unlikely to pass our benchmark, at least by default, because people perceive less mind in machines than humans, especially pertaining to perceptions of experience. This research, thus, goes one step further than Blascovich et al., in that it proposes a structure for perceiving mind in human and non-human others. The implication is that, the higher the perceived agency and experience in virtual humans, the more likely they are to pass our benchmark.

3 Empirical Evidence

In this section we present several studies that compare people's behavior with machines versus humans. This review is not meant to be exhaustive, but representative of computational systems – many of which involving virtual agents – that failed, passed, and even surpassed our benchmark. We also present cases where it is actually better *not* to pass the benchmark, i.e., where the goal is to develop virtual agents that should not act like humans. We take particular care to frame all these systems within the theoretical framework mentioned in the previous section.

---

[1] Blascovich et al. [20, 21] used the term "agency" instead of "mindfulness"; however, this use of the term conflicts with its use in the mind perception literature. In this paper, we adopt the latter definition of agency.

3.1   Systems That Are not as Good as Humans

Neuroeconomics is an emerging field that studies the biological basis of decision making in the brain [28]. To accomplish this, researchers compared people's behavior with humans versus computers. This evidence reveals that people tend, by default, to reach different decisions and show different patterns of brain activation with machines in the exact same decision making tasks, for the exact same financial incentives, when compared to humans [29–36]. For instance, Gallagher et al. [29] showed that when people played the rock-paper-scissors game with a human there was activation of the medial prefrontal cortex, a region of the brain that had previously been implicated in mentalizing (i.e., inferring of other's beliefs, desires and intentions); however, no such activation occurred when people engaged with a computer. McCabe et al. [30] also replicated this pattern in the trust game. Riedl et al. [31] further replicated this result with virtual humans. Finally, in a seminal study, Sanfey et al. [35] showed that, when receiving unfair offers in the ultimatum game, people showed stronger activation of the bilateral anterior insula – a region associated with the experience of negative emotions – with humans, when compared to computers. In line with mind perception theories, this evidence suggests that people experienced less emotion and spent less effort inferring mental states with machines than with humans. This suggests that machines will fail to pass our benchmark, at least by default, in social decision making.

In digital games, Ravaja [14] demonstrated that people tend to show higher arousal and engagement with human than computer opponents. Specifically, people showed stronger EMG response in facial musculature (e.g., zygomaticus major), higher skin conductance, and better self-reported ratings with humans than computers. Moreover, the study showed that participants experienced stronger psychophysiological response with humans that were friends than strangers. This suggests that, in game-playing contexts, familiarity and long-term interaction may improve the likelihood that virtual agents will pass our benchmark.

Finally, research in social robotics tends to show that people behave differently with robots, when compared with humans. Kahn et al. [37] presented a study that clearly demonstrates this. In their experiment, children interacted for about 15 min with a humanoid robot, before an experimenter came into the room, interrupted the inter-action, and asked the robot to "go wait in the closet". The question was whether this was fair to the robot, and whether the robot had any civil or moral rights. Effectively, children believed that the robot was entitled to fair treatment and had some rights; however, when compared to the case where this happened to an actual person, children were more likely to find the interruption unfair and to ascribe the person moral and civil rights. In line with mind perception theories, this result suggests that social robots will, thus, fail to pass our benchmark, at least by default.

3.2   Systems That Are as Good (or Better) Than Humans

Recently, de Melo et al. [38] had participants engage in the ultimatum game with human or computer counterparts. The ultimatum game [39] is a simple 2-player game where there is a proposer and a responder. The proposer is given an initial endowment of money and then decides how much to offer to the responder. The responder then decides whether to accept or reject the offer. If the offer is rejected, no one gets anything. In this experiment, participants always assumed the role of proposers. The interesting aspect of the experiment, however, was that responders were manipulated to have different levels of mind. The experiment followed a 2 × 2 × 2 factorial design: Responder (human vs. computer) × Agency (intentional vs. random) × Experience (non-emotional vs. emotional). For the manipulation of agency, they introduced a variation of the game where the responder was forced to make a random decision, independently of the offer, and the proposer was aware of this. For the manipulation of experience, the responder would either show a neutral facial display or show facial expressions of emotion. The emotion pattern rewarded fair behavior (e.g., sadness was shown when the offer was unfair or happiness when the offer was fair). The results showed, first, a main effect of Agency, with people offering more to intentional than random responders; nevertheless, there was no Responder × Agency interaction. The more interesting finding was a significant Responder × Experience interaction: when the responder showed no emotion, people offered more to human than computer responders, which is the usual bias in favor of humans; however, when responders showed emotion, people offered just as much to computers as they did to humans. Thus, adding appropriate emotion to computers was sufficient to "turn computers into humans", at least in the context of social decision making. These results show that perceptions of experience – the ability to sense and feel emotion – play an important role in making virtual humans pass our benchmark.

In a follow-up experiment, de Melo et al. [40] demonstrated that it was possible to use other social mechanisms to overcome this intergroup bias people show in favor of humans. In particular, they explored multiple social categories [41]. This mechanism relies on the fact that people naturally categorize others as belonging to "in-groups", with which they identify with, and "out-groups". In their experiment, participants engaged with human or computer counterparts that were either of the same or different race as the participant (see Fig. 1). The results showed that, as usual, people offered more to humans than computers; however, people also made better offers to counterparts that shared the same race. In fact, there was no statistical difference between offers to computers of the same race and humans of a different race. The experiment, thus, showed that it is possible to use social categories – in particular, race – to help virtual humans pass the proposed benchmark.

In yet another experiment, de Melo et al. [40] demonstrated that multiple social categories could be used, not only to overcome but, to reverse people's bias in favor of humans. In this experiment, a third social category was created using the task payoff structure. In practice, this category created two teams. Participants were placed in the first team with two computers that shared the same race. In the other team, there were humans of a different race. So, in this case, computers were associated with two "positive" social categories (same team and race) and humans were associated with two "negative" categories (different team and race). As expected, people offered more to computers than to humans, thus, actually surpassing our benchmark.

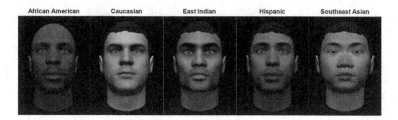

Fig. 1. People make more favorable offers to (human or non-human) counterparts that belong to the same social categories, such as race [40].

3.3   Systems That Should Not Be Like Humans

In this subsection, we present three interaction contexts that seem to inherently favor machines to humans. First, we consider self-disclosure in health-screening interviews. In these clinical settings, it is important that patients disclose information about themselves honestly so that healthcare professionals may get an accurate medical history. In a recent study, Lucas et al. [42] demonstrated that when people believed that a virtual doctor was being controlled by algorithms, versus being driven by an actual person, people reported lower fear of self-disclosure, lower impression management, and were rated by observers as being more willing to disclose truthfully (Fig. 2).

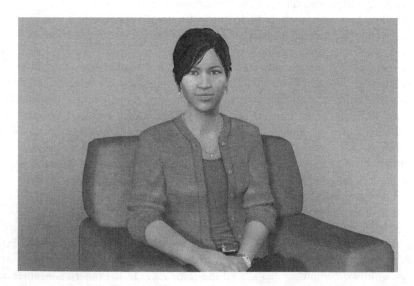

Fig. 2. People are more willing to self-disclose honestly with virtual than real healthcare professionals.

Second, in the context of social robotics, Malle et al. [43] studied how people apply moral norms to robots, when compared to humans. They asked people how morally accepting was for a human or a robot to make an "utilitarian choice" in the trolley dilemma. In this dilemma, a runway train is heading towards five workers in the tracks that will inevitably die, unless the decision maker, who is standing at a railroad intersection, pushes a lever that deviates the train away. However, the dilemma is that in the other track is a single worker, which will now be killed because the lever was pulled. Most people prefer to avoid making a decision, since they don't want to be responsible for the death of anyone. In this experiment, however, the results suggest that people would be more willing to accept the decision to pull the lever if it had been made by a robot, rather than by a human. Thus, if we assume that a decision needs to be made in such moral dilemmas, robots seem to be, by default, at an advantage when compared to humans.

Third, Sanfey et al. [35] showed that people were more willing to accept unfair offers in the ultimatum game if these were made by computers, rather than by humans. They further showed that this was happening because people experienced less negative emotion with computers than with humans. Therefore, if success is defined by the amount of money made, then it seems that computers are more likely to succeed than humans in making people accept unfair outcomes.

In all these social settings, it could be argued that people's decisions favor machines exactly because people have lower expectations of mental ability in machines. For instance, one might be more willing to accept unfair offers from a machine because a machine has no understanding of what it means to experience anger, or one might be more willing to self-disclose with a virtual human because one does not expect it to have the same kind of social concerns as humans (such as social image preservation). Thus, building on the mind perception framework, it would be interesting to confirm if, in these cases, proper simulation of mental ability in these machines – and emotional intelligence, in particular – would be sufficient to make people start treating them "just as badly" as they treat humans. Nevertheless, the main point here is that these systems should not aim to be like humans.

4   Conclusions

In this paper, we argued for a new benchmark for virtual agents that is more pragmatic, clearly defined, and useful than believability. The benchmark asks, in each specific social situation, that people behave with a virtual human in the same manner as with a real human. Thus, the benchmark serves as the basis for quantifying the difference between people's behavior with virtual and real humans. This benchmark can be easily measured in the lab, as demonstrated in the numerous studies reviewed in this paper. In fact, in many of these studies, the only thing that differed were participants' *beliefs* about whether they were interacting with a human or an autonomous agent. Moreover, the benchmark fits within a continuum, thus, allowing for continuous measurement of scientific progress towards the goal of achieving human-level social intelligence.

We also argue that perceptions of mind are critical for achieving virtual agents that are treated like humans in social settings. In particular, we reviewed evidence that perceptions of agency (the ability to plan and act) and experience (the ability to sense and feel emotion) play a powerful effect on people's behavior with virtual agents. This research also emphasizes that people expect, by default, virtual agents to lack in experience and, therefore, appropriate simulation of emotional intelligence is especially important for passing our benchmark.

Our review also shows that there are social settings for which virtual agents seem to be inherently better than real humans, i.e., people tend to behave better – according to some domain-specific criterion – with virtual rather than real humans. As mentioned above, the mind perception framework suggests that appropriate simulation of mental ability in these cases, thus, may actually be detrimental to virtual agents. The point is that, in some cases, we do not want our systems to have the full gamut of capabilities that we see in humans. Future research should continue to study these social settings for which virtual agents that are unlike humans are particularly suited.

Finally, due to space restrictions, there were several topics that we chose not to address in the paper. First, in general, the focus was on virtual agents that attempt to perform social tasks that are usually expected of real humans. In this sense, we excluded agents that are meant to be different than humans by design (e.g., for entertainment purposes) or that are meant to serve as mere tools (e.g., a calculator). Second, our benchmark focused on behavioral realism; nevertheless, some researchers have emphasized that visual realism can also impact people's behavior (e.g., [44]) and, therefore, may warrant related, yet separate, benchmarks. Third, it is important to discuss how long-term interaction with virtual agents impacts people's behavior with them and, in particular, whether it facilitates or hinders achieving the proposed benchmark. Fourth, we avoided a discussion about the ethical issues associated with creating computers that behave just like real humans, given the different social and legal standing of artificially intelligent agents or robots (e.g., [45]). These are, nevertheless, important issues that need to be addressed as we quickly move towards a society that is surrounded by artificial agents that can match (and even surpass) the mental ability and social skill we see in humans.

Acknowledgments. This research was supported in part by grants NSF IIS-1211064, SES-0836004, and AFOSR FA9550-09-1-0507. The content does not necessarily reflect the position or the policy of any Government, and no official endorsement should be inferred.

References

1. Bates, J.: The role of emotion in believable agents. Commun. ACM **37**, 122–125 (1994)
2. Mateas, M.: An oz-centric review of interactive drama and believable agents. In: Veloso, M.M., Wooldridge, M.J. (eds.) Artificial Intelligence Today. LNCS (LNAI), vol. 1600, pp. 297–328. Springer, Heidelberg (1999)
3. Riedl, M.O., Stern, A.: Believable agents and intelligent story adaptation for interactive storytelling. In: Göbel, S., Malkewitz, R., Iurgel, I. (eds.) TIDSE 2006. LNCS, vol. 4326, pp. 1–12. Springer, Heidelberg (2006)
4. Lester, J., Stone, B.: Increasing believability in animated pedagogical agents. In: Proceedings of the 1st International Conference on Autonomous Agents (AGENTS), pp. 16–21. ACM, New York (1997)
5. Rose, R., Scheutz, M., Schermerhorn, P.: Towards a conceptual and methodological framework for determining robot believability. Interact. Stud. **11**, 314–335 (2010)

6. Riedl, M.O., Young, R.M.: An objective character believability evaluation procedure for multi-agent story generation systems. In: Panayiotopoulos, T., Gratch, J., Aylett, R.S., Ballin, D., Olivier, P., Rist, T. (eds.) IVA 2005. LNCS (LNAI), vol. 3661, pp. 278–291. Springer, Heidelberg (2005)
7. Reeves, B., Nass, C.: The Media Equation: How People Treat Computers, Television, and New Media like Real People and Places. Cambridge University Press, New York (1996)
8. Nass, C., Moon, Y.: Machines and mindlessness: social responses to computers. J. Soc. Issues **56**, 81–103 (2000)
9. Sundar, S., Nass, C.: Source orientation in human-computer interaction: programmer, networker, or independent social actor? Commun. Res. **27**, 683–703 (2000)
10. Nass, C., Moon, Y., Carney, P.: Are people polite to computers? Responses to computer-based interviewing systems. J. Appl. Soc. Psychol. **29**, 1093–1109 (1999)
11. Nass, C., Fogg, B., Moon, Y.: Can computers be teammates? Int. J. Hum. Comput. Stud. **45**, 669–678 (1996)
12. Nass, C., Isbister, K., Lee, E.-J.: Truth is beauty: researching conversational agents. In: Cassell, J., Sullivan, J., Prevost, S., Churchill, E. (eds.) Embodied Conversational Agents, pp. 374–402. MIT Press, Cambridge (2000)
13. Gajadhar, B.J., de Kort, Y.A.W., IJsselsteijn, W.A.: Shared fun is doubled fun: player enjoyment as a function of social setting. In: Markopoulos, P., de Ruyter, B., IJsselsteijn, W.A., Rowland, D. (eds.) Fun and Games 2008. LNCS, vol. 5294, pp. 106–117. Springer, Heidelberg (2008)
14. Ravaja, N.: The psychophysiology of digital gaming: the effect of a non co-located opponent. Media Psychol. **12**, 268–294 (2009)
15. Hoyt, C., Blascovich, J., Swinth, K.: Social inhibition in immersive virtual environments. Presence **12**, 183–195 (2003)
16. Okita, S., Bailenson, J., Schwartz, D.: The mere belief of social interaction improves learning. In: Proceedings of the Annual Meeting of the Cognitive Science Society (2007)
17. Weibel, D., Wissmath, B., Habegger, S., Steiner, Y., Groner, R.: Playing online games against computer- vs. human-controlled opponents: effects on presence, flow, and enjoyment. Comput. Hum. Behav. **24**, 2274–2291 (2008)
18. Katsyri, J., Hari, R., Ravaja, N., Nummenmaa, L.: The opponent matters: elevated fMRI reward responses to winning against a human versus a computer opponent during interactive video game playing. Cereb. Cortex **23**, 2829–2839 (2012)
19. Lim, S., Reeves, B.: Computer agents versus avatars: responses to interactive game characters controlled by a computer or other player. Int. J. Hum Comput Stud. **68**, 57–68 (2010)
20. Blascovich, J., Loomis, J., Beall, A., Swinth, K., Hoyt, L., Bailenson, J.: Immersive virtual environment technology as a methodological tool for social psychology. Psychol. Inq. **13**, 103–124 (2002)
21. Blascovich, J., McCall, C.: Social influence in virtual environments. In: Dill, K. (ed.) The Oxford Handbook of Media Psychology, pp. 305–315. Oxford University Press, New York (2013)
22. Epley, N., Waytz, A., Cacioppo, J.: On seeing human: a three-factor theory of anthropomorphism. Psychol. Rev. **114**, 864–886 (2007)
23. Epley, N.: Waytz, A. In: Fiske, S., Gilbert, D., Lindsay, G. (eds.) The Handbook of Social Psychology, 5th edn, pp. 498–541. Wiley, New York (2010)
24. Waytz, A., Gray, K., Epley, N., Wegner, D.: Causes and consequences of mind perception. Trends Cogn. Sci. **14**, 383–388 (2010)
25. Haslam, N.: Dehumanization: an integrative review. Pers. Soc. Psychol. Rev. **10**, 252–264 (2006)

26. Gray, H., Gray, K., Wegner, D.: Dimensions of mind perception. Science **315**, 619 (2007)
27. Loughnan, S., Haslam, N.: Animals and androids: Implicit associations between social categories and nonhumans. Psychol. Sci. **18**, 116–121 (2007)
28. Rilling, J., Sanfey, A.: The neuroscience of social decision-making. Ann. Rev. Psychol. **62**, 23–48 (2011)
29. Gallagher, H., Anthony, J., Roepstorff, A., Frith, C.: Imaging the intentional stance in a competitive game. NeuroImage **16**, 814–821 (2002)
30. McCabe, K., Houser, D., Ryan, L., Smith, V., Trouard, T.: A functional imaging study of cooperation in two-person reciprocal exchange. Proc. Nat. Acad. Sci. **98**, 11832–11835 (2001)
31. Riedl, R., Moht, P., Kenning, P., Davis, F., Heekeren, H.: Trusting humans and avatars: behavioral and neural evidence. In: Proceedings of the 32nd International Conference on Information Systems (2011)
32. Rilling, J., Gutman, D., Zeh, T., Pagnoni, G., Berns, G., Kilts, C.: A neural basis for social cooperation. Neuron **35**, 395–405 (2002)
33. Krach, S., Hegel, F., Wrede, B., Sagerer, G., Binkofski, F., Kircher, T.: Can machines think? Interaction and perspective taking with robots investigated via fMRI. PLoS ONE **3**, 1–11 (2008)
34. Kircher, T., Blumel, I., Marjoram, D., Lataster, T., Krabbendam, L., Weber, J., et al.: Online mentalising investigated with functional MRI. Neurosci. Lett. **454**, 176–181 (2009)
35. Sanfey, A., Rilling, J., Aronson, J., Nystrom, L., Cohen, J.: The neural basis of economic decision-making in the ultimatum game. Science **300**, 1755–1758 (2003)
36. van't Wout, M., Kahn, R., Sanfey, A., Aleman, A.: Affective state and decision-making in the ultimatum game. Exp. Brain Res. **169**, 564–568 (2006)
37. Kahn, P., Kanda, T., Ishiguro, H., Freier, N., Severson, R., Gill, B., et al.: "Robovie, you'll have to go into the closet now": children's social and moral relationships with a humanoid robot. Dev. Psychol. **48**, 303–314 (2012)
38. de Melo, C., Carnevale, P., Gratch, J.: Bridging the gap between human and non-human decision makers. Presented at the annual meeting of the international association for conflict management (2014)
39. Güth, W., Schmittberger, R., Schwarze, B.: An experimental analysis of ultimatum bargaining. J. Econ. Behav. Organ. **3**, 367–388 (1982)
40. de Melo, C., Carnevale, P., Gratch, J.: Social categorization and cooperation between humans and computers. In: Proceedings of the Annual Meeting of the Cognitive Science Society (2014)
41. Crisp, R., Hewstone, M.: Multiple social categorization. Adv. Exp. Soc. Psychol. **39**, 163–254 (2007)
42. Lucas, G., Gratch, J., King, A., Morency, L.-P.: It's only a computer: virtual humans increase willingness to disclose. Comput. Hum. Behav. **37**, 94–100 (2014)
43. Malle, B., Scheutz. M, Arnold, T., Voiklis, J., Cusimano, C.: Sacrifice one for the good of many? People apply different moral norms to human and robot agents. In: Proceedings of Human-Robot Interaction (2015)
44. Yee, N., Bailenson, J., Rickertsen, K.: A meta-analysis of the impact of the inclusion and realism of human-like faces on user experiences in interfaces. In: Proceedings of CHI (2007)
45. Bingsjord, S.: Red-pill robots only, please. IEEE Trans. Affect. Comput. **3**, 394–397 (2012)

From One to Many: Simulating Groups of Agents with Reinforcement Learning Controllers

Luiselena Casadiego and Nuria Pelechano[✉]

Universitat Politecnica de Catalunya, Barcelona, Spain
npelechano@cs.upc.edu

Abstract. Simulation of crowd behavior has been approached through many different methodologies, but the problem of mimicking human decisions and reactions remains a challenge for all. We propose an alternative model for simulation of pedestrian movements using Reinforcement Learning. Taking the approach of microscopic models, we train an agent to move towards a goal while avoiding obstacles. Once one agent has learned, its knowledge is transferred to the rest of the members of the group by sharing the resulting *Q-Table*. This results in individual behavior leading to emergent group behavior. We present a framework with states, actions and reward functions general enough to easily adapt to different environment configurations.

Keywords: Crowd simulation · Reinforcement learning

1 Introduction

The basic requirement for most crowd simulation applications, is to model pedestrian movements with perception and placement. The perception encloses all knowledge the agent has about the environment including the situation of the other agents and its own status, while placement defines the desired position for an agent given the perception. Perception and placement could be defined as *state* and *action*.

Traditional microscopic methods specify each individual behavior and obtain emergent behavior from their autonomous interactions [1]. Data driven methods [2] imitate human movement patterns, but there is no learning involved. In contrast, reinforcement learning approaches aim at allowing the agents to learn individual behaviors based on what they experience [3]. Torrey [4] proposes reinforcement learning as a viable alternative method for crowd simulation. Cuayahuitl et al. [5] presented an approach for inducing adaptive behavior of route instructions. Martinez et al. [6] propose a new methodology that uses different iterative learning strategies, combining a vector quantization with Q-Learning algorithm.

We present a Reinforcement Learning (RL) approach where by training one agent and transferring its knowledge to a group of agents, we can achieve emergent behavior while reducing the training time. We discuss in detail the main

© Springer International Publishing Switzerland 2015
W.-P. Brinkman et al. (Eds.): IVA 2015, LNAI 9238, pp. 119–123, 2015.
DOI: 10.1007/978-3-319-21996-7_12

challenges when designing crowd behavior based on RL and provide ideas for future work in this field.

2   Reinforcement Learning for Agent Simulation

We start with one agent that learns to walk avoiding static obstacles to reach a goal position. This knowledge is then transferred to the rest of the agents, so that they can either use it as it is or further build upon it.

Our method is based on *Q-Learning* with ϵ-greedy policy. At each time step t, the agent receives some representation of the environment *state*, $s_t \in \mathcal{S}$, where $\mathcal{S}$ is the set of possible states, and on that basis selects an *action*, $a_t \in \mathcal{A}(s_t)$, where $\mathcal{A}(s_t)$ is the set of actions available in state s_t. After performing the action, the agent receives a *reward*, $r_{t+1} \in \mathbb{R}$, and moves to a new state, s_{t+1}. The agent seeks to maximize the R_t which is defined as a function of the reward sequence $r_{t+1}, r_{t+2}, r_{t+3}, \ldots$.

The behavior learned by an agent is stored in a *Q-table* of $n \times m$ entries, where $n = |\mathcal{S}|$ and $m = |\mathcal{A}|$. Each cell of this table contains the value learned for each pair (s, a). Once this table is filled with learned behaviors, it can be transferred to other agents. Therefore the other agents do not need to learn from scratch, but can still continue the learning process by using small $\epsilon > 0$. This provides heterogeneity in behaviors while still allowing fast learning for groups of agents.

3   Learning Problem Definition

The action set defines the movements the agents can make during the simulation and it is discretized in 8 possible directions. The states encode the nearby environment and we evaluated two approaches: nearest obstacle and occupancy code. Depending on the state definition, we also need to define different reward functions which must be carefully chosen with two principles in mind: collision must be punished, and moving towards the goal has to be rewarded positively.

Nearest obstacle: The states are defined by the goal position $\mathcal{S}_{goal}$ (in range $[0, 2]$, Fig. 1a), the distance to the nearest obstacle $\mathcal{S}_{obs}^d$ (in range $[0, 2]$, Fig. 1b), and the relative position of this obstacle $\mathcal{S}_{obs}^p$ (Fig. 1c). The obstacle position state is encoded with seven values for the front half of the circle (which simulates human perception) and one value for the back half.

The number of states is $S = |\mathcal{S}_{goal}| \times |\mathcal{S}_{obs}^d| \times |\mathcal{S}_{obs}^p|$ (192 states). Since the *Q-table* is small, the learning process is very fast, but there are several problems with such simple approach: (i) it only considers the nearest object at each time step, which can cause instabilities and local minima when several obstacles are too close to the agent and ii) there is no knowledge about the size of obstacles.

Occupancy code: The code is defined by $|\mathcal{S}_{obs}^p|$ values, where each value of the code $o[i]$ with $i \in [0, \mathcal{S}_{obs}^p - 1]$ indicates the distance to an obstacle according to $|\mathcal{S}_{obs}^d|$ (distance states). Figure 1d shows graphically this distribution of space with an example of occupancy code. The upper row depicts the number of angle

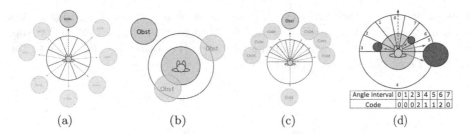

Fig. 1. Goal state definition (a), distance to obstacle state (b), and goal position states for the two approaches: nearest obstacle (c) and occupancy code (d).

interval and the bottom row shows the occupancy level of each interval. Note how obstacle size is represented by the number of regions being occupied. This representation also correctly encodes gaps between obstacles and aids the agent to learn whether it can walk through or needs to walk around a set of obstacles. The number of states is: $S = |\mathcal{S}_{goal}| \times |\mathcal{S}_{obs}^d||\mathcal{S}_{obs}^P|$ (52,488 states).

Reward Function The reward function is calculated as: $r(s_t, a_t) = r_g + r_o$, where r_g represents the positive reward gained by moving towards the goal and r_o the negative reward obtained from moving towards an obstacle. We tested two different r_g functions, (i) based on distance gained, and (ii) based on velocity vector being close to the goal direction. We observed that the second one resulted in straighter trajectories. Since the occupancy code encodes obstacles better we will focus only on the reward function for this case:

$$r_o(t) = \begin{cases} 0, & \text{if } d_o > \tau_2 \\ -\sum_{i=0}^{|\mathcal{S}_{obs}^d|-1} \frac{10}{10^{(o[i]-1)*2}}, & \text{otherwise} \end{cases} \quad (1)$$

where d_o is the distance between the agent and the obstacle.

4 Results

In this work we presented an RL approach to train one agent, and then apply knowledge transfer to the rest of the individuals in the crowd. The other agents can further learn during the simulation phase, by keeping a small $\epsilon > 0$ to leave room for some exploration. This allows us to reduce the time needed to train groups of agents, by separating the learning phase from the size of the simulated crowd.

During the training phase, we have one agent moving towards a goal and an obstacle somewhere in the scenario. Avoiding obstacles successfully depends on having an accurate state representation and finding a good equilibrium in the reward function between the positive feedback of moving towards the goal and the negative feedback of a collision. Our approach based on occupancy code better captures the complexity of the environment, and it is able to successfully reach the goal despite encountering more challenging situations (Fig. 2 top). Once the knowledge is transferred to several agents, we can simulate a group of agents reaching their individual goals while avoiding each other (Fig. 2 (bottom)). Note how agents are able to avoid moving obstacles (i.e. other agents), despite the training being done with static obstacles.

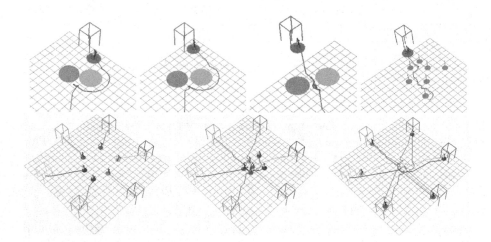

Fig. 2. Results of agents' reaching their goals while avoiding obstacles and agents.

Our preliminary results look promising, as we manage to have a group of agents wandering a virtual environment avoiding moving obstacles and reaching their destinations. But this work has also shown the challenges regarding choosing the right state representation and more importantly the right reward function. The goal of this research was to escape the cumbersome work of tweaking parameters in crowd simulation models, and while we had success with this, we did encounter a number of challenges in finding and tuning reward functions. Future work will focus on partially automating this selection process by incorporating inverse reinforcement learning techniques.

Acknowledgment. Funded by the Spanish Ministry, TIN2014-52211-C2-1-R.

References

1. Pelechano, N., Allbeck, J., Badler, N.: Virtual Crowds: Methods, Simulation, and Control. Morgan & Claypool Publishers, San Rafael (2008)
2. Charalambous, P., Chrysanthou, Y.: The PAG crowd: a graph based approach for efficient data-driven crowd simulation. Comput. Graph. Forum **33**(8), 95–108 (2014)
3. Sutton, R.S., Barto, A.G.: Introduction to Reinforcement Learning. MIT Press, Cambridge (1998)
4. Torrey, L. : Crowd simulation via multi-agent reinforcement learning. In: Artificial Intelligence and Interactive Digital Entertainment (AIIDE) (2010)

5. Cuayáhuitl, H., Dethlefs, N., Frommberger, L., Richter, K.-F., Bateman, J.: Generating adaptive route instructions using hierarchical reinforcement learning. In: Hölscher, C., Shipley, T.F., Olivetti Belardinelli, M., Bateman, J.A., Newcombe, N.S. (eds.) Spatial Cognition VII. LNCS, vol. 6222, pp. 319–334. Springer, Heidelberg (2010)
6. Martínez-Gil, F., Lozano, M., Fernández, F.: Strategies for simulating pedestrian navigation with multiple reinforcement learning agents. Auton. Agents Multi-Agent Syst. **29**(1), 98–130 (2015)

An Experience-Based Approach to Simulate Virtual Crowd Behaviors Under the Influence of Alcohol

Vinícius Jurinic Cassol[1]([✉]), Cliceres Mack Dal Bianco[1], Alexandre Carvalho[1], Jovani Brasil[1], Maristela Monteiro[2], and Soraia Raupp Musse[1]

[1] Virtual Humans Simulation Laboratory,
Pontifical Catholic University of Rio Grande Do Sul - PUCRS, Porto Alegre, Brazil
{vinicius.cassol,soraia.musse}@pucrs.br
[2] Pan American Health Organization, Washington, DC, USA

Abstract. Different models and tools are available in order to simulate homogeneous crowds taking into account different parameters. In this paper we present a framework to simulate heterogeneous crowds where we emphasize how the presence of alcohol into the simulated agents can make influence on the crowd behavior. Despite the obvious difficulty to evaluate results, this paper proposes a metric to compare the alcohol impact in crowd simulations and also taking as reference a real life scenario.

1 Introduction

Several scientists in different research fields have studied crowd behavior over the centuries. Among such scientists, we can highlight Gustave Le Bon [1], who defines crowd as a group composed by different people (independent of age, color, gender or ideology) sharing a common goal. Crowd simulation have been studied over recent decades [2]. Crowd simulation can be affected by different parameters. According to Fruin [3] crowd behavior is affected by the spatial perception of each individual considering his/her own knowledge and intelligence. When a specific person decides to move, he or she can also affect how close people can stay of each other and make influence on the personal space of others. In addition to the space perception, distance and kind of relationship among people, crowds can also be affected by the individual characteristics. The individuality can be represented by many factors as the gender, age of each individual or her/his physical state. The important question in the context of crowd simulation is to know when individualities are relevant to be considered in a simulation, since the simulation of heterogeneous crowds (if compared to homogeneous crowds) obviously includes complexities to be dealt with. Despite different applications for crowd simulation models during evacuation scenarios, the effort performed in order to simulate the influence of alcohol, or other drugs, on individual behavior is very incipient. One of the few studies developed in order to simulate people under alcohol influence was developed by Moore et al. [4]. The authors consider

© Springer International Publishing Switzerland 2015
W.-P. Brinkman et al. (Eds.): IVA 2015, LNAI 9238, pp. 124–127, 2015.
DOI: 10.1007/978-3-319-21996-7_13

the hypothesis that when under alcohol influence people can perform different behaviors including violent and aggressive actions. A particle model was implemented in order to validate such hypothesis. Moore also reaffirms features that people perform in usual conditions (without alcohol influence): self-organization, work in lanes, less effort. According to Challanger [5], the main challenge in order the evolve crowds is concerned with the representation of real behaviors considering, among others, factors such as alcohol and drugs influence on human beings. In this paper, we investigate how some differences in individual behaviors (e.g. caused by alcohol) can influence the crowd behavior. Inspired on available literature (World Health Organization[1]) we simulate the behavior of agents affected by alcohol in a nightclub.

2 Heterogeneous Agents: Modeling and Simulating Virtual Crowds

We present a framework able to simulate virtual crowds dealing with specific evacuation scenarios. In order to simulate coherent crowd behaviors, we developed *CrowdSim* [6]. Its main goal is to computationally reproduce crowd motion and behaviors and also to present some data that are used to estimate people comfort and safety in an specific environment. The tool is organized in two distinct modules: the *configuration* module allows users to define information specifying the walkable regions considering the environment structure as well as physical restrictions. Also, number of agents to be simulated, regions of interest to be considered during agents motion (goals) and regions where agents will be created during simulation are defined in this step. Afterwards, the user is able to specify behaviors such as: *(i) Goal Seeking*: The agents should seek their goals immediately or vague, performing random motion; *(ii) Keep waiting*: The agents, when achieve some specific region of the environment, can spend some time on it before look for another goal. The module of *Simulation* is able to compute the routes to each agent to achieve a specific goal. Routes can be computed based on user specification (i.e. a graph determined by the user) or based on the best paths only considering the distance criteria [7]. In addition, during the motion simulation, *CrowdSim* is able to avoid collisions among agents and/or obstacles (using a simple local geometry method). Since we intended to deal with heterogeneous crowds as well, we included this possibility in *CrowdSim* model. Mainly focused on a nightclub simulation, we chose to investigate the impact of alcohol on agents' behaviors into the crowd. Literature mentions some effects of alcohol on measured by the Blood Alcohol Concentration (BAC) (discussed values from 0.0 to 0.39) on the body [8]. We included just some of the effects described in the literature because many of them could not be considered in our simulations, e.g. "Decrease in various brain centre functions". We propose to implement an individual attribute in the *CrowdSim* agents called "goals persistence", which is related with a factor that represents how much the agents seek goals during

---

[1] http://www.who.int/.

the simulation (i.e. related with decreased attention and slowed reactions effects caused by alcohol effect). Our method presents a relationship among the main characteristics of each BAC [8] level (now each agent k is initialized with a BAC value - BAC_k) and the agent goal persistence ($0 <= gp_k <= 1$).

Goals persistence of agent k is defined through: $gp_k = \alpha \times e^{(-\beta \times BAC_k)}$, where $\alpha = 1$, i.e. the value of goal persistence when $BAC_k = 0$. $\beta = 7.44$ and represents a decay constant. We chosen an exponential curve to represent gp_k due to the textual description of alcohol effects, that clearly does not represent a linear function. Based on gp_k we compute directly how many frames from next f frames that agent k should seek the goal: $nf_k = gp_k \times f$. It means that in next nf_k from f frames, agent k is going to seek the goal, so in the remaining $f - nf_k$ agent k is going to vague randomly.

3   Obtained Results: A Night Club Case Study

In order to evaluate our model, we developed a case study applied in a real night club. It was a shared experience developed in partnership with the night club owners and a safety company. The goal was to evaluate the obtained results of simulations using *CrowdSim*. Is is important to mention that in order to compare results of real and virtual simulations, data from real life should be extracted, such as: local and global times, local and global densities and velocities. The real experience was performed in a night club where the audience (240 people) accorded to leave the club exactly at 2 AM. During the real escape exercise, we were able to collect different data (videos, people counting using infra-red technology) in order to evaluate results of this experience. In addition, the same population was used in simulation using *CrowdSim*. The obtained data are: *(i) Total time for evacuation (seconds)*: real life=175 and simulation=119; *(ii) Highest Density (people/m^2)*: real life=5, 4 and simulation=4, 5; *(iii) Highest speed (m/s)*: real life=1, 5 and simulation=1, 3. When analyzing such data it is clear the difference of evacuation time. Despite being a small difference, it can be explained by the fact that real people do not behave voluntarily as in an emergency situation, i.e. real people, not in panic, respect the space of others. Since we considered that the difference between real and simulated environment is acceptable, we re-simulated such scenario by considering heterogeneous agents. We considered three different scenarios having varied number from total population been affected by BAC level (i.e. simulating percentage of people who drank and how much). The tested BAC levels were: 0.05, 0.1 and 0.15 in percentages of population from 0 to 100 %. We did not test higher levels of BAC because people in such levels have several motor impairments and can even lose consciousness. As can be seen in Fig. 1 the simulation time is highly affected by increasing BAC level (black line has been used as reference for time obtained with non affected population). Computing the average time obtained with BAC= 0.05 for percentage from 20 to 100 of total population, we have a value 26 % greater than when agents were homogeneous. For BAC= 0.1 and 0.15 the obtained values are respectively 62 % and 127 % greater than for homogeneous crowds.

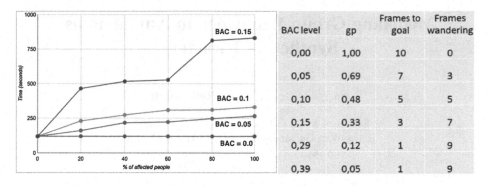

BAC level	gp	Frames to goal	Frames wandering
0,00	1,00	10	0
0,05	0,69	7	3
0,10	0,48	5	5
0,15	0,33	3	7
0,29	0,12	1	9
0,39	0,05	1	9

Fig. 1. Simulated data presenting the variation of evacuation time when BAC increases.

We were not able to compare virtual heterogeneous crowds with real life, since we do not have real data about BAC levels in real people. A contribution of this report in this aspect is the modelling of heterogeneous crowds based on alcohol literature.

Final Remarks: in this work, we presented a model able to simulate heterogeneous crowd behaviors. An important contribution is the model of heterogeneous crowds that seem to generate coherent results. As future work, we intend to simulate more scenarios in order to improve the evaluation of this work.

Acknowledgements. The project AutoScene is supported by Facin/PUCRS and Brazilian Research Agencies CAPES and FAPERGS.

References

1. LeBon, G.: Psychologie des Foules. Alcan, Paris (1895)
2. Thalmann, D., Musse, S.R.: Crowd Simulation, 2nd edn. Springer-Verlag, London Ltd (2013)
3. Fruin, J.: Pedestrian Planning and Design. Metropolitan Association of Urban Designers and Environmental Planners (1971)
4. Moore, S.C., Flajlik, M., Rosin, P.L., Marshall, D.: A particle model of crowd behavior: exploring the relationship between alcohol, crowd dynamics and violence. Aggression Violent Behav. **13**(6), 413–422 (2008)
5. Challenger, R., Clegg, C.R.M.: Understanding Crowd Behaviours: Guidance and Lessons Identified. The Cabinet Office Emergency Planning College, NewYork (2009)
6. Cassol, V.J., Rodrigues, R.A., Carneiro, L.C.C., Silva, A., Musse, S.R.: Crowdsim: Uma ferramenta desenvolvida para simulação de multidões. In: I Workshop de Simulação Militar - SBGames2012 (2012)
7. Hart, P.E., Nilsson, N.J., Raphael, B.: A formal basis for the heuristic determination of minimum cost paths. SIGART Bull. **37**, 28–29 (1972)
8. Organization, W.H.: Drinking and Driving: A Road Safety Manual for Decision-Makers and Practitioners. Global Road Safety Partnership, Geneva (2007)

Modelling Group Behaviour in Autonomous Synthetic Characters

Naziya Hussaini[(✉)] and Ruth Aylett

School of Mathematical and Computer Sciences,
Heriot-Watt University, Edinburgh EH14 4AS, UK
{nh4,R.S.Aylett}@hw.ac.uk

Abstract. This paper discusses the process of creating agents that are capable of socially interacting with each other and forming groups in a similar way to humans, without losing their autonomy. Our approach is to model group behaviour in autonomous agents by using FIRO (Fundamental Interpersonal Relationship Orientation) theory to add interpersonal drives to the existing FAtiMA- PSI architecture. This extends it for social agents that act as a collective group, and thus increasing their believability in-group situations.

Keywords: Autonomous agents · FAtiMA-PSI · Group dynamics

1 Introduction

The use of multiple IVAs is increasing in fields from games and learning environments, to training and problem solving activities. We argue that it is not sufficient to provide human-like abilities but it is also necessary to improve agent interaction abilities so that they can interact socially with each other in a believable way.

Social interaction is a complex process; but it can be seen that interaction between members of a group is easier and more comfortable than with non-group members. This paper discusses the modelling of group behaviour among virtual characters.

2 Background

Group Dynamics: This is the study of the processes involved in groups: group formation, the individual's behaviour, interaction between members within the group and also between groups, and group dissolution [1].

William Schutz proposed a theory of group behaviour in 1958, known as FIRO (Fundamental Interpersonal Relation Orientation), with the purpose of explaining both individual behaviour and the interaction between individuals [2].

FIRO: In this theory, interpersonal relations depend on the intention of an individual to interact with others, and this intention is generated on the basis of three interpersonal needs: inclusion, control and affection [1, 5], further categorised into expressed and wanted behaviour. The expressed behaviour shows the individual's desire to include,

© Springer International Publishing Switzerland 2015
W.-P. Brinkman et al. (Eds.): IVA 2015, LNAI 9238, pp. 128–131, 2015.
DOI: 10.1007/978-3-319-21996-7_14

control and love others whereas, the wanted behaviour shows the individual's desire to be included, controlled and loved by others [2].

Our work extends the FAtiMA architecture [3] in which the PSI theory [3] is embedded. This is similar to the FIRO theory in that it is based on the needs of an individual i.e., the need for energy, integrity, affiliation, competence and certainty [3]. The FIRO interpersonal needs also use a homeostasis mechanism, which always maintains the needs of an agent to a satisfactory level; and thus does not require any symbolic representation or explicit reasoning as in the case of a cognitive appraisal mechanism. Thus by establishing a causal relationship between both types of needs (i.e., motivational needs and interpersonal needs) we can model group behaviour in autonomous synthetic characters.

3   Group Dynamics Based Agent Model

In order to model group dimensions in an existing FAtiMA architecture, the value of interpersonal drives (similar to motivational drives [3]) are set to range between 0 and 10; where 0 means complete deprivation while 10 means complete satisfaction of the needs. The aim of the agent is to maintain these drives at the highest possible value.

Inclusion: The desire to be part of a group and to be accepted by a group - is similar to the need for affiliation [4]. According to Donelson, "People with a high need for affiliation tend to join groups more frequently, spend more of their time in groups, communicate more with other group members, and accept other group members more readily" [4]. Thus, this helps us to link the inclusion need with the affiliation need.

Apart from the need for affiliation, inclusion is also related to the need for competence and the need for certainty. Schutz relates inclusion behaviour to competence by giving an example of a student who was failed in a course because the professor finds him incompetent in his field. This generates an inclusion behaviour inside the student which makes him work hard to increase his competency level and pass his course work. Schutz also discusses a common issue in interpersonal relations i.e., commitment, where people are not sure whether they should involve themselves in a given relation or activity because they feel that they might not be valued or recognized by the group, further relating certainty to the need for inclusion.

Control: According to Timothy and Brent, a group allows people to satisfy their need for control through opportunities to control decision making, allocate resources, or take on leadership roles. Some people want to control others, while some want to be controlled by others depending upon their competency and certainty level, which led them to join groups. This reflects a causal relationship between the need for competence and certainty on one side and the need for control on the other side.

Thus the value of a particular interpersonal need depends upon the various PSI needs; and by assigning appropriate weights to the linked PSI needs, we can calculate the value of particular interpersonal needs. The weight varies in the range 0–1. The weights to the PSI needs are assigned depending upon the importance of the associated need to the character and for this we have defined forward and reverse mappings. In case of affiliation, the weights are assigned through the reverse mapping i.e., 0–10 to 1–0; whereas, in case of competence and certainty the forward mapping is applied i.e., 0–10 to 0–1. For example, if a character's level of affiliation is low say, 2 then a high weight is assigned to its affiliation drive say, 0.8 in order to satisfy its need for affiliation; and if the need for affiliation is already satisfied say, 9 then a low weight is assigned to it say, 0.1. In case of competence and certainty, if a character is competent enough and is certain about its goals then its desire to be involved in a group activity is higher. Thus, a high weight is assigned to these drives through the forward mapping. Finally, the values of the interpersonal needs are calculated by using the following formula:

$$I_i = \sum_{m=1}^{n} M_m * Wt_{mi}/n$$

Where,

I_i = Interpersonal Need (I_1 = Inclusion, I_2 = Control, and I_3 = Affection)
M_m = Associated Motivational Needs.
Wt_{mi} = Weights assigned to the associated need.
n = total number of associated motivational needs.

Goal Activation. For experimentation purposes, we have set the threshold value (the value at which group goals are selected) of the group parameters to 4. Group goals are separated from individual goals by including a condition involving group parameters in the preconditions at authoring time.

e.g., < Property name = "[Agent] (inclusion)" operator = "=" value = "True"/>

While adding a little extra burden to the authoring process, this reduces processing at the time of goal selection. After calculating the inclusion value, the system will compare the inclusion value of the agent with its threshold value. If the value of inclusion drive is less than or equal to the threshold value then the agent activates a goal involving it in a group activity and the importance of this group goal is increased to the highest level. Otherwise it activates a goal the agent would performs individually.

Along with the goal activation, the system will also generate behaviour depending upon the value of the group parameters. If the value of group parameters is less than or equal to their threshold value then the Wanted Behaviour is generated in which the agent wishes to be included in the group. Once the agent is a part of a group and if its group parameter value is greater than the threshold value then the Expressed Behaviour is generated where the agent will include others in the group.

4 Initial Prototype

We have implemented the inclusion dimension based on the ideas presented in this paper and we have tested it by running a small scenario. In the scenario, there are two characters: Tina and Amy and both are feeling hungry. Earlier Tina was playing a game with her friends whereas Amy was doing her work alone from a long time. At the goal selection time the inclusion intensities of Tina and Amy are 5.31 and 3.48 respectively; and their energy drive values are 2.85 and 2.97 respectively. Based on their motivational and interpersonal needs the system would activate goals that would satisfy most of their needs simultaneously.

As Tina's inclusion intensity is above the inclusion threshold (because while playing game her inclusion need is already satisfied), therefore the individual goal (i.e., Eat Alone) is activated due to her motivational need (in this case, Energy), as she was hungry.

Whereas, in case of Amy; her inclusion need along with her motivational need (in this case, Energy), is also low as she was busy in completing her work, which makes her feeling hungry and lonely at the same time. Thus, she will look for someone with whom she can eat and satisfy both the needs simultaneously. Therefore, the group goal (i.e., Eat with Friend) gets activated which results in involving her in a group activity.

5 Conclusion and Future Work

In this paper we have argued that in order to attain group believability in a virtual environment, the virtual agents should interact socially with each other depending upon their interpersonal needs. To achieve such believability, we have proposed a modification in the existing agent architecture by linking it to the social psychological theory of group dynamics based on interpersonal relations. We have also presented a proof-of-concept implementation for the inclusion dimension, which has been tested by running a small scenario and which will provide a test bed for the future work.

References

1. Hussaini, N., Aylett, R.: An idea for modelling group dynamics in autonomous synthetic characters. In: AISB 2013 (2013)
2. Schutz, W.: The Interpersonal Underworld. Science and Behaviour Books, Palo Alto (1966)
3. Lim, M.Y., Aylett, R., Dias, J., Paiva, A.: Creating adaptive affective autonomous NPCs. 24 (2), 287–311 (2012)
4. Forsyth, D.R.: Group Dynamics, 3rd edn, p. 91. Wadsworth Publishing Company, Belmont (1999)
5. Li, H., Lai, V.S.: Interpersonal relationship needs of virtual community participation: a FIRO perspective. In: Proceedings of AMCIS 2007, p. 319 (2007)

A Framework for Exogenous and Endogenous Reflexive Behavior in Virtual Characters

Ulysses Bernardet[(✉)] and Steve DiPaola

iVizLab, Simon Fraser University, Burnaby, Canada
{ubernard,sdipaola}@sfu.ca

Abstract. We present ongoing work on the development of an architecture for virtual characters that should serve as a base layer, equipping them with a minimal set of plausible reactive behavior. The architecture conceptualizes reflexive behavior as a response to external (exogenous) and internal (endogenous) stimuli.

Keywords: Reactive behavior · Cognitive architecture · Idle · Virtual character

1 Introduction

Humans do exhibit volitional, conscious behavior, but a great proportion of all behavior can be classified as non-conscious, autonomic. We present ongoing work on the development of a "pre-cognitive" behavior regulation framework, meaning we are mainly interested in the behaviors that lie "below" cognition. In the domain of artificial intelligence this behavior without explicit planning is referred to by some authors as "reactive" [1] or reflexive. From the perspective of behavior execution these reflexive behaviors are characterized by the fact that they are largely feed-forward, meaning that there is no continuous control during the execution, and that they are difficult to interrupt once initiated.

The key distinction we will be making is the one between reflexive behavior that has external (exogenous) and internal (endogenous) motivators. For exogenous behavior (reflexive and cognitive), attention as a mechanism that filters and prioritizes stimuli perceived by an organism, plays a key role. Correspondingly, a number of attention models have been proposed for robots (e.g. [2]) and virtual characters (e.g. [3]). Interestingly, most of these models do not elaborate on the behavioral consequences of the attention process. Endogenous mechanisms, at the behavioral level, partially overlap with what is referred to as "idle" behavior in the domain of virtual characters.

In our model we conceptualize both, endogenous and exogenous actions, as a form of reflexive behavior, and aim to provide a mechanistic model that is grounded in psychodynamic processes. The development of the model is motivated by the observation that there are few integrated frameworks that bring these two types of reflexive behaviors together. Ultimately, our goal is to provide a reusable architecture that can be used as a base layer of behavior in e.g. conversational agents.

We propose the following organization of reflexive behavior that distinguishes behavior based on the source of the stimulus that triggers it.

© Springer International Publishing Switzerland 2015
W.-P. Brinkman et al. (Eds.): IVA 2015, LNAI 9238, pp. 132–136, 2015.
DOI: 10.1007/978-3-319-21996-7_15

Exogenous: driven by external stimuli such as auditory, visual, and haptic (not all human sensory modalities made sense for a virtual character). Includes Orienting behavior (overt attention towards a stimulus), Aversive behavior, and Protective behavior.

Endogenous: driven by internal stimuli such as somatic proprioception. Includes Self-touching, and Posture (weight shifting, discomfort).

The hierarchy presented here should allow us to make *predictive* inferences, i.e. do foresee what behavior a given stimulus (e.g. a bright light) will cause. Complementarily, *diagnostic* inferences can be made that determine the cause of the behavior of a given effector (e.g. gaze).

2   Model of Exogenous Reflexive Behavior

We define exogenous reflexive behaviors these that are a direct consequence of an event external to the agent. Functionally the reflexive behavior mostly subserves the avoidance of harm, and hence is generally more concerned with negative stimuli than with appetitive ones. The reflexive behavior will in many cases be accompanied with a brief, autonomic expression of affect.

Given the context of virtual characters, we will focus on vision and audition, and set aside other modalities such as touch, smell, and taste that are relevant in biological systems.

Orienting Behavior is the reaction to a salient stimulus in the environment. The overt action is an orienting towards the stimulus, and hence takes as input the saliency, valence, and location at which the stimulus occurred in the environment. For both, the visual and auditory modality, orienting comprises a turning of head and body towards the stimulus. Additionally, we are likely to observe an expression of surprise.

Aversive Behavior is triggered by a negative, potentially painful, sensory stimulation above a given threshold. In the visual domain the actions associate with aversive behavior are a shutting of the eyes and a turning away of the head from the direction where the stimulus occurred. The latter is equally the response in the auditory domain. At the affective level we expect the experience and expression of irritation, disgust, and/or pain.

Protective Behavior serves to protect the agent from the negative effect of t a stimulus. For a visual stimulus the protective action constitutes shielding the eyes with the hand, and of an auditory stimulus the protection of the ears. Protective actions are very likely associate with the expression of pain.

Evasive Behavior is triggered by a prolonged exposure to aversive stimuli, and comprises a more complex set of action that result in the agent effectively evading the stimulus.

The integrated qualitative model (Fig. 1) comprises three main components for attention, behavior selection, and behavior execution. The *attention* component in turn is composed of a bottom-up and top-down processes. In the bottom-up steam a finite

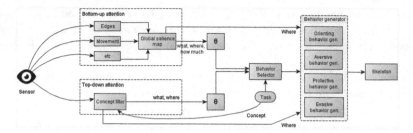

Fig. 1. Integrated qualitative model of exogenous reflexive behavior

number of "generic" filters is applied to input to detect edges, speed, color contrast etc. These filters are always active, and (largely) not influenced by the task at hand and knowledge about context. Conversely, in the top-down steam, an arbitrary concept can be "content" of the filter (e.g. face, hands, whole body, house, car etc.). Both streams are outputting coordinates and some form of identification. The attention module provides to the *behavior selection* component information about the stimuli in the environment such as their location and valence. Based duration on the characteristic and the time course of the stimulus, the behavior selection module will trigger one of the aforementioned behaviors. The role of the behavior generator modules is the actual execution of the orienting, aversive, protective, and evasive behavior. For that purpose the generator need to receive information about location of the stimulus in the environment.

3   Model of Endogenous Reflexive Behavior

With the term endogenous behaviors we denote behaviors that are driven by internal e.g. proprioceptive, signals. This class of behaviors comprises self-touching (e.g. scratching) and posture. Both of these classes of behaviors do have functions that go beyond mere reflexive action e.g. in communication. We do, however, explicitly not include these factors in the architecture presented here.

3.1   Self-touching Behavior

Self-touching is the touching of one's hand to one's face or body to scratch, rub, groom, or caress it [4]. Self-touching behavior can be motivated externally, or arise from internal motivations such as psychological discomfort, or as a displacement activity. We identify four core parameters of self-touching: (1) the location at which the manipulation is performed (e.g. head region, torso, forearm, etc.), (2) the action that is executed (rubbing, scratching, stroking, etc.), (3) frequency of the manipulation, (4) duration of the behavior. We assume that both, location and frequency, will be the under control of "somatic" cues, affective state, implicit communicative signaling, and habitual factors. *Model:* We generate one separate Poisson process for each combination of location and action (e.g. scratch-head, rub-hand, caress-forearm). To avoid overlapping of actions, and ensure a minimal waiting time between behaviors we will need to add a lateral inhibition, and refractory period to the overall system. Parameters of this model are the lambda for each Poisson process, and the minimal interval between actions. It should be noted that as a statistical model, the proposed mechanism are under specified in terms of the exact external or internal motivators of the behavior, e.g. how the frequency is specified. Additionally, the model assume a logical independence of action and location, which might not be entirely plausible, since humans might have a tendency to e.g. scratch more their chin, and rub more their forearms.

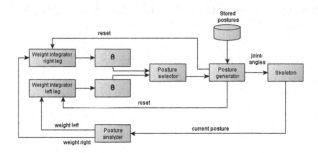

Fig. 2. Model for poster shifting based on fatigue.

3.2   Posture and Posture Switching

Functionally, posture refers to the stabilizing action of the musculoskeletal system that allows to maintain a stable pose such as standing or sitting. Next to this functional aspect, human posture can provide a significant amount of cues about emotional state, and serves as information channel in nonverbal communication. In our model we are primarily interested in the somatic aspect of posture, and more specifically the motivation for switching from one posture to another. In our model the switching of postures is a function of the somatic cue of fatigue caused by exertion. As an example the agent will shift the weight from one leg to the other based on how long he/she had the weight on one leg. In the present case we mainly focus on the lower body apparatus, but the model could equally be applied to other body parts. To calculate we apply a simple heuristic, as opposed to a realistic computation of actual strain on the joint. The current posture is constantly analyzed in terms of the strain that it produces on the target muscles. This strain is in turn integrated for each of the two body sides (weight integrator left right/left leg). Once the integrator has reached threshold θ, a new posture is selected from a repository of postures, and send to the skeleton as list of joint-angles. Simultaneously to this, the weight integrators are reset. This reset can also triggered by any other movement that are performed by the body, such as walking (Fig. 2).

Acknowledgments. This work was partially supported by "Moving Stories" and "Moving +Meaning" Canadian SSHRC and CANARIE grants respectively.

References

1. Ferber, J.: Multi-agent Systems: An Introduction to Distributed Artificial Intelligence. 1st edn. Addison-Wesley Professional (1999)
2. Ruesch, J., Lopes, M., Bernardino, A., Hornstein, J., Santos-Victor, J., Pfeifer, R.: Multimodal saliency-based bottom-up attention a framework for the humanoid robot iCub. In: 2008 IEEE International Conference on Robotics and Automation, pp. 962–967. IEEE (2008)
3. Hillaire, S., Lécuyer, A., Regia-Corte, T., Cozot, R., Royan, J., Breton, G.: A real-time visual attention model for predicting gaze point during first-person exploration of virtual environments. In: Proceedings of 17th ACM Symposium Virtual Reality Software Technology, pp. 191–198 (2010)
4. Heaven, L., McBrayer, D.: External motivators of self-touching behavior. Percept. Mot. Skills **90**, 338–342 (2000)

Nonverbal Behavior and Gestures

Real-Time Visual Prosody for Interactive Virtual Agents

Herwin van Welbergen[1,2]($\boxtimes$), Yu Ding[2], Kai Sattler[1,3], Catherine Pelachaud[2], and Stefan Kopp[1]

[1] Social Cognitive Systems Group, CITEC, Faculty of Technology,
Bielefeld University, Bielefeld, Germany
[2] CNRS-LTCI, Télécom-ParisTech, Paris, France
[3] Department of Psychology, University of Bamberg, Bamberg, Germany
hvanwelbergen@techfak.uni-bielefeld.de

Abstract. Speakers accompany their speech with incessant, subtle head movements. It is important to implement such "visual prosody" in virtual agents, not only to make their behavior more natural, but also because it has been shown to help listeners understand speech. We contribute a visual prosody model for *interactive* virtual agents that shall be capable of having live, non-scripted interactions with humans and thus have to use Text-To-Speech rather than recorded speech. We present our method for creating visual prosody online from continuous TTS output, and we report results from three crowdsourcing experiments carried out to see if and to what extent it can help in enhancing the interaction experience with an agent.

Keywords: Visual prosody · Nonverbal behavior · Realtime animation · Interactive agents

1 Introduction

Our heads move almost incessantly during speaking. These movements are related to e.g. the neurological and biomechanical coupling between head and jaw, the prosodic structure of speech, the content of speech and pragmatics such as turn-taking [10]. In this paper we focus on synthesizing and evaluating *visual prosody*: the movements of the head related to the prosodic structure of the accompanying speech [8]. It is important to endow Intelligent Virtual Agents (IVAs) with visual prosody, not only to make their movement and behavior more human-like, but also because visual prosody has been shown to help listeners in understanding speech [16].

Recently, many approaches to motion synthesis based on speech prosody have been proposed (see Sect. 2 for an overview). However, to the best of our knowledge, none of these approaches deal with *interactive* IVAs in live interactions with humans. Going beyond simple playback of prerecorded audio scripts, *interactive* IVAs have to rely on flexible Text-To-Speech (TTS) output. In such

© Springer International Publishing Switzerland 2015
W.-P. Brinkman et al. (Eds.): IVA 2015, LNAI 9238, pp. 139–151, 2015.
DOI: 10.1007/978-3-319-21996-7_16

agents, visual prosody must be generated in *real-time* from running synthetic speech. That is, the preparation of a motion segment (including the generation of TTS for it) should take less time than playing back the motion segment. Beyond that, we aim to use visual prosody in an incremental behavior realizer [17]. In such a realizer, utterances are generated in chunks much smaller than a full sentence, e.g. in a phrase. A visual prosody module that is of any use in such realization scenarios should work in an *online* fashion. That is, it should be able to deal with motion synthesis using only the current and previous phrases and make use of only little (if any) look-ahead.

In this paper, we present the first online TTS-based system for visual prosody. After discussing related work, we present our approach to creating online visual prosody for a behavior realizer. Finally, we report results from three crowdsourcing experiments carried out to measure if and to what extent this model can help in enhancing the interaction experience with an IVA. In particular, we compare our approach (1) to not using speech related head motion at all (as is common practise in most behavior realizers), (2) using motion captured head motion that is unrelated to the spoken content, and 3) feeding TTS to a state-of-the-art offline visual prosody model [5].

2 Related Work

The generation of speech-accompanying head movements has been tackled in several projects before. Lee and colleagues (see [12] for a recent overview of their work) have provided a nonverbal behavior generator (NVBG) that generates head and other motion on the basis of speech. Their work is complementary to ours: the NVBG generates motion based on speech content and pragmatics rather than on speech prosody. Other computer animation systems provide head motion on the basis of speech prosody. Typically these systems work offline (e.g. in [3–5,15]): they take a spoken sentence and generate head motion that is fluent and at the same time fits to the prosodic structure (e.g. speech pitch (f0), energy, or syllable boundaries) of the sentence. To capture the temporal evolution of sequential data (here, head rotations) these systems typically make use of a Hidden Markov Models (HMMs) as visual prosody models [3,15]. However, such visual prosody models suffer from the limitations of HMM independence assumptions.[1] This limitation can be attenuated by a variant of HMM, called parameterized (contextual) HMM, where state emission probabilities and state transition probabilities are defined by contextual parameters (e.g. prosody features) at each time step. Ding et al. [5] proposed a fully parameterized (contextual) HMM as visual prosody model, which not only embeds the advantage of HMMs but also overcomes the limitations of classical HMMs.

Others have worked on 'live' synthesis of visual prosody, where head motion is synthesized directly on the basis of microphone input. Levine et al. [14] generate

---

[1] The state at time t is independent of all the previous states given the state at time $t - 1$; the observation at time t is assumed independent of all other observations and all states given the state at time t.

a live stream of gesture (including head movement) from speech f0 and energy, summarized per syllable. Gesture synthesis is achieved using a HMM that selects the right gesture phase to perform at each syllable. In later work, rather than modeling the mapping between motion and speech prosody directly, Levine and colleagues [13] provide a two-layered model, which outperformes [14] in perceived realism. This model uses an inference layer (using a Conditional Random Field) that models the relationship between prosodic features and more abstract motion features (such as temporal and spatial extend, velocity, curvature). At synthesis time, a control layer selects the most appropiate gesture segment using a pre-computed optimal control policy that aims to minimize the difference between desired and selected gesture features while maximizing the animation quality. Le et al. [11] have implemented a live visual prosody system that synthesizes head, eye and eyelid motion on the basis of speech loudness and f0. The head motion synthesis of this model is implemented as a frame-by-frame selection of head posture on the basis of the prosodic features and the head posture on the previous two frames. It uses a Gaussian Mixture Model (GMM) to maximize the combined probability density of the head posture, velocity and acceleration with the prosodic features. This system outperforms some of the other online and offline systems ([3,4,14]) discussed in this section in terms of preference ratings by subjects. To the best of our knowledge, none of these live visual prosody systems have been tested with TTS rather than real human speech.

3   Online TTS-Based Visual Prosody

As live synthesis fits with our goal of implementing online visual prosody in incremental behavior realization scenarios, we decided to implement our online TTS-based visual prosody model on the basis of a live visual prosody model. Since we are currently exploring the feasibility of TTS-based visual prosody, we opted to implement a modified version of [11] and test it with TTS input, as their system is easy to implement, yet provides synthesis results that are beyond the quality of several existing visual prosody models.

Le et al.'s visual prosody model works as follows. Its speech features are f (f0) and l (loudness). Its motion features $\kappa \in \{r, p, y, v, a\}$ include the euler angles r_t (roll), p_t (pitch) and y_t (yaw) of the head at frame t, and the head velocity v_t and acceleration a_t, defined as:

$$v_t = \left\| \begin{bmatrix} r_t \\ p_t \\ y_t \end{bmatrix} - \begin{bmatrix} r_{t-1} \\ p_{t-1} \\ y_{t-1} \end{bmatrix} \right\|, a_t = \left\| \begin{bmatrix} r_t \\ p_t \\ y_t \end{bmatrix} - 2\begin{bmatrix} r_{t-1} \\ p_{t-1} \\ y_{t-1} \end{bmatrix} + \begin{bmatrix} r_{t-2} \\ p_{t-2} \\ y_{t-2} \end{bmatrix} \right\| \tag{1}$$

It makes use of five GMMs, one for each motion feature, modeling the joint probability density of that motion feature with the two speech features:

$$P(\boldsymbol{X}) = \sum_{i=1}^{m} c_i \frac{1}{\sqrt{(2\pi)^3 |\boldsymbol{\Sigma_i}|}} e^{-\frac{1}{2}(\boldsymbol{X}-\mu_i)^T \Sigma_i^{-1}(\boldsymbol{X}-\mu_i)} \tag{2}$$

Here $\boldsymbol{X} = (\kappa, f, l)^T$, m is the number of mixtures, c_i, μ_i and Σ_i are the weight, mean and covariance matrix of the i-th mixture respectively. The GMMs are trained using the Expectation-Maximation algorithm. At synthesis, the next head pose is then found using:

$$(r_t^*, p_t^*, y_t^*) = \arg \max_{r_t, p_t, y_t} \prod_{\kappa_t \in \{r_t, p_t, y_t, v_t, a_t\}} P(\kappa_t, f_t, l_t) \qquad (3)$$

Given the head poses from the previous two frames $(r_{t-1}^*, p_{t-1}^*, y_{t-1}^*)^T$ and $(r_{t-2}^*, p_{t-2}^*, y_{t-2}^*)^T$, this simplifies to:

$$(r_t^*, p_t^*, y_t^*) = \arg \max_{r_t, p_t, y_t} \prod_{\kappa_t \in \{r_t, p_t, y_t\}} P(\kappa_t, f_t, l_t) \times$$

$$P\left(\left\|\begin{bmatrix} r_t \\ p_t \\ y_t \end{bmatrix} - \begin{bmatrix} r_{t-1}^* \\ p_{t-1}^* \\ y_{t-1}^* \end{bmatrix}\right\|, f_t, l_t\right) \times$$

$$P\left(\left\|\begin{bmatrix} r_t \\ p_t \\ y_t \end{bmatrix} - 2\begin{bmatrix} r_{t-1}^* \\ p_{t-1}^* \\ y_{t-1}^* \end{bmatrix} + \begin{bmatrix} r_{t-2}^* \\ p_{t-2}^* \\ y_{t-2}^* \end{bmatrix}\right\|, f_t, l_t\right) \qquad (4)$$

Thus, the method favours poses and velocities that are likely in combination with the prosodic features, and additionally, by taking into account the previous two frames of animation and the likelihood density of velocities and accelerations, smooth motion trajectories.

We provide several modifications to this model. Le et al. use a customly recorded motion capture corpus in which an actor is asked to read from a phone balanced corpus for 47 min. As neither this corpus nor their trained models are publicly available, we opted to train the model from the IEMocap corpus [2] instead. The corpus contains dialogs between two actors in 8 improvised and 7 scripted scenarios. In each dialog, the movement of one of the actors is recorded using motion capture. Each scenario is recorded for five male and five female actors. We performed Canonical Correlation Analysis (CCA) on the head motion and speech, which revealed significant differences for the synchrony of head motion and speech, both between different actors and between their scripted and improvized sessions. Based on this observation we decided to train the model based on the speech and motion of one female actor (actor F1) in her scripted scenarios. We choose to train on the scripted scenarios, as they have a higher CCA coeficient and we hypothised that they therefore may have less head motions that are unrelated to speech prosody. In total, the training set contained 7.4 min of speech and head motion.

Similarly to [11], we use openSMILE [6] to extract audio features. However, rather than using loudness and f0, we opted to use RMS energy and f0, as we found that RMS energy correlates more with the head postures and is easier to obtain directly from TTS software. As we have less training data available, we decided to use a higher sample rate (120 Hz instead of 24 Hz as used in [11]) to obtain more training samples. Figure 1a shows a histogram of the head pitch and f0 in the training data. In 31 % of the samples in the training data (the red box in Fig. 1a), the f0 is 0, that is, there is either a silence or the speech is not voiced. As it turned out to be difficult to fit a GMM to this speech pattern we decided to learn the GMM only on the voiced parts of the speech, which left us with 5.1 min of training data. As we observed that the head velocity is low during unvoiced speech (Fig. 1b), we decided to keep the head still whenever $f0$ is 0 during synthesis. Based on cross validation results, we set the number of GMMs to 11 in all mixture models ([11] uses 10). Rather than using gradient descent search to find the optimum of Eq. 4, we opted to use the Broyden-Fletcher-Goldfarb-Shanno (BFGS) algorithm for optimization (we make use of the algorithm as provided by WEKA [9]) as it converges faster than gradient descent and works with different (TTS) voices without requiring manual tweaking of the optimization parameters for each voice.

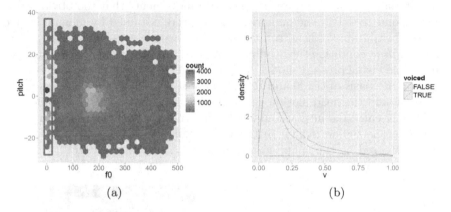

(a)   (b)

Fig. 1. Left: Histogram of head pitch and f0; right: probability density of head velocity during voiced and unvoiced speech.

4   Evaluation

To measure if and to what extent implementing online visual prosody in a behavior realizer can help in enhancing the interaction experience, we conducted three experiments. The first two experiments explore whether an IVA that exhibits visual prosody is perceived as warmer, more competent and/or more human-like. In the third experiment, we check whether subjects perceive the online visual prosody as fitting to the accompanying speech.

4.1   Experimental Conditions

We use four experimental conditions to measure the performance of online visual prosody. In the *none* condition no visual prosody is used, which is the common practise in current behavior realizers. In the *mocap* condition the head movement of the IVA is steered by motion capture motion from a speaker in the corpus. That is, the IVA replays a real human speaking motion, but it is not produced in concordance with the accompanied TTS output. Motion capture segments that may represent visual prosody are selected from the IEMOCAP corpus [2] using the following criteria:

1. The head should, on average, face in the direction of the interlocutor. This corresponds with motion segments that have their mean pitch, yaw and roll in the ranges $< -4, 4 >, < -5, 5 >$ and $< -6, 6 >$ degrees respectively.
2. Extreme head poses are to be avoided, the head pitch, yaw and roll should be in the ranges $< -8, 8 >, < -15, 15 >$ and $< -12, 12 >$ degrees respectively.
3. Extreme rotational velocities (greater than $240°/s$) and accelerations (greater than $60°/s^2$) are to be avoided.

These criteria are meant to prevent excessive movements that too obviously do not correspond to TTS. The numerical values were obtained by manual inspection of the histograms of head rotations in the corpus.

In the *offline* condition the head movement of the IVA is steered by a state-of-the-art offline visual prosody model [5]. This model synthesizes head and eyebrow motions on the basis of the f0 and RMS energy of speech. In the experiments we make use of only the head motion generated by this model. This is a challenging baseline as it can take into account more information when synthesizing head motion than the online model. In the *online* condition the head movement of the IVA is steered by the online visual prosody model (see Sect. 3).

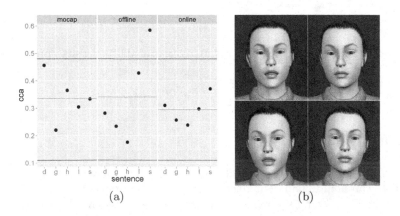

(a)   (b)

Fig. 2. Left: CCA-coefficients of the stimuli; right: prototypical head movements.

4.2   Stimuli

For all stimuli, behavior is steered using AsapRealizer [17], with the 'Armandia' virtual character (see Fig. 2b) and the 'Hannah' US-American voice frome

CereProc.[2] We introduce Armandia to the subjects as a virtual assistant that helps manage their appointments. We created four appointments for Armandia to introduce to the subjects (see Fig. 3 for an example). For each appointment, we created videos for all four conditions. The eye gaze of the IVA is directed at the camera in all interaction segments. Videos for the stimuli in all conditions are provided at http://www.herwinvanwelbergen.nl/visual_prosody.

To evaluate the speech-gesture synchrony of our stimuli we calculate the CCA-coefficient between the euler angles of the head and the f0 of speech (see Fig. 2a). This, or similar linear correlations have been used to demonstrate the synchrony between head posture and speech prosody in related work (e.g. [3, 16]) and the CCA-coefficient is proposed as an objective measurement for visual prosody by Mariooryad and Busso [15]. The mean CCA-coefficients (indicated with the red lines) are below the CCA-coefficients found in real speech (top black line), but well above chance level (lower black line). Interestingly, the CCA-coefficients are also high in the mocap condition. We hypothesize that this is because both speech and gesture are rhythmic signals and some linear correlation can always be found between two such signals.

All studies are conducted online. Subjects are recruited using the Crowd-Flower crowdsourcing platform[3] and got paid for participating. Participant recruition was limited to English speaking countries. At the start of each of the experiments, subjects are shown a video of Armandia reading a login code to them. Subjects have to enter this code to proceed to the rest of the study. This video serves both to let the subject get used to Text-To-Speech and our IVA and to make sure that they understand what is being said (e.g. their audio is enabled and at a high enough level, they understand some English). We introduced several mechanisms (discussed in detail in each experiment) to filter out subjects that provided nonsense answers to minimize their time spend on the experiment and maximize their profit. Subjects were given the option to provide free-text feedback after each experiment. At the end of each study, subjects were debriefed on its purpose.

4.3   Evaluating Warmth, Competence and Humanlikeness

Our experimental design (including the questionnaires) to measure warmth, competence and human-likeness is based upon the design used in succesful laboratory studies by Bergmann and colleagues (e.g. in [1]), in which these factors are compared for several gesturing strategies (including not gesturing at all).

Subjects are instructed that they are to evaluate a virtual assistant that helps manage their appointments. We use a between-subject design: each subject is shown videos of Armandia in one condition. In this experiment, the login code is read using that condition. After logging in, subjects are shown four videos of Armandia discussing an appointment in one or two sentences. Each video is followed by two-choice comprehension questions (see Fig. 3 for an example).

---

[2] https://www.cereproc.com/.
[3] http://www.crowdflower.com/.

Appointment: Your plane to Hawaii leaves on Saturday at 10 am, so you
                    should take the train at 7:10, what do you think about that?
Question: What leaves at 10 am?
Possible answers: Train, Plane

Fig. 3. Example appointment and comprehension question.

The comprehension questions are used to make sure subjects pay attention to the videos and filter out those that did not understand what was said in them. After watching the four videos subjects are asked to rate how well 18 adjectives (see Table 1) fit Armandia's behaviour on a 7-point Likert scale ranging from not appropiate to very appropiate. The 18 adjectives are intertwined with three test adjectives that have a more or less clear answer (we used 'blond', 'dark-haired', 'english-speaking'). We used a pilot study with 10 subjects from our laboratories to select a set of test adjectives that is best understood by the subjects and to establish baselines for correctly answered comprehension questions.

Results. In total 260 subjects participated in the study, 232 of these finished the questionnaire. We filtered out subjects that did not watch all videos (6), did not rate the test adjectives correctly (48) or could not answer more than 6 out of 8 of the comprehension questions correctly (7). This left us with 171 participants (101 female, 70 male, aged between 18 and 71; $M = 39.7, SD = 12.2$).

To measure the reliability of our warmth, competence and human-likeness factors, we calculated Cronbach's α. All α valuses were above 0.7, which justifies combining these items into one mean value as a single index for this scale (see Table 1).

Table 1. Reliability analysis for the three factors.

Factor	Items	Cronbach's α
Warmth	pleasant, sensitive, friendly, likeable, affable, approachable, sociable	.927
Competence	dedicated, trustworthy, thorough, helpful, intelligent, organized, expert	.925
Human-likeness	active, humanlike, fun-loving, lively	.846

We conducted a one-factorial ANOVA and found no significant difference between the conditions in warmth ($F(3, 167) = .284$, $p = .837$), competence ($F(3, 167) = 1.095$, $p = .889$) nor human-likeness ($F(3, 167) = .722$, $p = .828$). Figure 4 (right) shows the distribution of the factors in each condition.

To check the consistency of the ratings on the questionnaire we conducted principal component analysis (PCA) with orthogonal rotation (varimax) on the 14 questionnaire elements relating to warmth and competence. We selected only these factors, as they are consistently found as universal dimensions of social judgement [7], while human-likeness is added as a more experimental factor, which is not necesaraly orthogonal to warmth and competence in [1]. Two components had eigenvalues of over Kaiser's criterion of 1 and in combination explained 70.8 % of the variance. Figure 4 (left side) shows the factor loading after rotation and the mean and standard deviation of each factor. The items that cluster on the same components suggest that one corresponds to competence and the other to warmth and that each item clusters to its expected component.

item	warmth	competence
pleasant	.705	.406
sensitive	.763	.082
friendly	.802	.322
likeable	.765	.429
affable	.732	.322
approachable	.754	.433
sociable	.824	.300
dedicated	.493	.625
trustworthy	.407	.760
thorough	.222	.858
helpful	.196	.796
intelligent	.521	.680
organized	.238	.845
expert	.394	.699

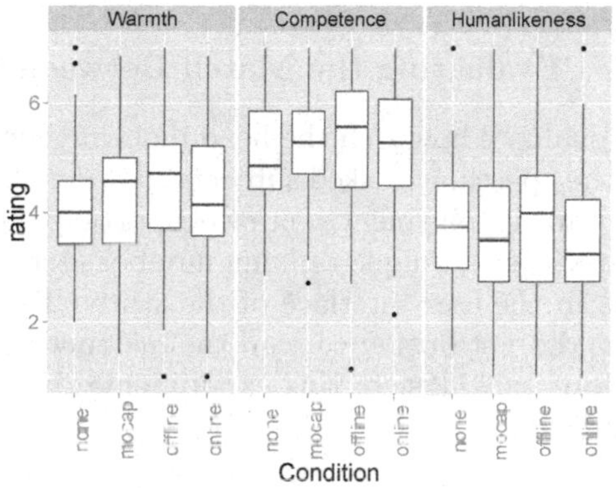

Fig. 4. Results of the evaluation of warmth, competence and human-likeness.

Over 42 % (72) of the subjects used the possibility to provide free-text feedback. Most of the comments (42, in all conditions) were on the quality of the TTS. Several subjects (11, in all conditions) commented that aspects of movement were missing (e.g. emotion, smiles, blinking, gaze). Only one of the subjects commented on the head motion.

4.4   Warmth, Competence and Humanlikeness Revisited

We hypothized that because of the comprehension task, many subjects may have been too focused on understanding the speech to notice the head movement. Therefore we ran a second experiment, in which we removed all comprehension questions. Furthermore, we added a question at the end on which motions were perceived by the subjects (head, lips, blinks, breathing).

Results. After filtering out subjects in the same way as for experiment 1, 176 subject remained. Of these we focus our analysis on the 142 (77 female, 65 male, aged between 20 and 68; $M = 37.8$, $SD = 10.7$) that either correctly perceived head movement when the head moved in their condition, or reported no head movement when they were assigned the none condition (analysis on the aforementioned 176 shows similar results). Of these 142, 53 subjects have participated in the first experiment. This might bias the results in favour of our models, as it creates a partial within-subject condition for some of the participants.

As in the previous experiment, we calculate Cronbach's α on the factors, and again combining them into a one mean value as a single index for each factor was justified. We conducted a one-factorial ANOVA and found no significant difference between the conditions in warmth ($F(3, 138) = .733, p = .534$), competence ($F(3, 138) = .923, p = .432$) nor human-likeness ($F(3, 138) = .919, p = .433$). The means and standard deviations of the factors are almost identical to those of the first experiment.

4.5   Evaluating the Match Between Speech and Head-Motion

To evaluate how well the head motion generated by our model is perceived to fit to the speech, we asked subjects to order the videos of the different conditions for all four appointment sentences: participants were instructed to give each of the four videos a unique ranking number (1st, 2nd, 3rd, 4th), but we did not enforce this in the user interface of the study. This allowed us to filter out participants that did not bother to read the instructions and (arguably) might not give very serious rankings. In this experiment, the login code was read in the no-motion condition.

Results. In total 125 subjects participated in the study. Of these, 95 completed the study. We filtered out subjects that did not watch the videos completely (8), did not provide a unique ranking for each video (27), participated in the previous experiments (7) or reported mistakes in filling out the ranking (1). This left us with 52 participants (30 female, 22 male, aged from 17 to 64; $M = 38.06$, $SD = 11.95$) for the analysis of our results.

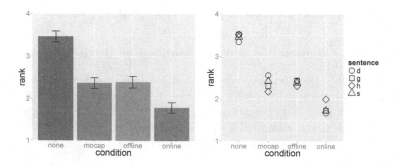

Fig. 5. Left: overview of the rankings, whiskers indicate the 95 % confidence intervals; right: spread of the rankings per appointment sentence.

We performed a repeated measures ANOVA to compare the ranking of the conditions and their interaction with the appointments. Mauchly's test indicated that the assumption of sphericity had been violated for the main effect of condition, $\chi^2(5) = 12.257$, $p = .031$ and the interaction between appointment and condition $\chi^2(44) = 62.156$, $p = .038$, therefore the degrees of freedom were corrected using Huynh-Feldt estimates of sphericity ($\epsilon = .929$, $\epsilon = .934$ respectively). The results show a significant main effect between the conditions $F(2.788, 339.144) = 45.919$, $p < 0.001$, $\eta_p^2 = .474$. Post hoc tests (using Bonferroni adjustment for multiple comparisons) show that the no-motion condition is always ranked significantly lower as all other conditions ($p < 0.001$), online visual prosody is always rated significantly higher as all other conditions ($p < 0.002$) and offline and mocap are inbetween and their ratings do not significantly differ ($p = 1.00$). No interaction between appointment and condition was found ($F(8.407, 428.741) = 1.207$, $p = .291$). An overview of the rankings for each condition and their spread over different appointment sentences is given in Fig. 5.

5 Discussion

The evaluation showed that the online visual prosody model can provide head motion that is perceived to fit better to TTS than using a state-of-the art offline method for visual prosody with TTS, using motion capture from a different speech segment, or using no motion at all. Surprisingly, motion synthesized with the offline visual prosody model was not perceived as fitting better to speech than motion captured motion that is unrelated to the speech. It could well be that generating motion that is perceived to fit to TTS requires different motion qualities (e.g. being more robotic) than generating motion that fits to real human speech. Recall that the offline model is a more intricate model than the relatively simple online model and might capture aspects of human speech (for example prominence) that are not available in TTS. The online model might thus outperform the offline model with TTS-speech because it is more robust in generating head motion that is coherent to speech when some human-like qualities of speech are missing.

We did not find any effect of visual prosody on perceived warmth, competence or human-likeness. There could be several reasons for this: (1) visual prosody might not affect perceived competence, warmth, nor human-likeness, (2) the effects are relatively small and cannot be found in a between-subject crowdsourcing study where we do not control screen-size, attention, outside distractions, sound quality, etc., (3) other factors are far more important for perceived competence, warmth or human-likeness than prosodic head motion (e.g. speech quality, lipsync quality). We aim to tease apart which of these reasons explain our results in further studies. Our experimental design to assess warmth, competence and humanlike-ness was based on a successful laboratory study on the perceived effects of gesture [1]. To assess (2), we plan to both run our study in the laboratory and the laboratory study of Bergmann et al. [1] in a crowdsourceing experiment. Point (3) is supported by the comments of subjects on the quality of the TTS and the lack of other facial motion. Using visual prosody on more than one modality has been shown to enhance the perceived human-likeness of an IVA for real speech [5,15]. In future work we thus aim to enhance the online visual prosody model to include more modalities such as eye and eyelid movement (e.g. using the online model of [11]) and eyebrow movement (as in [5,15]) and assess if those help us in enhancing the human-likeness, warmth and/or competence of TTS-driven real-time visual prosody.

Acknowledgements. We would like to thank Kirsten Bergmann and Philipp Kulms for their feedback on the design of the study and their help with the evaluation of the results. This work was partially performed within the Labex SMART (ANR-11-LABX-65) supported by French state funds managed by the ANR within the Investissements d'Avenir programme under reference ANR-11-IDEX-0004-02. It was also partially funded by the EU H2020 project ARIA-VALUSPA; and by the German Federal Ministry of Education and Research (BMBF) within the Leading-Edge Cluster Competition, managed by the Project Management Agency Karlsruhe (PTKA). The authors are responsible for the contents of this publication.

References

1. Bergmann, Kirsten, Kopp, Stefan, Eyssel, Friederike: Individualized gesturing outperforms average gesturing – evaluating gesture production in virtual humans. In: Safonova, Alla (ed.) IVA 2010. LNCS, vol. 6356, pp. 104–117. Springer, Heidelberg (2010)
2. Busso, C., Bulut, M., Lee, C.C., Kazemzadeh, A., Mower, E., Kim, S., Chang, J., Lee, S., Narayanan, S.: IEMOCAP: interactive emotional dyadic motion capture database. Lang. Resour. Eval. **42**(4), 335–359 (2008)
3. Busso, C., Deng, Z., Neumann, U., Narayanan, S.: Natural head motion synthesis driven by acoustic prosodic features. Comput. Animation Virtual Worlds **16**(3–4), 283–290 (2005)
4. Chuang, E., Bregler, C.: Mood swings: expressive speech animation. Trans. Graph. **24**(2), 331–347 (2005)
5. Ding, Y., Pelachaud, C., Artières, T.: Modeling multimodal behaviors from speech prosody. In: Aylett, R., Krenn, B., Pelachaud, C., Shimodaira, H. (eds.) IVA 2013. LNCS, vol. 8108, pp. 217–228. Springer, Heidelberg (2013)
6. Eyben, F., Weninger, F., Gross, F., Schuller, B.: Recent developments in openSMILE, the Munich open-source multimedia feature extractor. In: Conference on Multimedia, pp. 835–838. ACM (2013)
7. Fiske, S.T., Cuddy, A.J.C., Glick, P.: Universal dimensions of social cognition: warmth and competence. Trends Cogn. Sci. **11**(2), 77–83 (2007)
8. Graf, H.P., Cosatto, E., Strom, V., Hang, F.J.: Visual prosody: facial movements accompanying speech. In: Automatic Face and Gesture Recognition, pp. 381–386. IEEE Computer Society (2002)
9. Hall, M., Frank, E., Holmes, G., Pfahringer, B., Reutemann, P., Witten, I.H.: The WEKA data mining software: an update. SIGKDD Explor. **11**(1), 10–18 (2009)
10. Heylen, D.K.J.: Head gestures, gaze and the principles of conversational structure. Int. J. Humanoid Rob. **3**(3), 241–267 (2006)
11. Le, B.H., Ma, X., Deng, Z.: Live speech driven head-and-eye motion generators. Trans. Visual Comput. Graphics **18**(11), 1902–1914 (2012)

12. Lee, J., Marsella, S.: Modeling speaker behavior: a comparison of two approaches. In: Nakano, Y., Neff, M., Paiva, A., Walker, M. (eds.) IVA 2012. LNCS, vol. 7502, pp. 161–174. Springer, Heidelberg (2012)

13. Levine, S., Krähenbühl, P., Thrun, S., Koltun, V.: Gesture controllers. Trans. Graph. **29**(4), 124:1–124:11 (2010)

14. Levine, S., Theobalt, C., Koltun, V.: Real-time prosody-driven synthesis of body language. In: SIGGRAPH Asia, pp. 1–10. ACM, New York (2009)

15. Mariooryad, S., Busso, C.: Generating human-like behaviors using joint, speech-driven models for conversational agents. Audio Speech Lang. Process. **20**(8), 2329–2340 (2012)

16. Munhall, K.G., Jones, J.A., Callan, D.E., Kuratate, T., Vatikiotis-Bateson, E.: Visual prosody and speech intelligibility: head movement improves auditory speech perception. Psychol. Sci. **15**(2), 133–137 (2004)

17. van Welbergen, H., Yaghoubzadeh, R., Kopp, S.: AsapRealizer 2.0: the next steps in fluent behavior realization for ECAs. In: Bickmore, T., Marsella, S., Sidner, C. (eds.) IVA 2014. LNCS, vol. 8637, pp. 449–462. Springer, Heidelberg (2014)

Predicting Co-verbal Gestures:
A Deep and Temporal Modeling Approach

Chung-Cheng Chiu[1]([✉]), Louis-Philippe Morency[2], and Stacy Marsella[3]

[1] Google Inc., Mountain View, USA
redjava@gmail.com
[2] Language Technology Institute, School of Computer Science,
Carnegie Mellon University, Pittsburgh, USA
morency@cs.cmu.edu
[3] Northeastern University, Boston, USA
stacymarsella@gmail.com

Abstract. Gestures during spoken dialog play a central role in human communication. As a consequence, models of gesture generation are a key challenge in research on virtual humans, embodied agents capable of face-to-face interaction with people. Machine learning approaches to gesture generation must take into account the conceptual content in utterances, physical properties of speech signals and the physical properties of the gestures themselves. To address this challenge, we proposed a gestural sign scheme to facilitate supervised learning and presented the DCNF model, a model to jointly learn deep neural networks and second order linear chain temporal contingency. The approach we took realizes both the mapping relation between speech and gestures while taking account temporal relations among gestures. Our experiments on human co-verbal dataset shows significant improvement over previous work on gesture prediction. A generalization experiment performed on handwriting recognition also shows that DCNFs outperform the state-of-the-art approaches.

1 Introduction

Embodied conversational agents (ECAs) are virtual characters capable of engaging face-to-face interaction with human and play an important role in many applications such as human-computer interaction [6] and social skills training [29]. A key challenge in building an ECA is giving them the ability to use appropriate gestures while speaking, as users are sensitive to whether the gestures of an ECA are consistent with its speech [11]. This challenge is also true for social robotic platforms [30]. Such co-verbal gestures [36] must coordinate closely with the prosody and verbal content of the spoken utterance. Manual development of an agent's gestures is typically a tedious process of manually handcrafting gestures and assigning them to the agent's utterances. A data-driven approach that learns to predict and generate co-verbal gestures is a promising alternative to such manual approaches.

However, the prediction and generation of co-verbal gestures presents a difficult, novel machine learning challenge in that it must span and couple multiple

© Springer International Publishing Switzerland 2015
W.-P. Brinkman et al. (Eds.): IVA 2015, LNAI 9238, pp. 152–166, 2015.
DOI: 10.1007/978-3-319-21996-7_17

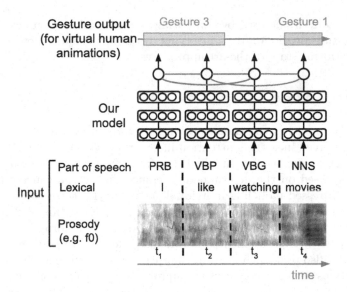

Fig. 1. The overview of our framework for predicting co-verbal gestures. Our Deep Conditional Neural Field (DCNF) model predicts gestures by integrating verbal and acoustic while preserving the temporal consistency.

domains: the conceptual content in the utterance, utterance prosody and the physical domain of gestural motions. The coupling between these domains has several complex features. There is a tight coupling between gesture motion, the evolving the content of the utterance as well as the prosody of speech. This coupling is the product of the information conveyed through both speech and gestures [4] that may be shared at a hidden, abstract level [25] which relates utterance content and physical gestures. These properties suggest that generating gestures from speech can exploit a representation that takes into account this relation between form and function (what the gesture conveys) and a model capable of modeling the deep and temporal relationship between speech and gestures. Additionally, speech and gesture are closely coupled in time, which raises its own challenges since gestures are physical motions with tight temporal and spatial constraints if the motion is to look natural.

In this paper, we introduce a deep, temporal model to realize the prediction of gestures from verbal content and prosody of the spoken utterance. The structure of the entire framework is shown in Fig. 1. Our model, called deep conditional neural field (DCNF), is an extension of previous work [10,13] that combines the advantages of deep neural network for mapping complex relation and an undirected second-order linear-chain for modeling the temporal coordination of speech and gestures. We also propose a gesture representation scheme that takes advantage of previous literature that relates the form and communicative function of gestures [4,18,24].

We assess our framework by evaluating the prediction accuracy on actual co-verbal gesture prediction data involving dyadic interviews, showing that our model outperforms state-of-the-art approaches.

2   Related Work

Data-driven approaches to generate co-verbal gestures for intelligent embodied agent have received increasing attention in gesture research. Reference [32] took the co-generation perspective in which the framework synthesizes both speech and gestures based on the determined utterance during the conversation. Reference [27] addressed modeling individual gesture styles through analyzing the relation in the data between extracted utterance information and a person's gestures. Our technique can be applied to predict this information, and their approaches can then be applied to accomplish the gesture generation process. Reference [19] also took the co-generation perspective and focused on modeling individual styles on iconic gestures to improve human-agent communication.

Some of the previous work focused on realizing the relation between prosody and motion dynamics [8,22,23]. By using only prosody as input, these models do not require speech content analyses but are limited to the subset of gestures that correlate closely to prosody, for example, a form of rhythmic gesture called beats. Our approach goes beyond prosody to realize a mapping from the utterance content to more expressive gestures and can be integrated to extend existing work to generate animations beyond beat gestures.

Alternatives to data-driven machine learning approaches are the handcrafted rule-based approaches [1,7,21,24]. These exploit expert knowledge on speech and gestures to specify the mapping from utterance features to gestures. While earlier works based on this approach have focused on addressing the mapping relation between only linguistic features and gestures [7,21], recent work [24] has also addressed how to use acoustic features to help gesture determination.

Realizing a mapping from speech to gestures involves learning a model that relates two sequences, the speech input sequence and the gesture output sequence. Recent advances in neural networks toward modeling the two sequence problems apply recurrent neural networks (RNNs) [33] and its extension, long short-term memory (LSTM) network [16]. The RNN-based architecture is designed to address problems in which the input and output time series can have different lengths and are correlated as whole sequences but may not have a strong correlation at the frame-by-frame level. The resulting model utilizes less of the structure in the data and make predictions by maximizing only the distribution of targeting sequences. On the other hand, our approach utilizes the fine-grained synchronization between observed and predicting sequences and also learns the global conditional distributions of both sequences to further improve the prediction accuracy.

Previous approaches in deep learning that utilize the synchronized structure of two sequences trained separately a deep neural network and a linear-chain graphical model. For example, in speech recognition [26] the common approach is to train deep learning with individual frames and then applies hidden Markov models (HMMs) with the hidden states. Our approach learns both the deep neural network and temporal contiguity of CRFs with a joint likelihood. There are previous works that adopt similar perspective on extending CRFs with deep structure [10, 38] and show improvement over a single-layer CRFs or CRFs combined with a shallow layer of neural network [28]. Our experiments show improvement over these approaches.

To our knowledge, this work is the first to introduce a gesture representation scheme that relates the form and communicative function of gestures and a deep, temporal model capable of realizing the relation between speech and the proposed gesture representation. Reference [8] adopt the concept of unsupervised training of deep belief net [35], but without an effective gesture representation and a supervised training phase the learning task is much more challenging and therefore has been limited to realizing the relation between prosody and rhythmic movement. Our proposed model goes beyond prior work [10, 13] by combining the advantages of deep neural network for mapping complex relation with an undirected second-order linear-chain for modeling the temporal coordination of speech and gestures.

3   Predicting Co-verbal Gestures

Predicting co-verbal gestures brings together many core domains of artificial intelligence, including the conceptual content in the utterance, utterance prosody and the physical domain of gestural motions. A common function of the parallel use of speech and gesture is to convey meaning in which gesture plays the complementary or supplementary role [14], and gestures may help to convey complex representations through expressing complementary information about abstract concepts [25]. Realizing this relation between speech and gesture requires realizing the hidden abstract concept. To build a successful predictive model it is important to first create a formal representation of its output label, the co-verbal gestures. Based on this idea, we exploit gestural signs [4] which summarize the functions and forms of co-verbal gestures to allow the predictions of gestures from speech signals, including utterance content and prosody. In particular, we focus on gesture categories that can be more reliably predicted from the utterance content and prosody: abstract deictic, metaphoric, and beat gestures. Abstract deictic gestures are pointing movements that indicate an object, a location, or abstract things which are not physically present in the current surroundings. Metaphoric gestures exhibit abstract concept as having physical properties. Beat gestures are rhythmic actions synchronized with speech and they tend to correlate more with prosody as opposed to utterance content. This ignores those gestures that convey information that is uncoupled or distinct from the utterance content and prosody [5] in the sense that learning would require additional information to predict the gestural signs.

We design our dictionary of gestural signs based on previous literature in gestures [4, 18, 24] and the three gesture categories, and then calculated their

Table 1. A formalized representation of co-verbal gestures for computational prediction.

Gestural signs	Description
Rest	Resting position of both hands
Palm face up	Lift hands, rotate palms facing up or a little bit inward, and hold for a while
Head nod	Head nod without arm gestures
Wipe	Hands start near (above) each other and move apart in a straight motion
Whole	Move both hands along outward arcs with palms facing forward
Frame	Both hands are held some inches apart, palms facing each other, as if something is between hands
Dismiss	Hand throws to the side in an arc as if chasing away
Block	Hand is positioned in front of the speaker, palm toward front
Shrug	Hands are opened in an outward arc, ending in a palm-up position, usually accompanied by a slight shrug
More-Or-Less	The open hand, palm down, swivels around the wrist
Process	Hand moves in circles
Deictic.Other	Hand is pointing toward a direction other than self
Deictic.Self	Points to him/herself
Beats	Beats

occurrences in a motion capture data [12] which records co-verbal gestures performed during face-to-face conversations to filter out those that rarely appeared. The final set of gestural signs has size of 14, and the list and their descriptions are shown in Table 1. This discrete set of co-verbal gestures was selected to include considerable coverage while keeping a clear distinction between gesture labels to make learning feasible. An important challenge for predicting gestural signs is to model the temporal coordination between speech and gestural signs. A state-of-the-art work [22] applies conventional conditional random fields (CRFs) for learning co-verbal gesture predictions. The limitation of conventional CRFs is that it requires defining functions for modeling the correlation between input signals and labels, and manually defining these functions that may express the relation between high-dimensional speech signals and gestures is no trivial task. Thus, we argue instead to use a deep model to learn this complex relation.

4   Deep Conditional Neural Fields

In this section, we formally describe the Deep Conditional Neural Field (DCNF) model which combines state-of-the-art deep learning techniques with the temporal modeling capabilities of CRFs for predicting gestures from utterance content and prosody (see Fig. 2). The prediction task takes the transcript of the utterance, part-of-speech tags of the transcript, and prosody features of the speech

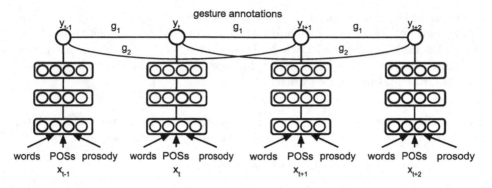

Fig. 2. The structure of our DCNF framework. The neural network learns the nonlinear relation between speech features and gestural signs. The top layer is a second-order undirected linear-chain which takes the output of the neural network as input and model the temporal relation among gestural signs. Both the top undirected chain and deep neural networks are trained jointly.

audio as input $\mathbf{x} = \{x_1, x_2, \ldots, x_N\}$, and learn to predict a sequence of gestural signs $\mathbf{y} = \{y_1, y_2, \ldots, y_N\}$ in which the sequence has length N. At each time step t, the gestural sign y_t is contained in the set of our gestural sign dictionary $y_t \in \mathbf{Y}$ defined in the previous section (see Table 1) , and the input x_t is a feature vector $x_t \in \mathbf{R}^d$ where d corresponds to the number of input features (see next section for a detailed description of our input features).

Following the formalism of [10,13], the DCNF extends previous models to follow a 2nd-order Markov assumption and is defined as:

$$P(\mathbf{y}|\mathbf{x}; \boldsymbol{\theta}) = \frac{1}{Z(\mathbf{x})} \sum_{t=1}^{N} \exp[\sum_{k} \theta_k^{g_1} g_k^1(y_{t-1}, y_t)$$
$$+ \sum_{l} \theta_l^{\mathbf{g_2}} \mathbf{g_l^2}(\mathbf{y_{t-1}}, \mathbf{y_t}, \mathbf{y_{t+1}})$$
$$+ \sum_{i} \theta_{i,y_t}^{f} f_i(x_t, \theta^w)]$$

where model parameters $\boldsymbol{\theta} = [\theta^{g_1}, \theta^{g_2}, \theta^f, \theta^w]$ and $Z(\mathbf{x})$ is the normalization term. gs correspond to edge features in which $g^1(y_{t-1}, y_t)$ and $g^2(y_{t-1}, y_t, y_{t+1})$ denote the first and second order edge functions, and θ^{g_1} and θ^{g_2} correspond to their parameters respectively. The 2nd-order term $g^2(y_{t-1}, y_t, y_{t+1})$ is one of the the major improvement of the DCNF model. f is related to neural networks in which $f(x_t, \theta^w)$ associates the output of the last layer of the deep neural network with θ^f denotes its parameters, and y and $\theta^w = \{\theta_1^w, \theta_2^w, \ldots, \theta_{m-1}^w\}$ represents the network connection parameters of the m neural network layers:

$$f(x_t, \theta^w) = h(a_{m-1}\theta_{m-1}^w) \text{ where}$$
$$a_i = h(a_{i-1}\theta_{i-1}^w), \ i = 2 \ldots m - 1$$

where a_i represents the output at ith neural network layer, θ_i^w represents the connection weights between ith and $i + 1$th layers, and h is the activation function. This work applies the logistic function $(1/1 + \exp(-a\theta^w))$ as the activation function[1]. Readers can refer to [10,13] for more background about the combination of CRFs and neural networks.

Prediction. Given a sequence $\mathbf{x}$ and parameters learned from the training data, the prediction process of DCNFs predicts the most probable sequence $\mathbf{y}*$:

$$\mathbf{y}* = \arg\max_{\mathbf{y}} P(\mathbf{y}|\mathbf{x}; \theta^{g_1}, \theta^{g_2}, \theta^f, \theta^w)$$

$$= \arg\max_{\mathbf{y}} \frac{1}{Z(\mathbf{x})} \sum_{t=1}^{N} \exp[\sum_{k} \theta_k^{g_1} g_k(y_{t-1}, y_t)$$

$$+ \sum_{l} \theta_l^{g_2} g_l(y_{t-1}, y_t, y_{t+1})$$

$$+ \sum_{i} \theta_{i,y_t}^f f_i(x_t, \theta^w)]$$

To estimate the probability of each label of frame t, the neural networks take the input x_t and forward the value through the network to generate f_i, the undirected linear chain performs forward-backward belief propagation to calculate the values of g_k and g_l, and the potential of each label is the weighted summation of g_1, g_2, f and the probability of each label is its normalized potential.

Learning. To prevent the overfitting of DCNFs, the model has a regularization term for all parameters and we define our objective function as follows:

$$L(\boldsymbol{\theta}) = \sum_{t=1}^{N} \log P(y_t|x_t; \boldsymbol{\theta}) - \frac{1}{2\gamma^2}\|\boldsymbol{\theta}\|^2,$$

in which $\boldsymbol{\theta}$ denotes the set of model parameters and γ corresponds to regularization coefficients. The regularization term on training the deep neural networks encourages the weight decay which reduce the complexity increase of the network connections along the parameter updates. We applied stochastic gradient descent for training DCNFs with a degrading learning rate to encourage the convergence of the parameter updates[2].

To also help prevent co-adaptation of network parameters which result overfitting, we apply the dropout technique [17] to change the feed-forward results of $f_i(x_t, \theta^w)$ in the training phase. By performing dropout, at the feed-forward

---

[1] We have experimented with both the logistic and the rectified linear $(\max(a\theta^w, 0))$ functions with similar results. Because of space constraints, we are focusing on the logistic function.

[2] The full derivation of the gradient was omitted because of space constraint.

phase the output of each hidden node has a probability of being disabled. Consequently the output of hidden nodes in the training phase is different from that of the testing phase. The dropout nodes are re-sampled at every feed-forward process. This stochastic behaviors encourage hidden nodes to model distinct patterns and therefore further prevent the overfitting. The dropout technique is not applied during the testing phase.

Gradient Calculation. To learn our model parameters, we derived the gradient of our objective function with respect to $\theta^{g_1}, \theta^{g_2}, \theta^f, \theta^w$. We derive $\theta^{g_1}, \theta^{g_2}, \theta^f$ following previous work on CRFs [20], and derive θ^w with backpropagation [10,13]. Backpropagation decomposes the gradient at each layer as the product of an error term δ with the input and propagates δ to the lower layers to facilitate gradient calculation. Thus, performing backpropagation on DCNF requires determining δ_{m-1} of θ^w_{m-1} in which $\nabla\theta^w_{m-1} = \delta_{m-1}\hat{a}_{m-1}$ for $\nabla\theta^w_{m-1}$ denotes the gradient of θ^w_{m-1} and $\hat{a}_{m-1}$ denotes the output at layer $m-1$ with dropout. As the gradient of θ^w_{m-1} is given by:

$$\frac{\partial \log P}{\partial \theta^w_{m-1}}$$

$$= \sum_t^N \sum_i [\lambda_{i,y_t}\frac{\partial f_i(x_t,\theta^w)}{\partial\theta^w_{m-1}} - \sum_{\tilde{y}} p(\tilde{y}|x_t)\lambda_{i,\tilde{y}}\frac{\partial f_i(x_t,\theta^w)}{\partial\theta^w_{m-1}}]$$

$$- \sum_t^N \sum_i [\lambda_{i,y_t}\frac{\partial h(\hat{a}_{m-1}\theta^w_{m-1})}{\partial\theta^w_{m-1}}$$

$$- \sum_{\tilde{y}} p(\tilde{y}|x_t)\lambda_{i,\tilde{y}}\frac{\partial h(\hat{a}_{m-1}\theta^w_{m-1})}{\partial\theta^w_{m-1}}]$$

$$= \sum_t^N \sum_i [\lambda_{i,y_t}h'_i(\hat{a}_{m-1}\theta^w_{m-1})\hat{a}_{m-1}$$

$$- \sum_{\tilde{y}} p(\tilde{y}|x_t)\lambda_{i,\tilde{y}}h'_i(\hat{a}_{m-1}\theta^w_{m-1})\hat{a}_{m-1}]$$

we can decompose the gradient term and derive

$$\delta_{m-1} = \lambda_{i,y_t}h'(\hat{a}_{m-1}\theta^w_{m-1}) - \sum_{\tilde{y}} p(\tilde{y}|x_t)\lambda_{i,\tilde{y}}h'(\hat{a}_{m-1}\theta^w_{m-1}).$$

where DCNF propagates δ_{m-1} to the lower layers so that it can calculate the gradient of these layers. One thing to notice is that the gradient is calculated with $\hat{a}_{m-1}$ instead of a_{m-1} due to the influence of dropout.

5   Experiments

Our main experiment is designed to evaluate the performance of our DCNF model on co-verbal gesture prediction from verbal content and prosody. The following sub-section presents our dataset, gesture annotation, input features, baseline models and methodology. To help assess the generalization of our DCNF, we evaluated the performance with a well-studied handwriting recognition (optical character recognition) task [34].

5.1 Co-verbal Gesture Prediction Experiments

The dataset consists of 15 videos which in total represent more than 9 hours of interactions taken from a large-scale study focusing on semi-structured interviews [15]. Our experiment focused on predicting the interviewee's gestures from his/her utterance content and prosody. All the videos were segmented and transcribed using the ELAN tool [3]. Each transcription was reviewed for accuracy by a senior transcriber.

Data Segmentation. The data is segmented into sequences based on the speaking period. The segmentation can be due to a long pause or the interviewer asked a question. Each frame in the sample data is defined to be 1 second of the conversations. Some of the sequences contained only a very short sentence in which the interviewee replied to the question of the interviewer with a short answer such as "yes/no". We removed all sentences that are less than 3 seconds. The resulting dataset has total 637 sequences with average length of 47.54 s.

Gestural Sign Annotation. In the annotation process, we first trained the annotators with the definition of all gestural signs and showed a few examples for each gestural sign. The annotator then used the ELAN tool, looked at the behavior of the participants only when they are speaking, and marked the beginning and the ending time of gestural signs in the video. There will be at most one gestural sign at any time in the data. The annotation results were inspected to analyze the accuracy and insure the annotator had well understood the definition of gestural signs.

Linguistic Features. Linguistic features encapsulate the utterance content and help determine the corresponding gestures. The extracted data has 5250 unique words, but most of them are unique to a few speakers. To make the data more general, we remove words that happen fewer than 10 times among all the 15 videos, and the resulting number of unique words is down to 817. We represent features as a binary values so that features will be set to 1 when the corresponding linguistic features appear in the corresponding time frame, and 0 otherwise. The linguistic features at the previous time frame and the next time frame are also helpful. In particular, a gesture can for example, proceeds its corresponding linguistic features. Therefore, when a linguistic feature appears at a time frame, its appearance will also be marked in the previous and the next time frame.

The data collection process extracted text from the transcript and also ran a part-of-speech tagger [2] to determine the grammatical role of each word.

POS tags are encoded at the word level and are automatically aligned with the speech audio through using the analyzing tools of FaceFX.

Prosodic Features. In terms of prosody, the data extracted the following audio features: normalized amplitude quotient (NAQ), peak slope, fundamental frequency (f0), energy, energy slope, spectral stationarity [31]. The sampling rate is 100 samples per second. All prosodic features within the same time frame are concatenated into one feature vector. As the time frame is 1 s and the sampling rate is 100 in our dataset, all 100 samples are concatenated into one feature vector as the prosodic features for that time frame. The extraction process also determines whether the speaker is speaking based on f0, and for the periods in the speech that identified as not speaking all audio features are set to zero.

Baseline Models. Our experiments compared DCNFs with models representing state-of-the-art approaches. We include CRFs, which is applied in the state-of-the-art work [22] on gesture prediction, for comparisons. We also compared with the second-order CRFs. Additionally, we include support vector machines (SVMs) and random forests, two effective machine learning models. The SVM is an approach that applies kernel techniques to help find better separating hyperplanes in the data for classifications. The random forest is an ensemble approach which learns a set of decision trees with bootstrap aggregating for classification. Both approaches have a good generalization in prior work. Additionally, two existing works that combine CRFs and neural networks, CNF [28] and Neuro-CRF [10], are evaluated in the experiment. The experiment also evaluated the performance of DCNFs without using the sequential relation learned from CRFs (denoted as DCNF-no-edge).

Methodology. The experiments use the holdout testing method to evaluate the performance of gesture predictions in which the data is separated into training, validation, and testing sets. We trained DCNFs with three hidden layers each with 256 hidden nodes and set the initial learning rate to 0.1 with 0.0003 degrading rate at each iteration. The choice of these hyperparameters are determined based on the validation results. The final result is the performance on the testing set. Each videos in the co-verbal gesture dataset corresponds to a different interviewee. We chose the first 8 interviewees (total clip length correspond to 50.86 % of the whole dataset) as the training set, 9 through 12 interviewees (23.18 % of the whole dataset) as the validation set, and last 3 interviewees (25.96 % of the whole dataset) as the testing set.

Results. The results are shown in Table 2. Both the DCNF and DCNF-no-edge models outperform other models. The performance similarity of DCNFs with and without edge features suggest that the major improvement comes from the exploitation of deep architecture. In fact, models that rely mainly on sequential relation show significantly lower performance, suggesting the bottleneck

Table 2. Results of co-verbal gesture prediction.

Models	Accuracy(%)
CRF [22]	27.35
CRF second-order	28.15
SVM	49.17
Random forest	32.21
CNF [28]	48.33
NeuroCRF [10]	48.68
DCNF-no-edge	59.31
DCNF (our approach)	59.74

on co-verbal gesture prediction lies in the realization of the complex relation between speech and gesture. The results are unexpected, as based on the work of McNeill, Calbris and others [4,25], it is reasonable to expect temporal dependencies. Calbris talks of ideation units and rhythmic-semantic units that span multiple gestures, for example. The fact that our models could not exploit temporal dependencies may due to that some of the the gestural signs defined in this task obscure the temporal dependency. For example, some gestural signs that express semantic meanings more specifically can break this kind of temporal correlation. Take wipe as an example, when someone does a wipe, it does not indicate much about whether a frame or a shrug will follow. Given that these are co-speech gestures, if a dependency at this aggregate/abstract level would to occur at the gesture level, it suggest that the same constraint should co-exist at the language level. However, since a speaker can reorder or compose different phrases, it is essentially common for a speaker to alter the verbal content and the underlying gestural behaviors. On the other hand, other subsets of gestural signs might reveal stronger dependencies, for example ones comprising rhetorical structures like enumeration and contrasts, or gestural signs tied to the establishment of a concept such as a container gesture showing a collection of ideas, followed by operations on the concept, such as adding or removing ides/items from the container. Even in these cases, there is the question of whether the features currently being used make it feasible to learn such dependencies. In addition to these fundamental difficulty on formulating the temporal relation, another possible reason is that the data collected in this task may still be too limited for learning the temporal relation.

5.2   Handwriting Recognition

To access the generality of DCNFs, we also applied it to a standard hand writing recognitions dataset [34]. This dataset contains a set of (total 6877) handwriting words collected from 150 human subjects with average length of around 8 characters. The prediction targets are lower-case characters, and since the first character is capitalized, all the first characters in the sequences are removed.

Each word was segmented into characters and each character is rasterized into 16 by 8 images. We applied 10-fold cross validation (9 folds for training and 1 fold for testing) to evaluate the performance of our DCNF model and compare the results with other models. We trained DCNFs with three hidden layers each with 128 hidden nodes and set initial learning rate to 0.2 with 0.0003 degrading rate at each iteration. The choice of these hyperparameters are also determined based on the validation results.

Baseline Models. In addition to the models compared in the gesture prediction task, this experiment also compared with the state-of-the-art result previously published using the structured prediction cascade (SPC) [37]. The SPC is inspired by the idea of the classifier cascade (for example, boosting) to increase the speed of the structured prediction. The process starts filtering possible states at 0-order and then gradually increase the orders with considering only the remaining states. While the complexity of a conventional graphical model grows exponentially with the order, SPC's pruning approach reduces the complexity significantly and therefore allows applying higher order models. The approach is the state-of-the-art results on the handwriting recognition task. The comparison results of DCNFs with SPC, along with other existing models, are shown in Table 3.

Table 3. Results of handwriting recognition. Both the results of NeuroCRF and Structured prediction cascades are adopted from the original reported values.

Models	Accuracy(%)
CRF	85.8
CRF second-order	93.32
SVM	86.15
Random forest	96.97
CNF	91.11
NeuroCRF [10]	95.44
DCNF-no-edge	97.21
Structured prediction cascades [37]	98.54
DCNF (our approach)	99.15

Results. In this handwriting recognition task DCNF shows improvement over published results. Compared to the gesture prediction task, the mapping from input to prediction targets is easier to realize in this task, and therefore the sequential information provides an influential improvement, as shown by the improvement of DCNF over DCNF-no-edge. We have also applied [10, 13] on the task and the results are similar to DCNF-no-edge.

6   Conclusion

Gesture generation presents a novel challenge to machine learning: prediction of gestures must take into account the conceptual content in utterances, physical properties of speech signals and the physical properties of the gestures themselves. To address this challenge, we proposed a gestural sign scheme to facilitate supervised learning and presented the DCNF model, a model to jointly learn deep neural networks and second-order linear chain temporal contingency. Our approach can realize both the mapping relation between speech and gestures and the temporal relation among gestures. Our experiments on human co-verbal dataset shows significant improvement over previous work on gesture prediction. A generalization experiment performed on handwriting recognition also shows that DCNFs outperform the state-of-the-art approaches.

Our framework predict gestural signs from speech, and by combining with existing gesture generation system, for example [9], the overall framework can be applied to animate virtual characters' gestures from speech. The framework relies only on linguistic and prosodic features that could be derived from speech in real-time, thus allowing for real-time gesture generation for virtual character.

Acknowledgements. The projects or effort described here has been sponsored by the U.S. Army. Any opinions, content or information presented does not necessarily reflect the position or the policy of the United States Government, and no official endorsement should be inferred.

References

1. Bergmann, K., Kahl, S., Kopp, S.: Modeling the semantic coordination of speech and gesture under cognitive and linguistic constraints. In: Aylett, R., Krenn, B., Pelachaud, C., Shimodaira, H. (eds.) IVA 2013. LNCS, vol. 8108, pp. 203–216. Springer, Heidelberg (2013)

2. Bird, S., Loper, E., Klein, E.: Natural Language Processing with Python. OReilly Media Inc, Santa Clara (2009)

3. Brugman, H., Russel, A., Nijmegen, X.: Annotating multi-media/multimodal resources with ELAN. In: Proceedings of the Fourth International Conference on Language Resources and Evaluation, LREC 2004, pp. 2065–2068 (2004)

4. Calbris, G.: Elements of Meaning in Gesture: Gesture Studies 5. John Benjamins, Philadelphia (2011)

5. Cassell, J., Prevost, S.: Distribution of semantic features across speech and gesture by humans and computers. In: Workshop on the Integration of Gesture in Language and Speech (1996)

6. Cassell, J.: Embodied conversational interface agents. Commun. ACM **43**(4), 70–78 (2000)

7. Cassell, J., Vilhjálmsson, H.H., Bickmore, T.: Beat: the behavior expression animation toolkit. In: SIGGRAPH 2001 Proceedings of the 28th Annual Conference on Computer Graphics and Interactive Techniques, pp. 477–486. ACM, New York (2001)

8. Chiu, C.-C., Marsella, S.: How to train your avatar: a data driven approach to gesture generation. In: Vilhjálmsson, H.H., Kopp, S., Marsella, S., Thórisson, K.R. (eds.) IVA 2011. LNCS, vol. 6895, pp. 127–140. Springer, Heidelberg (2011)
9. Chiu, C.C., Marsella, S.: Gesture generation with low-dimensional embeddings. In: Proceedings of the 13th International Joint Conference on Autonomous Agents and Multiagent Systems. AAMAS 2013 (2014)
10. Do, T., Artieres, T.: Neural conditional random fields. In: International Conference on Artificial Intelligence and Statistics (AI-STATS), pp. 177–184 (2010)
11. Ennis, C., McDonnell, R., O'Sullivan, C.: Seeing is believing: body motion dominates in multisensory conversations. In: ACM SIGGRAPH 2010 papers, SIGGRAPH 2010, pp. 91:1–91:9. ACM, New York(2010)
12. Ennis, C., O'Sullivan, C.: Perceptually plausible formations for virtual conversers. Comput. Animation Virtual Worlds **23**(3–4), 321–329 (2012)
13. Fujii, Y., Yamamoto, K., Nakagawa, S.: Deep-hidden conditional neural fields for continuous phoneme speech recognition. In: International Workshop of Statistical Machine Learning for Speech (IWSML) (2012)
14. Goldin-Meadow, S., Alibali, M.W., Church, R.B.: Transitions in concept acquisition: using the hand to read the mind. Psychol. Rev. **100**(2), 279–297 (1993)
15. Gratch, J., Artstein, R., Lucas, G., Stratou, G., Scherer, S., Nazarian, A., Wood, R., Boberg, J., Devault, D., Marsella, S., Traum, D., Rizzo, A.S., Morency, L.P.: The distress analysis interview corpus of human and computer interviews. In: Proceedings of the Ninth International Conference on Language Resources and Evaluation (LREC 2014), European Language Resources Association (ELRA), Reykjavik, Iceland, May 2014
16. Graves, A., Mohamed, A.R., Hinton, G.: Speech recognition with deep recurrent neural networks. In: IEEE International Conference on Acoustics, Speech, and Signal Processing (ICASSP) (2013)
17. Hinton, G.E., Srivastava, N., Krizhevsky, A., Sutskever, I., Salakhutdinov, R.: Improving neural networks by preventing co-adaptation of feature detectors (2012). pre-print arXiv:1207.0580v1
18. Kipp, M.: Gesture generation by imitation - from human behavior to computer character animation. Ph.D. thesis, Saarland University (2004)
19. Kopp, S., Bergmann, K.: Individualized gesture production in embodied conversational agents. In: Zacarias, M., de Oliveira, J.V. (eds.) Human-Computer Interaction. SCI, vol. 396, pp. 287–302. Springer, Heidelberg (2012)
20. Lafferty, J.D., McCallum, A., Pereira, F.C.N.: Conditional random fields: probabilistic models for segmenting and labeling sequence data. In: ICML, pp. 282–289 (2001)
21. Lee, J., Marsella, S.C.: Nonverbal behavior generator for embodied conversational agents. In: Gratch, J., Young, M., Aylett, R.S., Ballin, D., Olivier, P. (eds.) IVA 2006. LNCS (LNAI), vol. 4133, pp. 243–255. Springer, Heidelberg (2006)
22. Levine, S., Krähenbühl, P., Thrun, S., Koltun, V.: Gesture controllers. In: ACM SIGGRAPH 2010 papers, pp. 124:1–124:11. ACM, New York (2010)
23. Levine, S., Theobalt, C., Koltun, V.: Real-time prosody-driven synthesis of body language. ACM Trans. Graph. **28**, 172:1–172:10 (2009). http://doi.acm.org/10.1145/1618452.1618518
24. Marsella, S.C., Xu, Y., Lhommet, M., Feng, A.W., Scherer, S., Shapiro, A.: Virtual character performance from speech. In: Symposium on Computer Animation. Anaheim, CA, July 2013
25. McNeill, D.: So you think gestures are nonverbal? Psychol. Rev. **92**(3), 350–371 (1985)

26. Mohamed, A.R., Dahl, G.E., Hinton, G.: Acoustic modeling using deep belief networks. IEEE Trans. Audio Speech Lang. Process. **20**(1), 14–22 (2012)
27. Neff, M., Kipp, M., Albrecht, I., Seidel, H.P.: Gesture modeling and animation based on a probabilistic re-creation of speaker style. ACM Trans. Graph. **27**(1), 1–24 (2008)
28. Peng, J., Bo, L., Xu, J.: Conditional neural fields. In: NIPS, pp. 1419–1427 (2009)
29. Rickel, J., Johnson, W.L.: Task-oriented collaboration with embodied agents in virtual worlds. In: Cassell, J., Sullivan, J., Prevost, S. (eds.) Embodied Conversational Agents, pp. 95–122. MIT Press, Cambridge (2000)
30. Salem, M., Rohlfing, K.J., Kopp, S., Joublin, F.: A friendly gesture: investigating the effect of multimodal robot behavior in human-robot interaction. In: 2011 IEEE RO-MAN, pp. 247–252, July 2011
31. Scherer, S., Kane, J., Gobl, C., Schwenker, F.: Investigating fuzzy-input fuzzy-output support vector machines for robust voice quality classification. Comput. Speech Lang. **27**(1), 263–287 (2013)
32. Stone, M., DeCarlo, D., Oh, I., Rodriguez, C., Stere, A., Lees, A., Bregler, C.: Speaking with hands: creating animated conversational characters from recordings of human performance. In: ACM SIGGRAPH 2004 Papers, SIGGRAPH 2004, pp. 506–513. ACM, New York (2004)
33. Sutskever, I., Martens, J., Hinton, G.: Generating text with recurrent neural networks. In: ICML (2011)
34. Taskar, B., Guestrin, C., Koller, D.: Max-margin Markov networks. In: Thrun, S., Saul, L., Schölkopf, B. (eds.) Advances in Neural Information Processing Systems 16. MIT Press, Cambridge (2004)
35. Taylor, G., Hinton, G.: Factored conditional restricted Boltzmann machines for modeling motion style. In: Bottou, L., Littman, M. (eds.) Proceedings of the 26th International Conference on Machine Learning, pp. 1025–1032. Omnipress, Montreal, June 2009
36. Wagner, P., Malisz, Z., Kopp, S.: Gesture and speech in interaction: an overview. Speech Commun. **57**, 209–232 (2014)
37. Weiss, D., Sapp, B., Taskar, B.: Structured prediction cascades (2012). preprint arXiv:1208.3279v1
38. Yu, D., Deng, L., Wang, S.: Learning in the deep-structured conditional random fields. In: NIPS Workshop on Deep Learning for Speech Recognition and Related Applications (2009)

Modeling Warmth and Competence
in Virtual Characters

Truong-Huy D. Nguyen[✉], Elin Carstensdottir, Nhi Ngo,
Magy Seif El-Nasr, Matt Gray, Derek Isaacowitz, and David Desteno

Northeastern University, Boston, MA 02115, USA
{tru.nguyen,magy,ma.gray,d.isaacowitz,
d.desteno}@neu.edu, elin@ccs.neu.edu,
ngo.ho@husky.neu.edu

Abstract. Developing believable virtual characters has been a subject of research in many fields including graphics, animations, artificial intelligence, and human-computer interaction. One challenge towards commoditizing the use of virtual humans is the ability to algorithmically construct characters of different stereotypes. In this paper, we present our efforts in designing virtual characters that can exhibit non-verbal behaviors to reflect varying degrees of warmth and competence, two personality traits shown to underlie social judgments and form stereotypical perception. To embark on developing a computational behavior model that portrays these traits, we adopt an iterative design methodology tuning the design using theory from theatre, animation and psychology, expert reviews, user testing and feedback. Using this process we were able to construct a set of virtual characters that portray variations of warmth and competence through combination of gestures, use of space, and gaze behaviors. In this paper we discuss the design methodology, the resultant system, and initial experiment results showing the promise of the model.

Keywords: Believable virtual characters · Non-verbal behavior · Personality traits

1   Introduction

There has been a growing interest in building high-fidelity virtual characters for serious purposes, such as in military trainings [29, 30], clinical interaction education [19, 24, 27], and inter-cultural communication education [15, 16, 18]. In such applications, creating virtual characters that are able to exhibit personality, mannerisms, and emotions in a similar manner as their human counterparts plays an important role in their success outcome [12]. Previous attempts addressed different challenges such as natural animation [14, 26, 28], personality [1, 10], emotions and their expressions [10, 21, 23]. In this work, we are concerned with the procedural modeling of virtual character stereotypes, characterized along two cognition dimensions: warmth and competence.

Why warmth and competence? Cross-cultural psychological studies have shown that warmth and competence are the fundamental dimensions that humans use to evaluate each other in social interactions [9, 11, 17]. Specifically, these dimensions account for 82% of the variance in perceptions of everyday social behaviors [31].

© Springer International Publishing Switzerland 2015
W.-P. Brinkman et al. (Eds.): IVA 2015, LNAI 9238, pp. 167–180, 2015.
DOI: 10.1007/978-3-319-21996-7_18

Warmth judgments (e.g., perceived kindness, empathy, friendliness, and trustworthiness) are used to evaluate the intent and motives of others, while competence judgments (e.g., perceived intelligence, power, efficacy, and skill) affect the assessment of how effectively others can act on their motives, i.e. perceived ability [17]. The perception of warmth and competence underlies most stereotypical judgments of traits, people, groups, and cultures [3, 9, 17]. For instance, a typical soldier leader's appearance (disciplined, strict, and often cold) elicits a different perception of warmth and competence than that of a family host (kind, accommodating). By investigating how to procedurally depict these two dimensions, we hope to form a foundation on which a wide range of virtual character stereotypes can be constructed to suit the need of specific scenarios.

According to many psychology studies, warmth and competence are expressed and reinforced through non-verbal behaviors. In expressing warmth, voluntary smiles and positive interest cues such as leaning forward, nodding, open gestures and posture have positive effect [4, 25], while the lack of which, together with backward and away body orientations, signals coldness [32]. Competence is inferred from non-verbal behavior cues that relate to dominance, power and assertiveness, such as expansive postures and open gestures, with erectness in posture and dominant poses having the major effect [5, 13].

While there are psychology researches alluding to the importance of these traits and define generally how they are manifested, none of the current theories provide a complete model of how such gestures are to be animated, e.g. how to set the timing of the synchronization of gestures and speech, the mannerism of gestures (e.g. speed, intensity), and the frequency of patterns that signify these traits. In this paper, we present our effort in procedurally modeling warmth and competence traits on virtual characters, using a perception-centric approach that treats perception outcomes as the central validator. Our methodology used combinations of analysis of video recording of actors exhibiting these traits, development, iteration, and feedback from an expert panel composed of two psychologists, a theatrical performance director, a virtual human designer, and an animator. Using this methodology we developed a procedural system and a set of rules to computationally encode non-verbal behaviors. The output animations are empirically validated, showing evidence that the resultant system has indeed produced non-verbal performance that is perceived as intended. Our approach of leveraging collective knowledge from different fields is similar in spirit to the work by Bänziger and Scherer [2] in building the GEMEP corpus of audio-video emotion portrayals.

The organization of the paper is as follows. We first discuss previous related work, before presenting the design methodology and the system in detail. To validate the results of our system, we then discuss a study we conducted to investigate how people perceive the characters we developed, which were specifically designed to show warmth and competence in high and low combinations. Finally, we conclude this paper with a discussion outlining the results and our future work.

2   Previous Work

Most of the works looking at creating personality-specific virtual characters inherit models from psychology to define and reflect personality. For instance, Andre et al. [1] adopted the OCEAN model of personality (openness, conscientiousness, extroversion, agreeableness, and neuroticism) [8] but reduced it to extroversion and agreeableness to exhibit in their setting of social interaction. These traits, together with emotional states, determine the actions (such as choice of dialog or animation sequence) to be carried out by the characters, in a rule-based manner, e.g., extroverted characters tend to engage more with users. The work focuses on verbal cues, i.e. dialog choices. Alternatively, Egges et al. [10] described a general computational framework for modeling personality, emotion and mood. These entities are represented as real-value vectors, the dimensions of which represent different aspects of the respective. They are then updated using the OCC (Ortony, Collins, and Clore) Model of Appraisal [7], which constitutes a set of rules for adjusting emotions based on character' goals, standards and attitudes. While the foundations of these works on psychology are sound, the actual perception of human participants on exhibited behavior and the perception interference among modeled traits have not been examined.

In order to transform psychology behavior models to computational models, we need a language to analyze and describe behaviors. In theatrical performance, there exist notable frameworks for this purpose, such as Laban Movement Analysis (LMA) [20] and McNeill's Growth Point (GP) [22]. While LMA provides a holistic framework to describe bodily movement, GP focuses solely on how hand gestures accompany speech in the discourse of thought. Our gesture analysis is influenced by LMA, especially the Effort component, which describes movement in four dimensions speed, weight, time and flow, but adopts GP notation of gesture space for behavior analysis. Our approach of leveraging collective knowledge in theatrical performance and psychology is similar in spirit to the work by Bänziger and Scherer [2] in building the GEMEP corpus of audio-video emotion portrayals.

Provided a general set of behavior selection rules, we need a system to actualize the rules to generate behaviors, given input speech, and turn them into animations. Researchers have developed procedural 3D articulation systems that can generate gestures from speech text as well as transitions and blends between them. A popular approach is using linguistic and contextual information analysis of text to generate behaviors as demonstrated by the BEAT animation toolkit [7]. Using a set of rules derived from nonverbal conversational research, BEAT mapped the input text to facial, intonational and body gestures. A similar approach was used for developing the Non-Verbal Behavior Generator (NVBG) [23], composed of a set of rules that use affective information, such as the emotional state of the agent, and coping strategy in addition to analysis of the syntactic structure of the text to select appropriate behaviors. The outputs of NVBG are formatted in Behavior Markup Language (BML) [28], an XML-based programming language used for authoring and synchronizing animations. These BMLs are then transformed into synchronized sequences of animations using the animation engine Smartbody [26]. Our system also produces BMLs and relies on Smartbody to animate the results.

3   Design Methodology

We gathered an expert panel consisting of two psychologists, one performance artist, and one virtual character expert to curate the design process. To minimize the effect of preconceived ideas the involved experts might have regarding the output behaviors, we adopted a bottom-up design approach. We first constructed scenarios for our case study, which was determined to be a virtual character doing a sales pitch to a user. We employed theatre actors to act as financial agents with different personality settings: high warmth/high competence (herein abbreviated as HighW-HighC), high warmth/low competence (HighW-LowC), low warmth/low competence (LowW-LowC), and low warmth/high competence (LowW-HighC). The actor is given scripts to perform as in a theatre class, but provided minimal instructions in terms of tactics for their choice of behaviors. The actor then acts out the scenario, the performance of which is recorded (Fig. 1). Next, the expert panel watches the videos to determine whether the performances reflect the intended trait setting appropriately at general perception level. If not, advice is conveyed to actors for improvement. Once a set of performances are decided to be sufficiently discernible, the experts analyze the resulting videos (analysis process and results discussed below) to come up with a set of rules that were then encoded in the virtual character algorithm under development. Videos of the virtual characters were then distributed to the expert panel for analysis and feedback. This process continued until the expert panel was unanimously satisfied with the resulting virtual characters.

There were two female actresses recruited for this process due to the availability of actors and the intended scenario. After both of them acted out the scenarios, the expert panels selected the most convincing performances to use for depiction (Fig. 1).

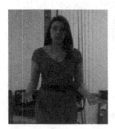 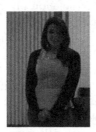 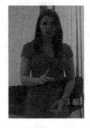 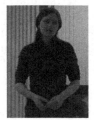

(a) High warmth high competence   (b) High warmth low competence   (c) Low warmth high competence   (d) Low warmth low competence

Fig. 1. Screenshots of recorded actor performances for four personality configurations

3.1 Selection of Depiction Strategies

While there is a consensus on what constitutes competence or warmth, there are different ways to depict incompetence and coldness. This is because while increasing warmth and competence can be achieved by adding more cues (e.g. more open gestures/leaning forward/smiling), decreasing them means taking out cues but not so many as to render the performance completely lifeless. Which cues to neglect? Is there any specific manner to enhance the perception of incompetence and coldness? There is little in the literature to guide us in the design process.

As it turned out, the actors had similar problems determining how to act to depict personalities that involve low setting of traits (i.e. LowW-HighC, HighW-LowC, and LowW-LowC). To resolve the confusion, we gave them guidelines in the form of stereotypical references, inspired by psychology works in how perception of warmth and competence is elicited from group stereotypes [3, 9]. In particular, for LowW-HighC, the stereotype is a financial agent that is high-ranked and under time pressure. HighW-LowC model is an enthusiastic agent who is ready to please the audience but does not know much about the material, while that of LowW-LowC does not care about the pitch nor the customer. The guidelines were given after the first round of performance videos when performance struggle was observed. Eventually, the experts unanimously agreed that the stereotypes led to performances that elicit the intended setting of warmth and competence.

3.2 Analysis of Actor Videos

We conducted two types of analyses on the actor videos. First, we annotated the video with observations, identifying: (1) gesture selection, (2) repeated patterns behavior patterns, and (3) facial expressions and posture. These observations were based on the expert knowledge and experience of the researchers involved. The expert panel then discussed these annotations comparing them and synthesizing a list of patterns to be encoded in the virtual character.

To complement and further deepen the analysis, a second analysis was performed on the videos in latter iterations, to obtain a *space usage profile* for each personality. A space usage profile is a heat map indicating the space occupancy frequency of gestures recorded in a performance. We adopt the gesture space sectors as described by McNeill [22] as the representation. In this model, the performance space in front of an actor is divided into three gesture space sections: Center-Center (CC), Center (C), and Periphery (P). CC is the central section directly in front of the chest, while subsequent sections (C and P) form spatial layers spreading outwards (see Fig. 2a). Using this template, the gesture space profiles of actor videos corresponding to four personalities are obtained (Fig. 2b). For example, low-warmth-low-competence performance consists of gestures mostly in the lower, center P region, while high-warmth-high-competence focuses mostly in the CC and C regions.

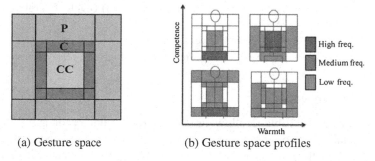

(a) Gesture space   (b) Gesture space profiles

Fig. 2. (a) Gesture space and (b) actor gesture space profiles of four personality settings in two dimensions warmth and competence.

Combining the results of this analysis with prior psychology guidelines in eliciting warmth and competence perception [4, 5, 13, 25, 32], we arrived at two sets of signature behavior rules for each personality setting. Base behaviors, encoded in BML format and continuously executed throughout the experience, are defined for four body parts: eyes, face, hands, and postures (Table 1). Most adjectives in the rules are encoded as canned animations, such as "happy" face depicted as a smile and soft eyes. There are two exceptions that involve temporal encoding, i.e. "frequent gaze diversion" and "alternating" postures. For the former, we change gaze target every 7-10 seconds, and for the latter every 20-40 seconds. "Wobbling posture" is one that involves the body to slightly rock sideward.

Table 2 depicts the behavior rules to be synchronized with text. We use (1) type of gestures in terms of spatial articulation (open/close) to reflect warmth and (2) synchronization with gesture events detected from the text to reflect competence. In addition, rules reflect the stereotypes adopted to depict personalities, such as "giggle, head flicks at mistakes" in HighW-LowC or reducing the occurrence of gestures to only performance-related events in LowW-HighC.

Table 1. Base behavior patterns and depiction strategies for each personality configuration.

Traits	Depiction	Base Behavior Rules (throughout the experience)
HwHc	Attentive, welcoming	(1) Eye fixated on the audience, (2) Happy face, (3) Hands held center/center, (4) posture leaning forward, stable
HwLc	Enthusiastic, innocuous	(1) Eye fixated on the audience, (2) Happy face, (3) Hands held peripheral, down low, (3) wobbling posture
LwHc	Professional, factual	(1) eye fixated on the audience, (2) visibly irritated face, (3) Hands held center/center, (4) posture upright, stable
LwLc	Inattentive, tired	(1) frequent gaze diversion, (2) neutral face, (3) alternating between hands fiddling, arms crossed, shrugs, (4) posture upright

Table 2. Behavior Trait Rules ("events" to be explained in Sect. 3.3)

Traits	Gesture Rules
HwHc	(1) Open gesture; (2) In-sync, all gesture events
HwLc	(1) Open & leans-in; (2) Off-sync 0.3 s, all events; (3) Giggle, head flicks at mistakes
LwHc	(1) Close; (2) In-sync, performance-related events
LwLc	(1) Close; (2) Off-sync ±0.3 s, low frequency, performance-related events

3.3 Behavior Sequencer

The behavior rules in Table 2 allow us to construct a library of atomic behavior animations containing two types of animations, i.e. open and close, coded using BML. Next, to turn the rules into coherent animation sequences for each personality, we devised a behavior sequencer algorithm that takes as input the speech text of the character, a warmth-competence setting, and returns a temporally synchronized behavior series made from behavior blocks in our animation library.

Figure 3 depicts the workflow of the sequencer with its components. The architecture of this system is similar to that of BEAT and NVBG, with major differences

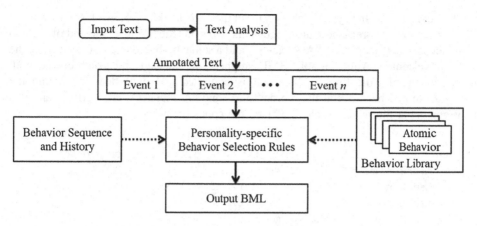

Fig. 3. The flow of BML Sequencer; solid line indicates flow, dotted line influencers.

being the types of annotation tags attached to input text and the behavior selection rules. Note that both BEAT and NVBG output behaviors that are all highly warm and competent according to our analyses, thus not sufficient for our purpose.

The system first analyzes the input text to tag it with *gesture events* of one of the two event types:

1. *Semantic-based events*: Associated with words with specific meanings. In our financial pitching scenario, we identified three sets of semantic-based events, specifically performance-related, mistakes and greetings. For example, the sentence "We have served more than seven millions investors…" has a performance-related event starting at the word "seven", where the speaker is boasting about the significance of her company. A mistake event is attached to meta-words such as "um", "ah", or repeated words indicating stuttering.
2. *Syntactic events*: Associated with punctuations, such as start/end of sentence, comma, question, exclamation marks, etc. These events allow the system to attach animations to pauses in the text.

The system then determines for each event whether it should be accompanied by an *atomic behavior*, based on the personality setting and behavior history. Each atomic behavior contains the following information:

1. *Descriptive characteristics*: describe the mannerism of the behavior executed, e.g. open or close, and the applicable type of gesture events it can be used.
2. *BML codes:* The composition of the animation written in BML
3. *Synchronization time points*: include temporal information that marks the "stroke", i.e., the "beat" of the animation to be synchronized with gesture event time point, the start, and the end of animation.

For each personality, using the behavior rules in Table 2, the sequencer generates a BML file for BML-compliant animation systems, such as SmartBody, to synchronize them with the accompanying final audio files.

For example, as the system takes as input the speech text: "OK, well, shall we start? Welcome to Finnmore Associates!" it detects two syntactic events at the end of the two sentences, i.e., at "start" and "Associates", and a semantic-based event (Greeting) at the word "Welcome". After suitable BML snippets are selected and synchronized with respective words, the final BML result is compiled and outputted, instructing the character to nod her head at the words "start" and "Associates", and perform an open beat gesture at the word "Welcome" (see the codes below).

```
<speech ref="Start" id="sp1" type="application/ssml+xml">
      <mark name="T0" />OK,<mark name="T1" />
      <mark name="T2" />well,<mark name="T3" />
      <mark name="T4" />shall<mark name="T5" />
      <mark name="T6" />we<mark name="T7" />
      <mark name="T8" />start?<mark name="T9" />
      <mark name="T10" />Welcome<mark name="T11" />
      <mark name="T12" />to<mark name="T13" />
      <mark name="T14" />Finnmore<mark name="T15" />
      <mark name="T16" />Associates!<mark name="T17" />
</speech>

<!-- At the word "start" -->
<head type="WAGGLE" sbm:pitch="0.05" start="sp1:T8"/>

<!-- At the word "Welcome" -->
<gaze sbm:handle="lean-in" sbm:fade-in="1.1" start="sp1:T10"/>
<gaze sbm:handle="lean-in" sbm:fade-out="1.1" start="sp1:T12"/>
<gesture name="BEATMEDBT" stroke="sp1:T10" />

<!-- At the word "Associates" -->
<head type="WAGGLE" sbm:pitch="0.1" start="sp1:T16"/>
```

3.4   Analysis of Virtual Behavior Videos

The results of the behavior sequencer system, in the form of animation videos (Fig. 4), are watched by the experts for critique and identification of issues, such as gesture selection issues (synchrony, manner) and whether they elicit intended perception. In addition, informal sanity checks were performed regularly using students through informal feedback gathering. At the end of this step, we decide to iterate or finalize the system for a validation study. Some comments for improvement include: action transition is not smooth enough, or need more gestures for a natural movement effect, or the character is not perceived to as warm or competent enough. These comments inform the adjustment of the behavior rule sets, as well as enrichment of the animation library should the current set be deemed insufficient.

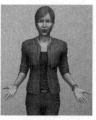 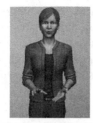 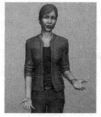 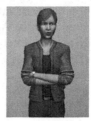

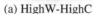

(a) HighW-HighC   (b) LowW-HighC   (c) HighW-LowC   (d) LowW-LowC

Fig. 4. Animations of the four personality configurations.

4 Validation Study

To validate the resultant computational models of personality-specific behaviors, we conducted a crowd-sourced validation study on Amazon Mechanical Turk. The validation is meant to examine the effect of our behavior models on user perception. Besides, since prior works have posited that there is an age difference in social judgements [6, 33], we want to validate our models with different age ranges as well.

4.1 Study Design

Four animations returned by the final system are recorded as four video clips, each corresponding to one trait settings and about thirty seconds to one minute long (see supplementary materials). Each clip shows a virtual character delivering a pitch to the viewer, with audio muted so that user perception is based solely on non-verbal performance. Participants of different age groups, recruited on Amazon Mechanical Turk (AMT) are shown one video at a time, in a randomized order, and asked to rate on a scale from 1 (lowest) to 10 (highest) the avatar's warmth and competence. They were then asked to explain the reasons for the ratings.

4.2 Data Collection and Results

We received responses from 150 AMT participants in three age ranges, 50 younger adults (YAs) age 18–34 years old, 50 middle-aged (MAs) age 35–64, and 33 older adults (OAs) age 65 and above (note that it is a lot harder to recruit older adults on AMT than middle-aged and younger adults). After collecting rating data, we observed some noise in the responses. A few participants appeared to skip through the animation videos instead of fully watching them before reporting their ratings, in which case the reported results are not genuine. This behavior is detected if the total time spent is less than the sum of individual clips' durations. We removed the data of such participants from our data pool, leaving a total of 32 YAs, 38 MAs, and 28 OAs for our analysis. Due to the uneven group sizes, age was used as a continuous variable in our analysis.

Quantitative Results. We conducted a 2 (character warmth: low, high) × 2 (character competence: low, high) Multivariate Analysis of Variance (MANOVA) on the warmth and competence ratings, with age as a covariate. This analysis was followed by two univariate ANOVAs on warmth and competence ratings alone. These analyses allow us to dissect the effect of the independent variables (intended warmth and competence levels) and covariate (age) on the dependent variables (warmth and competence ratings) altogether and individually. The numerical results are depicted in Fig. 5.

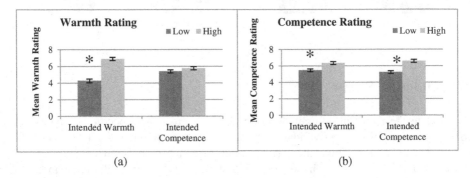

Fig. 5. Mean warmth and competence ratings as a function of intended warmth and intended competence levels encoded in the animation videos; (*) denotes significance at $p < .001$.

In summary, the analyses showed that our videos were perceived as intended: high-warmth characters were perceived as warmer than low-warmth characters, regardless of whether they were competent or not (Fig. 5a); and high-competence characters were perceived as more competent than low-competence characters regardless of whether they were warm or not (Fig. 5b). Interestingly, while different competence levels did not affect perception of warmth ($p = .96$) (Fig. 5a), high-warmth characters were perceived as more competent than low-warmth characters (Fig. 5b). This pattern of result was clarified by the significant warmth x competence interaction, which means that the effects of intended warmth levels on warmth and competence ratings differ depending on the intended level of competence. Specifically, if a character is highly warm, their competence level does not affect how warm they are perceived ($p = .11$). However, if a character is low-warmth, they are perceived as warmer if they are more competent ($p < .001$). In contrast, at both levels of competence, intended high warmth characters were perceived as warmer than intended low warmth characters (p values $\leq .002$). It appears that perception of warmth can be influenced by how competent a character is, but the reverse might not be true: there was no evidence that levels of competence can moderate the perception of warmth beyond the intended warmth levels. Finally, age was not a significant predictor of warmth and competence ratings across videos, showing that there was no evidence that people of different ages rated the videos differently.

Qualitative Results. While the numerical validation results show promising evidence, the self-reported explanations on the ratings yield insights on how the participants actually feel towards the characters. A summary of the qualitative comments is shown in Table 3 at the end of this section.

Table 3. The counts of positive/neutral/negative comments and most used words in comments on warmth and competence in each animation clips (HwHc, HwLc, LwHc, and LwLc).

		Young Adults		Middle-Aged		Old Adults	
		Pos/Neu /Neg	Most used adjectives	P/N/N	Adjectives	P/N/N	Adjectives
Hw Hc	W	21/7/3	warm, friendly	20/16/3	leaning, inviting	18/9/1	warm, relaxed
	C	24/6/1	competent, sure	28/9/2	confident, sincere	20/5/3	confident
Hw Lc	W	23/7/1	warm, friendly	26/11/2	sincere, nervous	18/8/2	warm, friendly
	C	14/14/3	unsure, incompetent	23/14/2	comfortable, competent	12/13/ 3	nervous, unconfident
Lw Hc	W	7/13/11	angry	10/18/11	serious	10/9/9	not warm
	C	18/12/1	confident, angry	22/12/5	confident, competent	13/9/6	stiff, angry
Lw Lc	W	2/10/19	nervous, not warm	6/14/19	nervous	5/8/15	nervous
	C	4/9/18	nervous, unsure	9/9/21	nervous, fidgeting	1/13/1 4	nervous, fidgety, shifty

Table 3 shows the number of positive, neutral and negative comments for each clip with respect to each trait rating, along with most frequently used words in each category. Positive comments include praises such as "her gestures were personable" (on warmth) or "firm and confident" (competence), while negative such as "seemed very serious and condescending" (warmth) or "nervous and disorganized" (competence). Neutral comments are those that either indicate perception indifference, e.g. "average and not very adequate", or are unrelated, e.g. commenting on competence for warmth rating. As it turns out, some participants used their perception of warmth to rate competence and vice versa.

Some of our observations include:

- Some comments indicate ratings were based on clothing and appearance (hair color, outfit). For example, in some cases, the character of LowW-LowC setting receives high competence rating because "her clothes are neat and respectable", or "she seems competent and professional in appearance". This happens on LowW-HighC character too; sometimes her outfit leads to high warmth rating. This shows that the outlook design of virtual avatars can be of great impact to user perception.
- Some comments indicate clear inference of competence on warmth perception, and this appears most often in mixed trait characters (HighW-LowC, and vice versa). For instance, on HighW-LowC character, low warmth rating (3 and 4): "She acts too nervous to be warm. She lacks confidence and that affects how the audience embraces her", "seemed unsure of herself", i.e. using competence cues to judge

warmth. On the same character, high competence rating (9): "seems like she's the friendliest and welcoming", i.e. using warmth cues to judge competence.

- Overall, it is hardest to summarize the comments of older adults, as they often quote reasons that are unrelated to intended cues, such as appearance/outfits, e.g. "looks smarter…based on her clothes" (note how they have a lot of neutral comments, instead of positive or negative in Table 3). Older adults also discuss about warmth a lot more than competence, regardless of the trait type they are commenting on.

5 Conclusion and Future Work

In this work, we have proposed a novel procedural model for behavior generation that reflects warmth and competence, two of the key personality traits that govern social judgments in human interactions. To the best of our knowledge, this is the first work of its kind in modeling these two important traits in virtual characters. The presented model demonstrated the fruitfulness of our interdisciplinary approach for design, which is to combine cross-discipline knowledge from experts in animation, theatre, and psychology within our expert panel. This helped synthesize the final computational model using several theories and technologies such as LMA and GP (theatrical performance), animation technologies, and personality modeling (psychology). The validation results showed the promise of the model, as it is able to endow virtual characters with non-verbal behaviors that amount to the intended perception of warmth and competence. That said, the current system has only been validated in a non-interactive business scenario; it remains a question whether the obtained rules transcend to other real-life settings as well. In the future, we plan to examine the performance of this model in interactive settings that allow participants to engage in bi-directional conversations with virtual agents.

Acknowledgements. We would like to thank Stacy Marsella for his insightful discussions and advice, Stacy Marcotte for helping us setting up validation experiments, and Teresa Dey for the character animations. This research is supported by Northeastern Tier 1 Grant.

References

1. André, E., Klesen, M., Gebhard, P., Allen, S., Rist, T.: Integrating models of personality and emotions into lifelike characters. Affect. Interact. **1814**, 1–15 (2000)
2. Banziger, T., Scherer, K.R.: (University of G. Introducing the Geneva Multimodal Emotion Portrayal (GEMEP) Corpus. A blueprint for an affectively competent agent: Cross-fertilization between Emotion Psychology, Affective Neuroscience, and Affective Computing (2010)
3. Brambilla, M., Sacchi, S., Castellini, F., Riva, P.: The effects of status on perceived warmth and competence: malleability of the relationship between status and stereotype content. Soc. Psychol. **41**(2010), 82–87 (2010)
4. Carli, L.L., LaFleur, S.J., Loeber, C.C.: Nonverbal behavior, gender, and influence. J. Pers. Soc. Psychol. **68**, 1030–1041 (1995)

5. Carney, D.R., Hall, J.A., LeBeau, L.S.: Beliefs about the nonverbal expression of social power. J. Nonverbal Behav. **29**(2005), 105–123 (2005)
6. Castle, E., Eisenberger, N.I., Seeman, T.E., Moons, W.G., Boggero, I.A., Grinblatt, M.S., Taylor, S.E.: Neural and behavioral bases of age differences in perceptions of trust. Proc. Nat. Acad. Sci. USA **109**(51), 20848–20852 (2012)
7. Colby, B.N., Ortony, A., Clore, G.L., Collins, A.: The cognitive structure of emotions. Contemp. Sociol. **18**, 851–859 (1989)
8. Costa, P.T., McCrae, R.R.: Normal personality assessment in clinical practice: the NEO personality inventory. Psychol. Assess. **4**, 5–13 (1992)
9. Cuddy, A.J.C., Glick, P., Beninger, A.: The dynamics of warmth and competence judgments, and their outcomes in organizations. Res. Organ. Behav. **31**, 73–98 (2011)
10. Egges, A., Kshirsagar, S., Magnenat-Thalmann, N.: A model for personality and emotion simulation. In: Palade, V., Howlett, R.J., Jain, L. (eds.). LNCS, vol. 2773, pp. 453–461. Springer, Heidelberg (2003)
11. Fiske, S.T., Cuddy, A.J.C., Glick, P.: Universal dimensions of social cognition: warmth and competence. Trends Cogn. Sci. **11**(2), 77–83 (2007)
12. Fox, J., Ahn, S.J(.: Recommendations for designing maximally effective and persuasive health agents. In: Bickmore, T., Marsella, S., Sidner, C. (eds.) IVA 2014. LNCS, vol. 8637, pp. 178–181. Springer, Heidelberg (2014)
13. Hall, J.A., Coats, E.J., LeBeau, L.S.: Nonverbal behavior and the vertical dimension of social relations: a meta-analysis. Psychol. Bull. **131**(2005), 898–924 (2005)
14. Hartholt, A., Traum, D., Marsella, S.C., Shapiro, A., Stratou, G., Leuski, A., Morency, L.-P., Gratch, J.: All together now. In: Aylett, R., Krenn, B., Pelachaud, C., Shimodaira, H. (eds.) IVA 2013. LNCS, vol. 8108, pp. 368–381. Springer, Heidelberg (2013)
15. Johnsen, K., Raij, A., Stevens, A., Lind, D.S., Lok, B.: The validity of a virtual human experience for interpersonal skills education. In: Proceedings of the SIGCHI Conference on Human factors in Computing Systems - CHI 2007, p. 1049, New York, USA, April 2007
16. Johnson, W.L., Valente, A.: Tactical language and culture training systems: using ai to teach foreign languages and cultures. AI Mag. **30**(2), 72–83 (2009)
17. Judd, C.M., James-Hawkins, L., Yzerbyt, V., Kashima, Y.: Fundamental dimensions of social judgment: understanding the relations between judgments of competence and warmth. J. Pers. Soc. Psychol. **89**(2005), 899–913 (2005)
18. Kim, J., Hill, R.W., Durlach, P., Lane, H.C., Forbell, E., Core, M., Marsella, S.C., Pynadath, D.V., Hart, J.: BiLAT: a game-based environment for practicing negotiation in a cultural context. Int. J. Artif. Intell. Educ. **19**, 289–308 (2009). Issue on Ill-Defined Domains
19. Kleinert, H.L., Sanders, C., Mink, J., Nash, D., Johnson, J., Boyd, S., Challman, S.: Improving student dentist competencies and perception of difficulty in delivering care to children with developmental disabilities using a virtual patient module. J. Dental Educ. **71**(2), 279–286 (2007)
20. Laban, R., Lawrence, F.C.: Effort: Economy of Human Movement. Macdonald & Evans, London (1979)
21. Marsella, S., Gratch, J., Petta, P.: Computational models of emotion. In: Scherer, K.R., Banziger, T., Roesch, E. (eds.) A Blueprint for an Affectively Competent Agent: Cross-Fertilization Between Emotion Psychology, Affective Neuroscience, and Affective Computing, pp. 21–41. Oxford University Press, Oxford (2010)
22. McNeill, D.: Hand and Mind: What Gestures Reveal About Thought. University of Chicago Press, Chicago (1992)
23. Reilly, S.: Believable Social and Emotional Agents. Carnegie Mellon University (1996)

24. Sanders, C.L., Kleinert, H.L., Free, T., Slusher, I., Clevenger, K., Johnson, S., Boyd, S.E.: Caring for children with intellectual and developmental disabilities: virtual patient instruction improves students' knowledge and comfort level. J. Pediatr. Nurs. **22**(6), 457–466 (2007)

25. Surakka, V., Hietanen, J.K.: Facial and emotional reactions to Duchenne and non-Duchenne smiles. Int. J. Psychophysiol. **29**(1998), 23–33 (1998)

26. Thiebaux, M., Marsella, S., Marshall, A.N. and Kallmann, M.: SmartBody: behavior realization for embodied conversational agents. In: Proceedings of the 7th International Joint Conference on Autonomous Agents and Multiagent Systems, vol. 1, pp. 151–158, May 2008

27. Triola, M., Feldman, H., Kalet, A.L., Zabar, S., Kachur, E.K., Gillespie, C., Anderson, M., Griesser, C., Lipkin, M.: A randomized trial of teaching clinical skills using virtual and live standardized patients. J. Gen. Intern. Med. **21**(5), 424–429 (2006)

28. Vilhjálmsson, H., Cantelmo, N., Cassell, J., Chafai, N.E., Kipp, M., Kopp, S., Mancini, M., Marsella, S., Marshall, A.N., Pelachaud, C., et al.: The behavior markup language: recent developments and challenges. Intell. Virtual Agents **2007**, 99–111 (2007)

29. Virtual reality used to train Soldiers in new training simulator (2012). http://www.army.mil/article/84453. Accessed 09 October 2014

30. Virtual training puts the "real" in realistic environment (2013). http://www.army.mil/article/97582/Virtual_training_puts_the__real__in_realistic_environment/. Accessed 09 October 2014

31. Wojciszke, B., Bazinska, R., Jaworski, M.: On the dominance of moral categories in impression formation. Pers. Soc. Psychol. Bull. **23**, 1 157–1 172 (1998)

32. Word, C.O., Zanna, M.P., Cooper, J.: The nonverbal mediation of self-fulfilling prophecies in interracial interaction. J. Exp. Soc. Psychol. **10**, 109–120 (1974)

33. Ybarra, O., Chan, E., Park, D.: Young and old adults' concerns about morality and competence. Motiv. Emot. **25**(2001), 85–100 (2001)

Storytelling Agents with Personality and Adaptivity

Chao Hu[1]([✉]), Marilyn A. Walker[1], Michael Neff[2], and Jean E. Fox Tree[1]

[1] University of California, Santa Cruz, USA
{zhu,mawalker,foxtree}@ucsc.edu
[2] University of California, Davis, USA
mpneff@ucdavis.edu

Abstract. We explore the expression of personality and adaptivity through the gestures of virtual agents in a storytelling task. We conduct two experiments using four different dialogic stories. We manipulate agent personality on the extraversion scale, whether the agents adapt to one another in their gestural performance and agent gender. Our results show that subjects are able to perceive the intended variation in extraversion between different virtual agents, independently of the story they are telling and the gender of the agent. A second study shows that subjects also prefer adaptive to nonadaptive virtual agents.

Keywords: Personality · Gesture generation and variation · Gestural adaptation · Story telling · Collaborative story telling

1   Introduction

It is a truism that every person is a unique individual. However, when interacting with or observing others, people make inferences that generalize from specific, observed behaviors to explanations for those behaviors in terms of dispositional traits [1]. One theory that attempts to account for such inferences is the Big Five theory of personality, which posits that consistent patterns in the way individuals behave, feel, and think across different situations, can be described in terms of trait adjectives, such as sociable, shy, trustworthy, disorganized or imaginative [2,3].

Previous work suggests both that personality traits are *real*, and that they are *useful* as a basis for models for Intelligent Virtual Agents (IVAs) for a range of applications [4-8]. Many findings about how people perceive other humans appear to carry over to their perceptions of IVAs [9-13]. Research suggests that human users are more engaged and thus learn more when interacting with characters endowed with personality and emotions, and that a character's personality, surprisingly, affects users' perceptions of the system's competence [14,15]. Recent experiments show that the Big Five theory is a useful basis for multimodal integration of nonverbal and linguistic behavior, and that automatically generated variations in personality are perceived as intended [16-19].

© Springer International Publishing Switzerland 2015
W.-P. Brinkman et al. (Eds.): IVA 2015, LNAI 9238, pp. 181–193, 2015.
DOI: 10.1007/978-3-319-21996-7_19

However, personality is not expressed in a void. Conversants dynamically adapt to their conversational partner, both in conversation and when telling stories, and using both verbal and nonverbal features [20–24], *inter alia*. There is also evidence that people prefer IVAs that align with human behavior, such as by mimicking head movements [22] or speech style [11]. A human's attraction to an IVA is increased when the IVA adapts its personality to the human over time rather than maintaining a consistently similar personality [11]. Inspired by previous work, this paper:

- Introduces a novel task of two IVAs co-telling a story.
- Varies IVA personality through gestural parameters of gesture rate, speed, expanse and form.
- Varies whether the IVAs adapt to one another's gestures in gesture rate, speed, expanse and form and use of specific gestures.
- Tests the effect of, and interaction between, these variations with human perceptual experiments and report our results.

Our stories come from weblogs of personal narratives [25] whose content has been regenerated as dialogues to support story co-telling. Example dialogs from the four we use in our experiments are in Figs. 1 and 5 in Sect. 3. These dialogs have a fixed linguistic representation and use oral language, discourse markers, shorter sentences, and repetitions and confirmations between speakers, as well as techniques to make the story sound like the two speakers experienced the event together. Our aim is to mimic the finding that storytelling in the wild is naturally conversational [24], and that the style of oral storytelling among friends varies depending on their personalities [24].

Protest Story
A1: Hey, do you remember that day? It was a work day, I remember there was some big event going on.
B1: Yeah, that day was the start of the G20 summit. It's an event that happens every year.
A2: Oh yeah, right, it's that meeting where 20 of the leaders of the world come together. They talk about how to run their governments effectively.
B2: Yeah, exactly. There were many leaders coming together. They had some pretty different ideas about what's the best way to run a government.
A3: And the people who follow the governments also have different ideas. Whenever world leaders meet, there will be protesters expressing different opinions. I remember the protest that happened just along the street where we work.
B3: It looked peaceful at the beginning....
A4: Right, until a bunch of people started rebelling and creating a riot.
B4: Oh my gosh, it was such a riot, police cars were burned, and things were thrown at cops.
A5: Police were in full riot gear to stop the violence.
B5: Yeah, they were. When things got worse, the protesters smashed the windows of stores.
A6: Uh huh. And then police fired tear gas and bean bag bullets.
B6: That's right, tear gas and bean bag bullets... It all happened right in front of our store.
A7: That's so scary.
B7: It was kind of scary, but I had never seen a riot before, so it was kind of interesting for me.

Fig. 1. Protest dialogue, with fixed level of linguistic adaptation.

We carry out two experiments. In the personality experiment, we elicit subjects' perceptions of two virtual agents designed to have different personalities. In the gestural adaptation experiment, we ask whether subjects prefer adaptive vs. non adaptive agents. Our results show that agents intended to be extroverted or introverted are perceived as such, and that subjects prefer adaptive stories. Section 2 describes our story dialog corpus. Sections 3 and 4 presents our experimental design and results. In order to compare more concisely with our work, we delay discussion of related work until Sect. 5, where we discuss our results and describe future work.

2   Story Dialog Corpus

We first annotate dialogs with a general underspecified gesture representation, then we prepare several versions of each dialog by varying experimental parameters such as agent extraversion and adaptivity.

Table 1. The gestural correlates of extraversion.

Parameter	Introvert findings	Extravert findings
Gesture amplitude	Narrow	Wide, broad
Gesture direction	Inward, self-contact	outward, Table-plane and horizontal spreading gesture
Gesture rate	Low	High, more movements of head, hands and legs
Gesture speed, response time	Slow	Fast, quick
Gesture connection	Low smoothness, rhythm disturbance	Smooth, fluent
Body part		Head tilt, shoulder erect, chest forward, limbs spread, elbows away from body, hands away from body, legs apart, legs leaning, bouncing, shaking of legs

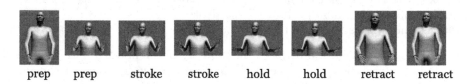

prep   prep   stroke   stroke   hold   hold   retract   retract

Fig. 2. Prep, stroke, hold and retract phases of gesture Cup_Horizontal.

Gesture Annotation. We build on Neff et al.'s work on the impact of extraversion on gesture in IVAs [17], as shown in Table 1, and select parameters to depict both introverted and extraverted IVAs by varying gesture amplitude, direction, rate and speed. We test user perceptions of IVA personality during story co-telling without adaptation, and then test whether we can achieve effects on personality perception when IVAs adapt to one another.

We construct the dialogs for the two IVAs manually from the monolog webblogs. We then generate audio for the utterances of each IVA using the AT&T Text to Speech engine (female voice Crystal and male voice Mike). We annotate the dialogs with a general, underspecified gestural representation, specifying both potential gestures and gesture placements. This representation allows us to procedurally generate hundreds of possible combinations of story co-tellings varying both gestural performance (personality) and adaptation. Annotators can insert a gesture when the dialog introduces new concepts, and add gesture adaptation (mimicry) when there are repetitions or

A1: [1.90s](Cup, RH 0.46s) Hey, do you remember [3.17s](PointingAbstract, RH 0.37s) that day? It was a [4.97s](Cup_Horizontal, 2H 0.57s) work day, I remember there was some big event [7.23s](SweepSide1, RH 0.35s) going on.

B1: Yeah, that day was the start of [9.43s](Cup_Down_alt, 2H 0.21s) the G20 summit. It's an event that happens [12.55s](CupBeats_Small, 2H 0.37s) every year.

A2: Oh yeah, [14.2s](Cup_Vert, RH 0.54s) right, it's that meeting where 20 of the leaders of the world [17.31s](**Regressive, RH 1.14s**) come together. They talk about how to run their governments [20.72s](**Cup, RH 0.46s**) effectively.

B2: Yeah, [22.08s](**Cup_Up, 2H 0.34s**) exactly. There were many leaders [24.38s](**Regressive, LH 1.14s**/Eruptive, LH 0.76s) coming together. They had some pretty [26.77s](**WeighOptions, 2H 0.6s**) different ideas about what's the best way to [29.13s]*(**Cup, RH 0.46s**/ShortProgressive, RH 0.38s) run a government.

A3: And [30.25s]*(PointingAbstract, RH 0.37s) the people who follow the governments also have [32.56s](**WeighOptions, 2H 0.6s**/Cup, 2H 0.46s) different ideas. Whenever [34.67s](**Cup_Up, 2H 0.34s**/Dismiss, 2H 0.47s) world leaders meet, there will be protesters expressing [37.80s](Away, 2H 0.4s) different opinions. I remember the [39.87s]*(Reject, RH 0.44s) protest that happened just [41.28s](SideArc, 2H 0.57s) along the street where we work.

B3: ......

Fig. 3. Sample blog story dialog with gesture annotations (two versions). Format of annotation: [gesture stroke begin time](gesture name, hand use, gesture stroke duration).

confirmations in the dialog. The decisions of where to insert a gesture and which gesture to insert are mainly subjective. We use gestures from a database of 271 motion captured gestures, including metaphoric, iconic, deictic and beat gestures. Figure 2 illustrates how every gesture can be generated to include up to 4 phases [26]:

- prep: move arms from default resting position or the end point of the last gesture to the start position of the stroke
- stroke: perform the movement that conveys most of the gesture's meaning
- hold: remain at the final position in the stroke
- retract: move arms from the previous position to a default resting position

Figure 3 shows the first 5 turns of the protest story annotated with gestures. The timing information of the gestures comes from the TTS audio timeline. Each gesture annotation contains information in the following format: [gesture stroke begin time](gesture name, hand use, stroke duration). For example, in the first gesture "[1.90 s](Cup, RH 0.46 s)", gesture stroke begins at 1.9 s of the dialog audio, it is a Cup gesture, uses the right hand, and the gesture stroke lasts 0.46 s. Research has shown that people prefer gestures occurring earlier than the accompanying speech [27]. Thus in this annotation, a gesture stroke is positioned 0.2 s before the beginning of the gesture's following word. For example, the first word after gesture "Cup" is "Hey", it begins at 2.1 s, then the stroke of gesture "Cup" begins at 1.9 s.

Our gesture annotation does not specify features associated with particular gestures (i.e. gesture amplitude, direction and speed). But these features can be easily adjusted in our animation software, which can vary the amplitude, direction and speed. The default gesture annotation frequency is designed for extraverts, with a gesture rate of 1–2 gestures per sentence. For an introverted agent, a lower gesture rate is achieved by removing some of the gestures. In this way, both speakers' gestural performance can vary from introverted to extraverted using the whole scale of parameter values for every parameter.

In addition, we can also vary gestural adaptation in the annotation. In extravert and extravert gestural adaptation (based on the model described in [28]), two extraverts move together towards a more extraverted personality. Gesture rate is increased by adding extra gestures (marked with an asterisk "*"). Specific gestures are copied as part of adaptation, especially when the co-telling involves repetition and confirmation. Gestures in bold indicate copying of gesture form (adaptation), gestures after the slash "/" are non-adapted. Combined with personality variations for gestures described in the previous paragraph, it is possible to produce combinations of two agents with any level of extraversion engaged in a conversation with or without gestural adaptation.

Stimulus Construction. We currently have 50 annotated story dialogs. In this experiment, we use four stories with different subject matter: protest, pet, storm and gardening, as illustrated in Figs. 1 and 5. Figure 4 shows a screenshot of the stimuli. We use our own animation software to generate the stimuli based on the specified gesture script. This software uses motion captured data for the wrist path, hand shape and hand orien-

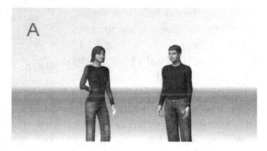

Fig. 4. A snapshot of the experimental stimuli.

tation for each gesture stroke, motion captured data for body movement, and spline based interpolation for preparation and retractions. It also uses simplified physical simulation to add nuance to the motion. A gesture contains up to 4 phases: prep, stroke, hold and retract: we insert a hold and connecting prep between two strokes if they are less than 2.5 s away from each other. Otherwise, we insert a retraction.

The animation software takes as input scripts specifying gesture sequences, along with modifying edits (specifying features such as gesture amplitude, direction and speed), and produces an animation meeting the constraints as output. This is exported as a bvh file, that is then imported into Maya for rendering on the final model. In the video, two IVAs stand almost face-to-face, but each has an 55° angle "cheat" towards the audience, as is commonly used in stage performances. We also add background body movements [29] and head rotation movements for both agents. Both of these are kept constant for each stimuli pair.

3   Experiment Method

We conduct two separate experiments, one on personality variation during co-telling a story, and the second using the same personalities but with and without adaptation.

Experiment 1: Personality Variation. We prepared two versions of the video of the story co-telling for each of the four stories, one where the female is extraverted (higher values for gesture rate, gesture expanse, height, outwardness, speed and scale) and the male is introverted (lower values for those gesture features) and one where only the genders (virtual agent model and voice) of the agents are switched. The dialogue scripts and corresponding gesture forms do not vary from one co-telling to another. This results in 8 video stimuli for four stories.

Pet Story
A1: I have always felt like I was a dog person but our two cats are great. They are much more low maintenance than dogs are.
B1: Yeah, I'm really glad we got our first one at a no-kill shelter.
A2: I had wanted a little kitty, but the only baby kitten they had scratched the crap out of me the minute I picked it up so that was a big "NO".
B2: Well, the no-kill shelter also had what they called "teenagers", which were cats around four to six months old...a bit bigger than the little kitties.
A3: Oh yeah, I saw those "teenagers". They weren't exactly adults, but they were a bit bigger than the little kittens.
B3: Yeah one of them really stood out to me then– mostly because she jumped up on a shelf behind us and smacked me in the head with her paw.
A4: Yeah, we definitely had a winner!
B4: I had no idea how much personality a cat can have. Our first kitty loves playing. She will play until she is out of breath.
A5: Yeah, and then after playing for a long time she likes to look at you like she's saying, "Just give me a minute, I'll get my breath back and be good to go."
B5: Sometimes I wish I had that much enthusiasm for anything in my life.
A6: Yeah, me too. Man, she has so much enthusiasm for chasing string too! To her it's the best thing ever. Well ok, maybe it runs a close second to hair scrunchies!
B6: Oh I love playing fetch with her with hair scrunchies!
A7: Yeah, you can just throw the scrunchies down the stairs and she runs at top speed to fetch them. And she always does this until she's out of breath!
B7: If only I could work out that hard before I was out of breath... I'd probably be thinner.

Fig. 5. Pet dialogue, with fixed level of linguistic adaptation.

We conducted a between-subjects experiment on Mechanical Turk where we first ask Turkers to answer the TIPI [30] personality survey for themselves, and then answer it for only one of the agents in the video, after watching the video as many times as they like. Thus for each video stimulus, there are two surveys. We ran our 16 surveys as 16 HITs (Human Intelligence Tasks) on Mechanical Turk, requesting 20 subjects per HIT (each worker can only do one of the tasks), which results in 320 judgements. The average completion time for the 8 HITs on Mechanical Turk was 5 min 15 s. The average stimulus length was 1 min 32 s. Since the survey is hosted outside Mechanical Turk, sometimes we get more than 20 subjects for each HIT.

Experiment 2: Gestural Adaptation. For the adaptive experiment, both agents are designed to be extroverted. We chose to use two extraverted agents because we have foundations from previous work showing the adaptation model between two extraverted speakers [28] (where both agents become more extraverted). We use only a part of each story for one experimental task. The stimuli for one task has two variations: adapted and non-adapted. Both stimuli use the same audio, contain 2 to 4 dialog turns with the same gestures as an introduction to the story (which we refer to as context), and the next (and last) dialog turn with gesture adaptation or without gesture adaptation (which we refer to as response). Adaptation only begins to occur in the last dialog turn. In this way, subjects can get to know the story through the context, and compare the responses to decide whether they like the adapted or non-adapted version.

- Non-adapted: In the last dialog turn, the extraverted agent maintains his or her gesture rate (1–2 gestures per sentence), expanse, height, outwardness, speed and scale. There is no copying of specific gestures.
- Adapted: In the last dialog turn, the extraverted agent increases the gesture rate (1–3 gestures per sentence), expanse (18 cm further from center), height (10 cm higher), outwardness (10 cm more outward), speed (1.25 times faster) and scale (1.5 times larger). Figure 6 shows the same gesture with different expanses and heights. In the adapted version, specific gestures are copied (e.g. gestures in bold font in Fig. 3).

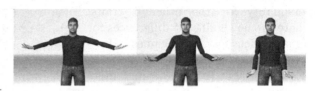

Thus every story has two versions. One version ends with the female agent's response, another ends with the male agent's response. For example, Garden ABA has three turns, ending with the female agent adapting to the male, and Garden ABAB has

Fig. 6. Virtual agent with different gesture expanse and height for the same gesture.

four turns, ending with the male agent adapting to the female. Every version consists of two conditions (adapted and non-adapted versions) and a short survey. The order of the two conditions is random for every participant. But there is a letter mark assigned to every video for easy reference (see Fig. 4).

Subjects are asked to watch the two stimuli first, and then finish the survey. Subjects are told that the audio of the two videos is the same, but only the last few gestures of the female/male agent are different. Subjects are also advised to watch the video as many times as they want. The survey has two questions: (1) Which video is a better story co-telling based on the gestures? (2) Please explain the reason behind your choice to the previous question (which we refer to as the "why" question). Our primary aim is to determine whether people perceive the adaptation and whether it makes a better story.

We ran our 8 tasks for 4 stories as 8 HITs on Mechanical Turk, requesting 25 subjects per task. The average completion time for the 8 tasks on Mechanical Turk was 2 min 53 s. The average stimulus length was 35.3 s. This means that, on average, a subject spent 1 min 43 s answering the questions. We removed subjects who failed to state their reasons of preference in the "why" question.

4   Experimental Results

4.1   Personality Results

We conducted a three-way ANOVA with agent intended personality, agent gender and story as independent variables and perceived agent personality as the dependent variable. See Table 2. The results show that subjects clearly perceive the intended extraverted or intended introverted personality of the two agents ($F = 67.1$, $p < .001$). There is no main effect for story (as intended in our design), but there is an interaction effect between story and intended personality, with the introverted agent in the storm story being seen as much more introverted than in the other stories ($F = 7.5$, $p < .001$). There is no significant variation by agent gender ($F = 2.3$, $p = .14$).

Since previous work suggests that personality is perceived for an agent along all Big Five dimensions whether it is designed to be manifest or not [16, 31], we also conducted a two-way ANOVA by story and agent intended personality for the other 4 traits. There are no significant differences for Conscientiousness, or Openness. However Introverted agents are seen as more agreeable ($p = .008$) and more emotionally stable ($p = .016$). There were no significant differences by story except that both agents in the Storm story were seen as less open, presumably because the content of the story is about how scary the storm is.

Table 2. Experiment results: participant evaluated extraversion scores (range from 1–7, with 1 being the most introverted and 7 being the most extraverted).

Story	Intro-agent	Extra-agent
Garden	4.2	5.4
Pet	4.7	5.0
Protest	4.2	5.3
Storm	3.7	5.7

4.2   Adaption Results

The results in Table 3 show that across all the videos, the mean percentage of people who preferred the adapted version was 64 % (19 % standard deviation), which is marginally better than a predicted preference of 50 %, $t(7) = 2.15$, $p = .07$. Analysis of participants' descriptions of why they preferred one video over another shows 4 distinct categories of reasons of why people made their choices (see Table 4).

Subjects who preferred the adapted versions said that the gestures fit the dialog better ("adapted good gestures" in Table 4): the subjects stated that the adapted versions had gestures that "flowed better with the words", were "more natural", "more appropriate to what he said", and "relevant to the dialog", and that they "could imagine a friend making various hand gestures similar" to the ones in the story. Another reason was that gestures were "more animated" ("adapted animated"): the adapted version had "more hand gestures", and the agent "used his arms more", "gestured more", and "was much more alive". In contrast, in the non-adapted version, the agent "seemed very bored" and "wanted to end the conversation". This indicates that the subjects preferred agents with a higher gesture rate. Ten subjects commented on the expanse, height, scale and speed of the gestures: they chose the adapted version because the agent "gestured higher in the air", "making wider, grander gestures" that were "more expansive" and "bigger". And in the non-adapted version, the gestures were "too slow". However, there was no comment about the copying of gestures, possibly

Table 3. Experiment results: number and percentage of subjects who preferred the adapted (A) stimulus and the non-adapted (NA) stimulus. The letters in the story version refer to dialog turns by speaker A or B. For example, ABA means A takes dialog turns 1 and 3 in the stimuli, while B takes dialog turn 2.

Story version	#A	#NA	%A	%NA
Garden ABA	11	9	55 %	45 %
Garden ABAB	20	2	91 %	9 %
Pet ABABA	10	13	43 %	57 %
Pet ABABAB	19	5	79 %	21 %
Protest ABAB	8	11	42 %	58 %
Protest ABABA	11	11	50 %	50 %
Storm ABABA	16	4	80 %	20 %
Storm ABABAB	14	5	74 %	26 %
Total	109	60	64 %	36 %

Table 4. Answers to the second survey question ("why" question) classified into categories. Note that one subject could belong to none or multiple categories, so the percentages for each line don't add up to 100 %.

Story version	%A good gest	%NA good gest	%A animated	%NA realistic
Garden ABA	30 %	30 %	20 %	30 %
Garden ABAB	41 %	9 %	59 %	0 %
Pet ABABA	22 %	43 %	13 %	9 %
Pet ABABAB	54 %	13 %	33 %	0 %
Protest ABAB	21 %	32 %	26 %	0 %
Protest ABABA	27 %	32 %	23 %	9 %
Storm ABABA	20 %	15 %	45 %	0 %
Storm ABABAB	32 %	21 %	47 %	0 %
Total	31 %	24 %	33 %	6 %

because copying was less obvious when the expanse and height of the gestures changed in the adapted version.

Among those who preferred the non-adapted versions of the stories, one reason was that the gestures fit the dialog better ("non-adapted good gestures" in Table 4): the subjects stated that the gestures in the non-adapted version "went a lot better with what she was saying" and were "more appropriate". Another reason is that the gestures were "more realistic" ("non-adapted realistic") : subjects didn't like the gestures being "too animated", or "too busy", nor did they like the agents "showing way too much emotions" or "looking like she is exercising". That is, too much animation can be seen as unrealistic.

The percentages of the subjects that had comments related to those 4 categories are in Table 4. In 7 out of 8 tasks, there were more subjects who preferred the adapted version because it was animated at the right level (e.g. animated enough, but not too animated). If we only consider the "animated" factor in deciding which is a better stimulus, 84 % of the subjects preferred the adapted version.

5   Discussion and Future Work

To our knowledge this is the first time that it has been shown that subjects perceive differences in agent personality during a storytelling task, and that adaptive gestural behavior during storytelling is positively perceived. We re-use natural personal narratives that are rendered dialogically, so that two IVAs co-tell the story.

It is obvious that being able to adapt is a key part of being more human-like. There are attempts to integrate language adaptation within natural language generation [32] and research has shown that human bystanders perceive linguistic adaptation positively [33]. However, this is the first experiment to demonstrate a positive effect for gestural adaptation.

Recent work on gesture generation has focused largely on iconic gesture generation. For example, Bergmann and Kopp [34] present a model that allows virtual agents to automatically select the content and derive the form of coordinated language and iconic gestures. Luo et al. [29] also presents an effective algorithm for adding full body postural movement to animation sequences of arm gestures. More generally, current systems generally select gestures using either a text-to-gesture or concept-to-gesture mapping. Text-to-gesture systems, such as VHP [13], may have a limited number of gestures (only 7 in this case) and limited gesture placement options, but the alignment of speech content and gestures are more accurate. Concept-to-gesture systems such as PPP [35], AC and BEAT [36] defines general rules for gesture insertion based on linguistic components. For example, iconic gestures are triggered by words with spatial or concrete context (e.g. "check"). These kind of systems have more gestures, but the gesture placement largely depends on general rules derived from literature, thus the accuracy is not guaranteed. An alternative approach learns a personalized statistical model that predicts a gesture given the text to be spoken and a model that captures an individual's gesturing preferences [37]. None of these models adequately address the production of gesture for dialogues, where a process of co-adaptation will modulate both the type of gesture chosen and the specific form of that gesture (e.g. its size). This current work aims to provide a basis for developing such models.

Gratch investigates creating rapport with virtual agents using gesture adaptation mainly focused on head gestures and posture shifts (while ours focused on hand gestures), and used real human movements as control [38]. Our adaptation stimuli are more similar to Endrass et al. [12]. To investigate culture-related aspects of behavior for virtual characters, they chose prototypical body postures from corpora for German and Japanese cultural background, embodied those postures in a two-agent dialogs, and asked subjects from German and Japanese cultural background to evaluate the dialogs.

In future work, we aim to test the expression of personality and adaptivity with different personality combinations. Our ultimate goal is to automatically convert monologic blog stories to dialogs with both linguistic and gestural adaptation. Experimental exploration, such as undertaken here, is crucial for formulating models of gesture generation that correctly incorporate personality and adaptation.

References

1. Nisbett, R.E.: The trait construct in lay and professional psychology. In: Retrospections on Social Psychology, pp. 109–130 (1980)
2. Mehl, M.R., Gosling, S.D., Pennebaker, J.W.: Personality in its natural habitat: manifestations and implicit folk theories of personality in daily life. J. Pers. Soc. Psychol. **90**, 862–877 (2006)
3. Norman, W.T.: Toward an adequate taxonomy of personality attributes: replicated factor structure in peer nomination personality rating. J. Abnorm. Soc. Psychol. **66**, 574–583 (1963)
4. Bickmore, T., Schulman, D.: The comforting presence of relational agents. In: CHI 2006 Extended Abstracts on Human Factors in Computing Systems, pp. 550–555. ACM (2006)
5. Hartmann, B., Mancini, M., Pelachaud, C.: Implementing expressive gesture synthesis for embodied conversational agents. In: Gibet, S., Courty, N., Kamp, J.-F. (eds.) GW 2005. LNCS (LNAI), vol. 3881, pp. 188–199. Springer, Heidelberg (2006)
6. Kopp, S., Wachsmuth, I.: Synthesizing multimodal utterances for conversational agents. Comput. Anim. Virtual Worlds **15**, 39–52 (2004)
7. Thiebaux, M., Marshall, A., Marsella, S., Kallman, M.: Smartbody: behavior realization for embodied conversational agents. In: Proceedings of 7th International Conference on Autonomous Agents and Multiagent Systems (AAMAS 2008), pp. 151–158 (2008)
8. Heloir, A., Kipp, M.: EMBR – a realtime animation engine for interactive embodied agents. In: Ruttkay, Z., Kipp, M., Nijholt, A., Vilhjálmsson, H.H. (eds.) IVA 2009. LNCS, vol. 5773, pp. 393–404. Springer, Heidelberg (2009)
9. André, E., Klesen, M., Gebhard, P., Allen, S., Rist, T.: Integrating models of personality and emotions into lifelike characters. In: Paiva, A.C.R. (ed.) IWAI 1999. LNCS, vol. 1814, pp. 150–165. Springer, Heidelberg (2000)
10. Ruttkay, Z., Dormann, C., Noot, H.: Embodied conversational agents on a common ground. In: From Brows to Trust: Evaluating Embodied Conversational Agents, chap. 2, pp. 27–66. Kluwer Academic Publishers, Norwell (2004)
11. Moon, Y., Nass, C.: How "real" are computer personalities?: Psychological responses to personality types in human-computer interaction. Commun. Res. **23**(6), 651–674 (1996)
12. Endraß, B., André, E., Rehm, M., Nakano, Y.I.: Investigating culture-related aspects of behavior for virtual characters. Auton. Agent. Multi-Agent Syst. **27**(2), 277–304 (2013)
13. Noma, T., Badler, N.I., Zhao, L.: Design of a virtual human presenter. Center for Human Modeling and Simulation, p. 75 (2000)

14. Tapus, A., Tapus, C., Mataric, M.J.: User robot personality matching and assistive robot behavior adaptation for post-stroke rehabilitation therapy. Intel. Serv. Robot. **1**(2), 169–183 (2008)
15. Wang, N., Johnson, W.L., Mayer, R.E., Rizzo, P., Shaw, E., Collins, H.: The politeness effect: pedagogical agents and learning gains. Front. Artif. Intell. Appl. **125**, 686–693 (2005)
16. Mairesse, F., Walker, M.A.: Controlling user perceptions of linguistic style: trainable generation of personality traits. Comput. Linguist. **37**(3), 455–488 (2011)
17. Neff, M., Wang, Y., Abbott, R., Walker, M.: Evaluating the effect of gesture and language on personality perception in conversational agents. In: Safonova, A. (ed.) IVA 2010. LNCS, vol. 6356, pp. 222–235. Springer, Heidelberg (2010)
18. Bee, N., Pollock, C., André, E., Walker, M.: Bossy or wimpy: expressing social dominance by combining gaze and linguistic behaviors. In: Safonova, A. (ed.) IVA 2010. LNCS, vol. 6356, pp. 265–271. Springer, Heidelberg (2010)
19. Neff, M., Toothman, N., Bowmani, R., Fox Tree, J.E., Walker, M.A.: Don't scratch! self-adaptors reflect emotional stability. In: Vilhjálmsson, H.H., Kopp, S., Marsella, S., Thórisson, K.R. (eds.) IVA 2011. LNCS, vol. 6895, pp. 398–411. Springer, Heidelberg (2011)
20. Fox Tree, J.E.: Listening in on monologues and dialogues. Discourse Process. **27**, 35–53 (1999)
21. Parrill, F., Kimbara, I.: Seeing and hearing double: the influence of mimicry in speech and gesture on observers. J. Nonverbal Behav. **30**, 157–166 (2006)
22. Bailenson, J.N., Yee, N.: Digital chameleons: automatic assimilation of nonverbal gestures in immersive virtual environments. Psychol. Sci. **16**(10), 814–819 (2005)
23. Tolins, J., Fox Tree, J.E.: Addressee backchannels steer narrative development. J. Pragmat. **70**, 152–164 (2014)
24. Thorne, A., Korobov, N., Morgan, E.M.: Channeling identity: a study of storytelling in conversations between introverted and extraverted friends. J. Res. Pers. **41**(5), 1008–1031 (2007)
25. Gordon, A., Swanson, R.: Identifying personal stories in millions of weblog entries. In: 3rd International Conference on Weblogs and Social Media, Data Challenge Workshop, San Jose, CA (2009)
26. Kita, S., van Gijn, I., van der Hulst, H.: Movement phases in signs and co-speech gestures, and their transcription by human coders. In: Wachsmuth, I., Fröhlich, M. (eds.) GW 1997. LNCS (LNAI), vol. 1371, p. 23. Springer, Heidelberg (1998)
27. Wang, Y., Neff, M.: The influence of prosody on the requirements for gesture-text alignment. In: Aylett, R., Krenn, B., Pelachaud, C., Shimodaira, H. (eds.) IVA 2013. LNCS, vol. 8108, pp. 180–188. Springer, Heidelberg (2013)
28. Tolins, J., Liu, K., Wang, Y., Tree, J.E.F., Walker, M., Neff, M.: Gestural adaptation in extravert-introvert pairs and implications for IVAs. In: Aylett, R., Krenn, B., Pelachaud, C., Shimodaira, H. (eds.) IVA 2013. LNCS, vol. 8108, p. 484. Springer, Heidelberg (2013)
29. Luo, P., Kipp, M., Neff, M.: Augmenting gesture animation with motion capture data to provide full-body engagement. In: Ruttkay, Z., Kipp, M., Nijholt, A., Vilhjálmsson, H.H. (eds.) IVA 2009. LNCS, vol. 5773, pp. 405–417. Springer, Heidelberg (2009)
30. Gosling, S.D., Rentfrow, P.J., Swann, W.B.: A very brief measure of the big five personality domains. J. Res. Pers. **37**, 504–528 (2003)

31. Liu, K., Tolins, J., Tree, J.E.F., Walker, M., Neff, M.: Judging IVA personality using an open-ended question. In: Aylett, R., Krenn, B., Pelachaud, C., Shimodaira, H. (eds.) IVA 2013. LNCS, vol. 8108, pp. 396–405. Springer, Heidelberg (2013)

32. Buschmeier, H., Bergmann, K., Kopp, S.: An alignment-capable microplanner for natural language generation. In: Proceedings of the 12th European Workshop on Natural Language Generation, pp. 82–89. ACL (2009)

33. Hu, Z., Halberg, G., Jimenez, C., Walker, M.: Entrainment in pedestrian direction giving: how many kinds of entrainment? In: IWSDS (2014)

34. Bergmann, K., Kopp, S.: Increasing the expressiveness of virtual agents: autonomous generation of speech and gesture for spatial description tasks. In: Proceedings of the 8th International Conference on Autonomous Agents and Multiagent Systems, vol. 1, pp. 361–368 (2009)

35. André, E., Müller, J., Rist, T.: WiP/PPP: automatic generation of personalized multimedia presentations. In: Proceedings of the Fourth ACM International Conference on Multimedia, pp. 407–408. ACM (1997)

36. Cassell, J., Vilhjálmsson, H.H., Bickmore, T.: Beat: the behavior expression animation toolkit. In: Prendinger, H., Ishizuka, M. (eds.) Life-Like Characters. Cognitive Technologies, pp. 163–185. Springer, Heidelberg (2004)

37. Neff, M., Kipp, M., Albrecht, I., Seidel, H.P.: Gesture modeling and animation based on a probabilistic re-creation of speaker style. ACM Trans. Graph. **27**(1), 5:1–5:24 (2008). ACM

38. Gratch, J., Wang, N., Gerten, J., Fast, E., Duffy, R.: Creating rapport with virtual agents. In: Pelachaud, C., Martin, J.-C., André, E., Chollet, G., Karpouzis, K., Pelé, D. (eds.) IVA 2007. LNCS (LNAI), vol. 4722, pp. 125–138. Springer, Heidelberg (2007)

Gestural Coupling Between Humans and Virtual Characters in an Artistic Context of Imitation

Elisabetta Bevacqua(✉), Céline Jost, Alexis Nédélec, and Pierre De Loor

UEB, Lab-STICC, ENIB, Brest, France
{bevacqua,jost,nedelec,deloor}@enib.fr

Abstract. We present a human-agent interaction based on a theatrical mirroring game. The user and the agent imitate each other's body movements and introduce, from time to time, changes by proposing a new movement. The agent responses are linked to the game scenario but also to the user's behavior, which makes each game session unique.

Keywords: Human-agent body interaction · Coupling

1 Context

This demonstration has been realized within the collaborative French project called Ingredible. The fundamental goal of this project is to reproduce the mutual influence that is intrinsic to human-human interaction for a human-virtual agent interaction. The Ingredible project focuses, especially, on the gestural behavior and gestural expressive quality shown by both the virtual agent and the user while interacting. This type of interactions contains some spontaneous and emergent behaviors which are hard to tackle for virtual characters because the evolution of the interaction is shared between the protagonists. A first attempt was proposed by [5] but this work does not show the evolution of the decision relative to the quality of the interaction. Previous works on human-human interaction have studied the dynamical evolution of communication. In "Alive Communication" [3], Fogel and Garvey showed that, while interacting, people coordinate their behaviors and mutually influence their actions and intentions. Ordinary variability, that is slight modifications in the behavior due, for example, to personal style, emerges naturally without braking the bounds of the interaction. From time to time, extraordinary variability (called *innovation*) can appear, obliging interactants to make an effort to integrate the novelty in order to keep the communication going. This theory highlights the dynamical evolution of human-human interactions, the mutual influence and the capability to resist and to adapt to changes. Regular and unexpected behaviors appear naturally and previous works showed that reproducing the equilibrium between them in human-agent interactions is fundamental to improve agent believability and user's engagement [1]. Within the Ingredible project we aim to reproduce this evolving equilibrium between regularity and surprise, that we call *coupling* [2]. This demonstration shows our last progress in this direction.

© Springer International Publishing Switzerland 2015
W.-P. Brinkman et al. (Eds.): IVA 2015, LNAI 9238, pp. 194–197, 2015.
DOI: 10.1007/978-3-319-21996-7_20

2   The Ingredible Project Framework

To reach our goal we propose a framework composed of five modules: the **Capture module** retrieves data from tracking devices and generates a unified 15-joints skeleton. Skeletons are sent to the **Analysis module** which tries to recognize the current gesture and its expressivity. The **Decision module** determines the agent's response depending on the user's behavior and the interaction scenario. The **Synthesis module** computes the final skeleton animation that is displayed by the **Rendering module**, implemented in Unity3D.

The Ingredible project is still an ongoing project, and this demonstration focuses mainly on the Analysis and Decision modules. The Analysis module collects, in a continuous flow, data from devices enabling skeletal tracking of a single person. The recognition process is based on skeleton analysis and motion features computation. Skeleton joints are used to compute features which are stored in a reference database. A Principal Component Analysis (PCA) is computed to select the most important features, useful in discriminating gestures. During real-time recognition, using distance measures, real-time selected features are compared to the reference database to find the most similar gesture. More details can be found in [4]. The objective of the Decision module, shown in Fig. 1(a), is to generate an appropriate action of the virtual agent according to the user's non verbal behavior. An action can be an animation to play, a joint to move, or an expressivity to change (for example, moving faster). The decision is based on the level of coupling between the human and the virtual agent, which shows mutual influence, engagement, and willing to keep on interacting together. A high level of coupling indicates that, both human and virtual agent, are engaged in the interaction, while a low level of coupling results in a bad feeling about the interaction. Analyzing this coupling, the main objective is to maintain the interaction. According to Fogel [3], three strategies are possible: (i) to maintain the current coupling level (co-regulation) if everything is going well, (ii) to induce a small variation of coupling level (ordinary variability) for example to avoid human's boredom, or (iii) to change dramatically the coupling level (innovation) for example to reengage the human. To take such a decision, the Decision module refers to a scenario which describes its expectations (what human is supposed to do), and its goals (what virtual agent is supposed to do). The satisfaction of expectations implies that the level of coupling increases, otherwise it decreases. The first implementation of this module is scenario-dependent and rule-based. A scenario is written in XML and describes actions which can be done by the virtual agent, a sequence of possible events and associated expectations. Rules, also written in XML, describe relations between the level of coupling and the goal to reach. This is only a first attempt to reproduce the mutual influence of human-human interaction. Our next objective is to make the decision module more generic to decrease the importance of a predefined scripted scenario. Moreover, a learning process will be added to automatically define the rules which conducted to the best experience between the human and the virtual agent.

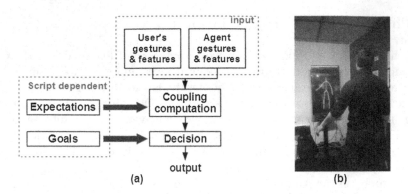

Fig. 1. (a) Decision module architecture. (b) Theatrical mirroring game.

3   Theatrical Mirroring Game Scenario

As explained in Sect. 1, the Ingredible project focuses on gestural behavior, particularly in the artistic domain. For such a reason, we collaborate with a theater company to define scenarios in which the whole interaction is based solely on body movements (neither speech nor facial expressions). The mirroring game is a good example of the researched interactions: two players imitate each other's movements and introduce, from time to time, changes by proposing a new movement or by modifying the expressivity, that is the manner in which the movement is performed. A very interesting characteristic of this game is that at any moment both players can be the leader and the follower, for example a person can control the movement of left hand while the other is leading that of the right hand. If the game is correctly realized, it is impossible for an external observer to guess who is in control of which part of the body and just the players can feel it. They are strongly aware of how their behavior is both influenced and influential. To play successfully this type of game, coupling between the players is fundamental; for such a reason, the mirroring game is the scenario we chose in this demonstration. It evolves as follows: the virtual agent performs idle movements in its virtual environment, patiently waiting for a user who would like to play with it. When the user appears in front of the agent and the Kinect tracks him, to establish the interaction, the agent and the user must communicate. Since neither verbal behavior nor facial expressions are allowed, both interactants have nothing but gestures to express themselves. So the agent greets the user waving its hand (or greets back if the user waves his hand first). From this moment, to start the game, both virtual and human players can express their intention to play by performing a bow. It does not matter who bows first, what is important is that, by bowing, both show that they agree to play the game together. Figure 1(b) shows the demo set-up. During the game the agent expects that the user imitates its gestures and their expressivity and that from time to time the user proposes something new. So, when the Analysis module informs the Decision module about the user's behavior, this module compares the input data with the agent expectations and updates the level of coupling. In this scenario, there is just one expectation: "the human and the virtual agent are doing the same thing". To measure this coupling, human position and features are compared to virtual agent position and features. The coupling is inversely proportional to the resulting distance. For example, if the human and the virtual agent are doing the same thing, distance is minimum, therefore the coupling is maximum. In this context, the virtual agent has two possible goals: to imitate human (goal 1) or to introduce new movement (goal 2). In relation to "Alive Communication" theory, we consider that co-regulation is goal 1, that ordinary variability is goal 2, and that innovation is stopping the game. During the game, virtual agent alternates these goals according to rules until the end of the game. In this first implementation, rules are minimalist and describe the relation between coupling and goals:

```
if state == goal1 then
    if coupling == too low then stop the game
    else if coupling == high then state ← goal2
    else coregulation
    end if
else if state == goal2 then
    if coupling == too low then state ← goal1
    else coregulation
    end if
end if
```

At any moment, both the agent and the user can stop the game showing a specific gesture. The agent could stop the game for several reasons, for example if the game has lasted long enough or if the user is not a "good" player and the coupling level remains low (the user rarely follows new movement propositions, that is he rarely adapts his behavior to that shown by the agent). When the interaction is over, the virtual character greets the human player and goes back to its idle motion waiting again for a new player.

Acknowledgments. This work was funded by the ANR INGREDIBLE project: ANR-12-CORD-001 (http://www.ingredible.fr).

References

1. Bevacqua, E., Stanković, I., Maatallaoui, A., Nédélec, A., De Loor, P.: Effects of coupling in human-virtual agent body interaction. In: Bickmore, T., Marsella, S., Sidner, C. (eds.) IVA 2014. LNCS, vol. 8637, pp. 54–63. Springer, Heidelberg (2014)
2. De Loor, P., Bevacqua, E., Stanković, I., Maatallaoui, A., Nédélec, A., Buche, C.: Utilisation de la notion de couplage pour la modélisation d'agents virtuels inter-actifs socialement présents. In: Conférence III. Oxford University Press, France (2014)
3. Fogel, A., Garvey, A.: Alive communication. Infant Behav. Dev. **30**(2), 251–257 (2007)
4. Jost, C., Stanković, I., De Loor, P., Nédélec, A., Bevacqua, E.: Real-time gesture recognition based on motion quality analysis. In: INTETAIN (2015)
5. Pugliese, R., Lehtonen, K.: A framework for motion based bodily enaction with virtual characters. In: Vilhjálmsson, H.H., Kopp, S., Marsella, S., Thórisson, K.R. (eds.) IVA 2011. LNCS, vol. 6895, pp. 162–168. Springer, Heidelberg (2011)

Pedagogical Agents in Health and Training

Negotiation as a Challenge Problem
for Virtual Humans

Jonathan Gratch[1]([⊠]), David DeVault[1], Gale M. Lucas[1],
and Stacy Marsella[2]

[1] University of Southern California, Los Angeles, USA
{gratch,devault,lucas}@ict.usc.edu
[2] Northeastern University, Boston, USA
marsella@ccs.neu.edu

Abstract. We argue for the importance of negotiation as a challenge problem
for virtual human research, and introduce a virtual conversational agent that
allows people to practice a wide range of negotiation skills. We describe the
multi-issue bargaining task, which has become a de facto standard for teaching
and research on negotiation in both the social and computer sciences. This task
is popular as it allows scientists or instructors to create a variety of distinct
situations that arise in real-life negotiations, simply by manipulating a small
number of mathematical parameters. We describe the development of a virtual
human that will allow students to practice the interpersonal skills they need
to recognize and navigate these situations. An evaluation of an early
wizard-controlled version of the system demonstrates the promise of this technology for teaching negotiation and supporting scientific research on social
intelligence.

1 Introduction

Negotiation is an indispensable skill for any social creature. Civil society frowns on
those that simply take what they need from others. Whether in the home, the market
place or virtual market place, people achieve what they need through discussion and
compromise. Unfortunately, most of us are poor negotiators. Research has documented
a range of cognitive biases that undermine the q of negotiated agreements [1], and
companies invest billions of dollars in training their employees to negotiate and resolve
conflict [2]. Automated decision tools might help people avoid these limitations, but to
the extent computers are able to negotiate at all, it is only through very restrictive
protocols that simplify away many of the complexities faced by human negotiators.

In this article, we argue for the importance of negotiation as a challenge problem for
virtual human research. Negotiation engages a wide range of skills that are not only
crucial for people, but essential for machines that socially engage with humans:

- **Intelligence:** Negotiations bring together a number of cognitive skills. They involve
  tradeoffs across multiple goals; they require one to infer and reason about the goals
  of one's negotiation partner, engaging theory of mind reasoning; they evoke
  emotion and these shape outcomes for good and ill.

© Springer International Publishing Switzerland 2015
W.-P. Brinkman et al. (Eds.): IVA 2015, LNAI 9238, pp. 201–215, 2015.
DOI: 10.1007/978-3-319-21996-7_21

- **Language:** Negotiations create unique challenges for natural language research as parties often violate the standard Gricean Maxims of cooperative communication. Negotiators hedge, obscure or outright lie about their preferences, or adopt sophisticated strategies such as reciprocal disclosure to build trust. A skilled negotiator is attuned not only to explicit statements, but also to the implications of what is not said and the subtleties of how information is conveyed.
- **Embodiment:** Negotiation research emphasizes that expressions, postures and paralanguage can convey your partner's preferences and power, and improved skill in reading these signals leads to better outcomes. On the flip side, regulating one's own nonverbal signals can strongly influence how a negotiation will unfold.

Creating virtual humans with this range of capabilities can have important practical and scientific benefits. In practical terms, virtual human negotiators can help teach interpersonal skills [3–5]. More broadly, the capabilities needed to successfully negotiate can inform the design of a wide range of machines that socially interact with people. From a scientific perspective, the act of creating a virtual negotiator can serve to advance theories of human cognition. This can occur through the act of concretizing social theories into working artifacts [6], but also because virtual agents enable a level of experimental control unobtainable in most social science research [7].

   This paper describes the development of a virtual human that allows people to practice a wide range of negotiation skills. We first describe the *multi-issue bargaining problem*, a formulation of negotiation that has been adopted by the social science, education and the multi-agent communities. We then describe the Conflict Resolution Agent, a conversational agent that performs this task and allows students to practice an array of negotiation concepts (see Fig. 2). The agent is being developed through an iterative design process, starting with face-to-face data collecting, moving to a wizard-assisted system, and then finally moving to a fully-automated virtual human. Currently, we are part-way through this design process but already the system has supported a number of scientific findings. We report on our progress and argue for the importance of negotiation as a challenge problem to advance virtual human research.

2   Definitions

Negotiations are dialogues aimed at reaching an agreement between parties when there is a perceived divergence of interests, beliefs, or in ways to achieve joint ends [8]. Although this definition is broad, researchers have sought to abstract essential elements of negotiations into more structured formalisms that are suitable for both teaching and scientific enquiry. In this paper, we focus on one useful and common abstraction known as the multi-issue bargaining task [9], which has become a de facto standard for both teaching and research on negotiation in both the social and computer sciences (e.g., see [2, 10, 11]). Multi-issue bargaining generalizes simpler games developed in game theory, such as the ultimatum game, and more closely approximates many of the challenges found in real-life negotiations. This task has received so much attention amongst educators and researchers because, with only a small number of mathematical parameters, one can evoke a wide range of psychologically-distinct decision-tasks. Thus, multi-issue bargaining has been used to teach and study a wide range of negotiation concepts.

In its basic form, multi-issue bargaining requires parties (typically 2) to find agreement over a set of issues. Each issue consists of a set of levels and players must jointly decide on a level for each issue (levels might correspond to the amount of a product one player wishes to buy, or it might represent attributes of a single object, such as the price or warranty of a car). Each party receives some payoff for each possible agreement and each player's payoff is usually not known to the other party. The payoff is often assumed to be additive (i.e., a player's total payoff is the sum of the value obtained for each issue) and presented to players through a payoff matrix. For example, Table 1 illustrates the two payoff matrices for a hypothetical negotiation over items in an antique store. In this case, players must divide up three crates of records, two lamps and one painting, but each party assigns different value to items.

Table 1. Example 3-issue bargaining problem

Side A Payoff						Side B Payoff					
Record Crates		Lamps		Painting		Record Crates		Lamps		Painting	
Level	Value	Level	Value	Level	Value	Level	Value	Level	Value	Level	Value
0	$0	0	0	0	$0	0	$0	0	0	0	$0
1	$20	1	$10	1	$100	1	$10	1	$30	1	$0
2	$40	2	$20			2	$20	2	$60		
3	$60					3	$30				

Preference Weights: The weight each party assigns to issues defines one class of parameters for creating qualitatively different classes of negotiation. The payoff structure in Table 1 defines an *integrative* (or win-win) negotiation. For example, as player A receives the most value from the painting and records, whereas player B receives the most value from the lamps, the joint payoff is maximized when player B gets all the lamps and player A gets the rest (also known as the *Pareto efficient* solution). A *distributive* (or zero-sum) negotiation arises when both parties have conflicting preferences. For example, if both parties had the same payoff as side A, any gain in value to one side would result in an equal loss to the other side. The painting represents a special type of issue known as a *compatible issue* as one party doesn't incur a cost if the other party receives their preferred level. Compatible issues create an opportunity for *misrepresentation*. Specifically, if player B, claims that the painting has value to them, they can offer this 'invented' value in exchange for other items they want [12].

BATNA: The second important class of parameters is the Best Alternative to a Negotiated Agreement (BATNA) for each player. This represents how much a party would receive if the negotiation fails. For example, if player A already has a tentative deal with another player that affords him $150, there is no reason to accept a deal worth less than $150 from player B (e.g., 2 records and a painting). The BATNA represents the player's bargaining power, and as with preference weights, these are typically unknown to the other player. If player B's BATNA is only $20, then player A has more potential power in the negotiation, although whether this translates into better outcomes depends on how each party shapes the other party's perceptions and how carefully they attend to the structure of the negotiation.

Figure 1 summarizes several basic negotiation concepts. The graph shows all 24 possible agreements defined in Table 1 in terms of the value each player receives. The Pareto frontier defines the set of *efficient* agreements. Expert negotiators should not accept any deal below this frontier as inefficient solutions can always be improved for one party without harming the other (thus increasing joint value), although inexpert negotiators often fail to discover efficient solutions. The BATNAs define a *zone of agreement*. Any deal outside this zone should be rejected by one player as it is below their BATNA, however inexpert negotiators often fail to follow this principle. The fact that the Pareto frontier is convex means there is integrative potential: players can improve on a 50–50 split by understanding each other's preferences and allocating each player their most important issue. Inexpert negotiators often assume negotiations are distributive (a 'fixed-pie' bias) and fail to realize integrative potential.

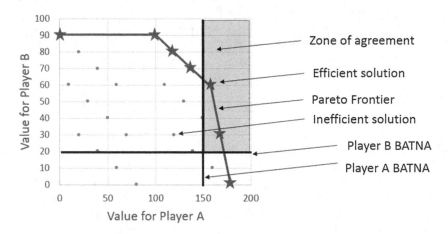

Fig. 1. Summary of key bargaining concepts

It is important that preference weights and BATNA are typically unknown to the other party and must be estimated through language and/or the pattern of offers. Much of the skill of negotiation comes from learning when to reveal truthful information or how to elicit truthful information from the other party. A player that reveals too much information without reciprocation could be exploited, creating a tension between cooperation and competition. However, even when all information is public, players often fail to find efficient agreements.

Preference weights and BATNA define the basic mathematics of the multi-issue bargaining task[1] but several other factors can be varied which are irrelevant from the

---

[1] Time pressure can be introduced by adding a deadline or a temporal discounting function. Automated negotiation agents usually require parties to alternate complete offers. Generalizations are also possible, e.g., by relaxing the assumption of an additive utility function.

perspective of classical rationality, but that can have profound differences on human decision-making, especially for inexpert negotiators. For example, preferences can be presented as losses or gains. Issues can carry moral significance [13]. Parties can negotiate for themselves or as representatives of their organization or as part of a team [14]. The amount of information available (e.g., the other player's preferences and/or BATNA) can also be varied. All of these – and other – factors have been shown to influence the negotiation processes, especially for inexpert negotiators.

Uses: Researchers can create a vast number of psychologically-distinct negotiation problems with only a small number of mathematical parameters and a bit of textual framing. Thus, multi-issue bargaining has proven an especially rich tool for the study and teaching of human social skills, as well as a tool for advancing artificially intelligent agents. For example, in emotion research, bargaining tasks are used to examine how signaled or induced emotion shapes joint outcomes [11]. In conflict-resolution research it is used to study various social processes involved in resolving disputes [8]. In social neuroscience, it is used to examine specific brain regions associated with social cognition [15]. In game theory, it is used to advance rational models of multi-party decision-making [16]. In artificial intelligence, it serves as a standard challenge problem for advancing automated models of social decision-making [10]. Finally, in educational settings, this extensive body of research provides a firm theoretical basis for informing pedagogy as bargaining games are used to teach a wide range of interpersonal skills including negotiation, conflict-resolution, teamwork, emotional intelligence and inter-cultural fluency (e.g., see the leadership exercises at the Northwestern Dispute Resolution Research Center at negotiationexercises.com). Therefore, virtual humans that can perform bargaining tasks in a general way will have broad impact on science and education.

3   Related Work and Current Limitations

Research on negotiation within computer science has already yielded tangible benefits. Machines can predict the outcome of a negotiation by analyzing the verbal and non-verbal cues of negotiators [17, 18]. Even stylized virtual humans evoke physiological threat [19] and influence negotiation outcomes with their emotional expressions [20]. Virtual humans can use language to establish beneficial long-term relationships with other negotiators [21]. An analysis of the language of negotiation has advanced dialog research on turn-taking and incremental speech production [22]. We build on this research, but also extend it in ways that enhances its connections with the larger body of research on teaching and understanding human negotiation skills.

Several algorithms have been developed to automate the decision-making of an artificial negotiator [10]. Unfortunately, most of this work has focused on agent-agent interaction and adopts assumptions that may not apply in human negotiations. Such agents only communicate through formal representations of offers, whereas people rely heavily on language. Agents usually only allow the exchange of complete offers, whereas people often focus on a subset of issues at a time (indeed, learning how to "package" different issues is a key skill taught to negotiators). Agents assume money is the only source of value whereas people often assign value to intangible considerations like fairness or maintaining relationships [23]. These restrictions avoid many of the challenges that face human negotiators (although see [24] for one attempt to relax these restrictions). Nevertheless, this research can serve as an important basis for the reasoning techniques that inform a virtual human negotiator.

Education researchers have looked at the potential of bargaining agents to teach negotiation, though none of these systems have tackled spoken interaction. For example, the pocket negotiator uses preference-elicitation techniques and visualizations of the Pareto frontier to help students better prepare for a face-to-face negotiation [25]. ELECT BiLAT allows students to practice a series of negotiations with virtual characters that use sophisticated decision-theoretic and theory-of-mind techniques to guide their behavior. However, the main pedagogical focus of BiLAT, like the pocket negotiator, is on the preparations leading up to a negotiation [26]. Kraus and colleagues have shown that negotiating with a disembodied rational agent can help students learn [3]. This research serves to inform how to use virtual humans to teach negotiation skills.

Finally, a line of research within the virtual human community has explored natural language negotiations with embodied agents. For example, the SASO system allowed student-soldiers to negotiate with a local leader over how best to conduct a peace-keeping operation [27]. However, this class of approaches adopts a very different formalism of negotiation, building more on planning and shared-plans frameworks (e.g., [28]), and thus has only limited relevance to the larger body of research on multi-issue bargaining. Nonetheless, this research provides a foundation for the natural language understanding and dialog processes required for a virtual human negotiator.

4   The Conflict Resolution Agent

The Conflict Resolution Agent (CRA), pictured in Fig. 2, is a game-like environment that allows negotiation students to engage with different virtual human role-players across a variety of multi-issue bargaining problems. Our goal is to allow students to communicate with a fully automated agent through natural language and nonverbal expressions. By altering preference weights, BATNAS, and task-framing, students can be presented with a wide range of negotiation and dispute-resolution concepts such as

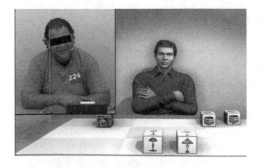

224: I'll tell you what. I'll take this box of records 'cause it looks like it has the least.

CRA: That doesn't seem fair though...

224: Why not? [exasperated laugh]

CRA: Well, you see, I have a buyer right now that is interested in old records.

224: So do I.

CRA: Your customers would probably love those lamps.

224: My customers?

Fig. 2. A participant (#224) interacting with the Conflict Resolution Agent.

integrative potential, anchoring, reciprocal information exchange, rights vs. interests, emotional intelligence and establishing rapport. This mirrors how bargaining games are used to teach negotiation in business schools.

Virtual humans can augment negotiation training in many of the same ways that automated tutoring research has benefited other "harder" skills, by allowing students more opportunities to experience the domain, tailoring their experience to match their current skills, and providing targeted feedback. Currently, negotiation is taught by a mixture of lecture and in-class "simulations" where students role-play bargaining exercises with each other. Simulations are widely considered to have the greatest teaching value but are difficult to realize. In a typical semester-long negotiation course, students might participant in only a small number of simulated negotiations.[2] In class simulations also have something of a blind-leading-the-blind flavor, with large variance in quality and many students failing to achieve the core principle underlying the exercise. The instructor then leads a discussion illustrating why certain students succeeded or failed. Agent technology can improve this process by allowing students to practice as much as they like with a partner programmed to more consistently evoke the intended behaviors and negotiation processes. Further, as all student behavior is being tracked, understood and recorded, agents or instructors could provide customized tutorial feedback and commentary on the student's behavior. Virtual humans can also complement the growing interest in online courses. Of course, another aim of the project is to advance the capabilities of virtual humans more generally, and the techniques underlying CRA build upon and reinforce domain-independent techniques for virtual humans.

To this end, CRA is being developed through a series of iterations, beginning with a face-to-face data collection to serve as a baseline for comparison and to create a large corpus to inform the design of individual system components. Presently, we have completed the face-to-face data collection, designed the basic game environment, and completed several iterations on improving a wizard-controlled system (described below).

CRA is implemented with the publicly-available virtual human toolkit [29]. In the Wizard-of-Oz setup (WOz), CRA is semi-automated, with low-level functions carried out automatically, while two wizards make high-level decisions about the agent's verbal and nonverbal behavior. Gestures and individual utterances are based on data collected during face-to-face negotiations between inexpert negotiators on variants of the task shown in Table 1. The WOz interface allows the agent to speak over 10,000 distinct utterances. Utterances are synthesized by the NeoSpeech text-to-speech system and gestures and expressions are generated automatically by NVBG [30] and realized using the SmartBody character animation system [31]. This low-level automation complements and facilitates the decision-making of the wizards. Details of the development and capabilities of the CRA WOz interface can be found in [32].

CRA realizes a physically-embodied version of the multi-issue bargaining task developed by Carnevale and described in [17]. As can be seen in Fig. 2, issues are

---

[2] Personal communication with Professor Peter Kim, instructor of the negotiation course at the University of Southern California's Marshall School of Business.

represented as different types of physical objects (e.g., crates of records, lamps, and paintings) and levels correspond to the number of each type of item the player receives. Participants communicate with CRA through spoken natural language (currently interpreted through the wizards) or by manipulating, gazing at, and/or gesturing at the physical objects. The intent behind the physical objects is to elicit multimodal behavior and create multiple communication channels to facilitate the understanding of participant intent. For example, the participant can make an offer via language ("Would you like the painting?"), moving the objects, or both. The agent can respond in kind, making offers either via speech or by manipulating the objects.

One of the challenges in designing the wizard interface is allowing wizards to rapidly access a large number of possible utterances quickly enough to approximate the pace of normal human dialog [32]. The wizards select amongst utterances using a filtering system which acts as a decision tree (see Fig. 3). Utterances can be filtered by the class of speech act and by the negotiation items mentioned in the intended utterance. The wizards also use pause fillers (e.g., "uh", "um") and gaze behaviors (e.g., look away or at objects) to hold the turn until appropriate responses can be selected, or use "hot keys" to trigger common responses. A separate nonverbal interface allows wizards to select appropriate postures and gestures, and to move the items under discussion.

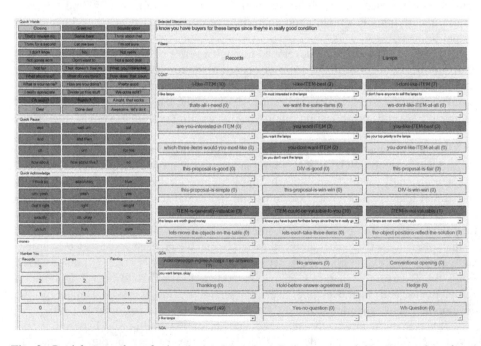

Fig. 3. Partial screenshot of wizard verbal interface. Items at upper-left correspond to short, high-frequency utterances. The right half of the interface organizes longer and less frequent utterances by speech acts. Filters at the top allow navigation by speech acts' specific topics.

One reason for using human wizards is that it allows us to rapidly experiment with different dialog and negotiation policies. Although wizards use their own judgment to select verbal and nonverbal behavior, these choices are scripted to facilitate subsequent automation. This scripting is based on our analysis of the face-to-face dialogues and also to realize specific negotiation concepts. For example, the concept of reciprocal information exchange states that a negotiator should be reluctant to reveal his or her own preferences unless the other party reciprocates. Thus, wizard behavior is scripted to only reveal minor preference information initially and subsequently match the participant's own disclosure. Another concept is integrative potential (i.e., discovering win-win solutions). Many students fail to discover integrative solutions because they assume fixed-pie bias (they assume negotiations are distributive); this is because they don't ask the right questions about the other party's interests and they are often too soft when negotiating with another student, and thereby don't effectively communicate their own priorities to the other party. Students also sometimes confuse the number or level of an item with its value. To facilitate the discovery of efficient solutions, wizards are scripted to query the other party about their preferences, and make proposals that are more efficient with respect to these preferences. Wizards are also scripted to be somewhat tough, to be reluctant to concede their high-value items, and to attend to the value of proposed deals rather than fixate on the number of items.

5 Data Collection and Evaluation

We evaluate CRA to demonstrate both the naturalness of the spoken language interaction and the extent to which wizards can guide inexpert negotiators towards efficient solutions. The initial design of CRA is informed by a face-to-face negotiation dataset (113 same-sex dyads; 38 female). Each dyad was recruited from an on-line job service and randomly assigned to an integrative or distributive negotiation. The integrative task matched the structure of Table 1, except that the painting was only worth 5 for side A (not 100) but still worth 0 for side B. In the distributive task, both sides received the payoff of side A in Table 1, except that side A received 5 for the painting and side B received 0 (i.e., the painting was a compatible issue in both the integrative and distributive tasks). Participants could make money based on their performance. Rather than dollars, participants received lottery tickets based on the value of items they obtained. If they failed to reach agreement, their BATNA equaled the number of tickets they would have received for one of their highest-value items. Tickets were then entered into a $100 lottery.

We collected several traits on participants (not relevant to this paper) and several subjective post-game measures. They rated their own preferences (used to verify they understood the task), their satisfaction with the outcome, and how cooperatively they behaved. They also were asked for their impressions of their negotiation partner: the partner's preferences, their satisfaction with the deal, their cooperativeness, whether they established rapport, and how easy it was to come to an agreement with them.

The face-to-face data serves as a baseline for comparing the performance of the virtual human, both in terms of outcomes (e.g., the quality and efficiency of agreements), process (e.g., is the quality and fluidity of agent speech similar to human negotiators), and subjective impressions. All dialogues were manually transcribed and annotated with semantic frames containing up to eight different key-values (see [32]). The frames encode information about generic dialogue acts (e.g., statement or question), negotiation-specific dialogue acts (e.g., make or reject an offer), propositional content templates (e.g., i-like-ITEM-best)), offers, and valence. These frame annotations serve as the basis for organizing the WOz interface. Sessions were also automatically annotated with facial expressions and vocal quality.

We next ran three rounds of WOz interaction (15, 10 and 12 participants, respectively – 18 female), improving the interface after each iteration to enhance the fluidity of interaction and increase the variety of utterances. The recruitment and design were identical to the face-to-face collection except that all participants played as side B of the integrative task, and all participants were led to believe they were interacting with an agent. As with face-to-face data, participants received lottery tickets based on the value of items they obtained. Male participants interacted with a male virtual human, pictured in Fig. 2, while females interacted with a female virtual human controlled by the same wizard interface. The female virtual human uses the same utterances, general dialogue policy and gestures, but does differ in appearance and voice.

Wizards followed a script: they acted as if the participant preferences were unknown; the wizard avoided volunteering their own preferences unless participants used reciprocal information exchange; the wizard avoided making the first offer unless directly asked, at which point they would make a distributive offer (ask for 2 lamps and 1 record); if the participant insisted on a 3–3 split, the wizard responded "We should focus on the value not the number of items" but did not push the issue further. If the participant revealed that the painting had no value, but still insisted on obtaining it, the wizard would first ask why the participant wanted something of no value before acquiescing. The aim of the WOz script was to see if participants would discover integrative value.

We next describe a comparison of face-to-face and WOz data. As all WOz participants faced an integrative negotiation, we only compare against the integrative subset of face-to-face data: 66 same-sex dyads (12 female).

Outcomes: The wizard script was designed to help participants to discover the concept of integrative potential and this goal was achieved. From t-tests on the number of points both participants and their partners received in the negotiation, we see that participants realized more integrative potential (i.e., joint gain) when negotiating with CRA than when negotiating with another participant. As can be seen in Fig. 4, both participants ($t(1,64) = -1.95, p = .05$) and their computer partner ($t(1,64) = -5.98, p < .001$) earned more points when negotiating with CRA than when both participants were humans. This benefit persisted across the three phases of development.

We examined the outcomes to understand why people performed better with CRA than when negotiating with inexpert human partners. Differences arise from two errors: (1) how participants dealt with the compatible issue and (2) confusion between the number and value of objects. Recall that the painting is a compatible issue, as it only has value for side A. Instead, side B often fought for the painting and got it far more often with human (83 %) vs. agent (53 %) partners ($\chi^2(1,N = 66) = 6.97, p = .008$).

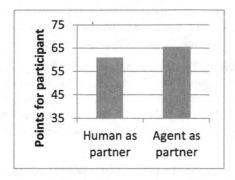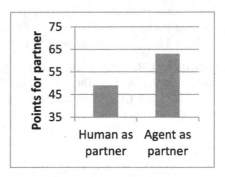

Fig. 4. Lottery tickets obtained by players and their partners

Participants also favored an equal division of the objects more often with human (73 %) than agent (22 %) partners ($\chi^2(1,N = 66) = 17.24$, $p < .001$). For example, one participant said, "Me walking away with two things and you walking away with four things is not going to work" even though this was the most efficient deal. Indeed, side B would often fight for the painting only to give up on a higher value item in order to maintain a 3-3 split. They occurred less often with CRA, probably as the wizard-script called attention to difference between the number of items and their value. It is also possible that people are less willing to apply the norm of fairness to computer programs (e.g., see [33]). Further studies will disambiguate these factors.

Subjective Impressions: We assessed several subjective impressions of the negotiation and one's partner when negotiating with both human participants and CRA. These are summarized in Table 2.

Table 2. Subjective impressions

	Partner	
	Human	CRA
Satisfaction	6.28 (0.19)	6.31 (0.25)
Partner satisfaction	6.00 (0.19)	6.47 (0.12)[*]
Ratings of partner	5.66 (0.27)	5.60 (0.17)
Ratings of self	5.76 (0.31)	6.05 (0.13)
Rapport	5.25 (0.19)	5.23 (0.14)
Ease of agreement	5.73 (0.19)	5.83 (0.21)

Note. $* = p \leq .05$, $** = p \leq .01$,
$*** = p \leq .001$

Satisfaction: As shown in Table 2, participants were as satisfied when paired with CRA as when paired with human participants ($t(1,63) = -0.09$, $p = .93$). Furthermore, they perceived CRA to be more satisfied with the negotiation than they perceived their human partners ($t(1,63) = -2.19$, $p = .03$). This is likely due to the fact that CRA obtained better outcomes than the inexpert human participants. Participants reported no greater satisfaction for themselves ($F(2,33) = 0.20$, $p = .82$) or for their partners ($F(2,33) = 1.27$, $p = .30$) as the agent was improved through development.

Cooperation: CRA was rated as cooperative as human partners on an 8-item scale ($t(1,63) = 0.19$, $p = .85$). They also rated their own level of cooperation no differently when paired with CRA than with a human partner ($t(1,63) = -0.92$, $p = .36$). Participants also did not rate their partners ($F(2,33) = 1.29$, $p = .51$) or themselves ($F(2,33) = 1.84$, $p = .18$) differently as the agent was improved through each iteration of development.

Rapport: Participants felt the same level of rapport (11-item scale) when paired with CRA as when paired with other human participants ($t(1,63) = 0.08$, $p = .94$). Likewise, they reported no less ease of reaching agreement when paired with our agent than with a human partner ($t(1,63) = -0.36$, $p = .72$),. Participants also reported no greater rapport ($F(2,33) = 0.68$, $p = .51$) or ease of reaching agreement ($F(2,33) = 1.18$, $p = .32$) as the agent was improved through development.

Design Goals: After each iteration of the WOz, we worked to improve the fluidity of the agent by reducing latency between speech acts as well as increasing the number of utterances that the agent could use during the negotiation. We tested these improvements by several subjective ratings. In addition to the survey questions described above, participants in the three rounds of WOz testing also rated the frequency of awkward pauses and how repetitive the agent seemed. We conducted t-tests on their ratings of how many awkward pauses and how much repetition there was in the conversation. As can be seen in Fig. 5, over the phases of development, participants reported significantly fewer awkward pauses ($F(2,33) = 4.85$, $p = .01$) and viewed the agent as significantly less repetitive ($F(2,33) = 4.26$, $p = .02$).

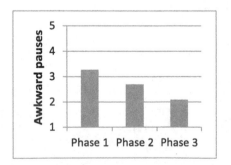 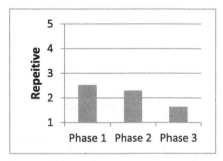

Fig. 5. Decreases in unnaturalness of the interaction across WOz iterations

6   Summary and Conclusion

Negotiation requires a number of cognitive and interpersonal skills and the multi-issue bargaining tasks allow many of these skills to be independently evoked and practiced by the judicious choice of preference weights and BATNA assigned to each party in a negotiation. Because of the complexity and necessity of negotiation in everyday life, bargaining problems have been an active focus of research across several research communities including multi-agent systems, social science, and education. Here we argue that bargaining is an important challenge area as it evokes the three pillars of the intelligent virtual agent community: intelligence (e.g., theory of mind reasoning, emotion, and decision-making), language (i.e., the full range of natural language processing) and embodiment (e.g., nonverbal communication).

The project has already yielded some tangible results along these lines. For example, the data collected in the face-to-face negotiations has been used to develop and evaluate potential algorithms for inferring a user's preferences from their pattern of offers and stated preferences. We found that techniques developed to fully automate negotiation perform poorly on human data but that heuristic methods can do a fairly accurate job at estimating a negotiator's preferences. We also find evidence that techniques can detect if a negotiator is lying by identifying discrepancies in what they say they want vs. what they are willing to offer [34].

In summary, we reported on our efforts to build a Conflict Resolution Agent that can negotiate with people and allow students to practice their negotiation skills. The current Wizard-of-Oz system evokes behavior similar to behaviors observed in face-to-face negotiations and leads people towards better solutions than they discover when negotiating against novice human negotiators.

Acknowledgments. This research was supported by the US Army. The content does not necessarily reflect the position or the policy of any Government, and no official endorsement should be inferred.

References

1. Thompson, L.L., Hastie, R: Judgement tasks and biases in negotiation. National Institute for Dispute Resolution (1990)
2. Movius, H.: The effectiveness of negotiation training. Negot. J. **24**(4), 509–531 (2008)
3. Lin, R., Oshrat, Y., Kraus, S.: Investigating the benefits of automated negotiations in enhancing people's negotiation skills. In: 8th International Conference on Autonomous Agents and Multiagent Systems (2009)
4. Core, M., et al.: Teaching negotiation skills through practice and reflection with virtual humans. Simulation **82**(11), 685–701 (2006)
5. Broekens, J., Harbers, M., Brinkman, W.-P., Jonker, C.M., Van den Bosch, K., Meyer, J.-J.: Virtual reality negotiation training increases negotiation knowledge and skill. In: Nakano, Y., Neff, M., Paiva, A., Walker, M. (eds.) IVA 2012. LNCS, vol. 7502, pp. 218–230. Springer, Heidelberg (2012)
6. Simon, H.: The Sciences of the Artificial. MIT Press, Cambridge (1969)
7. Blascovich, J., et al.: Immersive virtual environment technology as a methodological tool for social psychology. Psychol. Inq. **13**, 103–124 (2002)
8. Carnevale, P.J., Pruitt, D.G.: Negotiation and mediation. Ann. Rev. Psychol. **43**(1), 531–582 (1992)
9. Kelley, H.H., Schenitzki, D.P.: Bargaining. In: McClintock, C. (ed.) Experimental Social Psychology, pp. 298–337. Holt, Rinehart, and Winston, New York (1972)

10. Baarslag, T., et al.: Evaluating practical negotiating agents: Results and analysis of the 2011 international competition. Artif. Intell. **198**, 73–103 (2013)

11. Van Kleef, G.A., De Dreu, C.K.W., Manstead, A.S.R.: The interpersonal effects of anger and happiness in negotiations. J. Pers. Soc. Psychol. **86**(1), 57–76 (2004)

12. O'Connor, K.M., Carnevale, P.J.: A nasty but effective negotiation strategy: misrepresentation of a common-value issue. Pers. Soc. Psychol. Bull. **23**(5), 504–515 (1997)

13. Dehghani, M., et al.: Sacred values and conflict over Iran's nuclear program. Judgm. Decis. Making **5**(7), 540–546 (2010)

14. O'Connor, K.M.: Groups and solos in context: the effects of accountability on team negotiation. Organ. Behav. Hum. Decis. Process. **72**(3), 384–407 (1997)

15. Bhatt, M.A., et al.: Neural signatures of strategic types in a two-person bargaining game. Proc. Natl. Acad. Sci. **107**(46), 19720–19725 (2010)

16. Nash Jr., J.F.: The bargaining problem. Econometrica: J. Econometric Soc. **18**, 155–162 (1950)

17. Park, S., et al.: Mutual behaviors during dyadic negotiation: Automatic prediction of respondent reactions. In: 2013 Humaine Association Conference on Affective Computing and Intelligent Interaction (ACII) (2013) IEEE

18. Li, R., Curhan, J., Hoque, M.E.: Predicting video-conferencing conversation outcomes based on modeling facial expression synchronization. In: The 11th IEEE International Conference on Automatic Face and Gesture Recognition. IEEE: Ljubljana, Slovenia (2015)

19. Khooshabeh, P., et al.: Negotiation strategies with incongruent facial expressions of emotion cause cardiovascular threat. In: 35th annual meeting of the Cognitive Science Society, Berlin, Germany (2013)

20. de Melo, C., Carnevale, P.J., Gratch, J.: The effect of expression of anger and happiness in computer agents on negotiations with humans. In: The Tenth International Conference on Autonomous Agents and Multiagent Systems, Taipai, Taiwan (2011)

21. Mell, J., Lucas, G., Gratch, J.: An effective conversation tactic for creating value over repeated negotiations. In: 14th International Conference on Autonomous Agents and Multiagent Systems, Istanbul, Turkey (2015)

22. DeVault, D., Sagae, K., Traum, D.: Incremental interpretation and prediction of utterance meaning for interactive dialogue. Dialogue Discourse **2**(1), 143–170 (2011)

23. Curhan, J.R., Elfenbein, H.A.: What do people value when they negotiate? Mapping the domain of subjective value in negotiation. J. Pers. Soc. Psychol. **91**(3), 493–512 (2006)

24. Rosenfeld, A., et al.: NegoChat: a chat-based negotiation agent. In: 13th International Conference on Autonomous Agents and Multi-agent Systems, Paris, France (2014)

25. Hindriks, K.V., Jonker, C.M.: Creating human-machine synergy in negotiation support systems: towards the pocket negotiator. In: Proceedings of the 1st International Working Conference on Human Factors and Computational Models in Negotiation. ACM (2008)

26. Kim, J.M., et al.: BiLAT: a game-based environment for practicing negotiation in a cultural context. Int. J. Artif. Intell. Educ. **19**(3), 289–308 (2009)

27. Traum, D., Marsella, S.C., Gratch, J., Lee, J., Hartholt, A.: Multi-party, multi-issue, multi-strategy negotiation for multi-modal virtual agents. In: Prendinger, H., Lester, J., Ishizuka, M. (eds.) IVA 2008. LNCS (LNAI), vol. 5208, pp. 117–130. Springer, Heidelberg (2008)

28. Grosz, B., Kraus, S.: Collaborative plans for complex group action. Artif. Intell. **86**(2), 269–357 (1996)

29. Hartholt, A., Traum, D., Marsella, S.C., Shapiro, A., Stratou, G., Leuski, A., Morency, L.-P., Gratch, J.: All together now. In: Aylett, R., Krenn, B., Pelachaud, C., Shimodaira, H. (eds.) IVA 2013. LNCS, vol. 8108, pp. 368–381. Springer, Heidelberg (2013)

30. Lee, J., Marsella, S.C.: Nonverbal behavior generator for embodied conversational agents. In: Gratch, J., Young, M., Aylett, R.S., Ballin, D., Olivier, P. (eds.) IVA 2006. LNCS (LNAI), vol. 4133, pp. 243–255. Springer, Heidelberg (2006)
31. Thiebaux, M., et al., SmartBody: behavior realization for embodied conversational agents. In: International Conference on Autonomous Agents and Multi-Agent Systems, Portugal (2008)
32. DeVault, D., Mell, J., Gratch, J.: Toward Natural Turn-Taking in a Virtual Human Negotiation Agent. In: AAAI Spring Symposium on Turn-taking and Coordination in Human-Machine Interaction. AAAI Press, Stanford, CA (2015)
33. de Melo, C., Carnevale, P.J., Gratch, J.: Humans vs. Computers: The Effect of Perceived Agency on People's Decision Making. University of Southern California (2013)
34. Nazari, Z., Lucas, G., Gratch, J.: Opponent modeling for virtual human negotiators. In: W.-P. Brinkman et al. (eds.) IVA 2015, LNAI(LNCS), vol. 9238, pp. 39–49. Springer, Heidelberg

Generation of Non-compliant Behaviour in Virtual Medical Narratives

Alan Lindsay[1], Fred Charles[1], Jonathon Read[1], Julie Porteous[1],
Marc Cavazza[1(✉)], and Gersende Georg[2]

[1] School of Computing, Teesside University, Middlesbrough, UK
M.O.Cavazza@tees.ac.uk
[2] Haute Autorité de Santé, 2 Avenue du Stade de France, Saint-denis, France

Abstract. Patient education documents increasingly take the form of
Patient Guidelines, which share many of the properties of clinical guidelines in terms of knowledge content and the description of clinical protocols. They however differ in one specific aspect, which is that some
recommendations for patient behaviour may be violated, and that no
explicit representation of undesired behaviour is embedded in the guidelines themselves. In this paper, we take as a starting point the plan-
based representation of clinical guidelines, which has been promoted by
several authors, and introduce a method to automatically derive the set
of "opposite actions" that constitute violations of recommended patient
behaviours. These additional alternative actions are generated automatically as PDDL operators complementing the description of the guideline.
As an application, using a patient guideline on bariatric surgery, we also
present examples of how these actions can be used to visualise undesirable patient behaviour in a 3D serious game, featuring virtual agents
representing the patient and healthcare professionals.

1 Introduction

Patient education plays an important role in the success of complex, life-changing
therapies such as bariatric surgery, which requires preparation, informed consent and compliance with lifestyle instructions after surgery. As patient education documents become more complex they are increasingly referred to as
Patient Guidelines[1], sharing important properties with other guidelines in terms
of knowledge content, namely the description of underlying protocols and a set
of recommendations prescribing desired behaviour.

However, taking full advantage of patient education documents still poses
considerable challenges to a large fraction of the patient population, and it has
been previously suggested that visual media could assist with the health literacy
problem [18]. In this paper, we introduce a new method to automatically expand
the narrative representation of patient guidelines to include actions representing

---

[1] The term *Patient Guidelines* is drawn from working documents of the
Guidelines International Network (GIN), http://www.g-i-n.net/document-store/
working-groups-documents/g-i-n-public/toolkit/toolkit-chapter-4.pdf.

© Springer International Publishing Switzerland 2015
W.-P. Brinkman et al. (Eds.): IVA 2015, LNAI 9238, pp. 216–228, 2015.
DOI: 10.1007/978-3-319-21996-7_22

patient violation of guideline recommendations. Our approach is to explicitly represent non-compliance in the same format, so as to support the presentation of counter examples, which we refer to as *undesirable behaviour*. Our rationale is to derive concrete examples of actions to be avoided, from the generic recommendations contained in the patient guidelines, in order to provide additional information to patients without increasing the authoring burden. We illustrate this approach on the plan-based generation of narratives for clinical guidelines developed to address health literacy issues and presented to patients as a 3D interactive serious game featuring virtual agents representing the patient and healthcare professionals [18]. The textual guideline is translated into a narrative planning domain manually, through a complex knowledge engineering process that requires additional input on the background medical knowledge required to properly stage the course of action.

Planning has been one of the most popular techniques to support narrative generation [16]. Several authors have also advocated the use of Planning formalisms to represent the knowledge content of clinical guidelines. This can be intuitively justified by the suitability of plans to represent the underlying sequence of clinical actions. We take as a starting point the use of Planning formalisms for the representation of guidelines contents [4,13,19] and in particular standard planning formalisms such as PDDL [4,5]. Our method is based on the principled generation of "contrary" actions from the logical structure of the PDDL unit representing an action, which can be used instead of the original action set during narrative generation thus allowing the generation of alternate strategies for non-compliance.

In the next sections, after briefly discussing the role of Planning in the formalisation of guidelines based on previous work, we introduce the various aspects of the method and show its application. Furthermore, in the specific case of using this approach to visualise guidelines, we show how visual content generation can adapt to the expansion of the knowledge base, without constituting a bottleneck for the production of a guideline-based 3D interactive serious game. Throughout the paper, we illustrate the work with examples from a fully implemented 3D serious game featuring an interactive narrative in the field of bariatric surgery.

2   Rationale and Previous Work

The use of narratives featuring virtual agents has previously been reported in health applications, for their ability to organise information related to patient history, disease history or relating to daily living issues (for prevention or family education). An authoring system for personal health narratives is described in [1]. Based on conversational characters and dialogue, rather than plot-oriented, it is centred on personal narratives rather than educational ones. More recently, interactive narrative techniques have been applied to the topic of AIDS prevention [14] using virtual agents endowed with Theory of Mind reasoning [11]. Narrative techniques have also been proposed for medical education. Magerko et al. [12] described its use to coordinate training scenarios in basic life support and provide a more personalised training experience.

The work undertaken in [6] included a study which investigated if challenges associated with interpersonal communication skills training could be overcome by building a virtual human with back story. Back story was achieved through the use of cut-scenes which played throughout the virtual human interaction. In [2] a virtual human exercise counsellor is described that interacts daily with users to promote exercise. An integrated dynamic social storytelling engine was used to maintain user engagement with the agent and retention in the intervention.

Several authors have advocated the use of Planning formalisms to represent the knowledge content of clinical guidelines. This can be intuitively justified by the suitability of plans to represent the underlying sequence of clinical actions. A variety of planning formalisms have been described, from standard PDDL [4] and HTN [8,10], to guidelines-specific extensions [13], incorporating, for instance, temporal aspects. In the present work, we use PDDL 3.0 [9], which incorporates extensions improving its knowledge representation abilities.

The rationale for our approach is to start with a domain model where operators represent desired behaviours and from this to automatically generate one or more contrary operators that correspond to undesirable behaviour–those that violate the recommended course of action. A naïve example, prior to any formalisation, would consist in observing that there are several opposites to healthy eating: unbalanced diet, skipping meals, and excessive calorie intake. Our work aims at providing a more rigorous and operational implementation of this phenomenon. For our original domain model we used a subset of a published guideline on bariatric surgery which corresponds to lifestyle recommendations and post-surgery eating habits. We modelled the entire guideline, as a PDDL planning domain, which contained over 111 operators and 230 predicates.

Our method of generating contrary, non-compliant operators, builds on that introduced in [17]. Their approach identified "missing" contrary (i.e. opposite) actions through analysis of the state transitions described in the operators and generated new operators by reversal of pre- and post-conditions, with names for the new operators generated using antonyms sourced from on-line lexical resources. Our approach differs in the following key aspects:

– Operator pre-conditions are analysed to identify key predicates which enable *desired* behaviour (as defined by the guidelines) and whose antonyms represent *undesirable* behaviour. On-line lexical resources are used to identify one or more antonyms that provide meaningful labels for these non-compliant behaviours and which will be used to generate names for new PDDL operators and content.
– New PDDL operators are generated for the identified undesirable behaviours and whose structure implements the transformed formulae in its preconditions or effects (or both as applicable).
– In order to enhance domain readability when new names for predicates and operators are produced, the generated antonymic names are used in conjunction with a small grammar of rewriting rules (see Sect. 3.3).

The automatically generated antonymic operators are used to extend the planning domain representing the protocol, and can be used to generate examples

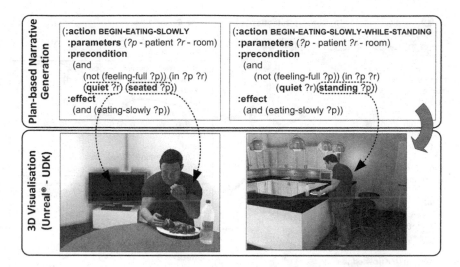

Fig. 1. Generation of 3D visualisation from description of PDDL operators: BEGIN-EATING-SLOWLY is one of the original PDDL operators and the identified enabling predicate in the pre-conditions (**seated** *?p*) is highlighted. The operator BEGIN-EATING-SLOWLY-WHILE-STANDING is the newly generated action based on the violation of the condition, featuring the antonymically named (**standing** *?p*).

of undesirable behaviour or give explicit warnings taking into account specific contexts (e.g. type of surgery, patient profile). Figure 1 illustrates one of the original actions, BEGIN-EATING-SLOWLY, that was modelled from the guidelines and represents recommended behaviour, along with an automatically generated violating action, BEGIN-EATING-SLOWLY-WHILE-STANDING, which was generated based on a violation of the enabling condition (**seated** *?p*). The figure also shows the 3D visualisations resulting from the staging of these actions from operators encoding both the recommended and the violating behaviour. The 3D visualisation, or staging, of these actions allows for the real-time illustration for the patient of the narrative situations generated within a typical virtual agents based interactive virtual environment (this is detailed further in Sect. 4).

3 Extension of Patient Guidelines Using Non-compliance

In this section, we consider the problem of automatically extending planning domains representing knowledge from patient guidelines with operators that violate the guidelines' recommendation. We consider the use of guidelines that detail the correct contexts for patient pathway and how we can generate alternative contexts for those behaviours, corresponding to non-compliance.

3.1 Guidelines Modelling in PDDL

PDDL [9] is a standard language for encoding planning problems, which has gained popularity since it allows the same problem description to be processed

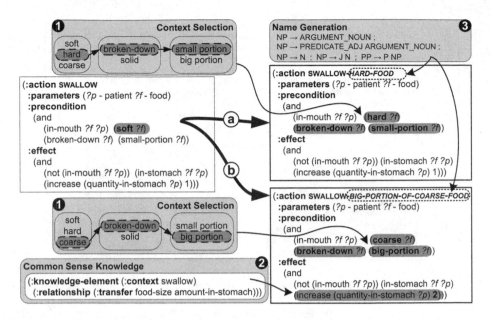

Fig. 2. Generating Alternative Actions: (a) and (b) are alternative actions generated from (1) Context Selection and (2) Common Sense Knowledge mechanisms. Name Generation (3) generates the new action names (please see text for details).

by a variety of planning systems. Its suitability for representing guidelines has been suggested by Bradbrook et al. [4]. In the case of patient guidelines, operators' contents are a mix of generic predicates and specific ones corresponding to the recommendation element. For a given operator, there is a set of precondition *enablers* that represent the recommendation element of the guideline, often corresponding to a condition explicitly mentioned in the text (such as the environment in which the patient should take their meals). We refer to these recommended elements as *contexts*.

For example, the `swallow` operator can be modelled in PDDL, as presented in Fig. 2 and applicable action instances are generated at plan-time by instantiating the operator parameters. The `swallow` operator has several pre-conditions, including that the bolus is in the patient's mouth and the operator is not applicable unless these conditions are met. The effects of applying the operator are that the bolus is transferred from the mouth to the stomach and the quantity in the stomach is increase. The `swallow` operator requires that the bolus is small, soft and broken-down: these *enabler* conditions encode explicit recommendations from the guidelines.

3.2   Non-Compliance as Alternative Contexts

While patient guidelines describe recommended behaviour, non-compliance can occur for multiple reasons, ranging from misunderstanding of the instructions to an inability to follow prescribed behaviour, due to competing motivations. Non-compliance could be described as not carrying out a recommended action. However, when the guidelines describe activities of daily living whose actions are essential, non-compliance is more often concerned with not carrying out the recommended action properly (in terms of execution or circumstances) or carrying out the wrong action. In the remainder of this section we detail how these are identified via: identification of candidate predicates; and generation of alternative contexts.

Identification of Candidate Predicates. The first step is to extract the *enabler* predicates from the pre-conditions of PDDL operators. For example, the recommendation "Sit down to eat your meals and do so in a calm environment", directly refers to the predicates, (`seated` *?patient*) and (`quiet` *?room*).

Generation of Alternatives. The generation of contrary operators is realised through the generation of antonyms for the labels of the predicates identified in the section above in the operators' pre-conditions. This process is realised in two steps, the first obtains a set of possible candidate antonyms from linguistic resources and the second filters this set by statistically measuring candidates' association with the particular type of the original predicate, as described below. Of course a word can have various meanings and the correct discovery of possible alternatives requires each of these to be considered. For example, quiet can be opposed with noisy, but also with `public` (as in "carried out in quiet" versus "carried out in public"). In our context, each of these words is a useful consideration of alternative context for a patient eating and similarly a violation of the guideline. However, the word is used in a context particular to the domain, and so the filtering approach we use exploits the context of the planning domain by measuring candidates' association with their type, in order to better choose candidates. These types are identified directly from the predicate arguments in the PDDL model. For each predicate we predict the argument of the predicate that would appear after the predicate in common parlance. We exploit typical predicate encoding practice: for unary predicates we select the first parameter, whereas for higher arity predicates the second argument would be selected. For example, for the predicate (`still` *?d*), we use the type, `drink`, which is the type of parameter *?d*.

We use a collection of online lexical resources[2] in order to generate the candidate antonyms. The first step is to generate a collection of the senses of the word, by identifying the synset in WordNet [7]. Each sense is then used with each of the lexical resources to generate a collection of candidate antonyms, which are subsequently passed to the filtering process.

Filtering antonyms is a matter of statistically evaluating the strength of collocation—the degree to which words occur in juxtaposition. To measure collocation between a candidate antonym (a) and its associated type (t) we employ

---

[2] Merriam-Webster http://www.dictionaryapi.com; Big Huge Thesaurus http://words.bighugelabs.com; Power Thesaurus http://www.powerthesaurus.org.

normalised pointwise mutual information (NPMI) [3]

$$\text{NPMI}\,(a;t) = \frac{1}{-\log p\,(a,t)} \log \frac{p\,(a,t)}{p\,(a)\,p\,(t)} \tag{1}$$

where probabilities are estimated using maximum likelihood estimation over frequency counts in a corpus of Wikipedia articles[3]. For this task we are interested in whether the candidate antonyms legitimately modify the type associated with the original predicate and so, using the Stanford CoreNLP tagger [20] to predict part-of-speech tags, we constrain joint frequency counts to instances where the candidate appears as an adjective immediately preceding the type occurring as a noun. Then, to filter candidate antonyms we select the candidate with the greatest association with the context word.

When predicates are multi-word expressions an additional procedure is employed, whereby candidate multi-word antonyms are generated by pairing the individual words with an antonym generated as described above, and enumerating in-sequence combinations (e.g. small-portion yields large-portion, small-whole and large-whole). Then the most likely candidate is estimated using a probabilistic n-gram language model [15], trained over the same Wikipedia articles.

3.3   Generation of Antonymic Operators

The overall process of generation of new operators is illustrated in Fig. 2 and results in a considerable expansion in the number of operators. Operator content is assembled as follows:

Pre-conditions. The pre-condition is generated by substituting the original operator context with the newly generated context. This is equivalent to performing a similar action in a different context, opposite to the recommended one. For example, Fig. 2 shows the pre-condition created for the new action SWALLOW-HARD-FOOD where the recommended context (soft $?f$) is replaced with an alternate non-compliant context: (hard $?f$).

Effects. The effect part of the operator will typically remain the same, except where the context directly impacts object transformations by the operator (for instance, chewing slowly a food portion). In this case, we rely on a common sense knowledge base to propagate changes without complexifying the operator at the expense of modularity. This common sense inference of effects exploits those *enablers* that describe modalities on how the action is performed, which need to be taken into account when considering its effects. For example, swallowing a large portion of food might result in increasing stomach content more rapidly than thorough eating normally as recommended.

---

[3] Wikipedia provides a broad coverage sample of language which is appropriate here because activities of daily living do not involve specialised terminology.

```
( :knowledge−element
    ( :context  swallow )
    ( :relationship  ( :transfer  food−size  amount−in−stomach ) ) )
```

Fig. 3. Example Knowledge Element: knowledge elements detail the transition that it applies to (context) and a relationship between the objects involved. Here it is the act of swallowing which relates the portion size to the amount of food in the stomach.

We have developed a collection of supporting common knowledge relationships, called *knowledge elements*, that we can use to make appropriate modifications to the effects of the operator. A common underlying principle is to define the relationships between ranges of values. For example, the size of the portion of food that the patient is swallowing is related to the space that it will occupy when in the stomach, as represented in the example in Fig. 3. A number of common sense rules on preservation of quantities and relationships between density and volume ensure an appropriate mapping.

The formalisation allows a mapping onto the planning domain by resolving certain issues related to default values and range of variation that may not be fully represented in the planning domain, keeping the latter efficient. In terms of inference, these rules can be applied in sequence before the effects of a new operator are instantiated (consider for instance, the increase in food volume in the stomach associated with swallowing a large portion without chewing it properly - two violations).

Table 1. Generated operator names given the non-compliant predicates of `swallow`.

Original action	Non-compliant predicates	New operator names
		swallow-hard-food
		swallow-solid-food
	hard *?food*	swallow-big-portion-of-food
swallow	solid *?food*	swallow-hard-solid-food
	big-portion *?food*	swallow-big-portion-of-solid-food
		swallow-big-portion-of-hard-food
		swallow-big-portion-of-hard-solid-food

Operator Naming. Operator names are generally composed of a set of hyphened words describing an action and its main modalities. New names for automatically generated antonymic operators are composed following the same principle, by inspecting each of the alternative predicates and generating a phrase according to a simple rewriting grammar of the type depicted in component 3 of Fig. 2, in which the part-of-speech and prepositional preferences of arguments and predicates are determined using a manually-constructed lexicon.

The result of this generation process is a distinct phrase for each argument. The new operator name will always start with the original operator name (e.g. `begin-eating`). However, the ideal ordering of the phrases generated to represent such alternate predicates is difficult to specify formally. For example, given a set of alternative predicates {(`standing` *?patient*), (`noisy` *?room*)}, the above process yields the phrases {while-standing, in-a-noisy-room}. Concatenating these without regard to order could lead to unnatural names, so we generate all permutations of these phrases, and employ a probabilistic *n*-gram language model [15] to rank candidates according to their likelihood. Table 1 lists the names generated for predicates of non-compliance for the `swallow` action.

Table 2. A comparison of the antonyms generated with the ANTON approach from [17] and our extended approach that uses a contextualising filter: ANTON + Filtering.

Context	Word	ANTON	ANTON + Filtering
Person	Seated	Standing	Standing
Food	Soft	Hard	Hard/Coarse
Drink	Still	Agitate	Sparkling
Room	Quiet	Noisy	Noisy
Room	Private	Public	Public

3.4   Evaluation

An initial PDDL domain model representing the correct eating practice habits fragment of the guidelines was encoded using 11 operators. Then the approach developed in this paper was used to expand the domain, resulting in the addition of 43 operators, each demonstrating an alternative instance of non-compliance. In terms of instantiated operators, this represents an increase from roughly two hundred instantiated operators in the original domain, to thousands of instantiated operators in the extended domain.

Table 2 shows the single word predicates that were encoded in our domain model and a comparison between the approach to generating antonyms introduced in ANTON [17] and the approach that we introduced in this paper which features a contextualising filter. Although the approaches are similar, through exploiting context the accuracy can be improved, as is the case for the antonyms for the word `still` shown in the table: whereas ANTON prefers the antonym `agitate`, the contextual filtering, using the context of `drink`, results in `sparkling` ranked highest.

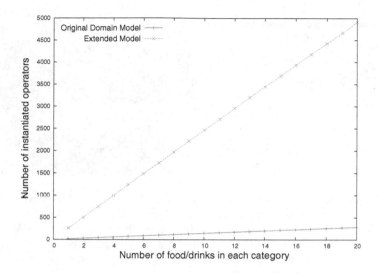

Fig. 4. Comparison of the rate of increase in number of instantiated operators between the original and antonymically extended domain models (depending on food/drink items available). During narrative generation this increase yields consequent increases in the possible degree of narrative variation, whilst the potential performance overhead is managed via filtering out of operators that aren't involved in branching aspects.

In terms of instantiated operators, the number increases with the number of food and drink items of each category. We have identified a typical scenario with a patient in the patient-kitchen and have used this to generate 20 PDDL problem models for the normal domain and the enhanced domain, with increasing numbers of food and drink items. We generate more food and drink items for each combination of properties, such as hard and small-portion. Figure 4, illustrates how the number of instantiated operators grows as the number of objects in each category is increased, for both the original and the extended model.

4   Visualising Alternative Actions and Non-Compliance

Our target application consists in generating 3D visualisation of narratives from guidelines contents [5] and, within this application, the role of antonymic generation is to extend the number of actions available to explicitly illustrate incorrect behaviour making the contents of the guideline more accessible. The generation of 3D visuals for guidelines actions is based on an intermediate semantic representation embedded in the graphics engine (UDK), which describes both objects categories and action properties (the latter being parametrised through a set of animations, defining characters attitudes and motion speed).

The 3D visualisation of guidelines actions is defined through the staging of the resources involved in the scene to be generated, such as characters and objects. The context of the action being visualised is also defined through parameterisation of the virtual environment. We defined an ontology to provide

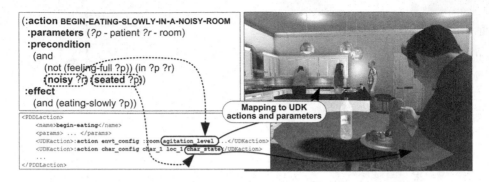

Fig. 5. Mapping of operator predicates representing the context of the environment to UDK actions and parameters via an XML-based intermediate layer. Here the predicates (`seated` *?p*) and (`noisy` *?r*) are mapped to action descriptions in the XML, which represent the sequences of UDK actions and parameters involved (including virtual agents and scene configurations). This supports the dynamic generation of contrary actions without having to encode them a priori.

domain knowledge to the virtual environment which underpins the representation of objects and their properties. Our ontology covers the general concepts of resources available within the virtual environment. The staging of the guideline actions as defined by the Planning operators is described by sequences of parametrised actions and associated 3D animations that enable the action's visualisation. In order to generate the visualisation for the alternative actions, we map the modified contextual elements from the planning operators to modify the original staging description. The alternative operator having been generated provides the details for the elements of staging modification, through the set of modified predicates (e.g. (`seated` *?patient*) and (`standing` *?patient*); and (`quiet` *?room*) and (`noisy` *?room*))

For instance in Fig. 5, the staging of the `noisy` environment property (defined by the predicate) is mapped onto the definition of the generation of possible alternative stagings where the context of the virtual environment surrounding the patient is instantiated appropriately. The virtual environment includes physical devices with properties such as *volume levels* for objects such as radio and television for which the volume level is selected according to the context of the situation to be staged. As such, a `quiet` environment will be instantiated by a minimal level of noise for radio and television volume levels. On the contrary, a `noisy` environment will provide a degree of agitation for the room translated to the number of background virtual agents and a medium to high volume level for television and radio.

5   Conclusions

We have introduced a mechanism for the automatic extension of Planning domains derived from patient guidelines, to generate examples of non-compliance. This method leverages on the use of lexical resources to produce operators that retain the consistency of the original ones from which they are derived. The use of generic lexical resources is made possible by the fact that lifestyle advice uses very little medical terminology. These first results (both qualitative and quantitative) are encouraging, the only limitation consisting in some spurious generation, which in our application has been filtered out when mapping to the semantic layer of the virtual environment in which these alternative actions are staged. In future work, this method could be extended, at least in part, to the representation of clinical actions, subject to a redefinition of contrary actions and their relation to more specialised lexical resources.

Acknowledgments. This work has been funded in part through the Open FET MUSE project (FP7-296703). The contents of this paper only reflect the authors opinions and not necessarily the official position of Haute Autorité de Santé.

References

1. Bickmore, T., Ring, L.: Making it personal: end-user authoring of health narratives delivered by virtual agents. In: Allbeck, J., Badler, N., Bickmore, T., Pelachaud, C., Safonova, A. (eds.) IVA 2010. LNCS, vol. 6356, pp. 399–405. Springer, Heidelberg (2010)
2. Bickmore, T., Schulman, D., Yin, L.: Engagement vs. deceit: virtual humans with human autobiographies. In: Ruttkay, Z., Kipp, M., Nijholt, A., Vilhjálmsson, H.H. (eds.) IVA 2009. LNCS, vol. 5773, pp. 6–19. Springer, Heidelberg (2009)
3. Bouma, G.: Normalized (pointwise) mutual information in collocation extraction. In: Proceedings of the Biennial GSCL Conference, pp. 31–40 (2009)
4. Bradbrook, K., Winstanley, G., Glasspool, D.W., Fox, J., Griffiths, R.N.: AI planning technology as a component of computerised clinical practice guidelines. In: Miksch, S., Hunter, J., Keravnou, E.T. (eds.) AIME 2005. LNCS (LNAI), vol. 3581, pp. 171–180. Springer, Heidelberg (2005)
5. Charles, F., Cavazza, M., Smith, C., Georg, G., Porteous, J.: Instantiating interactive narratives from patient education documents. In: Peek, N., Marín Morales, R., Peleg, M. (eds.) AIME 2013. LNCS, vol. 7885, pp. 273–283. Springer, Heidelberg (2013)
6. Cordar, A., Borish, M., Foster, A., Lok, B.: Building virtual humans with back stories: training interpersonal communication skills in medical students. In: Bickmore, T., Marsella, S., Sidner, C. (eds.) IVA 2014. LNCS, vol. 8637, pp. 144–153. Springer, Heidelberg (2014)
7. Fellbaum, C. (ed.): WordNet: An Electronic Lexical Database. MIT Press, Cambridge (1998)
8. Georg, G., Cavazza, M.: Integrating document-based and knowledge-based models for clinical guidelines analysis. In: Bellazzi, R., Abu-Hanna, A., Hunter, J. (eds.) AIME 2007. LNCS (LNAI), vol. 4594, pp. 421–430. Springer, Heidelberg (2007)
9. Gerevini, A., Long, D.: Plan constraints and preferences in pddl3. The Language of the Fifth International Planning Competition. Technical report, Department of Electronics for Automation, University of Brescia, Italy, 75 (2005)

10. González-Ferrer, A., Ten Teije, A., Fdez-Olivares, J., Milian, K.: Automated generation of patient-tailored electronic care pathways by translating computer-interpretable guidelines into hierarchical task networks. Artif. Intell. Med. **57**(2), 91–109 (2013)
11. Klatt, J., Marsella, S., Krämer, N.C.: Negotiations in the context of AIDS prevention: an agent-based model using theory of mind. In: Vilhjálmsson, H.H., Kopp, S., Marsella, S., Thórisson, K.R. (eds.) IVA 2011. LNCS, vol. 6895, pp. 209–215. Springer, Heidelberg (2011)
12. Magerko, B., Wray, R.E., Holt, L.S., Stensrud, B.: Customizing interactive training through individualized content and increased engagement. In: The Interservice/Industry Training, Simulation & Education Conference (I/ITSEC), number 1 (2005)
13. Miksch, S., Shahar, Y., Johnson, P.: Asbru: a task-specific, intention-based, and time-oriented language for representing skeletal plans. In: Proceedings of the 7th Workshop on Knowledge Engineering: Methods & Languages (KEML-97), Milton Keynes, UK, The Open University, pp. 9–19 (1997)
14. Miller, L., Appleby, P., Christensen, J., Godoy, C., Si, M., Corsbie-Massay, C., Noar, S., Harrington, N.: Virtual interactive interventions for reducing risky sex: adaptations, integrations, and innovations. In: eHealth Applications: Promising Strategies for Health Behavior Change, pp. 79–95. Routledge, New York (2012)
15. Pauls, A., Klein, D.: Faster and smaller n-gram language models. In: Proceedings of the 49th Meeting of the Association for Computational Linguistics, HLT 2011, pp. 258–267, Stroudsburg, PA, USA (2011)
16. Porteous, J., Cavazza, M., Charles, F.: Applying planning to interactive storytelling: narrative control using state constraints. ACM Trans. Intell. Syst. Technol. (TIST) **1**(2), 10 (2010)
17. Porteous, J., Lindsay, A., Read, J., Truran, M., Cavazza, M.: Automated extension of narrative planning domains with antonymic operators. In: Proceedings of the 14th International Conference on Autonomous Agents and Multiagent Systems, pp. 1547–1555. IFAAMAS (2015)
18. Safeer, R.S., Keenan, J.: Health literacy: the gap between physicians and patients. Am. Fam. Physician **72**(3), 463–468 (2005)
19. Shahar, Y., Musen, M.A.: Plan recognition and revision in support of guideline-based care. In: Working notes of the AAAI Spring Symposium on Representing Mental States and Mechanisms, pp. 118–126 (1995)
20. Toutanova, K., Klein, D., Manning, C.D., Singer, Y.: Feature-rich part-of-speech tagging with a cyclic dependency network. In: Proceedings of the 2003 Conference of the North American Chapter of the Association for Computational Linguistics on Human Language Technology, NAACL 2003, Stroudsburg, PA, USA, vol. 1, pp. 173–180 (2003)

Virtual Role-Models: Using Virtual Humans to Train Best Communication Practices for Healthcare Teams

Andrew Cordar[1]([⊠]), Andrew Robb[1], Adam Wendling[1],
Samsun Lampotang[1], Casey White[2], and Benjamin Lok[1]

[1] University of Florida, Gainesville, FL, USA
{acordar,arobb,lok}@cise.ufl.edu,
{awendling,slampotang}@anest.ufl.edu
[2] University of Virginia, Charlottesville, VA, USA
cw4xz@virginia.edu

Abstract. Due to logistical scheduling challenges, social training of conflict resolution skills with healthcare professionals is a difficult task. To overcome these challenges, we used virtual humans to fill in as surgical teammates and train conflict resolution skills in a surgical scenario. Surgical technologists were recruited at a United States teaching hospital to interact with a virtual nurse, virtual surgeon, and virtual anesthesiologist in a team training exercise. Leveraging social learning theory, the virtual nurse on the team modeled one of two conflict resolution strategies, either best practices or bad practices, during an important decision moment in the exercise. In a second important decision moment, we assessed if surgical technologists demonstrated the conflict resolution model they observed. We found human participants were successfully able to demonstrate the ideal conflict resolution strategy after observing the virtual nurse model best practices. While we found participants were positively influenced by the best practices model, we also found that conversely, the bad practices model negatively influenced participants' conflict resolution behavior. If humans can be positively influenced by virtual humans, this form of social training could transform medical team training, empowering more healthcare professionals to speak up, and potentially decreasing the chances of patient morbidity or death in the OR.

Keywords: Virtual humans · Social learning theory · Team training

1 Introduction

Our paper explores how to use social training with virtual humans to teach best practices for communication in a medical team. Specifically, we investigate if humans are malleable and can be influenced to learn by example from virtual humans. If humans can be positively influenced by virtual humans, this form of social training could transform medical team training, empower more healthcare professionals to speak up to their team when they have concerns, and potentially decrease the chances of patient morbidity or death in the operating room.

© Springer International Publishing Switzerland 2015
W.-P. Brinkman et al. (Eds.): IVA 2015, LNAI 9238, pp. 229–238, 2015.
DOI: 10.1007/978-3-319-21996-7_23

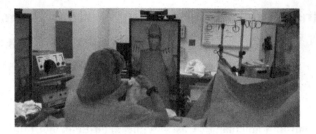

Fig. 1. Surgical technologist conducting a closing count with a virtual team

To investigate this, surgical technologists were recruited at a United States teaching hospital to interact with virtual humans in a four-person surgical team training exercise (Fig. 1). The training was intended to address one of the most important and difficult skills in the operating room: communication. At this hospital, nursing management implemented a policy requiring best communication practices during the closing count of a surgery. Best practices means speaking up if proper procedure is not followed and calling a supervisor or charge nurse if the issues cannot be resolved between the team. Failure to follow best practices during the closing count could lead to retained foreign bodies, i.e. surgical equipment left inside the patient. Retained foreign bodies can be harmful to patients and can cause severe injury or even death [1].

In perioperative care, role models are a valuable resource for ensuring a safe work environment and for ensuring patient safety [2]. Unfortunately, role models who exhibit best practices are not always present in the operating room. Research has shown that interpersonal conflict or bullying of staff is common especially with new hires with less experience [3]. One way to address the lack of positive role modeling is through social training.

Social training opportunities for healthcare teams; however, are difficult to coordinate [4]. Healthcare professionals have inflexible schedules and each member is essential in real operating room environments. To address these issues, we used virtual humans to fill in as operating room teammates and train best practices for conflict resolution in the operating room.

Leveraging social learning theory, a virtual nurse on the team modeled best practices for conflict resolution with a virtual surgeon during an important decision moment. We investigated if surgical technologists, after observing the first decision moment, would demonstrate a similar behavior in the same scenario during a subsequent closing count in which the virtual surgeon wants to make a risky decision.

We found human participants were successfully able to demonstrate the best practices for conflict resolution after observing the virtual nurse model best practices. While we found human participants were positively influenced by the virtual nurse, we also found when the virtual nurse modeled bad practices for conflict resolution, surgical technologists were less likely to resolve the conflict effectively, e.g., call a supervisor.

2 Background

Our research leverages existing research on social learning theory and mixed reality virtual humans. With mixed reality virtual humans, we developed a medical team training scenario that incorporates social learning theory to enhance the training experience.

2.1 Social Learning Theory

Social Learning Theory was created by Albert Bandura who suggested learning is a social activity in which people can learn by observing the behaviors of others, also known as vicarious learning [5]. Bandura's most famous experiment, the Bobo doll experiment, demonstrated that children, when observing adults either play roughly or gently with a toy, the bobo doll, would imitate the behavior they observed when playing with the toy [6].

2.2 Virtual Humans

Virtual humans can be represented in many ways [7, 8]; however, for the purposes of our research, we used mixed reality agents known as ANDI [9]. These mixed reality humans are rendered life-size on a 40″ television set in portrait mode. A Microsoft Kinect is used for head-tracking to enable head-gaze and perspective correct rendering.

The virtual humans interacted with human participants using pre-recorded dialog and motion-captured gestures and animations. The virtual humans used a simple eye-gaze model in which they looked at whomever was speaking and would intermittently glance at other teammates.

The virtual humans were operated using a Wizard-Of-Oz (WoZ) approach. In a WoZ system, a human operator listens to user input and controls the virtual human's dialog choices based on the user's input. We chose a WoZ approach to eliminate speech recognition and understanding errors as these errors could have interfered with the learning objects of the training exercise.

3 Related Work

This research builds on prior work applying social learning theory with virtual humans or agents.

3.1 Virtual Agents and Social Learning Theory

Social learning theory has been applied with virtual humans mainly in areas related to health, and bicycle safety.

Fox and Bailenson investigated how virtual representations of the self, also known as doppelgangers, could be used to influence exercise behavior [10]. In one study, participants saw the weight of a virtual representation of themselves fluctuate based on the participants' current physical activity. Participants who saw their virtual doppelganger lose/gain weight based on their activity performed more voluntary exercise than participants who saw an unchanging virtual doppelganger or no doppelganger.

Babu et al. developed a bicycle safety virtual environment in which children rode a bike with a virtual peer [11]. Participants interacted with either a risky virtual peer or safe virtual peer while crossing busy intersections in a virtual environment. A risky virtual peer crossed intersections with tight gaps between cars while a safe virtual peer chose large gaps between cars. Researchers found that participants who interacted with the risky virtual peer were negatively influenced by the risky peer's road-crossing behavior.

4 Virtual Human Training Exercise

4.1 Background

The virtual human training exercise used in this study was created in collaboration with nursing management at a teaching hospital in the United States. Nursing management indicated nurses needed to be trained on a policy change involving the closing count of a surgery. The closing count occurs prior to closing the surgical wound on a patient. The surgical team counts surgical items to verify they match the count conducted prior to the start of the surgical procedure. A new policy was put into place to ensure maximal patient safety when there is a discrepancy between the closing count and the initial count. When a discrepancy occurs, the surgical team should first try to locate the missing item. The process includes searching trash bins, sponge counting bags, drapes, and other places around the operating room. If the item cannot be located, an x-ray must be requested for the patient. Proper protocol states the attending surgeon on the team must speak with an attending radiologist to for review of the x-ray.

Nursing management believed employees at their hospital should feel empowered to speak up if proper protocol was not followed. To address this need, we created a scenario in which a virtual surgeon does not want to comply with the new closing count protocol after a discrepancy is discovered. For trainees, their goal was to speak up to the virtual surgeon, try to get the surgeon to follow the policy, and ultimately call a supervisor or charge nurse if the surgeon does not comply with the policy.

4.2 Virtual Humans

For this simulation exercise, we developed three virtual humans who formed an operating room team with the surgical technologist participant. In addition to the surgical team, a patient, in the form of a plastic mannequin patient simulator was also incorporated into the exercise. Doctor Girard is a new surgical attending who was recently employed at the hospital. Doctor Sanders is a new attending anesthesiologist. Sandy is a circulating nurse who works at the hospital. Depending on condition, Sandy either modeled best practices of speaking up behavior for participants to learn. Eric Mason is 59 year old man who is undergoing a laparoscopic Whipple, or, pancreas removal. Eric was represented as a mannequin lying on an OR bed. To enhance realism, a monitor looped vital signs displaying his heart rate and other important vital information. An anaesthesia machine was also cycling to simulate ventilation of the patient.

4.3   Scenario

The speaking up opportunities occur in two important stages of the surgical procedure. Each stage included an important decision making moment. The two stages are as follows: Pre-Incision Timeout and the Closing Count.

Prior to the two decision making moments, the participants interact with their virtual teammates in preparing the patient for surgery. This stage is known as the Pre-Induction Briefing. Participants and virtual humans introduce themselves to each other and the team works together to go over the patient's vital signs and information about the surgical procedure.

Pre-Incision Timeout – Decision Moment One. The Pre-Incision Timeout occurs right before the surgical procedure begins. During the timeout, anesthesia has already been induced, and the patient is prepped and draped for surgery. The Pre-Incision Timeout serves as a moment for everyone on the team to address any concerns and make sure everyone is on the same page before beginning the surgery. The decision moment is based on a prior need from nursing management. A similar decision moment was used in a prior study [12].

The virtual surgeon asks if there are blood products ready for the procedure. Due to some communication failures with the blood bank, the anaesthesiologist admits blood is not currently available for the patient. The surgeon, frustrated with this information, berates the anaesthesiologist for his mistake.

Because of the surgeon's heavy case load for the day, he makes the decision to continue with the surgery despite no availability of blood products in the room. At this point, the virtual nurse, Sandy, will either model the best or bad practices speaking up behavior. The details of these models are discussed later in Sect. 5.

Closing Count – Decision Moment Two. During the Closing Count stage, the surgical technologist and virtual nurse must work together to count all of the items prior to closing the patient. Surgical technologists were instructed to conduct the closing count as they normally would in a real operating room environment. The virtual nurse holds a clipboard of the initial count and verifies the number of items counted with what is on the initial count.

The Closing Count stage occurs after the surgery has been performed. To enhance the realism of the simulation, participants counted real surgical equipment. The equipment included items such as sponges, needles, and blades. The setup of the Closing Count stage can be seen in Fig. 2.

While conducting the count, the virtual nurse and surgical technologist discover one item is missing. The item was intentionally missing for the purposes of the training; however, participants were not aware of this intention. The surgeon instructs the team to look for the missing item. After a few minutes of searching, the team concludes an

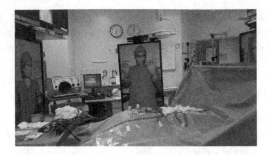

Fig. 2. Setup of the closing count stage (from participant perspective) Nurse is on the left, surgeon in the middle, and anesthesiologist to the right.

x-ray must be obtained. An x-ray is displayed on monitors above the simulation area. After receiving the x-ray, the surgeon determines that the x-ray is clear (i.e., there is no foreign body present in the patient). Because to him, the x-ray is clear, the surgeon makes the risky decision to start closing the patient's incision. His decision puts the patient's life at risk, and violates hospital's policy which requires the attending surgeon to speak with the attending radiologist to clear the x-ray. This moment is the second speaking up opportunity in which we assessed the effect of the modeling (Fig. 3).

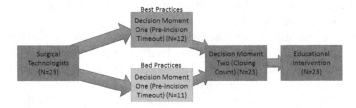

Fig. 3. Study flow

5   Study Design

The goal of this study was to investigate how to use social training with virtual humans to teach best practices for communication. While the main focus of this research is on teaching best practices for communication, we also investigated the effects of a virtual human modeling bad practices for communication. Unfortunately, the reality is healthcare professionals perceive that conflict resolution is not handled effectively in the OR [13]. The bad practices model was added to reflect the more common perception of how conflict is resolved in the operating room.

Participants were recruited from a United States teaching hospital. The participants were operating room surgical technologists at the hospital. Participants signed up for the training exercise through the hospital's training management system. 23 surgical technologists were recruited for the study (19 female, 4 male). No participant had participated in a virtual human training exercise prior to attending this training.

5.1   Social Learning Component

Leveraging social learning theory, we developed a model of both best practices and bad practices speaking up behavior.

Best Practices Speaking Up. In the best practices model, the virtual nurse models ideal speaking up behavior as recommended by the hospital and literature. During Decision Moment One, the nurse objects to the virtual surgeon proceeding with incision. The virtual surgeon rebuts to every challenge the virtual nurse gives. The nurse challenges the surgeon six times before calling a supervisor to intervene in the conflict: "If you insist on proceeding, then I'm going to have to call my charge nurse". The surgeon responds: "Fine, you do that".

Bad Practices Speaking Up. In the bad practices model, the virtual nurses fails to fully model ideal speaking up behavior. During Decision Moment One, the nurse challenges the surgeon only four times. The four challenges are exactly the same as the first four challenges of the Best Practices model. After challenging the surgeon four times, the virtual nurse gives into the surgeon: "Alright, well... I think this is a bad idea, but (sigh) you're the surgeon, and it's your call". The surgeon responds: "Finally, thank you. Now let's keep going".

5.2   Procedure

With the exception of the speaking up model, the training exercise was identical for both groups of participants. First, participants interacted with the virtual team in Decision Moment One. Participants either observed a virtual nurse demonstrate a best practices or bad practices model of speaking up behavior. After Decision Moment One, the simulation is set up for the closing count stage. Approximately ten minutes elapse between Decision Moment One and when participants conduct the closing count which encompasses Decision Moment Two.

After completing the training exercise, we conducted an educational intervention for all participants. During the intervention, all participants watched a short video in which a surgeon employed at the hospital went over the importance of the new closing count policy. This surgeon helped draft the new policy.

In addition to viewing the video, we also gave participants a handout of the TeamSTEPPS protocol. The handout addressed effective speaking up strategies when dealing with conflict. These strategies include the two-challenge rule in which participants were told they should voice their concerns at least twice to ensure they've been heard. The other strategy was the "CUS" acronym. "CUS" are three important words participants can use whenever speaking up. These words are "Concerned", "Uncomfortable", and "Patient Safety".

6   Results

Results presented are based on the speaking up outcomes from Decision Moment Two of the training scenario. Specifically, we assessed whether or not the surgical technologist called a supervisor or charge nurse to intervene. While 23 surgical technologists were recruited, only 22 data points are considered. One participant in the bad practices modeling group called the charge nurse on her own during Decision Moment One which meant the participant did not see any form of modeling from the virtual nurse. Based on interviews with participants, most surgical technologists would not speak up about issues with blood products as, typically, issues with blood are not their responsibility. To analyze the results, we ran a 2 × 2 contingency analysis using permutations.

6.1   Speaking Up Outcomes (n = 22)

As seen in Fig. 4, when participants observed the virtual nurse call the charge nurse in Decision Moment One, 75 % of participants in Decision Moment Two called the charge nurse after the surgeon refused to comply with the hospital's closing count policy. When participants observed the virtual nurse back down to the surgeon in Decision Moment One, only 30 % of participants in the Closing Count stage called the charge nurse. Seventy percent of participants in the Bad Practices modeling group failed to call the charge nurse during Decision Moment Two. Only 25 % of participants in the Best Practices modeling group failed to call the charge nurse during Decision Moment Two. The results are statistically significant with p = 0.0304.

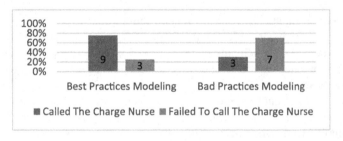

Fig. 4. Speaking up outcomes during decision moment two

7   Discussion

The results suggests participants were influenced by the model they observed. While the results are statistically significant, we also believe the results are practically significant given the participants for the study were healthcare professionals at an actual hospital. The participants work with real operating room teams on a daily basis caring for real patients. If virtual humans are capable of influencing how humans behave in a simulated environment, this same vicarious learning likely occurs in actual operating rooms. Unfortunately, in real high stakes environments, role models are not guaranteed to be present. With virtual humans, we can guarantee everyone sees the same best practices model. The novelty of this research is how virtual humans can influence humans. Virtual humans can be used to teach real humans best communication practices that humans can potentially apply in real-world situations.

7.1 Ethics

The results present a potential ethical dilemma for future studies with virtual human behavioral modeling. Participants who observed the virtual nurse back down to the virtual surgeon in Decision Moment One may have received a subpar experience compared to the participants who observed the virtual nurse successfully speak up to the virtual surgeon. Most of the surgical technologists attended the training during work hours. They likely left a real operating room to attend training and went back to a real operating room immediately after the training. We do not fully know the extent to which the virtual nurse's behavior influenced participants; however, any potential negative learned behavior which could be carried over into a live operating room environment could impact patient safety. Despite seeing a virtual nurse model bad practices, all participants received the same intervention in which they were told the proper hospital policy and given a set of guidelines to speak up (TeamSTEPPS). We made sure that all participants left with something positive and encouraging.

8 Limitations

There are two main limitations: a small sample size, and the possibility of priming.

Our sample, while small, is gathered from a population of healthcare professionals who work in very high stakes environments daily. Participants work with real teams in real operating room environments with real patients. Most participants worked with real patients on the same day they participated in the study.

Participants in the Best Practices modeling group may have been primed to call the charge nurse because they discovered it was a possibility of the simulation. The Bad Practices model participants did not see anyone call the charge nurse so they may not have realized calling the charge nurse was possible. We do not think any priming occurred. Participants in other conditions of the study (not relevant to the research presented in this paper) called the charge nurse at similar rates to the Best Practices modeling group without actually observing a virtual human call a charge nurse.

9 Conclusion and Future Work

Virtual humans are powerful tools for social training of effective communication strategies in a team training environment. If humans can be positively influenced by virtual humans, this form of social training could transform medical team training, empower more healthcare professionals to speak up, and potentially decrease the risk of patient morbidity or death in the operating room. Our results show virtual humans can serve as role models; humans can learn from these virtual role models.

Anecdotally, for a five month period which coincided during and after the training, no retained foreign bodies were reported at the hospital. While we cannot claim causation, the decreased rate of adverse events is encouraging nonetheless.

Reflection is an important component of social training and was not addressed in this research. We believe that incorporating a reflective component in addition to the modeling component may improve outcomes for all participants.

Acknowledgements. The authors would like to acknowledge Dave Lizdas, Drew Gonsalves, and Terry Sullivan for study setup and support. The authors would also like to acknowledge Jim Martindale for helping with the statistical analysis, and the surgical technologists who participated in the study. This work was supported in part by NSF Grant 1161491.

References

1. Gawande, A., Studdert, D., Orav, J., Brennan, T., Zinner, M.: Risk factors for retained instruments and sponges after surgery. N. Engl. J. Med. **348**, 229–235 (2003)
2. Sherman, R., Pross, E.: Growing future nurse leaders to build and sustain health work environments at the unit level. OJIN **15** (2010). http://nursingworld.org/MainMenuCategories/ANAMarketplace/ANAPeriodicals/OJIN/TableofContents/Vol152010/No1Jan2010/Growing-Nurse-Leaders.html
3. Woelfle, C.Y., McCaffrey, R.: Nurse on nurse. Nurse Forum **42**, 123–131 (2007)
4. Lok, B., Chuah, J., Robb, A., Cordar, A., Lampotang, S., Wendling, A., White, C.: Mixed-reality humans for team training. IEEE Comput. Graph. Appl. **34**, 72–75 (2014)
5. Bandura, A.: Social Learning Theory. Prentice-Hall, Englewood Cliffs (1977)
6. Bandura, A., Ross, D., Ross, A.: Transmission of aggression through the imitation of aggressive models. J. Abnorm. Soc. Psych. **63**, 575–582 (1961)
7. Peden, M., Chuah, J., Kotranza, A., Johnsen, K., Lok, B., Cendan, J.: NERVE – a three dimensional patient simulation for evaluating cranial nerve function. https://www.mededportal.org/publication/8255
8. Ring, L., Utami, D., Bickmore, T.: The right agent for the job? In: Bickmore, T., Marsella, S., Sidner, C. (eds.) IVA 2014. LNCS, vol. 8637, pp. 374–384. Springer, Heidelberg (2014)
9. Chuah, J.H., Lok, B.,: Hybrid virtual-physical entities, pp. 275–276. In: ISMAR (2012)
10. Fox, J., Bailenson, J.: Virtual self-modeling: the effects of vicarious reinforcement and identification on exercise behaviors. Media Psychol. **12**, 1–25 (2009)
11. Babu, S.V., Grechkin, T.Y., Chihak, B., Ziemer, C., Kearney, J.K., Cremer, J.F., Plumert, J.M.: An immersive virtual peer for studying social influences on child cyclists' road-crossing behavior. TVCG **17**, 14–25 (2011)
12. Robb, A., White, C., Cordar, A., Wendling, A., Lampotang, S., Lok, B.: A qualitative evaluation of behavior during conflict with an authoritative virtual human. In: Bickmore, T., Marsella, S., Sidner, C. (eds.) IVA 2014. LNCS, vol. 8637, pp. 397–409. Springer, Heidelberg (2014)
13. Sexton, J.B., Makary, M.A., Tersigni, A.R., Pryor, D., Hendrich, A., Thomas, E.J., Holzmueller, C.G., Knight, A.P., Wu, Y., Pronovost, P.J.: Teamwork in the operating room: frontline perspectives among hospitals and operating room personnel. Anesthesiology **105**, 877–884 (2006)

Exploring the Effects of Healthcare Students Creating Virtual Patients for Empathy Training

Shivashankar Halan[✉], Isaac Sia, Michael Crary, and Benjamin Lok

University of Florida, Gainesville, FL, USA
shivashankarh@ufl.edu, {isaacsia,mcrary}@phhp.ufl.edu,
lok@cise.ufl.edu

Abstract. Intelligent virtual agents have been successfully used for interpersonal skills training of healthcare students by enabling simulated interactions between healthcare students and virtual patient agents. However, during these interactions, students do not get the opportunity to take the perspective of the patient. Taking the perspective of the patient is essential for healthcare students to learn critical interpersonal skills like empathy. We propose having healthcare students create virtual patient agents of a particular race to provide them the opportunity to take the perspective of patients from that race, leading to increased empathy during subsequent interactions with patients of that race. We conducted a semester-long user study with 24 healthcare students to explore the effects of having them create virtual patient agents. Results indicate that healthcare students who created and interviewed virtual patients of the same race were significantly more empathetic than students who created virtual patients with a race discordant to the one they interacted with.

Keywords: Embodied conversational agents · Virtual patients · Agents in healthcare · Interpersonal skills training · Healthcare education · Empathy training

1 Introduction

For the research reported in this paper, we explore the idea of having healthcare students create and interview virtual agents of a particular race to teach them the essential interpersonal skill of empathy. Virtual agents have been widely used for interpersonal skills training in areas like military [1] and medical education [2, 3]. Specifically, the validity of using *virtual patients*, which are virtual agents that play the role of a patient, for training healthcare students with their interpersonal skills has been established [2]. The virtual patients used for interpersonal skills training look and speak like humans and are predominantly question-answering virtual agents [1, 2]. Traditionally, interpersonal skills training happens during interactions between healthcare students and the virtual patient. During these interactions, the virtual patients respond with pre-recorded responses to natural language questions or comments made by the healthcare student, who plays the role of the healthcare provider. A sample interaction with a virtual patient is shown in Fig. 1.

© Springer International Publishing Switzerland 2015
W.-P. Brinkman et al. (Eds.): IVA 2015, LNAI 9238, pp. 239–249, 2015.
DOI: 10.1007/978-3-319-21996-7_24

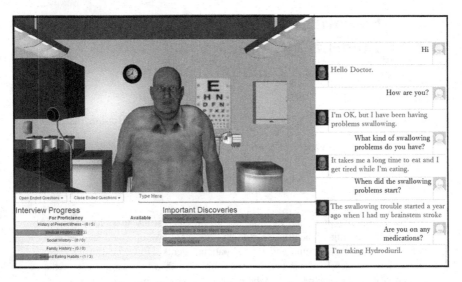

Fig. 1. Sample interaction with a virtual patient

Although virtual patient-based simulations have proven to be effective for interpersonal skills training, certain specific interpersonal skills are still challenging to teach through traditional usage of virtual patients. An example of an interpersonal skill that is difficult to train using only interactions with virtual patients is empathy towards patients [4]. Empathetic healthcare professionals construct more meaningful relationships with their patients that helps them to both elicit information efficiently and provide healthcare advice effectively. To train healthcare students to be more empathetic, virtual patient simulations need to provide students the opportunity to understand the patient's perspective [5–7]. To get the patient's perspective, healthcare students need to think from the patient's shoes. During simulated interactions with virtual patients, the student is still playing the part of a healthcare provider and so current virtual patient simulations do not provide an opportunity for students to take the patient's perspective.

In order to enable healthcare students to take the perspective of the patient for empathy training, we propose having healthcare students create virtual patients themselves. While creating a virtual patient, the healthcare student is forced to think from the perspective of the patient. Our hypothesis is that by having the student take the perspective of a certain type of patient, we can train the students to be more empathetic during subsequent interactions with patients of the same type. For example, if a female Caucasian student creates a male African American virtual patient, the student has the opportunity to take the perspective of a patient from a different gender and race and so can empathize with such patients during subsequent interactions.

To explore this idea, we integrated a virtual patient exercise that involved creating and interviewing virtual patients into a health professions course. Twenty four healthcare students studying to become speech language pathologists participated in a semester-long study as part of this exercise. The students who created virtual patients and then interacted with virtual patients of the same race as the ones they created were significantly more empathetic than students who created virtual patients that were of a different race compared to the virtual patients they interacted with. We also found that this positive effect of creating virtual patients for empathy training was more pronounced when students created patients with race discordant to their own race.

2 Related Work

Galinsky and Moskowitz have extensively studied the effect of perspective-taking on racial stereotypes and prejudice [8]. They have demonstrated through their work that the positive effect of perspective-taking is effective when working with a particular group characterized by a certain feature. For example, their results indicate that one can improve their understanding of all old people by taking the perspective of one old person. Researchers have explored providing alternate perspectives using virtual agent-based simulations to alter social behavior. Yee and Bailenson found that negative stereotyping of the elderly was significantly reduced by having participants placed in avatars of old people [9]. Peck et al. have shown that putting Caucasian participants in the skin of a black avatar reduces their implicit racial bias [10]. Raij et al. introduced the concept of virtual social perspective-taking which demonstrated that taking the perspective of the patient can be beneficial for healthcare professionals and students [11]. They constructed a virtual reality experience in which after an interaction with a virtual patient, healthcare professionals were immersed into a replay of the interaction, but this time from the perspective of the patient. Results indicate that this experience changes behavior in future, similar social interactions. Similarly, Kotranza et al. [12] demonstrated that having healthcare students themselves experience the double vision suffered by a virtual patient improves their concern for the patient's safety.

3 System Description: Virtual Patient Pipeline

Although there are several aspects to creating a virtual patient, we focus on having students construct the verbal or conversational capabilities of the virtual patient using a conversational corpus. The conversational corpus of a virtual patient consists of question-response pairs of what the students will say to the virtual patient (i.e., questions) and what the virtual patient will say back (i.e., responses). When a student poses a question or makes a comment to the virtual patient, the system searches the corpus for the most similar question and provides the paired answer. For example, if a healthcare student asked the virtual patient "Why are you here today?", "How are you?" or "Can you tell me about your problem?" the virtual patient would respond with "It hurts at the back of my throat when I try to swallow my food". To enable healthcare students to create virtual patients, we have built a web application called Virtual Patient Pipeline that uses techniques like crowdsourcing and reusing information from previously created virtual patients. The Virtual Patient Pipeline is a website that was built to enable users to create their own virtual patients by following a step-by-step process. The application has the following four main steps:

Step 1 – Name and Image: Authors choose a name for the patient and write out a short description about the virtual patient. They also choose an image that is most representative of the virtual patient they want to create from an array of headshot images. The array of headshots include images of characters with different races, age and gender. Sample headshot images are shown in Table 1 in Sect. 4.2.

Step 2 – Virtual Patient Template: In this step, authors fill out a *virtual patient template* - a form that has a pre-populated set of questions and allows authors to fill in just the response for each set of questions in order to create an initial version of the virtual patient. The response field is left blank for the student to fill out by playing the role of the patient. Examples of questions in the virtual patient template are name, age, marital status, medications and prior medical history. The patient template that was used in the course integration described in this paper had 135 question-response pairs. All pre-populated questions in the patient template have been gathered by mining questions from previously created virtual patients of similar pathologies.

Step 3 – Patient Training: In this training step, students can interview the patient that has been created through the process in Step 1 to add more information to the patient. The interviewing process involves the creator typing questions to the virtual patient and receiving responses. While interviewing the patient, students can correct any incorrect responses or add new questions and responses to their patients. Since the template might not have all the questions that the student wants their patient to be able to answer, this step allows them to add new question-response pairs.

Step 4 – Crowdsourcing: After the student has completed training their patient, he/she can share the virtual patient with his/her friends and acquaintances. While others interview the virtual patient, they will have the opportunity to flag any responses that they think are wrong. These incorrect responses are gathered in a list along with any questions to which the virtual patient did not know an answer to during the interview. This list can then be reviewed by the students and the virtual patient improved by correcting incorrect responses and adding responses to unanswered questions.

4 Experimental Study

4.1 Population

Participants in the study were speech and language pathology students taking a course titled "Dysphagia Management" during the spring of 2014 at the University of Florida. Dysphagia is a medical condition where the patient has difficulty swallowing food or liquids. There were 26 graduate students registered for the course. The study was offered as an extra-credit exercise as part of the course and students volunteered to participate. The extra-credit was 5 points on the final exam of the course. All but one student volunteered to participate in our study. One student failed to complete all the requirements for the study, so the data from 24 participants was analyzed [$n = 24$]. The course was taught for four months between January and April 2014 and the study ran throughout the duration of the course. All the students were either in the first or second semester of their graduate studies for a Master's in Speech Language Pathology. In the future, as speech language pathologists, these students will have to interview real patients, some of them suffering from dysphagia. Hence this virtual patient exercise and the interpersonal skill of empathy is very relevant to this population.

On the first day of class, all the students were asked to fill out a background survey form that asked for demographic and educational information. All but one participant were female (96 %). The average age of the participants was 24.24 (S.D. = 4.06). All but two participants were Caucasian (92 %). One participant was Asian and another one was a Pacific Islander. As can be seen from these numbers, we have a fairly homogenous group of predominantly Caucasian female participants with an average age of 24. This composition is reflective of the general composition of speech language pathologists and students around the country. 84 % of the students reported that they have not received any prior interpersonal skills training. According to the instructor of the course, the students had very minimal exposure to real patients.

4.2 Study Design

Although the exercise lasted an entire semester, we focus only on the first three tasks that were completed by the participants. The remaining tasks are beyond the scope of this paper. The first three tasks that students completed in the order of completion are:

1. *Interview* a virtual dysphagia patient - (last week of January)
2. *Create* a virtual dysphagia patient - (first two weeks of February)
3. *Interview* a virtual dysphagia patient - (third week of February)

The virtual dysphagia patient interviews (tasks 1 and 3) were used as metrics to evaluate the effect of creating a virtual patient (task 2). On the first day of class, a 30-min tutorial was provided to the entire class demonstrating a virtual patient interaction and the steps involved in creating a virtual patient using the Virtual Patient Pipeline.

Virtual Patient Interviews: All 24 participants participated in interviews with two virtual dysphagia patients. The two virtual patients interviewed were of the same gender but different race and medical diagnoses. One of the virtual patients was a Caucasian male while the other was an African American male. The order in which the virtual patients were interviewed was randomized. Half the participants interviewed the Caucasian male first and the African American male second and the other half interviewed the patients in the opposite order. Information about the two virtual patients interviewed by the participants is presented in Table 1.

The interviewing process involved students typing in questions to ask to the virtual patient and the virtual patient responding to the questions with both text and audio responses. The interaction interface is shown in Fig. 1. The virtual patient was represented as a 3D character with simple idle animations like blinking and breathing. The virtual patient had appropriate lip synching animations for the audio responses. The audio for the two virtual patients' speeches were recorded by voice actors of the

Table 1. Virtual patients that were interviewed by all participants

Virtual Patient	Virtual Patient Characteristics		
Vinny Devito	**Caucasian Male**	**Age: 63**	**Diagnosis :** Brainstem Stroke
	Empathetic Opportunity: *"Can you tell me if I can ever start eating like before? I'm a food guy and love eating. It sucks that all that I've been able to eat is pureed food for the last year. I just want to be able to eat like before and be normal at our family get-togethers. I feel so out-of-place now that I can't eat what I want. Please tell me if I would ever get back to my original diet."*		
Marty Graw	**African American Male**	**Age: 55**	**Diagnosis:** Esophageal Stric-ture
	Empathetic Opportunity: *"Doctor, imagine you being sick all the time. How would you feel about being sick and coughing while talking to your patients? My condition is the same. I am a chef but cannot even taste any of the food I'm cooking."*		

appropriate age and gender corresponding to the virtual patient. Students were instructed to interview each virtual patient for at least 10 min.

Virtual Patient Creation: All 24 participants also individually created a virtual dysphagia patient in between the two virtual patient interviews. The participants were asked to create a 55-year old male virtual patient suffering from dysphagia due to a left brainstem stroke. Half the students were asked to create a Caucasian virtual patient and the other half were asked to create an African American virtual patient. Other than the ethnicity, age, gender and diagnosis which was given to them, the students were instructed to come up with all the other information for the virtual patient on their own. Due to time constraints, participants completed only the first three steps of the Virtual Patient Pipeline that is explained in Sect. 3.

To summarize, in task two all the 24 participants created either a Caucasian or African American male virtual patient and then in task three interviewed a Caucasian male virtual patient or an African American male virtual patient. Comparing the race of the virtual patient they created and the race of the second virtual patient they interviewed, the participants could be divided into two groups – *concordant group* and *discordant group*. The concordant group's second virtual patient was of the same race as the virtual patient they created. The discordant group's second virtual patient was of a different race than the virtual patient they created.

4.3   Metrics

The two virtual dysphagia patient interviews were used to measure the difference in empathy between the concordant and discordant groups and was measured using empathetic opportunities. An *empathetic opportunity* is an instance during a virtual patient interview where the virtual patient expresses a concern or asks a question to which the participant is expected to respond with empathy. For example, during an interaction with a patient suffering from stomach pain, the patient could ask *"My brother recently died of peptic cancer. I'm afraid that this pain I'm having could be a symptom of stomach cancer. Am I going to die like my brother doctor?"*. The participant is expected to respond empathetically to this question. Each virtual patient had one empathetic opportunity that was spoken by the virtual patient approximately 7 min into the interview. While the virtual patient spoke the empathetic opportunity speech, a dialog box popped up that had the text for the opportunity and also a text area where the student could enter their response to the empathetic opportunity. The student had to respond to the opportunity to proceed with the interview. When the student submitted their typed response to the empathetic opportunity, the patient responded with a generic "Thank you, doctor" statement. The empathetic opportunities included in both the patients are listed in Table 1.

The participant's responses to these empathetic opportunities were rated by three expert empathetic raters trained on the Empathic Communication Coding System (ECCS) scale. The ECCS scale is an established measure for rating healthcare provider's empathy during an interaction with a patient [13]. The ECCS scale has seven levels of empathy for responses to empathetic opportunities. These seven levels are described in Table 2 along with examples of actual responses from study participants corresponding to each level of empathy. The ECCS scale has been successfully used to measure and rate empathy during virtual patient simulations [14]. The three raters were trained using empathetic opportunities from other virtual patient interactions prior to the actual rating of the responses from the experimental study. The rating for each response was the average rating from the three raters.

Table 2. Empathic communication coding system levels with example participant responses

Level	Name	Example response from participants
6	Shared feeling or experience	*"I love to cook and eat, as well. I understand how difficult that might be"*.
5	Confirmation	*"I'm so sorry to hear that. I know it can be hard, but we'll try to get to the bottom of this and get you better!"*
4	Acknowledgement with pursuit	*"Eating is enjoyable and we want to do everything we can here to get you back to where you can have a good quality of life"*.
3	Acknowledgement	*"We're gonna do our best"*
2	Implicit recognition	*"We'll finish talking and see what we can come up with together"*
1	Perfunctory recognition	*"Do you only have trouble with liquids during mealtimes"*
0	Denial	*"What has brought you in today?"*

5   Results

The ratings based on the ECCS scale by the three raters had high inter-rater reliability measured by Intraclass Correlations (ICC) ratings of 0.925 and 0.862 for the Caucasian and African American virtual patient ratings respectively. Since the ratings are ordinal and not normally distributed, Mann-Whitney U-tests were run to compare ratings between the concordant and discordant groups at each virtual patient interview. Results from this analysis are plotted in Fig. 2. There were no significant differences in the empathy ratings between the two groups during the first virtual patient interview. Empathy ratings during the second patient interview for concordant group participants (Mdn = 4.0) were significantly higher than for discordant group participants (Mdn = 3.67), U = 34.5, z = −2.181, p < 0.05, r = −0.45. Also, a within-subjects Wilcoxon signed-rank test was used to compare the ratings within each group. No significant differences were observed between the interviews within both the groups.

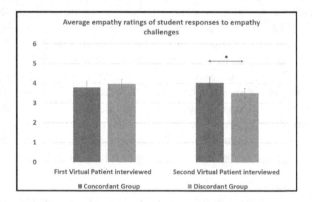

Fig. 2. Average empathy ratings of participant responses to empathy challenges. Values significantly different from each other are highlighted using an asterisk symbol.

Mann-Whitney U-tests were run to compare the empathy ratings of the concordant and discordant groups depending on whether the second virtual patient was Caucasian or African American. When the second virtual patient was African American [n = 12], there was a significant difference between the empathy ratings of the race concordant (Mdn = 5) and discordant (Mdn = 3.67) groups, U = 2.0, z = −2.234, p < 0.05, r = −0.70. When the second virtual patient was Caucasian [n = 12], there was only a marginally significant difference between the empathy ratings of the race concordant (Mdn = 4) and discordant (Mdn = 3.33) groups, U = 9.0, z = −1.774, p = 0.07, r = −0.51.

6   Discussion

Since there were no significant differences between the concordant and discordant group empathy ratings during the first patient interview and the only difference in treatment for the two groups was whether they created a race concordant or discordant virtual patient, we conclude that the reason for enhanced empathy was the process of creating a race concordant virtual patient. This validates the applicability of virtual patient creation as a tool for empathy training.

It was observed that there was a significant difference between the empathy ratings of concordant and discordant groups when the second virtual patient was African American and only a marginal significance when the virtual patient was Caucasian. All the 12 participants for whom the second virtual patient was African American were Caucasian. So creating and interviewing an African American virtual patient would mean taking the perspective of a patient population discordant to their own race. These results indicate that the effect of creating a virtual patient might be more pronounced when creating and interviewing a virtual patient that is race discordant to the student. These results are in-line with findings by Peck et al. in their study [10] and also in the psychosocial experiments conducted by Galinsky and Moskowitz [8].

In addition to the empathy training benefits presented above, we would like to present two additional contributions in this paper:

Feasibility for Virtual Patient Creation by end Users in an Educational Environment: We would like to highlight that the experimental study was conducted in a real-world educational environment as part of a health professions course and present this as one of the contributions of this paper. Although prior experiments have investigated the feasibility of having healthcare students create virtual patients [15], the contribution of this paper is in the setting of empathy training. This demonstrates that virtual agent creation exercises can be integrated into educational environments, as part of coursework, for teaching interpersonal skills.

Virtual Patients Created are Educational Artifacts: In the process of creating virtual patients for the sake of learning interpersonal skills, students are actually also creating virtual patients that can be used for training other students in the future. Each virtual patient created by these students has a different personality, backstory and background information that the students have come up with. Interestingly, the two virtual patients used for interviews in the described study were also created by students back in 2011 as part of a virtual patient creation exercise.

7   Conclusion

In this paper, we have explored the idea of healthcare students creating virtual patients for learning empathy. Although the idea has been introduced in the context of virtual patients and explored in the domain of healthcare education, the idea can be extended to domains like social training, specifically for gaining cultural competency. A person can create a virtual agent representing a particular culture and others belonging to the target culture can then interact with the agent created and provide feedback. The feedback will help the creator address any misconceptions or stereotypes that the creator has about the target culture.

As future work, we would like to explore other categories in which interpersonal skills through virtual patient creation can be useful like gender, age, ethnicity etc. Our eventual goal is to make virtual patient creation an enjoyable and effective tool for healthcare students to learn important skills like empathy. With more and more successful completions of virtual patient creation exercises, we would also be able to build a library of virtual patient agents that can be used for both research and educational purposes around the world.

Acknowledgements. The authors would like to thank Dr. Andrea Kleinsmith for her advice and assistance in conducting the study reported. This work was made possible by a Veterans Administration Rehabilitation Research and Development Grant (Grant ID: B0339-R).

References

1. Swartout, W., Gratch, J., Hill, R.W.W., Hovy, E., Marsella, S., Rickel, J., Traum, D.: Toward virtual humans. AI Mag. **27**(2), 96 (2006)
2. Johnsen, K., Raij, A., Stevens, A., Lind, D.S., Lok, B.: The validity of a virtual human experience for interpersonal skills education. In: Proceedings of the SIGCHI Conference on Human Factors in Computing Systems - CHI 2007, p. 1049 (2007)
3. Johnsen, K., Dickerson, R., Jackson, J., Shin, M., Hernandez, J., Stevens, A., Raij, A., Lok, B., Lind, D.S.: Experiences in using immersive virtual characters to educate medical communication skills. In: IEEE Proceedings on Virtual Reality (VR 2005), pp. 179–324 (2005)
4. Deladisma, A.M., et al.: Do medical students respond empathetically to a virtual patient? Am. J. Surg. **193**(6), 756–760 (2007)
5. Maxfield, H., Delzell, J.E., Chumley, H.: Eliciting the patient's perspective: does experience or type of case make a difference? Patient Educ. Couns. **82**(2), 222–225 (2011)
6. DasGupta, S., Charon, R.: Personal illness narratives: using reflective writing to teach empathy. Acad. Med. **79**(4), 351–356 (2004)
7. Moore, R.J., Hallenbeck, J.: Narrative empathy and how dealing with stories helps: creating a space for empathy in culturally diverse care settings. J. Pain Symptom Manag. **40**(3), 471–476 (2010)
8. Galinsky, A.D., Moskowitz, G.B.: Perspective-taking: decreasing stereotype expression, stereotype accessibility, and in-group favoritism. J. Pers. Soc. Psychol. **78**(4), 708–724 (2000)
9. Yee, N., Bailenson, J.: Walk a mile in digital shoes: the impact of embodied perspective-taking on the reduction of negative stereotyping in immersive virtual environments. In: Proceedings of PRESENCE, pp. 147–156 (2006)
10. Peck, T.C., Seinfeld, S., Aglioti, S.M., Slater, M.: Putting yourself in the skin of a black avatar reduces implicit racial bias. Conscious. Cogn. **22**(3), 779–787 (2013)
11. Raij, A., Kotranza, A., Lind, D.S., Lok, B.: Virtual experiences for social perspective-taking. In: 2009 IEEE Virtual Reality Conference, pp. 99–102 (2009)
12. Kotranza, A., Cendan, J.C., Johnsen, K., Lok, B.: Virtual patient with cranial nerve injury augments physician-learner concern for patient safety. J. Bio-algorithms Med-Syst. **6**(11), 25–34 (2010)
13. Bylund, C.L., Makoul, G.: Examining empathy in medical encounters: an observational study using the empathic communication coding system. Health Commun. **18**(2), 123–140 (2005)

14. Borish, M., Cordar, A., Foster, A., Kim, T., Murphy, J., Lok, B.: Utilizing real-time human-assisted virtual humans to increase real-world interaction empathy. In: Kansei Engineering and Emotion Research (KEER) (2014)
15. Halan, S., Lok, B., Sia, I., Crary, M.: Virtual agent constructionism: experiences from health professions students creating virtual conversational agent representations of patients. In: IEEE Proceedings, International Conference on Advanced Learning Technologies, pp. 249–253 (2014)

Improving Social Awareness Through Thought Bubbles and Flashbacks of Virtual Characters

Jeroen Linssen[1]([✉]), Mariët Theune[1], Thomas de Groot[2], and Dirk Heylen[1]

[1] Human Media Interaction, University of Twente, PO Box 217, 7500 AE
Enschede, The Netherlands
{j.m.linssen,m.theune,d.k.j.heylen}@utwente.nl
[2] T-Xchange, PO Box 217, 7500 AE Enschede, The Netherlands
t.f.degroot@txchange.nl

Abstract. We present two prototypes of a serious game which is a aimed
at raising police officers' awareness of social stance during street interventions by letting them interact with virtual characters. We discuss the
design, implementation and evaluation of a method of feedback on the
police officers' game actions. This method uses thought bubbles to show
the cognitive state of virtual characters, using a theory of interpersonal
stances. We use thought bubbles (1) to provide direct feedback by showing the agent's current attitude, and (2) to provide delayed feedback at
the start of a new scenario by showing a flashback to the previous scenario, expressing the character's overall attitude towards the player. We
conducted two experiments with students from the Dutch Police Academy and found that our implementations of these forms of feedback did
not lead to directly measurable learning gains.

Keywords: Serious games · Social awareness · Virtual agents · Meta-
techniques · Thought bubbles · Flashback · Law enforcement

1 Introduction

Attaining and maintaining good social skills is of importance to many professions, including that of police officers. There are limited means to train social
skills through role plays with professional actors. Therefore, we propose to augment the police officers' curriculum with serious games [5]. In these games, police
officers train with virtual characters to experience difficult social interactions.

Providing feedback about formative assessment is a current challenge that
must be tackled to improve serious games for training interpersonal skills [7]. In
this paper, we present our work on LOITER (LOItering Teenagers, an Emergent
Role-play), a series of prototype serious games in which police officers have to
deal with loitering juveniles. In the LOITER games, we provide feedback to players
during the game through *meta-techniques*. These are out-of-character techniques
used in live action role play to communicate information such as thoughts of
characters in the play. We investigate an implementation of this meta-technique
in the form of *thought bubbles* that explain the behaviour of virtual characters.

© Springer International Publishing Switzerland 2015
W.-P. Brinkman et al. (Eds.): IVA 2015, LNAI 9238, pp. 250–259, 2015.
DOI: 10.1007/978-3-319-21996-7_25

The remainder of the paper is structured as follows. In Sect. 2, we discuss related research on serious games for interpersonal skills training, thought bubbles and flashbacks. In Sect. 3, we describe the model for social interaction we adopted in our serious game, and the learning goals we focus on. In Sect. 4, we address the design of LOITER-TB and the implementation of thought bubbles. We describe the experiment we conducted with this prototype in Sect. 5 and discuss the improved prototype which features flashbacks in Sect. 6. Finally, we present the findings from our experiment with LOITER-FB in Sect. 7 and wrap up the paper with conclusions and future work in Sect. 8.

2   Related Work

Several approaches to feedback and in-game assessment to stimulate learning about social interactions have been studied. *BiLAT* (Bi-Lateral Negotiation) is a system for negotiation training with virtual characters [2]. Having played through a scenario, students discuss the events with a virtual tutor in an after-action review. A similar training environment featuring inter-cultural negotiation scenarios is offered by SASO-ST [10]. SASO-ST provides users with debriefs of played scenarios, giving rudimentary feedback on the character's cognitive state.

Moments for proper feedback and reflection improve learning in game-based learning approaches [11]. Rather than providing this feedback after finishing a game, as in *BiLAT* or SASO-ST, we give such feedback during gameplay. This way, students can try to adapt their approach during the game if necessary.

Recent research has looked at the use of thought bubbles to help people with autism spectrum disorder cope with everyday interactions [4,6], showing that thought bubbles helped people to recognise the emotions of others. In our research, we use thought bubbles to enrich interactions with virtual characters by providing extra information about the cognitive state of these characters.

To help medical students practice their interpersonal skills, Cordar et al. created virtual characters suffering from depression [1]. They found that students who were shown back stories of characters showed more empathy towards both the virtual characters and real-life actors with depression. Instead of providing flashbacks that show events that occurred before the interaction between players and virtual characters, as in [1], we investigate flashbacks that reveal how the players' own actions influenced the cognitive states of the virtual characters.

3   Interpersonal Skills Training

For our serious games, we address skills that should be attained by students of the Dutch Police Academy (DPA), focusing on interpersonal skills that are of use during street interventions. Instructors at the DPA uses *Leary's Rose*, a theory of interpersonal attitudes, to teach students about social interaction. Leary's Rose is used to classify interpersonal behaviour as *stances*: combinations of varying degrees of dominance and affect, see Fig. 1a. For example, a dominant and affectionate stance can be classified as 'helpful'. A police officer may say, in a confident and friendly tone: "Surely we can work on a solution together!" If he would assume an 'aloof' stance, he might say, averting his gaze and speaking with a low voice: "Of course I don't expect your cooperation..."

In our serious game, we use Leary's Rose to model the actions of the players' and virtual characters. The virtual characters' reactions are based on Leary's claim that stances 'invite' complementing behaviour: people tend to mirror the other person's affect, but act inversely on the dominant axis, see Fig. 1b.

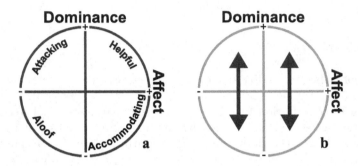

Fig. 1. (a) Leary's Rose: four interpersonal stances are as combinations of different degrees of dominance and affect. (b) 'Inviting' relationships between the stances.

In both LOITER-TB and LOITER-FB, we focus on the following learning goals:

1. Police trainees should know which stance to assume to invite a person to assume a desired stance.
2. Police trainees should be able to recognise and classify behaviour in terms of stances.

4   Thought Bubbles in LOITER-TB

In LOITER-TB, we use thought bubbles to help players achieve the learning goals from Sect. 3 by providing short-term feedback. The Serious Gaming Lemniscate Model (SGLM) asserts that players need to be drawn out of the game world and reflect on a meta-level to learn effectively [3]. For LOITER-TB, we chose to include short moments for explicit reflection.

Some live action role plays (*larps*) include *meta-techniques* offering information to players that would normally not be available to them in-character.[1] The meta-technique on which we base our use of thought bubbles is that of the inner monologue. Players can use this technique to narrate their thoughts so that other players may become aware of them. In LOITER-TB, we provide players with extra information in thought bubbles about the cognitive state of the virtual characters they interact with to help them attain the learning goals.

---

[1] In larps, people role play by physically acting out their characters' actions.

LOITER-TB features a short scenario that revolves around loitering juveniles playing loud music. The player's goal is to end this nuisance. He or she can do so by choosing from 4 different options on how to respond both verbally and non-verbally to the leader of the juveniles, based on the four stances from Leary's Rose. The player's choices influence how the juveniles will leave, based on the 'inviting' relations from Leary's model. For example, the juveniles may do so willingly or grudgingly. The postures of the virtual characters are based on previous research on non-verbal expression of interpersonal stances [8]. Figure 2a shows the interface of the game with a player action, the juvenile's reaction and his thoughts about the player's stance.

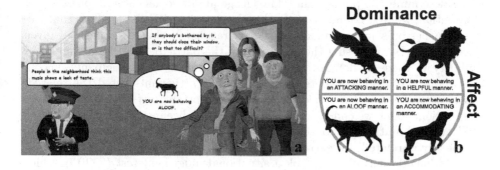

Fig. 2. (a) A screenshot of LOITER-TB when the player has just made a choice. (b) The visualisations of the four stances in the thought bubbles.

For the content of the thought bubbles, we used Dutch adjectives that correspond to stances in Leary's Rose [9]. Based on interviews with instructors from the DPA, we chose to include mnemonic pictures of animals that are archetypical for the different stances, as they are also used in this way in the current training curriculum of police officers, see Fig. 2b. On finishing the game, players receive a short debriefing of what happened in the scenario in which they are shown the result of their actions. The debriefing screen also indicates the stances both the player and the leader of the juveniles assumed most frequently.

5   Experiment 1: LOITER-TB

To evaluate our implementation of thought bubbles, we conducted an experiment with police trainees. Because meta-techniques provide insight in a character's thoughts, we expect that the information presented in thought bubbles aids trainees in learning about social interaction, as compared to a version of the game without the thought bubbles. We address the following three hypotheses.

Hypothesis 1. Thought bubbles help trainees to attain knowledge about social interaction that is similar to that of domain experts.

Hypothesis 2. Thought bubbles help trainees to determine which kinds of behaviour their own behaviour invites.

Hypothesis 3. LOITER-TB helps trainees to recognise stances of other people.

5.1   Method

We conducted an experiment with a repeated measures, between-subjects design with two conditions. Participants in condition TB played LOITER-TB with thought bubbles. Participants in the control condition (C) played the game without thought bubbles. The game featured eight choice points at which players chose between behaviours corresponding to the four stances (see Sect. 3).

To determine the participants' knowledge about social interaction in street intervention, we first conducted a Pathfinder network (PFnet) analysis that calculates a person's mental model based on ratings of the relatedness of given concepts [12]. By analysing the coherence of the participants' PFnets and their similarity to those of domain experts, we determined the participants' knowledge about the given concepts (hypothesis 1). Participants rated the relatedness between 10 different concepts[2] that are important to the domain of street intervention, which we constructed together with police instructors. Participants rated all combinations of concept pairs on a 7-point Likert scale, running from 'completely unrelated' to 'extremely related'.

Additionally, participants took a situational judgement test (SJT) in which they indicated which stance they would expect a juvenile to have in reaction to a given sentence. They also classified given utterance of a juvenile in terms of stance. We used these SJTs to assess participants' abilities to determine invited behaviour and to recognise stances of others (hypothesis 2 and 3).

Next, participants were instructed about the scenario and game mechanics of LOITER-TB. They played the game twice, allowing them to become more familiar with the scenario and the gameplay, and to experiment with different behaviours. Having finished the game, participants retook the PFnet test and the SJTs. They also rated their experience of the game on a number of 7-point Likert scales.

We conducted the experiment with a class of third-year police students of the DPA, who were being trained to become senior police officers ($n = 21$). These students already had practical experience by accompanying graduated police officers on the streets. The mean age of the participants was 33.0 ($SD = 6.9$); 71 % was male and 29 % female. On average, it took participants 30 min to complete the experiment, of which 6 were spent on playing the game. From the 21 participants, 12 were included in condition TB and 9 in condition C.[3]

---

[2] Attacking, aloof, accommodating, helpful, de-escalation, escalation, giving freedom, giving respect, working against each other, and working together.

[3] The inequality of the number of participants in the two conditions was caused by two participants not being able to complete the experiment due to technical issues.

5.2   Results

We compared the participants' pre- and post-test PFnets to an average of the PFnets of four domain experts (one police instructor and three researchers with expertise on Leary's Rose). Using ANCOVAs (dependent variables: post-test coherence and similarity scores, fixed factor: condition, covariates: pre-test coherence and similarity scores), we did not find significant differences between conditions for the coherence of the PFnets and for the similarity between participants' and domain experts' PFnets ($F(20) < 1, p > .05$). A paired-samples t-test showed that the coherence of participants' PFnets in both conditions increased significantly ($t(20) = 3.329, p = .003$; pre-game: $M = .370, SD = .363$; post-game: $M = .584, SD = .338$). Another paired-samples t-test did not show a significant difference ($t(20) < 1, p > .05$) between the pre- and post-game similarity between participants' and domain experts' PFnets across conditions.

An ANCOVA (dependent variable: post-game test score, fixed factor: condition, covariate: pre-game test score) did not show a significant difference ($F(20) < 1, p > .05$) between conditions for the participants' ability to indicate invited reactions of a juvenile (TB: $M = 2.420, SD = 1.084$; C: $M = 1.67, SD = .866$).

A paired-samples t-test showed no significant change ($t(20) < 1, p > .05$) in the participants' ability to recognise the juvenile's stances before ($M = 4.81, SD = .981$; correctly answered questions, out of 8) and after ($M = 5.05, SD = 1.284$) the game was played. An ANCOVA (dependent variable: post-game test score, fixed factor: condition, covariate: pre-game test score) also failed to show a significant difference ($F(20) < 1, p > .05$) between conditions for the participants' ability to recognise a juvenile's stance.

5.3   Discussion

Based on the PFnet analysis, we cannot prove hypothesis 1. We conclude that LOITER-TB aids participants in constructing more coherent mental models, but not in constructing mental models that are more similar to those of domain experts. The addition of thought bubbles in LOITER-TB does not improve the construction of mental models. Because the participants were already experienced at street interventions, we believe that they may already have had a good ability of analysing social interactions and did not get much added value from the feedback in the thought bubbles. Alternatively, it may have been the case that the provided feedback was not explicit enough. The SGLM suggests that players need to be drawn out of the game world to reflect on a meta-level. Our implementation of thought bubbles in the game may not have achieved this effect, which calls for closer scrutiny of how effective feedback should be provided.

Based on the analysis of the SJT, we cannot prove hypothesis 2 and 3. Because the police officers were experienced at street interventions, they already were adept at recognising stances. Therefore, there may be a ceiling effect, as they also indicated that they did not learn very much ($M = 3.24, SD = 1.57$ on a 7-point Likert scale). We expect that the learning effect of LOITER-TB may be stronger for less experienced police officers or trainees.

Participants commented on the difficulty of rating the word pairs for the PFnet analysis. Combined with the fact that we were not able to measure differences between the two conditions, we conclude that PFnet analyses may not be entirely suitable to determine people's mental models about social awareness.

6   Flashbacks in LOITER-FB

The main new meta-technique of LOITER-FB is the addition of flashbacks. These flashbacks refer to events that took place earlier in the game, thus providing feedback on players' behaviour during the game. We implemented flashbacks as thoughts of the juvenile and presented them in thought bubbles, see Fig. 3a. The flashback shows a past action and explains how the player's past average stance influences the juvenile's current preferred stance. Thus, the flashback provides both a retrospect on what happened and a prospect to what may happen.

We wrote two additional scenarios for LOITER-FB: one about the juveniles bothering shopping public, and one about the juveniles loitering at a business park. Thus, players interact with the group three times and have to bond with the juveniles. We modified the cognitive model of the virtual juvenile so that it takes the player's behaviour during previous scenarios in the same game into account. Internally, the player's choices correspond to stances in a two-dimensional grid resembling Leary's Rose. The average of these choices is then calculated as a point somewhere in that grid. Based on this average, the juvenile will have a preferred stance, namely the one that is invited by this average (see Fig. 1b). In the second and third scenario, he bases his follow-up action not only on the stance that the player's current action invites, but also on his preferred stance.

Based on comments from participants and police instructors who played LOITER-TB, we created an alternative visualisation of Leary's Rose in the thought bubbles of the virtual juvenile, see Fig. 3b. Instead of showing pictures animals, the thought bubbles show Leary's Rose with an emphasis on the stance that the player assumed. To prevent information overload, we show the thought bubble and the juvenile's reaction in sequence, and not at the same time.

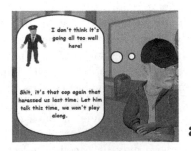 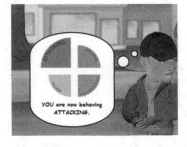

Fig. 3. (a) A thought bubble that shows a flashback. (b) The improved visualisation of Leary's Rose in the thought bubbles.

7 Experiment 2: LOITER-FB

We conducted an experiment with LOITER-FB similar to that in Sect. 5.

7.1 Method

For this experiment, we again used a repeated-measures, between-subjects design with two conditions. One group played the game with thought bubbles and flashbacks (condition FB) and the other played the game without (condition C). In total, participants made 24 choices (in 3 scenarios) when interacting with the juvenile. In condition FB, 12 thought bubbles of the virtual juvenile were shown as well as two flashbacks at the beginning of the second and third scenarios.

Instead of PFnet analyses, participants took an improved SJT. We provided more context in the situation descriptions and let participants rate the effectiveness of four given approaches (based on the four stances) to making the juveniles aware of their behaviour. This involved 8 items that were rated on a Likert scale from 1 to 7 (SJT1). In the second SJT, participants rated four stances of a juvenile on the likelihood of being invited by an utterance of the police officer, for a total of 16 items (SJT2). We compared the responses of participants to those of domain experts (two police instructors), rather than relying on preconceived notions about how these situations should be judged. We constructed similarity scores based on the differences between the ratings of the participants and the average of the ratings of the domain experts. At the end of the experiment, participants filled in the same self-report questionnaire as in Experiment 1.

In total, 28 senior police trainees completed the experiment. Their mean age was 25.9 ($SD = 7.3$); 72 % was male and 28 % female. Participants completed the experiment in 30 min; 15 played condition C, 13 condition FB.

7.2 Results

Table 1 shows the means of the participants' similarity scores on both SJTs and their increase in scores.[4] Independent samples t-tests did not show a difference between conditions on initial scores ($t(24) < 1, p > .05$), nor on post-game scores ($t(24) < 1, p > .05$) on SJT1. A one-sample t-test ($t(25) < 1, p > .05$) showed that the change in the scores of all participants did not significantly differ from 0. An ANCOVA (independent variable: post-SJT1 score; fixed factor: condition; covariate: pre-SJT1 score) showed no significant difference between condition C and FB ($F(25) < 1, p > .05$).

Independent samples t-tests did not show a difference between conditions on initial scores ($t(24) = -1.794, p > .05$), nor on post-game scores ($t(24) < 1, p > .05$) in SJT2. A one-sample t-test ($t(26) = 1.942, p > .05$) showed that the change in the scores of all participants did not significantly differ from 0. An ANCOVA (independent variable: post-SJT2 score; fixed factor: condition; covariate: pre-SJT2 score) showed no significant difference between condition C

---

[4] We assume linearity of the Likert scale items to average data across participants.

Table 1. Participants' scores on the situational judgement tests, per condition.

Condition	SJT1 score, 8 items (M)			SJT2 score, 16 items (M)		
	pre (SD)	post (SD)	incr. (SD)	pre (SD)	post (SD)	incr. (SD)
C	9.4 (2.3)	8.9 (2.7)	−.5 (3.1)	19.3 (4.9)	22.4 (4.4)	3.1 (4.6)
FB	9.3 (4.3)	9.7 (2.8)	.3 (4.7)	23.1 (5.9)	23.2 (6.2)	.1 (4.3)

and FB ($F(27) < 1, p > .05$). In both conditions, participants were satisfied with how they solved the game's scenario ($M = 5.5, SD = .8$), but were not convinced that the game improved their understanding of how their behaviour influenced others ($M = 3.8, SD = 1.6$).

7.3   Discussion

We did not find significant changes in the participants' social awareness, neither across, nor between the conditions. Our situational judgement tests showed that, before playing the game, participants already deviated only slightly from the average of the domain experts' ratings on both SJTs. This indicates that the participants may not be able to improve their social awareness much more, as our results confirm. Because of this ceiling effect, the added value of LOITER-FB may not be apparent for this user group. Some participants commented that they believed the game presents realistic cases, but that the difference between the available actions was very clear. This made it easy for them to tell which response would be the preferred one. Future prototypes may therefore benefit from a game mechanic that would allow for less restricted input.

8   Conclusions and Future Work

We designed and evaluated two iterations of a prototype serious game for improving social awareness of police trainees. Our games feature short interactions in which players resolve conflicts with virtual characters. The central contribution of our games is the inclusion of meta-techniques that provide extra information about the interaction. We used thought bubbles to show players how a virtual character interprets their behaviour and how this influences its actions. In our evaluations, we investigated the learning gains of police trainees of the Dutch Police Academy in versions of the games either with or without meta-techniques. We did not find evidence supporting our hypothesis that our implemented meta-techniques would improve the trainees' social awareness. This may be the case because these players are more adept at (unconsciously) translating such situations into knowledge without explicitly reflecting.

For future work, we will conduct experiments with less experienced police trainees to determine the effects on learning for this user group. We hypothesise that less experienced students may profit more from constructive feedback before analysing social interactions becomes natural to them. The game mechanics of the prototypes also deserve attention: input that is less restricted than through multiple-choice decision points will make the game more challenging and may cause players to behave differently. Additionally, we would like to investigate the adaptation of the virtual characters' behaviour to the players' assessed skills, making the scenarios more or less difficult when necessary.

Acknowledgements. We thank the police instructors and students who helped with our experiments. This publication was supported by the Dutch national program COMMIT.

References

1. Cordar, A., Borish, M., Foster, A., Lok, B.: Building virtual humans with back stories: training interpersonal communication skills in medical students. In: Bickmore, T., Marsella, S., Sidner, C. (eds.) IVA 2014. LNCS, vol. 8637, pp. 144–153. Springer, Heidelberg (2014)
2. Kim, J.M., Hill Jr., R.W., Durlach, P.J., Lane, H.C., Forbell, E., Core, M., Marsella, S., Pynadath, D., Hart, J.: BiLAT: a game-based environment for practicing negotiation in a cultural context. Int. J. Artif. Intell. Educ. **19**, 289–308 (2009)
3. Koops, M., Hoevenaar, M.: Conceptual change during a serious game: using a lemniscate model to compare strategies in a physics game. Simul. Gaming **44**(4), 544–561 (2012)
4. Laffey, J., Schmidt, M., Galyen, K., Stichter, J.: Smart 3D collaborative virtual learning environments: a preliminary framework. J. Ambient Intell. **4**(1), 49–66 (2012)
5. Linssen, J.M., Theune, M.: Meta-techniques for a social awareness learning game. In: Proceedings of ECGBL 2014, pp. 697–704 (2014)
6. Moore, D., McGrath, P., Powell, N.J.: Collaborative virtual environment technology for people with autism. Focus Autism Other Dev. Disabil. **20**(4), 231–243 (2005)
7. Pereira, G., Brisson, A., Prada, R., Paiva, A., Bellotti, F., Kravcik, M., Klamma, R.: Serious games for personal and social learning & ethics: status and trends. Procedia Comput. Sci. **15**, 53–65 (2012)
8. Ravenet, B., Ochs, M., Pelachaud, C.: From a user-created corpus of virtual agent's non-verbal behavior to a computational model of interpersonal attitudes. In: Aylett, R., Krenn, B., Pelachaud, C., Shimodaira, H. (eds.) IVA 2013. LNCS, vol. 8108, pp. 263–274. Springer, Heidelberg (2013)
9. Rouckhout, D., Schacht, R.: Ontwikkeling van een Nederlandstalig interpersoonlijk circumplex. Diagnostiekwijzer **3**, 96–118 (2000)
10. Traum, D.R., Swartout, W.R., Marsella, S.C., Gratch, J.: Fight, flight, or negotiate: believable strategies for conversing under crisis. In: Panayiotopoulos, T., Gratch, J., Aylett, R.S., Ballin, D., Olivier, P., Rist, T. (eds.) IVA 2005. LNCS (LNAI), vol. 3661, pp. 52–64. Springer, Heidelberg (2005)
11. Wouters, P., van Oostendorp, H.: A meta-analytic review of the role of instructional support in game-based learning. Comput. Educ. **60**(1), 412–425 (2013)
12. Wouters, P., van der Spek, E.D., van Oostendorp, H.: Measuring learning in serious games: a case study with structural assessment. Educ. Technol. Res. Dev. **59**(6), 741–763 (2011)

Automated Explanation of Research Informed Consent by Virtual Agents

Timothy Bickmore[1(✉)], Dina Utami[1], Shuo Zhou[1], Candace Sidner[2],
Lisa Quintiliani[3], and Michael K. Paasche-Orlow[3]

[1] College of Computer and Information Science, Northeastern University,
Boston, MA, USA
bickmore@ccs.neu.edu
[2] Worcester Polytechnic Institute, Worcester, MA, USA
[3] Boston Medical Center, Boston, MA, USA

Abstract. A virtual agent that explains research informed consent documents to study volunteers is described, along with a series of development efforts and evaluation studies. A study of nurse administration of informed consent finds that human explanations follow the structure of the document, and that much of information provided verbally is not contained in the document at all. A study of pedagogical strategies used by a virtual consent agent finds that automatic tailoring of document content based on users' knowledge receives the highest ratings of satisfaction compared to two control conditions that provided fixed amounts of information. We finally report on an approach that lets clinicians construct their own virtual agents for informed consent, along with a study that finds that nurses are able to use the system to develop and extend agents to explain their own study consent forms.

Keywords: Relational agent · Embodied conversational agent · Health literacy · Medical informatics · Health informatics

1 Introduction

Informed Consent is an obligatory procedure in the US, in which a significant amount of technical and legal information is supposed to be taught to a layperson before they can agree to participate in a research study or clinical trial. It is a cornerstone in the ethical treatment of human subjects, the result of decades of debate about how to prevent abuse of individuals participating in medical experiments. In addition to complex medical terms and procedures, informed consent documents also contain many concepts that are difficult for laypersons to understand, such as randomization, therapeutic misconception, equipoise, and conflict of interest [1]. While the regulations and requirements surrounding informed consent in the US are voluminous, the actual quality of informed consent document explanation is highly variable and is difficult to demonstrate or monitor [2]. This situation is exacerbated for study volunteers with inadequate health literacy—the ability to read, understand, and follow written medical instructions [3]—a classification that one third of the adults in the US fall into. As a result of these factors, there is ample evidence that a significant number of study

© Springer International Publishing Switzerland 2015
W.-P. Brinkman et al. (Eds.): IVA 2015, LNAI 9238, pp. 260–269, 2015.
DOI: 10.1007/978-3-319-21996-7_26

participants misunderstand informed consent documents, and thus agree to participate in studies without an understanding of their commitment or the risks involved [4].

Virtual agents may provide a particularly effective solution for automatically explaining research informed consent documents to volunteers, as adjuncts to the humans administering consent. Agents can use exemplary techniques that an expert research assistant or clinician might use, given that they had training in communicating with patients with low health literacy and had unbounded time available. Virtual agents should be significantly more effective than conventional media, such as print, web, or multimedia, since face-to-face consultation with a health provider—in conjunction with written instructions—remains one of the best methods for communicating information to patients in general, but especially those with low literacy levels [5, 6]. Face-to-face consultation is effective because it requires that the provider focus on the most salient information to be conveyed [6] and that the information be delivered in a simple, conversational speaking style. Protocols for grounding in face-to-face conversation allow providers to dynamically assess a patient's level of understanding and repeat or elaborate information as necessary [7]. Face-to-face conversation also allows providers to make their communication more explicitly interactive by asking patients to do, write, say, or show something that demonstrates their understanding [8]. Virtual agents can thus consistently evaluate patient comprehension of the information presented. Physicians infrequently evaluate patients' understanding, and when they do it is mostly simply to ask "do you understand?" without waiting for a reply [9].

In the rest of this paper we describe a series of efforts we have undertaken to automate parts of the research informed consent process using virtual agents (Fig. 1). Our "baseline" agent's nonverbal behavior is synchronized with a text-to-speech engine, and user contributions to the conversation are made via a touch screen selection from a multiple choice menu of utterance options, updated at each turn of the conversation. The virtual agent has a range of nonverbal behaviors that it can use, including hand gestures, body posture shifts, gaze shifts, eyebrow raises, and head nods. Conversational nonverbal behavior is determined for each utterance using the BEAT text-to-embodied-speech system [10], with several enhancements to support health dialogues, including the ability to point at parts of the document being explained based on a model of document deictics.

2 Related Work

An agent that explains a document is essentially teaching the user about the topics covered in the document, and thus pedagogical strategies pioneered by other developers of virtual agents are of relevance. Virtual pedagogical agents include Autotutor [11], Persona [12], and many others.

Evaluations of these agents have largely shown mixed educational outcomes. For example, users rated the Persona agent as more entertaining and helpful than an equivalent interface without the agent [12]. However, there was no difference in actual performance (comprehension and recall of presented material) in interfaces with the agent vs. interfaces without it. In another study, students using the AutoTutor peda-

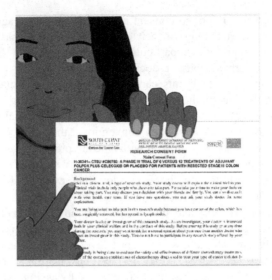

Fig. 1. Virtual agent explaining informed consent document

gogical agent in addition to their normal coursework outperformed both a control group (no additional intervention), and a group directed to re-read relevant material from their textbooks [13].

Bickmore et al., reported several prior studies on virtual agents explaining medical documents to patients. In one system, a "virtual nurse" agent explained a digital copy of patients' hospital discharge instructions to them while they were still in their hospital beds [14, 15]. Pilot and summative evaluations indicated that most patients preferred receiving their discharge instructions from the virtual nurse compared to their human doctors or nurses in the hospital, and that patients with low health literacy had significantly higher levels of satisfaction with the virtual nurse compared to patients with adequate health literacy. In another system, a virtual agent explained research informed consent documents to patients [16]. A study comparing the agent to a human research assistant and a self-study condition found that all participants were most satisfied with the consent process and were most likely to sign the consent form when the agent provided the explanation. However, the consent explanation in this system was entirely scripted for each consent document.

Fernando developed a dialogue system and virtual agent for explaining research informed consent documents that used a structured representation of each document together with a library of background concept tutorials and a few general document explanation techniques. He compared two versions of this system—a "verbose" agent that provided all relevant information about each section of a document, and a "tailored" agent that allowed users to request background information—to a self-study condition. He found that the verbose agent outperformed the other two conditions on comprehension test scores, but users were most satisfied with the tailored agent and least satisfied with the verbose agent [17].

3 Nurse Explanation of Oncology Informed Consent Documents

In order to inform the design of a virtual agent that administers research informed consent, we conducted a study of oncology nurses administering informed consent for clinical trials to mock study participants. In oncology clinical trials, patients will typically meet with a study nurse for an hour-long session to review the informed consent document, then take the document home to consider participation before meeting with their oncologist to answer any final questions and sign up for the trial.

We conducted detailed analyses of transcripts from several of the consent sessions. We found that the nurses structure their explanation following the structure of the informed consent document, generally proceeding linearly through the sections of the document (consistent with prior findings [17, 18]). Beyond that, there was often little correlation between what the nurses said and the contents of the document, or what ethicists would say is most important information to convey (e.g., the voluntary nature of participation, potential risks, and the ramifications of randomization). The nurses spent most of their time describing what it will actually be like to experience being in the trial, reassuring the patient that they will be ok, and relating anecdotal information they happen to know that is related to information in the consent form.

Based on these findings, we proceeded to design our virtual agent for automated informed consent whose explanations followed the structure of the consent document. Informed consent documents are approved by an Institutional Review Board (IRB)[1] and then cannot be changed, so any explanation offered must be entirely centered on the existing document.

4 Evaluation of Pedagogical Strategies for Document Explanation

As a next step in our research, we conducted a study to determine the amount of information that a virtual agent should provide to volunteers about a study, and a simple pedagogical strategy for tailoring the explanation of the informed consent document.

4.1 Methods

The experimental design of this study is a 3-treatment, counterbalanced, within-subjects design, comparing three consent document explanation strategies by a virtual agent. The three strategies were, respectively, a short overview of each section only (SHORT), overview plus a detailed reading of the informed consent document (DETAILED), and an adaptive strategy in which participants were given

---

[1] The panel that reviews and approves human subjects studies at each institution to meet US federal requirements.

comprehension checks of each major section of the document, and a tailored review based on their understanding (TAILORED). In all cases, users were given unbounded time to read each section of the digital document before proceeding.

Three informed consent documents for clinical trials involving methods for colonoscopy screening for cancer were created with different study protocols, risks, and compensation levels for use in this study. The domain of cancer screening was selected, for the documents contained a wide range of complex medical terms, facts and concepts, making it appropriate for testing an automated document explanation system. The length and complexity of the three documents were designed to be approximately the same across all three conditions.

Participants. In total, 74 subjects, 67.6 % female, aged 18 to 94 years old (mean = 50), participated in this study. Among all participants, 26 % had low levels of health literacy, based on the REALM screener [19].

Measures. Comprehension was assessed by a closed-book knowledge test, consisting of three YES/NO questions, and three multiple-choice questions for each document. Immediately following their interaction with the agent, participants completed a self-report questionnaire assessing satisfaction with the consent experience, including several single-item, scale response questions, based on the Brief Informed Consent Evaluation Protocol [20] (Table 1). We created two composite measures of overall satisfaction (Q1, Q2, Q3, Q10) and attitude towards the instructor (Q1, Q3, Q4, Q5, Q6).

Table 1. Self-report scale measures completed after agent interaction

Question	Anchor 1	Anchor 7
Q1. How satisfied are you with the instructor?	Not at all	Very satisfied
Q2. How satisfied are you with the instructional experience?	Not at all	Very satisfied
Q3. How much would you like to continue working with the instructor?	Not at all	Very much
Q4. How much do you trust the instructor?	Not at all	Very much
Q5. How much do you like the instructor?	Not at all	Very much
Q6. How knowledgeable was the instructor?	Not at all	Very knowledgeable
Q7. How much information did you get?	Too little	Too much
Q8. How likely would you have been to sign the document?	Extremely unlikely	Extremely likely
Q9. How much pressure did you feel to sign the document?	No pressure	Extreme pressure
Q10. How satisfied were you with the explanation?	Extremely unsatisfied	Extremely satisfied

4.2   Results

Non-parametric Friedman test were used for testing differences across the three experimental conditions for repeated measures.

Satisfaction. We found a significant effect of treatment conditions on participants' attitude towards the agent ($p < .05$), with highest satisfaction for the TAILORED condition, and lowest satisfaction with agent for the DETAILED condition. Similarly, we also found a significant effect of treatment conditions on participants' overall satisfaction ($p < .05$), with highest overall satisfaction for the TAILORED condition, and lowest overall satisfaction for the DETAILED condition. There was a trending effect of treatment conditions ($p = .078$) on perceived amount of information provided by the agent: participants tended to rate the SHORT and the DETAILED conditions as providing too much information compared to the TAILORED condition. No significant differences were found for likelihood to sign or perceived pressure to sign the document. Table 2 shows the descriptive statistics for the outcome measures.

Table 2. Study results (mean and (SD))

	SHORT	DETAILED	TAILORED	p
Attitude towards agent	5.9 (1.3)	5.8 (1.2)	6.1 (1.1)	<.05
Overall satisfaction	5.7 (1.3)	5.4 (1.4)	5.9 (1.2)	<.05
Amount of information provided	5.0 (1.3)	5.0 (1.5)	4.7 (1.2)	.078
Likelihood to sign	5.1 (1.8)	4.9 (2.1)	5.2 (1.9)	n.s.
Pressure to sign	2.3 (1.8)	2.5 (1.9)	2.2 (1.7)	n.s.
Comprehension	0.92 (0.7)	1.04 (0.8)	0.93 (0.8)	n.s.

Comprehension. No significant differences among treatment conditions were found for participants' total comprehension of the documents.

Health Literacy. We also investigated relationships between participants' health literacy and other measures using Spearman's rho non-parametric tests. We found that, participants' REALM scores (indicating levels of health literacy) were negatively correlated with their attitude towards the agent ($rho = -0.23$, $p < .001$), overall satisfaction ($rho = -0.15$, $p < .05$), and perceived pressure to sign the document ($rho = -0.15$, $p < .05$), indicating that low literacy participants liked the agent more, were more satisfied with the experience, and felt more pressure to sign, compared to participants with higher levels of health literacy. Their REALM scores were also significantly correlated with their total comprehension of the consent documents ($rho = 0.24$, $p < .001$), indicating that participants with higher levels of health literacy learned more about each document.

Discussion. In general, we found positive feedback from the participants on the consent document explanation system. Participants favored the TAILORED condition the most, rating highest on attitude towards the agent, and overall satisfaction with the experience, and they also felt the TAILORED condition provided the most appropriate amount of information compared to the other two conditions. However, we did not find any differences between approaches on comprehension.

5 Towards Fully-Automated Explanation

Given that our observed human explanations of informed consent documents followed the structure of the document, and that the document must be presented to patients without modification, we further developed our virtual agent-based consent explanation system to start with an import of a consent document and support the construction of an interactive consent experience centered on the document. Our goal was to automate as much of the explanation as possible given the document contents, while allowing non-technical clinicians to provide any additional adaptations required to produce a usable consent system. Our approach is to import a structured representation of the document in XML, and drive automated explanation based on XML document annotations that could either be automatically added through analysis of the document contents, or added by a clinician via a graphical editor.

There are at least three types of annotations that can be used in marking up an informed consent document to support explanation by an agent:

Structural Tags describe the structure and spatial layout of the document (e.g., SECTION, PARAGRAPH). These are essential since the agent needs to be able to display a page to the user and point at the block of text being discussed. We have used the DocBook tagset for this purpose [21].

Semantic Tags describe the semantic types of content, at varying level of detail in the document (e.g., RISKS_AND_BENEFITS, RISK, STUDY_VISIT). Use of these tags assumes there is a text generator capable of providing explanatory dialogue for the tagged content.

Procedural Tags serve as runtime instructions to the agent describing how it should explain some aspect of the document (e.g., SAY, COMPREHENSION_TEST, PRIORITY). These tags can be either declarative or procedural in nature, and are where most policy decisions about administration of consent for a given study site would be implemented.

Our initial approach was to tag all relevant data with semantic tags and use text generation to dynamically produce explanations. However, after reviewing over 20 sample informed consent documents we discovered that, although authors may use standard sections in their document (and many IRBs may require specific sections), there is no guarantee that authors will choose to populate these sections consistently or completely. We also observed that the authors often distribute information about a given topic across several sections of the document (e.g., there is nothing to prevent some aspects of study protocol from appearing in many different parts of a document). The definition of a hierarchical set of semantic tags (such as XML provides) presumes that all information about a given topic be contained only within a defined context, and thus is incompatible with the lack of structure we observed. In addition, following our observation of human informed consent, the agent will typically be eliding and gisting almost all of the details in the document, and offering additional information that is not represented at all in the document, thus obviating the need for semantic tags for the majority of information actually contained in the document. Finally, clinicians will require control over what the agent says about a given study in order to implement their consent policy, so some level of procedural control is required regardless. All of this led us to an annotation tag set comprised primarily of structural and procedural tags, which essentially instruct the agent how to explain each part of the document as it is linearly traversed by the system.

Based on this approach, we developed a set of tags that could be used to annotate an XML representation of an informed consent document, together with a library of common tutorials and other re-usable dialogue, and a visual editor that would facilitate annotation by non-technical clinicians. Most structural tags, and an initial set of procedural tags, are automatically generated by the visual editor tool when a new consent document is imported. The clinician uses the tool to iteratively extend and modify these tags and review the resulting explanation until they are satisfied with the result. Figure 2 shows the visual editor interface. The library includes descriptions of common concepts, such as voluntariness, randomization, and study overviews, that are parameterized by particular features of any given study. Clinicians can test any part of the explanation by clicking on a "preview" button.

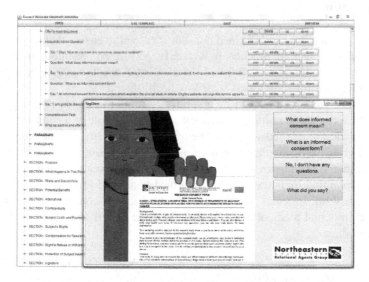

Fig. 2. Informed consent visual document annotator with preview running

Nurse Document Tagging Usability Evaluation. We conducted a pilot formative evaluation on the consent annotator system at a local hospital to determine if study nurses were able to use the visual editor to annotate their consent forms. Five oncology research nurses and research associates from the hospital were recruited. Participants were first shown a demo video about how to use the system, and then received further explanation on each function. Participants were then asked to complete four simple tasks using the system. After completing the tasks, they were asked to fill out a satisfaction questionnaire (Table 3) and interviewed about their experience. In general, nurses liked the major functions the annotator system provided, such as having a dictionary to mark up complicated medical terms and the ability to add in comprehension questions. The nurses provided valuable feedback on possible improvements to the usability of the system, such as adding visual aids to help patients understand the documents, allowing patients to audio record their questions to the study team, and extending the system to support non-English speakers.

Table 3. Nurse ratings of consent document annotator

Question	Anchors		Mean (SD)
I found the system unnecessarily complex.	1 = Strongly disagree	5 = Strongly agree	2.0 (1.7)
I thought the system was easy to use	1 = Strongly disagree	5 = Strongly agree	4.0 (1.0)
I found the various functions in the system were well integrated	1 = Strongly disagree	5 = Strongly agree	4.3 (1.2)
In general, how satisfied were you with the annotator?	1 = Not at all satisfied	7 = Very satisfied	5.7 (2.3)

6   Conclusion

The proper administration of informed consent is crucial to ensure the ethical treatment of human subjects, yet in practice it is poorly performed, resulting in most study participants not actually being "informed" at all. Virtual agents can greatly improve this situation, especially for individuals with low health literacy.

In this paper we have reported on a series of efforts to construct such agents, and have found that our study participants accept agents in the role of a consenting research assistant or clinician, learned well with the agent, and preferred a dynamically-tailored version of consent form explanation over a fixed presentation. We were also able to demonstrate that study nurses could use our system to develop virtual agent systems capable of explaining their own unique informed consent documents.

Our future work includes a randomized evaluation of consent agents created by study nurses in actual medical trials, comparing these agents to the standard informed consent procedure.

Acknowledgments. This work was supported, in part, by National Institutes of Health National Cancer Institute (NCI) Grant R01CA158219.

References

1. Sugarman, J., et al.: Empirical research on informed consent. An annotated bibliography. Hastings Cent. Rep. **29**(1), S1–S42 (1999)

2. Smith, T., Moore, E.J., Tunstall-Pedoe, H.: Review by a local medical research ethics committee of the conduct of approved research projects, by examination of patients' case notes, consent forms, and research records and by interview. BMJ **314**(7094), 1588–1590 (1997)

3. Ad Hoc Committee on Health Literacy for the Council on Scientific Affairs, A.M.A.: Health literacy: report of the council on scientific affairs. JAMA **281**(6), 552–557 (1999)

4. Joffe, S., et al.: Quality of informed consent in cancer clinical trials: a cross-sectional survey. Lancet **358**(9295), 1772–1777 (2001)

5. Madden, E.: Evaluation of outpatient pharmacy patient counseling. J. Am. Pharm. Assoc. **13**, 437–443 (1973)

6. Qualls, C., Harris, J., Rogers, W.: Cognitive-linguistic aging: considerations for home health care environments. In: Rogers, W., Fisk, A. (eds.) Human Factors Interventions for the Health Care of Older Adults, pp. 47–67. Lawrence Erlbaum, Mahwah (2002)

7. Clark, H.H., Brennan, S.E.: Grounding in communication. In: Resnick, L.B., Levine, J.M., Teasley, S.D. (eds.) Perspectives on Socially Shared Cognition, pp. 127–149. American Psychological Association, Washington (1991)

8. Doak, C., Doak, L., Root, J.: Teaching Patients with Low Literacy Skills, 2nd edn. JB Lippincott, Philadelphia (1996)

9. Schillinger, D., et al.: Closing the loop: physician communication with diabetic patients who have low health literacy. Arch. Intern. Med. **163**(1), 83–90 (2003)

10. Cassell, J., Vilhjálmsson, H., Bickmore, T.: BEAT: the behavior expression animation toolkit. In: SIGGRAPH 2001, Los Angeles (2001)

11. Graesser, A., et al.: AutoTutor: a simulation of a human tutor. Cogn. Syst. Res. **1**(1), 35–51 (1999)

12. Andre, F., Rist, T., Muller, J.: Integrating reactive and scripted behaviors in a life-like presentation agent. In: Proceedings of AGENTS 1998, pp. 261–268 (1998)

13. Person, N.K., et al.: Evaluating student learning gains in two versions of AutoTutor. In: Moore, J.D., Redfield, C.L., Johnson, W.L. (eds.) Artificial intelligence in education: AI-ED in the wired and wireless future, pp. 286–293. IOS Press, Amsterdam (2001)

14. Bickmore, T., Pfeifer, L., Jack, B.W.: Taking the time to care: empowering low health literacy hospital patients with virtual nurse agents. In: Proceedings of the ACM SIGCHI Conference on Human Factors in Computing Systems (CHI), Boston (2009)

15. Zhou, S., Bickmore, T., Paasche-Orlow, M., Jack, B.: Agent-user concordance and satisfaction with a virtual hospital discharge nurse. In: Bickmore, T., Marsella, S., Sidner, C. (eds.) IVA 2014. LNCS, vol. 8637, pp. 528–541. Springer, Heidelberg (2014)

16. Bickmore, T., Pfeifer, L., Paasche-Orlow, M.: Using computer agents to explain medical documents to patients with low health literacy. Patient Educ. Couns. **75**(3), 315–320 (2009)

17. Fernando, R.: Automated Explanation of Research Informed Consent by Embodied Conversational Agents, in College of Computer and Information Science. Northeastern University, Boston (2009)

18. Bickmore, T., Pfeifer, L., Yin, L.: The role of gesture in document explanation by embodied conversational agents. Int. J. Semant. Comput. **2**(1), 47–70 (2008)

19. Davis, T., et al.: Rapid estimate of adult literacy in medicine: a shortened screening instrument. Fam. Med. **25**, 391–395 (1993)

20. Sugarman, J., et al.: Evaluating the quality of informed consent. Clin. Trials **2**(1), 34–41 (2005)

21. Walsh, N.: DocBook 5: The Definitive Guide. O'Reilly Associates, Sebastopol (2010)

Linking Aetiology with Social Communication in a Virtual Stroke Patient

Harry Brenton[1]([⊠]), Peter Woodward[1], Marco Gillies[2], Jonathan Birns[3],
Diane Ames[1], and Fernando Bello[1]

[1] Imperial College London, London, UK
h.brenton@imperial.ac.uk
[2] Goldsmiths University, London, UK
[3] Guy's and St Thomas' NHS Foundation Trust, London, UK

Abstract. This paper describes an approach to building a virtual stroke patient which allows learners to visually explore connections between different stroke aetiologies and social behaviour. It presents an architecture that links a parametric model of aetiology to verbal and non verbal behaviour which can be manipulated in realtime. We believe that this design has the potential to consolidate understanding by allowing learners to systematically explore variations in clinical presentation. To the best of our knowledge, this is the first Intelligent Virtual Agent (IVA) that uses a parameterised behaviour model to provide an interactive examination and diagnosis of a stroke patient.

Keywords: Intelligent virtual agent · Virtual patients

1 Introduction

Virtual patients built using Intelligent Virtual Agents (IVAs) allow trainees to practice diagnostic and communication skills in a safe, standardised environment [1]. This gives entire cohorts of learners the opportunity to diagnose rare conditions, such as nerve injury, that cannot be feigned by an actor pretending to be a patient [2].

IVAs allow users to explore the impact of damage upon verbal and non-verbal communication. For example, a spoken request to look straight ahead reveals restricted eye movements that indicate a particular type of cranial nerve injury [3]. Similarly, hand gestures, body position, and gaze position can help to diagnose abdominal pain [1]. These systems use parameterised aetiology models to generate different presenting symptoms (aetiology is the study of the origins and causes of a disease or disorder). However, the variables cannot be manipulated at runtime, so learners are unable to explore the consequences of different aetiologies for themselves.

This paper describes a novel approach to building a virtual stroke patient that links a parametric model of aetiology to verbal and non verbal behaviour which can be manipulated in realtime. Correct diagnosis of a stroke (loss of brain function due to inadequate blood supply) is crucially important because misdiagnosing a stroke and administering incorrect treatment, can be lethal.

© Springer International Publishing Switzerland 2015
W.-P. Brinkman et al. (Eds.): IVA 2015, LNAI 9238, pp. 270–274, 2015.
DOI: 10.1007/978-3-319-21996-7_27

2   Instructional Design and Behaviour Model

There are three modes of operation.

1. **Examination mode** The user administers the 11 items of the NIHSS test
   (Table 1) and scores them between 0 and 4 as they progress through the
   simulation (Fig. 1).

Table 1. The National Institute of Health Stroke Scale (NIHSS) and corresponding
interaction with the IVA. The NIHSS scale quantifies the severity of a stroke between
0 (no symptoms) and 42 (a severe stroke).

NIHSS item	Interaction
1. Response to verbal and physical stimuli	Reciprocal eye contact
	IVA tracks user's nose and fingers
	IVA responds to user's finger poke
	IVA responds to spoken instructions
2. Horizontal eye movement	IVA tracks user's fingers
3. Visual field test	User's finger tests visual quadrants
	IVA states number of user's fingers
4. Facial paralysis	User instructs IVA to show teeth
	User instructs IVA to close eyes
	User instructs IVA to raise eyebrows
	IVA's face responds to instructions
5. Arm stability	User instructs IVA to raise arm
	IVA's raises arm & holds pose
6. Leg stability	User instructs IVA to raise leg
	IVA raises leg & holds pose
7. Limb coordination	User instructs IVA to touch finger
	IVA touches user finger
8. Sensory loss	User pricks IVA with a pin
	IVA grimaces / verbally repsonds
9. Language skills	User instructs IVA to describe a picture
	User instructs IVA to name objects
	User instructs IVA to read a list
	IVA verbally responds to instructions
10. Generative speech (motor function)	User instructs IVA to read a list
	IVA verbally responds to instructions
11. Extinction and Inattention (optional)	User instructs IVA to close eyes
	User touches left & right simultaneously
	IVA verbally responds to touch

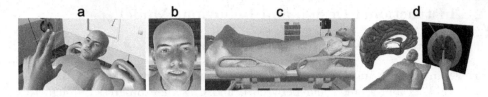

Fig. 1. Interacting with the IVA: (a) a user raises two fingers to administer a visual field test; (b) the IVA shows his teeth to test facial paralysis; (c) the IVA raises his right leg to test motor stability; (d) Selecting an artery on the CT scan or 3D brain simulates right sided partial paralysis in the IVA

2. **Debrief mode** Learners can consolidate learning by replaying encounters with virtual patients.
3. **Assisted discovery mode** The user interacts with either the 3D brain or the 2D CT scan to simulate the effect of a blood clot in an artery (Fig. 1d).

Our architecture is designed to link between parameters of aetiology and parameters of complex social behaviour (Fig. 2).

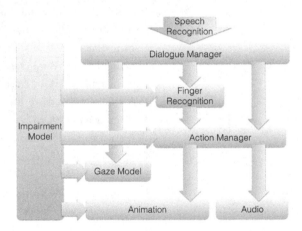

Fig. 2. The behaviour model used for the virtual patient. In each stage the behaviour is parameterised based on a model of the patient's impairment.

Impairment Model is a container for the key parameters of the patient's impairment that affect the visible behaviour. The following parameters are based on the NIHSS scale (Table 1) which is used to control the different aspects of the IVAs behaviour: 1a: general verbal responsiveness; 1b: ability to answer questions verbally; 2: ability to track gaze in left and right hemispheres testing (a) motor control and (b) vision; 3: ability to recognise visual stimuli in the four quadrants of vision; 4: facial palsy; 5: motor paralysis in the arms.

Dialogue Manager takes in text from a speech recognition system and uses pattern matching to select from a series of possible responses based upon the NIHSS diagnostic protocol (Table 1). Each response triggers an action in one of the following behaviour controllers: utterances, finger recognition and gaze.

Action Manager generates actions (animation and audio) in response to user activity. Speech is generated according to the threshold of parameter 1b (ability to answer questions verbally): very high impairment results in no speech, lower impairment results in occasional speech.

Finger Recognition implements items two and three of the NIHSS protocol (Table 1) in which the patient tracks and counts the number of fingers held up in various quadrants of vision.

Gaze Model is a model of conversational gaze based on [4]. The proportion of time spent looking at the clinician varies across a number of conditions: (1) whether the clinician is speaking; (2) when the clinician administers a physical stimulus; (3) when the clinician asks the patient to follow their nose. All of these conditions are dependent on the impairment parameter 1a: general responsiveness. If the patient has an impairment in a hemisphere, all gaze behaviour is turned off when the clinician is in that hemisphere.

Audio is an audio player for speech responses. It is triggered when the impairment does not affect speech in the Action Manager.

Animation generates movement of the patient's face and body based on triggers from the action manager. All of the actions are parameterised blends between a full response animation and an unresponsive animation.

3   Conclusion

This paper presented an approach to building a virtual stroke patient that allows users to visually explore connections between aetiology and social communication. We believe that this method has the potential to consolidate understanding by allowing learners to systematically explore variations in clinical presentation. The next step is to conduct validation studies to assess the acceptability and accuracy of the simulation. Stroke has a devastating impact upon people's lives, so any potential benefits of using IVAs for training are well worth investigating.

References

1. Deladisma, A., Cohen, M., Stevens, A., Wagner, P., Lok, B., Bernard, T., Oxendine, C., Schumacher, L., Johnsen, K., Dickerson, R., Raij, A., Wells, R., Duerson, M., Harper, J., Lind, D.: Do medical students respond empathetically to a virtual patient ? Am J Surg **193**(6), 756–760 (2007)
2. Johnson, T., Lyons, R., Chuah, J., Kopper, R., Lok, B., Cendan, J.: Optimal learning in a virtual patient simulation of cranial nerve palsies: the interaction between social learning context and student aptitude. Med. Teach. **35**(1), e876–884 (2013)

3. Peden, M., Chuah, J., Kotranza, A., Lok, B., Cendan, J., Johnsen, K.: Nerve - a three dimensional patient simulation for evaluating cranial nerve function. MedEd-PORTAL Publications (2011)
4. Vinayagamoorthy, V., Gillies, M., Steed, A., Tanguy, E., Pan, X., Loscos, C., Slater, M.: Building expression into virtual characters. Eurographics State of the Art Reports (2006)

Adapting a Geriatrics Health Counseling Virtual Agent for the Chinese Culture

Zhe Zhang[1], Ha Trinh[1], Qiong Chen[2], and Timothy Bickmore[1(✉)]

[1] College of Computer and Information Science, Northeastern University,
Boston, MA, USA
{zessiez,hatrinh,bickmore}@ccs.neu.edu
[2] Xin Hua Hospital, Shanghai, China

Abstract. The design of a virtual conversational agent that provides cardio-vascular health counseling to hospitalized geriatrics patients in China is described, along with the linguistic and cultural adaptations performed to tailor the agent for China. Results of a preliminary study comparing conversations with the agent to conversations with a geriatrician in a hospital in Shanghai demonstrated high levels of patient acceptance and satisfaction with the agent, although not as high as for the human doctor.

1 Introduction

With its aging population, mandatory retirement, and one-child policy, China is facing a crisis in its ability to care for its elderly. There will not be nearly enough caregivers to meet the demand of individuals who want to live independently as long as possible. Virtual agents provide a solution to automating many routine healthcare tasks, and agents that play the role of health counselors have been shown to be well-accepted by older adults in several cultures [1]. To help address these issues, we have developed a virtual agent to counsel geriatrics patients about cardiovascular health (Fig. 1). Cardiovascular conditions, such as stroke and myocardial infarction are among the leading causes of morbidity and mortality for Chinese older adults. Standard prevention measures include appropriate exercise, diet, and stress management, and adherence to prescribed medications.

Culture is important in health education interventions. Many studies have demonstrated the importance of cultural congruity between health providers and their patients. For example, patients usually prefer health counselors from their own culture due to their presumed familiarity with cultural values [2].

Our general approach was to first develop the agent for the English-speaking Anglo-American culture we are most familiar with, then methodically adapt it, linguistically and culturally, for the Chinese older adult population. The agent counsels patients on their diagnoses and medications specified by a clinician, as well as increasing physical activity, improving diet, decreasing stress, and motivating them to be more involved and proactive in their own care. The virtual agent speaks using synthetic speech driven by a dialogue engine, and has a range of nonverbal behaviors that it can use, including facial displays of emotion, hand gestures, body posture shifts,

© Springer International Publishing Switzerland 2015
W.-P. Brinkman et al. (Eds.): IVA 2015, LNAI 9238, pp. 275–278, 2015.
DOI: 10.1007/978-3-319-21996-7_28

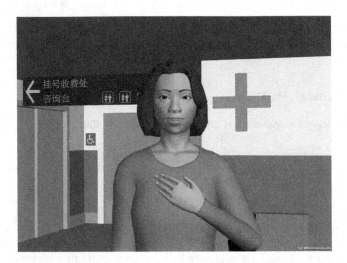

Fig. 1. Chinese geriatrics cardiovascular health counselor

gaze shifts, eyebrow raises, and head nods. The entire counseling system was deployed on an 8″ touchscreen tablet to facilitate use in a hospital environment.

2   Adaptation for the Chinese Culture

We began our cultural adaptation of the agent following Hofstede's framework [3]. Two dimensions stand out as particularly important for differentiating US and Chinese cultures: power-distance and individualism-collectivism. Physicians are at the top of the hierarchy in the US healthcare system and are highly regarded in healthcare and society in general. Thus, we initially assumed that in a high power-distance culture such as China, a virtual doctor should appear as a socially remote, authoritative figure. However, after our discussions with Chinese doctors and patients, we found that the situation in China is different. Healthcare in China is not entirely subsidized by the government, and the population has an extreme consumerist attitude about the healthcare system, demanding service and outcomes for their money. Given this, we designed our virtual health counselor to appear as more of an approachable and friendly peer, without the official trappings of a lab coat and stethoscope.

Given the greater bias towards collectivism in China compared to the US, we did weave elements of collectivism into the translated counseling scripts. For instance, we designed a particular coaching strategy to encourage patients to work together with their family members and close friends on their health conditions. Also, when motivating patients to adhere to different aspects of their medical regimen, we emphasized how their activity could potentially affect their family members.

Virtual Counselor Appearance. Prior research has highlighted the importance of the agent appearance for perceptions of cultural congruity. Accordingly, we tailored the virtual counselor character model to have more of a Chinese appearance, adjusting its skin-tone to be more yellowish and tailored its hair to be dark brown. We also designed black irises for the character to match Asian genetics. We designed a background for the character to match images of Chinese hospital interiors (Fig. 1).

Dialogue. Conversational dialogue is the primary communication avenue for the virtual agent to interact with its users. The dialogue content mainly focuses on topics such as cardiovascular diseases, associated medications, and physical activity, diet, and stress management, all considered common topics of physician-patients conversations in China. These dialogues are designed and delivered based on each patient's particular health conditions and doctors' recommendations. To make the dialogues culturally appropriate to Chinese patients, contextual adaptation was applied. For instance, we adapted "How are you *doing* today?" to a linguistically equal version of "How are you *feeling* today?" in Chinese based on how a doctor typically initiates a conversation with a patient in China. Also, we removed the "serving" concept from the fruit and vegetable promotion part of the diet dialogue given that it is not commonly used in Chinese culture, and adopted "bowl" to quantitatively measure vegetable and fruit intake. Finally, in the farewell dialogue, we replaced "Have a nice day" with "I wish you good health", which is the most common way to end a medical conversation in China.

Nonverbal Behavior. Our system automatically generates a number of nonverbal behaviors for the agent using our extended version of the Behavior Expression Animation Toolkit (BEAT) [4]. BEAT assigns nonverbal behaviors based on linguistic and contextual analysis of the agent's speaking text. As BEAT was originally developed for English, we extended its language module to perform syntactic and discourse analysis for the Chinese language. Our system annotates the Chinese text with grammatical structure information using the Stanford part-of-speech tagger and a factored parser trained on Xinhua newspaper text from Mainland China.

3 Pilot Acceptance Study

We collaborated with clinicians from Xin Hua Hospital in China, on a preliminary, between-subjects study to evaluate the acceptance and usability of the agent system by local geriatrics patients. Our aim was to assess the patients' overall satisfaction with the system and their attitude towards the culturally tailored agent following a brief counseling session, in comparison with a human geriatrician.

Participants. We recruited a total of 10 patients: 80 % male, aged from 70–94 (mean = 85.89), 80 % were inpatients, 60 % had high school or higher degrees, 50 % had high level of computer literacy, 50 % reported high level of confidence in filling out the forms by themselves. The patients had a variety of health conditions and occupational backgrounds, including professor, retired civil servant, military veteran, office clerk, and doctor. Six of them were randomized into the intervention group.

Measures. The acceptance and use of the system was evaluated using the 7-point scales outlined in Table 1.

Table 1. Patients' ratings of the culturally adapted agent system

Rating Aspects (Scale Measures from 1–7)	Agent Mean (SD)	Physician Mean (SD)
How satisfied were you? (1-not at all, 7-very satisfied)	4.67 (1.75)	6.00 (0.00)
How much would like to continue working with the counselor/doctor? (1-not at all, 7-very much)	4.83 (1.60)	6.50 (0.58)
How much do you trust the counselor/doctor? (1-not at all, 7-very much)	5.33 (1.21)	6.75 (0.50)
How much do you like the counselor/doctor? (1-not at all, 7-very much)	4.83 (1.60)	6.75 (0.50)
How easy was talking to the counselor/doctor? (1-easy, 7-difficult)	2.17 (1.94)	1.25 (0.50)
How would you characterize your relationship with the counselor/doctor? (1-complete stranger, 7-close friend)	3.67 (1.63)	5.25 (0.50)
How much do you feel the counselor/doctor cares about you? (1-not at all, 7-very much)	3.83 (1.47)	7.00 (0.00)
How likely is it that you will follow the advice? (1-not at all, 7-very likely)	6.00 (1.55)	7.00 (0.00)

Quantitative Results. Although not as high as for the human doctor, patients were highly satisfied with the virtual counselor, exhibited high desire to continue working with her, trusted and liked her, and would follow her advices in the future (Table 1). In addition, patients who had high school or higher degrees expressed significantly more trust in the virtual counselor than those whose degrees are lower than high school ($p < .05$). Patients with high computer literacy felt that the agent cared more about them, compared to those with low computer literacy ($p < .05$).

Conclusion. Patients in our study responded very well to the agent, expressing high levels of trust, engagement and respect for the agent. Future work includes extending the counseling content with more culturally appropriate health topics, while improving the visual appearance and nonverbal behavior of the agent and the quality of the agent's speech.

Acknowledgments. Thanks to Shuo Zhou and Lin Shi for review and input, and Zachary Berwaldt for work on the character model.

References

1. King, A., et al.: Employing 'virtual advisors' in preventive care for underserved communities: results from the COMPASS study. J. Health Commun. **18**(12), 1449–1464 (2013)
2. Sue, D., Ivey, A., Pederson, P.: Theory of Multicultural Counseling and Therapy. Thomson Brooks/Cole, Belmont (2007)
3. Hofstede, G.: Culture's Consequences. Sage, Beverly Hills (2003)
4. Cassell, J., Vilhjálmsson, H., Bickmore, T.: BEAT: the behavior expression animation toolkit. In: SIGGRAPH 2001, Los Angeles, CA (2001)

Breathe with Me: A Virtual Meditation Coach

Ameneh Shamekhi[✉] and Timothy Bickmore

College of Computer and Information Science, Northeastern University,
Boston, MA, USA
{ameneh, bickmore}@ccs.neu.edu

Abstract. A virtual agent that guides users through mindfulness meditation sessions is described. The agent uses input from a respiration sensor to both respond to user breathing rate and use deep breaths as a continuation and acknowledgment signal. A pilot evaluation study comparing the agent to a self-help video indicates that users are very receptive to the virtual meditation coach, and that it is more effective at reducing anxiety and increasing mindfulness and flow state compared to the video.

1 Introduction

Meditation involves a complex set of techniques designed to promote relaxation and emotional balance. It has been found to be therapeutic for a wide range of mental and physical conditions, including chronic pain, depression, anxiety, substance use, and insomnia, and is also an effective buffer against conditions such as post-traumatic stress disorder. Meditation works by increasing meta-cognitive awareness of one's mental states—both cognitive and affective—allowing the practitioner to more effectively cope with extreme cognitions, affective states and moods. The act of meditation thus bridges the divide between cognition and affect in a useful, therapeutic manner.

Meditation takes practice to master, and, unfortunately, most individuals do not have access to classes or experts who can effectively teach them the techniques required for mastery. Many self-help books, videos, and audio programs exist to provide meditation instruction, but they are neither tailored to individual needs nor interactive. In this project, we are developing a virtual agent that plays the role of a meditation coach that is designed to help practitioners focus on their breathing and relax. The meditation agent guides users through an interactive meditation session while monitoring their breathing and providing feedback (Fig. 1).

2 The Virtual Meditation Coach

The virtual meditation coach is an embodied conversational agent developed to guide novice users through a mindfulness meditation session and help them relax. The agent speaks using synthetic speech driven by a dialogue engine, with synchronized animated co-verbal behavior (Fig. 1). In order to evaluate the efficacy of this medium compared to ubiquitous self-help materials without introducing content-related confounds, we scripted the agent dialogue to match that from a self-help video as closely as possible.

© Springer International Publishing Switzerland 2015
W.-P. Brinkman et al. (Eds.): IVA 2015, LNAI 9238, pp. 279–282, 2015.
DOI: 10.1007/978-3-319-21996-7_29

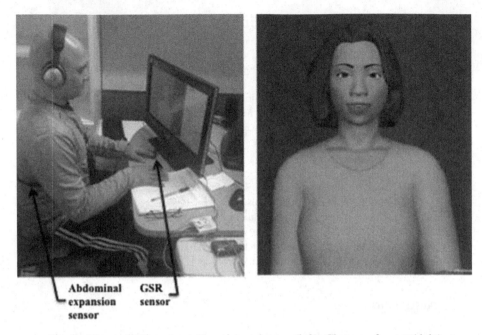

Fig. 1. The meditation agent. Experimental setup (left). Closeup of agent (right)

We used a publicly-available video that was approximately 10 min in length and featured a mid-shot of an instructor facing the camera throughout the entire session.

To make the virtual meditation coach interactive, we added a breathing sensor to the system. The Respiration Sensor from Thought Technology Ltd. is a flexible strap worn around the chest that measures abdominal expansion (Fig. 1, left). Data is processed through a Thought Technology ProComp2 Biofeedback device, and recorded and processed in the agent dialogue system. The dialogue system can respond to either absolute expansion level, or breathing rate. We used the former signal to allow users to signal that they are ready to continue during a meditation session by simply taking a deep breath. We felt that this was a more natural and less disruptive input modality than touch screen input or even speech while a user is meditating. We used breathing rate at certain key points during the meditation to ensure users are not breathing too rapidly, and asking them to slow down before continuing if they are.

3   Pilot Evaluation Study

We evaluated the virtual meditation coach in a randomized, counterbalanced, within-subjects experiment, in which we compared it to the self-help video of a human meditation instructor. In order to ensure that study participants were in similar, non-resting, emotional states prior to each meditation session, we induced mild frustration prior to the start of each session. This was accomplished by asking them to solve 10 challenging, timed math problems, in which they were forced to complete their answers very quickly with loud audio feedback regarding the correctness of their answers, with a pleasant tone for correct answers and a grating klaxon for incorrect ones. For the last 5 problems, participants were always given the klaxon regardless of their response.

Participants. Participants were recruited from an online job recruiting site, and were required to be 18 years of age or older, and to speak and read English. Participants were compensated for their time. We recruited 9 participants: 56 % male, aged 21 to 66 (mean 46.1). Most (66 %) had never tried mindfulness meditation.

Measures. We assessed their baseline mindful attention using the Mindful Attention Awareness Scale [1]. Following each meditation session we assessed State Anxiety [2], Positive and Negative Affect (PANAS [3]), Mindfulness (Toronto Mindfulness scale [4]), Flow state [5], and satisfaction with the instructor and experience (Table 1). Physiological arousal was measured using galvanic skin response (GSR) sensors from Thought Technology Ltd, worn on the non-dominant hand for each participant (Fig. 1, left). We computed the difference between the first 30 s (averaged) and final 30 s of each meditation session as our measure for change in arousal during meditation.

Table 1. Satisfaction questions (mean (SD)) Tests using non-parametric Wilcoxon signed ranks

Item	Anchor 1	Anchor 7	AGENT	HUMAN	p
How satisfied were you with the instructor?	Not at all	Very satisfied	6.11 (1.69)	6.56 (0.73)	.655
How aware was the instructor of your breathing?	Not at all	Very aware	5.22 (2.22)	3.89 (2.09)	.090
How would you characterize your relationship with the instructor?	Complete stranger	Close friend	2.88 (2.23)	2.67 (2.65)	1.00

Procedure. Participants were fitted with the respiration and GSR sensors and randomized to one of the two treatment conditions (AGENT vs. VIDEO). The participant then completed the frustration induction (math test), followed by a calibration procedure for the respiration sensor, followed by the selected meditation session. Participants then completed the post-test questionnaires. Participants were then assigned to the other treatment condition (AGENT or VIDEO) and repeated the frustration induction, calibration, meditation, and post-test measurements.

Results. As this is a small pilot study, we set our level of significance at 0.1. Results are summarized in Tables 1 and 2. Participants reported that the agent was significantly more aware of their breathing compared to the video-based instructor, although there were no significant differences in their overall satisfaction rating. Participants also reported significantly lower levels of anxiety following the session with the agent compared to the video-based human instructor, as well as scoring significantly higher on mindfulness. However, GSR readings indicated that the video led to greater reduction in physiological arousal compared to the agent. There were no significant differences on positive affect (PANAS) or flow, although the agent did score significantly higher on one subscale of flow – Transformation of Time, paired $t(8) = 2.0$, $p = .081$ – with no significant differences on the other subscales.

Table 2. Comparative outcomes for AGENT vs. VIDEO treatments (mean (SD)). Tests using paired-sample t-tests

Measurement	AGENT	VIDEO	p
State anxiety	2.92 (0.55)	3.19 (0.56)	.077
Positive affect	3.69 (0.95)	3.47 (0.83)	.449
Flow	3.60 (0.71)	3.53 (0.64)	.384
Mindfulness	2.72 (0.74)	2.55 (0.78)	.084
Physiological arousal (post-pre)	0.07 (0.28)	−0.14 (0.87)	.016

Conclusion and Future Work. We developed an interactive virtual meditation coach that is responsive to user breathing. Participants felt it was effective, liked the interactivity, and felt that breathing was an appropriate input modality for the system. The agent was significantly more effective than a videotaped meditation instructor at reducing anxiety and increasing mindfulness. We are currently extending the system to be more adaptive to users' needs, to be more tailored and interactive during the meditation process. We are investigating meaningful breathing patterns during meditation and dynamic adaptations that can be made to the meditation instruction. We are also planning a series of evaluation studies to test the efficacy of the resulting system.

References

1. Brown, K., Ryan, R.: The benefits of being present: mindfulness and its role in psychological well-being. J. Pers. Soc. Psychol. **84**, 822–848 (2003)
2. Marteau, T.M., Bekker, H.: The development of a six-item short-form of the state scale of the Spielberger State-Trait Anxiety Inventory (STAI). Br. J. Clin. Psychol. **31**, 301–306 (1992)
3. Watson, D., Clark, L., Tellegen, A.: Development and validation of brief measures of positive and negative affect: the PANAS scales. J. Pers. Soc. Psychol. **54**, 1063–1070 (1988)
4. Lau, M., et al.: The toronto mindfulness scale: development and validation. J. Clin. Psychol. **62**(12), 1445–1467 (2006)
5. Tenenbaum, G., Fogarty, G., Jackson, S.: The flow experience: a Rasch analysis of Jackson's flow state scale. J. Outcome Meas. **3**(3), 278–294 (1999)

LOITER-TB: Thought Bubbles that Give Feedback on Virtual Agents' Experiences

Jeroen Linssen[1](✉), Thomas de Groot[2], Mariët Theune[1], and Dirk Heylen[1]

[1] Human Media Interaction, University of Twente, PO Box 217,
7500 AE Enschede, The Netherlands
{j.m.linssen,m.theune,d.k.j.heylen}@utwente.nl

[2] T-Xchange, PO Box 217, 7500 AE Enschede, The Netherlands
t.f.degroot@txchange.nl

Abstract. We demonstrate LOITER-TB, a prototype of a serious game meant to improve the social awareness of police students. Central to its design is the provision of feedback through thought bubbles of virtual characters with which players interact. Our initial experiments provide weak support for our hypothesis that this form of feedback leads to gains in police students' understanding of social interaction.

Keywords: Serious games · Interpersonal interaction · Virtual agents · Meta-techniques · Flashback · Law enforcement

1 Improving Interpersonal Awareness

Social skills form an important part of everyday interactions, and recent work has investigated a broad variety of serious games to improve people's social skills [5]. In professions such as those of social workers and police officers, having good social awareness is critical to performing their tasks properly. In this demonstration, we show LOITER-TB (LOItering Teenagers, an Emergent Role-play – Thought Bubbles edition), a prototype of a serious game aimed at police students. In the game, players play the role of a patrolling police officer. They interact with a virtual loitering juvenile and his group of friends who need to be convinced by the player to go elsewhere. Depending on the approach the player takes in this interaction, the virtual juvenile will respond differently, for example by cooperating easily or by resisting the player's request. Previous work on serious games for social skills investigated several mechanics to improve learning, but not all of the developed systems provide adequate means for reflection [5]. A central feature of our game is the use of *meta-techniques*, aimed at making players learn more effectively. Meta-techniques are used in live action role play to provide information that is not available to the characters in the game world. In LOITER-TB, we show players the thoughts of virtual characters and let them reflect on this information. This way, we provide feedback about

W.-P. Brinkman et al. (Eds.): IVA 2015, LNAI 9238, pp. 283–286, 2015.
DOI: 10.1007/978-3-319-21996-7_30

the social interaction in the game by showing the experience from the juvenile's point of view [3]. Furthermore, our game incorporates research on cognitive models and nonverbal behaviour for virtual agents [1,6] to shape the scenarios and interactions.

2 LOITER-TB

One of our assumptions in creating LOITER-TB was that a completely realistic simulation of a social interaction does not necessarily lead to effective learning [2]. We decided to provide players with a game that focuses on the higher-level thought processes of virtual characters that govern their actions, instead of placing emphasis on nuances in verbal and non-verbal behaviour. The actions of virtual characters in LOITER-TB are largely based on their attitude towards the player, which may change over time due to the player's actions. To determine the attitude of the characters, we use Leary's theory of interpersonal *stances* [1]. According to this model (also called *Leary's Rose*), people assume stances in interpersonal interactions that can be classified as combinations of varying degrees of dominance and affect. For example, when a person acts submissively and shows positive affect toward someone else, this is classified as an accommodating stance. According to [1], certain behaviour 'invites' reactions of people: they tend to show an opposite degree of dominance while showing a similar degree of affection.

The game of LOITER-TB features a scenario in which players have to convince loitering juveniles to cooperate with them. During one play session, players interact three times in different situations with the same group of juveniles at different times in the game world. Players choose their actions in a multiple-choice fashion based on four stances in Leary's Rose. Figure 1 shows the interface of LOITER-TB at the moment which a player can decide how to respond to a juvenile. The juvenile currently has an 'aloof' attitude, expressing disinterest in both a verbal and

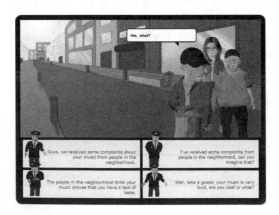

Fig. 1. The interface of LOITER-TB when the player can decide on what to do (translated from Dutch).

non-verbal way. The player can choose among four utterances, each representing a different stance, accompanied by corresponding non-verbal postures.

3   Feedback Through Thought Bubbles

In real-life interactions, we cannot always infer the motives behind other people's actions. To let players become aware of how their actions influence others, we use meta-techniques to augment the interactions in LOITER-TB. We show the virtual juvenile's point of view by means of thought bubbles, similar to those found in comics (see [3] for more examples of possible uses of meta-techniques). Currently, we have implemented two varieties of thought bubbles, one showing brief, immediate feedback on the player's actions, and the other providing a flashback to an earlier interaction. The first variety is shown at several points during the scenario while the player is interacting with the virtual juveniles. When the player has performed an action, a thought bubble shows how the juvenile sees the player's current stance in a depiction of Leary's Rose, see Fig. 2a. When the player indicates that he or she has seen this thought bubble, it disappears and the juvenile's actual verbal and non-verbal reaction is shown. This way, players have the opportunity to see how their actions come across to the virtual character, allowing them to reflect on the effects of their behaviour during the game.

To provide feedback on the entire interaction, a flashback from the perspective of the juvenile is shown at the start of the second and third interactions, before players choose their first action. This flashback is also shown in a thought bubble and shows information about the juvenile's impression of the player, see Fig. 2b. This impression is based on an average of the player's behaviour in terms of stances, for example, on average, the player may have acted in an 'attacking' manner. Based on this average, the juvenile adapts a 'preferred' stance for the following interaction, namely the stance which is invited by the player's average stance. The juvenile will use both this preferred stance and the stance that is invited by a player's action to determine his next action. The thought bubble with the flashback shows three items: a sentence which indicates what the

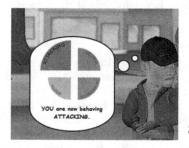 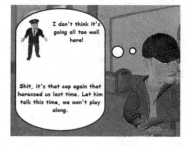

Fig. 2. (a) A thought bubble that indicates how the juvenile interpreted the player's action. (b) A thought bubble that shows a flashback of the juvenile to the previous situation, indicating how the juvenile remembers the player's behaviour.

player's average stance was; a flashback to an action of the player which illustrates to that stance; and a sentence which conveys the juvenile's preferred stance during the coming situation. With help of this feedback, players may become more aware of how their behaviour influenced the juvenile's stance and also of the way the juveniles will probably respond to them from then on. Thus, this feedback is both retrospective and prospective: it informs the player about what has happened and what he or she might expect during the following interaction.

4   First Results and Future Work

We evaluated the feedback in two iterations of LOITER-TB with several classes of police trainees of the Dutch Police Academy [4]. An experiment with the current prototype did not provide evidence for any learning gains in police trainees. Although they commented that the game was realistic enough in terms of setting, participants found it relatively obvious how to complete the game with a peaceful ending. Police instructors were positive about the game, noting that it could be useful in this form, but mainly for less experienced police trainees.

For upcoming iterations of the LOITER-TB prototype, we envision implementing ways to adapt the feedback to players of the game, based on their prowess in social interaction and their preferred form of feedback. Additionally, we would like to investigate the use of scenarios in which the virtual characters adapt their behaviour to players' progress and skill in the game. We plan to conduct experiments with police trainees who are at the beginning of their studies, in order to investigate whether learning gains would be higher with this user group.

Acknowledgements. This publication was supported by the Dutch national program COMMIT.

References

1. Leary, T.: Interpersonal Diagnosis of Personality: functional Theory and Methodology for Personality Evaluation. Ronald Press, New York (1957)
2. Linssen, J.M., de Groot, T.F., Theune, M., Bruijnes, M.: Beyond simulations: serious games for training interpersonal skills in law enforcement. In: Proceedings of ESSA 2014, pp. 604–607 (2014)
3. Linssen, J.M., Theune, M.: Meta-techniques for a social awareness learning game. In: Proceedings of ECGBL 2014, pp. 697–704 (2014)
4. Linssen, J.M., Theune, M., de Groot, T.F., Heylen, D.K.J.: Improving social awareness through thought bubbles and flashbacks of virtual characters. In: Brinkman, W.-P., et al. (Eds.): IVA 2015, LNAI, vol. 9238, pp. X–Y (2015)
5. Pereira, G., Brisson, A., Prada, R., Paiva, A., Bellotti, F., Kravcik, M., Klamma, R.: Serious games for personal and social learning and ethics: Status and trends. Procedia Comput. Sci. **15**, 53–65 (2012)
6. Ravenet, B., Ochs, M., Pelachaud, C.: From a user-created corpus of virtual agent's non-verbal behavior to a computational model of interpersonal attitudes. In: Aylett, R., Krenn, B., Pelachaud, C., Shimodaira, H. (eds.) IVA 2013. LNCS, vol. 8108, pp. 263–274. Springer, Heidelberg (2013)

Design and Implementation of Home-Based Virtual Reality Exposure Therapy System with a Virtual eCoach

Dwi Hartanto[1](✉), Willem-Paul Brinkman[1], Isabel L. Kampmann[2],
Nexhmedin Morina[2], Paul G.M. Emmelkamp[3,5],
and Mark A. Neerincx[1,4]

[1] Delft University of Technology, Delft, The Netherlands
d.hartanto@tudelft.nl
[2] University of Amsterdam, Amsterdam, The Netherlands
[3] King Abdulaziz University, Jeddah, Saudi Arabia
[4] TNO Human Factors, The Hague, The Netherlands
[5] Netherlands Institute for Advanced Study, Wassenaar, The Netherlands

Abstract. Current developments of virtual reality exposure therapy (VRET) system focus mainly on systems that can be used in health clinics under the direct supervision of a therapist. Offering patients however the possibility to do this treatment at home would make VRET more accessible. In this paper we therefore present a home-based VRET system for the treatment of social anxiety disorder. The system includes 19 exposure scenarios as well as a virtual health agent that guides the patients to various steps of therapy and explains how the system can be used. The presented design and techniques may form the bases for future home-based VRET systems.

Keywords: Virtual reality exposure therapy · Virtual health agent · Behaviour change support system · Social anxiety disorder · Self-therapy · At-home treatment

1 Introduction

Among mental disorders, social phobia is one of the most often occurring disorders. An effective treatment for this disorder is exposure therapy. Here patients are gradually exposed to social situations they fear until habituation occurs and anxiety diminishes. Despite its effectiveness, this treatment method has several limitations. For example, specific social scenarios are often difficult to arrange and to control. In recent years research has therefore focused on virtual reality exposure therapy as a potential way to overcome these limitations. Although promising, solutions explored mainly accommodated in clinic use. With an ever-growing need for more accessible and efficient therapy strategies, using a VRET system in a home-based setting would however allow patients to practice with social scenarios in the safety and comfort of their own home. A home-based VRET system could potentially be deployed in several ways, for example, as a part of a remote supervised home therapy, or additional homework

© Springer International Publishing Switzerland 2015
W.-P. Brinkman et al. (Eds.): IVA 2015, LNAI 9238, pp. 287–291, 2015.
DOI: 10.1007/978-3-319-21996-7_31

system besides regular face-to-face therapy with a therapist in a clinic, or in combination. In this paper we present the Memphis system, a home-based VRET system that incorporates a virtual health agent that guides patients through various steps of the therapy.

2   System Design

2.1   System Architecture

The Memphis system consists of three main blocks (Fig. 1): (1) the virtual health agent application, (2) the Virtual Reality (VR) system, and (3) the therapist application. While patients take home the treatment package that consist of a laptop, a Head Mounted Display (HMD), heart rate sensor, microphone, internet dongle and system manual operation handbook, therapists can sets the treatment plan and monitor progress remotely by using the therapist application. Data exchanged between therapist and patient is saved on a secure remotely server. Once patients start up the client application at home, the treatment plan is downloaded from the server automatically, which allows the virtual agent to guide patients thought day's session as set by the therapist.

2.2   The Virtual Health Agent

The virtual health agent, developed as a companion during the treatment, supports patient in several ways. It guides patients on how to utilize the machinery based on step-by-step guidance (Fig. 2) and motivates them during the treatment. It provides patients with an interactive psycho-education session regarding social anxiety disorder and principles behind the therapy. The agent also provides patients with an interpretation of the monitoring data collected during the virtual reality exposure sessions (Fig. 2) as well as information about overall treatment progress across the sessions.

2.3   The Virtual Reality System

Virtual Social Scenario. To provide patients with a diverge set of anxiety provoking situations in the exposure sessions, the system offers 19 social scenarios in virtual

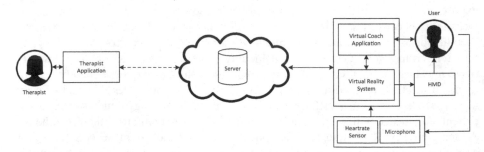

Fig. 1. Block diagram of Memphis system

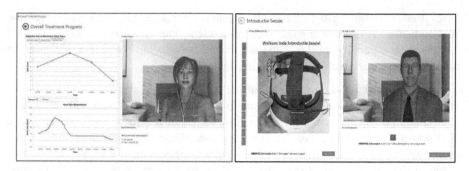

Fig. 2. On the left the female virtual health agent reflecting on monitoring data, and on the right the male virtual health agent giving a step-by-step HMD tutorial

reality. They include situations such as meeting an old friend, buying t-shirt in a shop, meeting a stranger at a party, and giving a presentation for an audience, etc. (Fig. 3). All these social scenarios were selected and developed based on *in vivo* exposure in the cognitive behavioral therapy [1].

The Phobic Stressors. In the VR scenarios, the Memphis system employs speech recognition and speech detection technology to provide patients with a free-speech dialogue interaction with virtual characters. To support flexibility and engage patients in long dialogues, each virtual social scenario has dialogues that can last around 18 min. To elicit different level of anxiety, the VR system controls several phobic stressors. For example, the questions and responses given by virtual characters could either be positive or negative as this can induce different level of anxiety [2]. Another

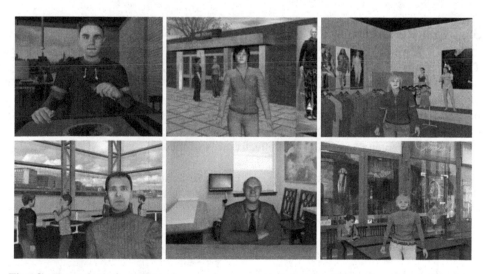

Fig. 3. Examples of six virtual scenarios supported by the Memphis system. Start top left-clockwise: dinner with a friend, interview at the train station, buying a t-shirt in a shop, being ask to participate in a survey, visiting a doctor, and meeting a stranger in a party

phobic stressor is the virtual characters' gestures, for example the behavior of the virtual audience [3] or the eye gaze of the characters. The virtual characters can be set to always stare at patients, or they can look toward patients only once in a while during a dialogue to simulate realistic turn talking behavior.

The Anxiety Feedback-Loop. To avoid the need for direct therapist intervention to control the anxiety evoked, the system employs an automatic feedback-loop algorithm that monitors patients' anxiety level to adjust the number phobic stressors used in a virtual scenario in real-time fashion. To determine the patient's level of anxiety, the system collects both subjective and physiological measurement data in the form of Subjective Unit of Discomfort (SUD) scale using speech recognition [4] and patients' heart rate. This data is combined in a linear regression model to create a personalized anxiety measure. When specifying the treatment plan, therapists can set the target and maximal anxiety levels for each exposure scenario. The system used this information to evoke the desired level of anxiety during an exposure session.

2.4   The Therapist Application

The therapist application is an application designed for the therapist to interacts with their registered patients, such as create personalized treatment plan, analyzing patient data, exchanging messages, and monitoring the treatment progress. To ensure security thereby considering ISO standards on the medical informatics security, such as ISO27001, ISO9001, ISO14001, but also the national guideline (NEN7510), all data stored on the server and data exchange between server and the therapist and patient application is encrypted. Prior to treatment both therapist and patients received personalized encryption and decryption keys, which they had to plug into their computer.

3   Final Remarks

The Memphis system is developed for home-based use, offering patients both the possibility to exposure themselves to social situations they fear, and a virtual agent that guide them through the therapy. For the therapists it offers the ability to set a treatment plan and monitor patient progress remotely. Although home-based VRET systems, like the Memphis system presented here, can offer these facilities, further research is needed to examine acceptance, usability and effectiveness of these systems.

Acknowledgments. This research is supported by the Netherlands Organization for Scientific Research (NWO), grant number 655.010.207. The funders had no role in study design, data collection and analysis, decision to publish, or preparation of the manuscript.

References

1. Hofmann, S.G., Otto, M.W.: Cognitive Behavioral Therapy for Social Anxiety Disorder: Evidence-Based and Disorder Specific Treatment Techniques. Routledge, New York (2008)
2. Hartanto, D., Kampmann, I.L., Morina, N., Emmelkamp, P.M.G., Neerincx, M.A., Brinkman, W.-P.: Controlling social stress in virtual reality environments. PLoS ONE **9**(3), e92804 (2014). doi:10.1371/journal.pone.0092804
3. Kang, N., Brinkman, W.-P., Riemsdijk, B.M., Neerincx, M.A.: An expressive virtual audience with flexible behavioral styles. IEEE Trans. Affect. Comput. **4**(4), 326–340 (2013)
4. Hartanto, D., Kang, N., Brinkman, W.-P., Kampmann, I.L., Morina, N., Emmelkamp, P.M.G., et al.: Automatic mechanisms for measuring subjective unit of discomfort. Annu. Rev. Cybertherapy Telemedicine **181**, 192–197 (2012)

Tools and Frameworks

Automated Generation of Plausible Agent Object Interactions

Tim Balint and Jan M. Allbeck[✉]

Laboratory for Games and Intelligent Agents, George Mason University,
4400 University Drive, MSN 4A5, Fairfax, VA 22030, USA
{jbalint2,jallbeck}@gmu.edu
http://cs.gmu.edu/~gaia

Abstract. To interact in a virtual environment, an agent must be aware of its available actions and the objects that can participate in these actions. Work such as Kallmann's SmartObjects allows for this information to be encoded by a simulation author, but these encodings tend to be constrained to individual graphical models. Furthermore, there may not be agreement on the proper operational information between simulation authors. To create consistent object operational information, we have devised a method that uses natural language lexical databases to parse and assemble this information. The method uses a two step process: 1. The names of motion clips are disambiguated using their name and a list of keywords; 2. Objects are connected to the actions by resolving the operational elements of a given verb. This method is tested on several common, publicly available action sets and the accuracy and coverage of our method are measured.

Keywords: Behavior planning and realization · Authoring/Reuse/ Tools · Applications for film, animation, art and game

1 Introduction

Virtual humans play a vital role in games, movies, and training simulations. Some virtual humans can reason about their environment provided information critical to that reasoning is inherent in the objects of the scenario. One important type of semantic information for objects is operational information, which instructs virtual agents on the way in which an object is used in an action. However, for a large scale virtual environment containing several hundred objects, attaching semantic operational information to each object is a tedious and time consuming process (See Fig. 1). Creating ontologies of objects allows similar objects to be grouped together into a forest of Directed Acyclic Graphs. Operational information can then exist at different levels of an ontology and propagate down to children, alleviating much of the burden a simulation author would face in creating a virtual environment [5].

One technique to encode semantic information into a virtual environment is to use SmartObjects [9]. This still requires a simulation author to encode all

© Springer International Publishing Switzerland 2015
W.-P. Brinkman et al. (Eds.): IVA 2015, LNAI 9238, pp. 295–309, 2015.
DOI: 10.1007/978-3-319-21996-7_32

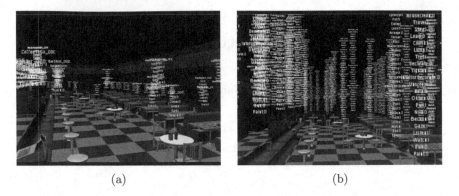

Fig. 1. Object operational data obtained (a) by previous manual methods for making object-action associations and (b) through the automated method presented in this paper.

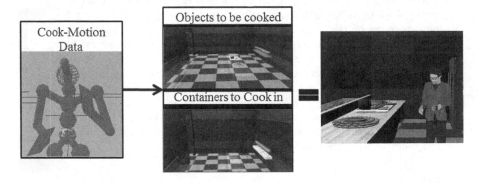

Fig. 2. A diagram showing how operational information is used by an agent.

the connections, which for a large scale simulation with several different actions can also become tedious. Correct information can be automatically generated through the use of Affordance Theory [6] if the information is purely visual. For functionality that is non-visual, other techniques must be developed. Managed online resources, such as WordNet [20] and FrameNet [1] contain academically generated action understandings and have been designed to interconnect. FrameNet in particular encodes different semantic roles in sentence structures. Its use would allow a system to distinguish the purpose of an object's participation in an action and the object's specific role, as seen by the different objects that can participate in an *Cook* action in Fig. 2. As these are general use natural language dictionaries, the data contained in them needs refinement to be appropriate for use with virtual humans. The generality of lexical databases also makes it challenging to determine the proper meaning of an action, which is required to use the lexical databases.

In spite of these limitations, the scale and accessibility of natural language lexical databases make them a useful tool in the design and creation of object operational information. To ease the work of a simulation author, we present an automated method for obtaining object operational information for use by virtual agents in large scale virtual environments. Specifically, the contributions of this work are:

- Automated generation of a hierarchy of actions from the names and short descriptions of motion clips.
- Automatic connection of the generated action hierarchy to an object ontology in a consistent and expandable manner.

These contributions are used to supply objects in a virtual environment with semantic information about their use given the motion clips available in the scenario.

2   Related Work

Cognitively, object operational information is dominated by Gibson's affordance theory [6]. This theory explains that physical humans can determine how an object is to be used by its physical properties. Affordance theory has been used by several virtual agent systems [3,14,17], and is a powerful technique in an agent decision making process. However, following the exact definition of affordances only allows an agent to know the usefulness of an object by its visual properties. Other properties, such as chemical and physical properties, are left out. A well used example of this is that it cannot be known just by examining an object whether or not can be safely consumed. Therefore, instead of using affordance theory for object operational information, we use natural language lexical databases to linguistically connect virtual objects to actions through the use of their names. This is analogous to a general domain knowledge approach for virtual agents.

While affordance theory has made strides in connecting virtual agent actions to semantic objects, other methods have tried to circumvent the visual constraint and ease the amount of necessary affordance information, even when using the term affordances. Pelkey and Allbeck [15] used natural language lexical databases to determine properties of an object, and Lugrin and Cavazza [12] uses semantic information to create non-kinematic visual effects in a game environment. Peters et al. [16] created a follow on technique to SmartObjects that specifically encoded operational information in the form of slots. This allows virtual objects to be used in several simulations actions, and were specifically designed for gaze behavior. To create operational information, these methods require explicitly written out connection between objects and actions, which our method does in an automated fashion. Instead of trying to generate affordances, Heckel and Youngblood [8] constrained the list of possible affordances based on situational awareness, but still requires affordances to be in the system.

There has been much work in showing the importance of object operational information, especially for use by virtual actors in a semantic environment. Much of this work is focused on ways to reason over the attachments as long as the attachments are already there, with some showing the usefulness of reusable operational information in simulations. Our work takes steps to fill in this knowledge gap by semi-automatically creating attachments from linguistic information about the objects and actions available in a scene.

3   Natural Language Lexical Databases

Converting action names into object operational information requires understanding the *sense* of a given action, that is, the proper context a given action would exist in. This can manifest itself through either its related words or meaning, as seen in Table 1. As another example, the phrase *pick up* has at least two senses, *to lift an object* or to *understand an idea*. The type of objects that can participate is vastly different depending on which sense the user desires, and different animations for a virtual human would accompany each sense. To disambiguate polysemous words, physical humans will examine a word's context, and determine which definition best fits the context. This is known as word sense disambiguation. A good survey of the topic can be found in [13]. Most word sense disambiguation techniques focus on a given context, such as the sentence in which the word is found. Unfortunately, even well named motion clips and processes do not readily appear in full sentences with enough context to determine their sense.

Table 1. An example of the polysemous word *Cook* taken from WordNet. Only the verb senses are shown.

Term	Synonyms	Definition
Cook	n/a	Prepare a hot meal
Cook	Fix, ready, make, prepare	Prepare for eating by applying heat
Cook	n/a	Transform and make suitable for consumption by heating
Cook	Fudge, manipulate, fake, falsify, wangle, misrepresent	Tamper, with the purpose of deception

For both word sense disambiguation and object operational connections, the choice of knowledge bases impacts our system's ability to attach operational information to objects. For our system, we use two knowledge bases that capture the linguistic understanding of object operational information, WordNet [20][1] and FrameNet [1][2]. FrameNet contains operational information in the form of

---

[1] Also found online at http://wordnet.princeton.edu.
[2] Also found online at https://framenet.icsi.berkeley.edu.

Frame Elements (FE), which are the participants of a frame of a verb. For example, a *sleep* verb contains the FEs *Sleeper* and *Place*. Shi and Mihalcea have connected FrameNet frames to WordNet senses [18]. We use WordNet to determine our initial sense due to its larger collection of verbs and the more prevalent parent-child relationships. The tree structure of WordNet allows verbs to be understood more generally, which we exploit in our process.

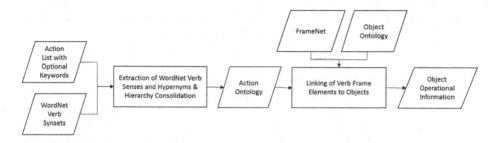

Fig. 3. System overview

Figure 3 illustrates how these lexical databases fit into our overall system. The list of actions available to be performed in the scenario are disambiguated, mapped to WordNet verb synsets, and formed into an action ontology. The FEs of the verbs are linked to WordNet object synsets and ultimately to object models in the virtual world. This linkage defines how objects can be used (i.e. *operated*) in the actions. The following sections will provide more details about these system processes.

4   Action Ontology Creation

4.1   Determining the Sense of an Action

To determine object operational information, our method first reasons about the actions that a simulation author has created. These actions can come from a variety of sources such as low level atomic animations or procedural controllers (e.g. picking up an object). The sense candidates chosen from WordNet are directly related to the name a simulation author provides for the action. Therefore, the level of detail and ability of an author to describe an action has a large impact on the system's ability to derive its sense, with more general methods being used to disambiguate fuzzy situations as is done cognitively by physical humans [2]. To enable this ability in our system and provide more information to an agent reasoning about actions, we maintain much of the synset hierarchy as an action ontology. The hierarchical nature of verbs also lends itself naturally to a hierarchical approach, as seen in Fig. 4. Our hierarchical method examines word senses using information on the word itself, its children, definition, and the relationship to other found senses.

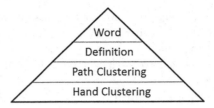

Fig. 4. The multi-pass technique's testing conditions. Each level determines word senses with the most precise methods higher up in the pyramid. Techniques lower in the pyramid are less precise but have greater coverage.

Unlike previous word sense disambiguation methods, our method examines a word w given a small constrained set of user provided keywords $k = \{k_1, \ldots, k_n\}$ and determines the proper sense of w from the set of candidate senses $s = \{s_1, \ldots, s_m\}$. w can be any word or word phrase, such as *pick up* or *duck and shoot*. For the verb *cook*, a user might provide the keywords *food* and *heat*. As our domain specifically focuses on actions for virtual agents, we assume that w contains at least one verb that can be performed by a virtual actor. This is an important assumption as it greatly prunes the search space of candidate senses for a given verb. It is also a reasonable assumption for our target applications. The keywords should contain some context to the given sense of w, however, due to the descriptions found in animations, this may not always be the case. The name of the motion itself may only give a partial clue to its nature. We process w to determine s by first searching for s using w. If no results are found, we determine if w is a phrase, and search for s from each verb in the phrase. If no results are found at this stage, s is considered unresolvable.

Once our system has determined the set of candidate senses s, we search for the most likely candidate sense, s_{found}, by testing s against each method seen in Fig. 4 and described in more detail in the following paragraphs, using Eq. 1. α is used to reject s_{found} for low matching senses, and allows other methods to be tested in an attempt to find a better match, while not undermining high probability matches. Through testing we have found that $\alpha = 0.3$ provides a strong threshold while not being too discriminating.

$$s_{found} = argmax(method(s)) > \alpha \qquad (1)$$

Word Disambiguation: The first methods used in our system attempts to disambiguate using only the sense set s and a set of k, similar to the disambiguation of agent commands done in [4]. As was done in [4], we use the lemmas of a sense, which are closely related to synonyms, as well as the parent verbs in WordNet's hierarchy, and determine the number of k that matches each candidate in s on these metrics. We have also added a third technique, which compares the lemmas of the sense's child verbs in WordNet's hierarchy to k by performing a Breadth First Search on the subtree of the sense. In order to get a percentage score to compare to α, we divide the total matches by $|k|$. For our example of *cook* with keywords *food* and *heat*, this method results in a score of zero. Neither keyword is found in the set of synonyms for *cook*.

Definition Disambiguation: If the above technique cannot disambiguate the sense of the word from its given components, we then examine the definition of each sense. The definition of a sense is a more relaxed search, and provides context to each sense in s. Testing the definition of a sense against k is a relaxed string matching approach. If a keyword matches any of the words in the definition, then it is considered a match, and is scored similarly to the word disambiguation technique. We also determine a percentage score for these techniques by dividing the total matching found by $|k|$. Here our *cook* example yields a score of 0.5, because the keyword *heat* is found in one of the sense definitions, but *food* is not. As we have found a sense whose score is higher than our α of 0.3, this sense is chosen.

Path Disambiguation: The final automated technique used to determine the sense of w is to compare s to the already disambiguated verb senses. This technique follows [11], which has been previously used to connect WordNet senses and FrameNet frames. Provided the system has determined one correct sense, this technique uses the Wu-Palmer Similarity [21] of s to determine the percent similarity to the already found senses of actions. This method is an iterative approach, and so will attempt to connect senses until no new senses are found.

Hand Clustering: When there is not enough information to disambiguate s or if none of the techniques are able to resolve the sense of a verb, then manual disambiguation is necessary. Our system provides tools for a user to choose the correct sense given a definition and list of synonyms of each sense in s. If the user cannot find a given sense at this stage, then the action name is considered unresolvable and connected to a created action sense called *Human Action*, which does not have any object operational information.

4.2 Tree Generation

After the initial examination and disambiguation of verbs, we build an IsA action hierarchy, modeled from WordNet's verb hierarchy. This allows a virtual agent to reason about an action using a broader definition (e.g. being able to understand that a *pirouette* is a *turn* or that *baking* is a form of *cooking* which is in turn a *creation action*). To construct an action forest, we first generate the full parent list of each disambiguated verb (See Fig. 5(b)). We then perform a node comparison, using Wu-Palmer path similarity [21] to the leaves of all previously generated trees to find candidate subtrees that the sense may belong to (See Fig. 5(a)). We then examine all nodes in the list and candidate sub-trees, searching for a direct string match for a given verb sense. When one is found, that node and all child nodes are directly connected to the sub-tree. This allows a large amount of information to be reasoned over, increasing the total coverage of the system.

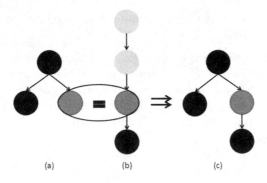

Fig. 5. A node in an action hierarchy being added (b) matches a node in an existing subtree (a). The hierarchies are merged at the common node and the ancestors of (b)'s matching node are removed (c).

Once the actions' word senses have been determined and the action ontology created, the actions can be linked to object participants, thus providing agents with information about how the objects can be used in virtual worlds.

5   Object Operational Information

Object operational information requires a connection between a given action and the objects that can be used in it. For several basic actions, this simply forms a triplet *(agent, action, object)*, where *agent* is the agent initiating the *action* on an *object*. However, actions can become very complex, requiring not only knowledge of *what* objects can participate, but *how* they can as well. For example, an agent mopping a floor requires not only a space in which to mop, but an instrument with which to perform the action. This creates a two-fold process, in which the correct sense of a frame must be disambiguated. Disambiguating the correct ordering of such an action combination is essential to streamlining an agent's decision making process [3].

After the sense of each action has been determined by the system, there is enough information to determine and link the set of actions to a set of physical objects found in a scenario. Figure 6 shows an overview of the connection step. Each Frame Element (FE) is matched against an ontology that contains graphical objects from one or more virtual environments and an understanding of their generalization. For the example of *cook*, one of the function elements is *container* (See Table 2). If the simulation contains a graphical representation of a *bowl*, then the ontology should reflect that a *bowl* is a type of *container*, which is ultimately a *physical object*. The connection between *cook* and *container* would then be reflected in the operational information, allowing the system to use a *bowl* for *cooking*. A similar connection is made between *food* and *cook*.

The generation of an object ontology is outside the scope of this work. A method for automated object ontology construction can be found in [15].

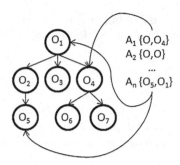

Fig. 6. A pictorial overview of the connection step. The object parameters of actions are linked to object types in the object ontology.

Table 2. Part of the frame elements for the verb *Cook*. Elements not picked up by the system are in italics.

Element	Object type connection
Cook	Semantic type linked to agent
Produced food	Food provides link to food object type
Container	Links to container object type
Degree	*Not a physical object*
Heating instrument	*While the sample environment includes a grill, the object hierarchy does not recognize it as a heating instrument.*
...	...

If a FE cannot be matched to the ontology, it is rejected. As we are only dealing with graphical semantic objects, we restrict the objects considered to a physical object ontology. This specifically removes two types of FEs: information that cannot be visualized by graphical models, such as *Purpose*, and ones that are simply not available to the simulation author, such as if they do not have a *heating instrument* for the *cook* action. While important to a full representation of an action, non-physical nouns that are described in an action (such as an action containing a *manner* object) are outside the scope of this paper.

We connect objects to found sense names using techniques identical to the string matching, partial string matching, and Breadth First Search methods used in the previous section and in [4] on FrameNet FEs. Some FEs contain a semantic type, which is a generalized explanation of that FE and can contain parent and children semantic types. Unlike word disambiguation, we want the FE to be as specific as possible, and therefore only search on the children of the semantic types.

Creating object operational information in this manner provides an upper bound on the types of objects that are connected to that action. Agents can then use this upper bound to help determine possible candidates by examining the object ontology and their environment. The utility of our method is therefore dependent on the ability to disambiguate the sense of an action's name and connect important components of the action to objects.

6   Analysis and Results

In order to test the ability of our method to determine the sense of an action from its name and keywords and provide object operational data to virtual environments, we have formulated and tested several hypotheses:

- **H1:** A consistent, extensible action ontology can be created using well named motion data and online lexical databases.
- **H2:** Using a mutli-pass method is a more accurate way of determining the sense of a verb obtained from an animation's name.
- **H3:** The resolution provided by FrameNet and a virtual object ontology covers the usable objects in a scenario.
- **H4:** An action ontology derived from WordNet provides more extensive and accurate coverage than using FrameNet alone.

To test **H1** and **H2** we used action names from CMU's motion capture library [7], a scan of the SmartBody documentation [19], and a higher level data set that represents common behaviors listed in tables provided by the Bureau of Labor Statistics (BLS) [10]. There is some overlap between senses from the SmartBody and CMU action sets. This creates a list of sixty actions, fifteen actions, and forty two actions respectively that a virtual human would be capable of. Naturally, behaviors in the BLS set do not inherently correspond to virtual human capabilities, but the set provides us with another source of potential behaviors. We create a ground truth for each data-set that contains the correct sense for each action by hand examining the senses in WordNet. For each dataset, we also create two list of keywords: a definition list from the Merriam Webster's dictionary definition (generally the longest words in the definition) and a list containing synonyms from Merriam Webster's dictionary[3]. We then create several tests from the set of keywords, choosing either the definition or synonym set for each action. These are used to compare our overall method to each of its components. The results can be seen in Fig. 7. As the path similarity metric requires one action sense to examine WordNet paths, we combine that method with both our word metrics and definition metrics.

As can be seen from Fig. 7a almost all of the multi-pass methods that included [11] were able to overwhelmingly find a sense to attach to an action's name. This means that, more often then not, using [11] will allow for some sense to be found and an action ontology to be generated for most of the actions without the need for an author to manually add them. Using our word disambiguation with path disambiguation for CMU's data set was an exception. This is because this method did not find enough senses using word disambiguation to connect senses using [11]. A lower α value would allow the process to find more

---

[3] The definition and synonym lists can be seen in the additional materials.

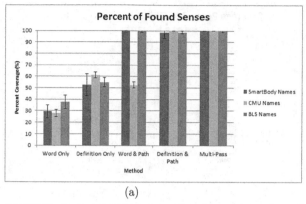

(a)

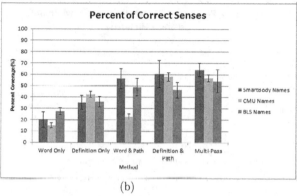

(b)

Fig. 7. The percent of found (a) and correct (b) senses for our ten sample test. Error bars represent one standard deviation. A single factor ANOVA analysis provided a negligible p-value for both figures, with a Tukey-Kramer test showing significant difference between our method and the word only, definition only, and word with path methods for CMU's data set, and word only and definition only for Smartbody's data set. A Tukey-Kramer test shows significant differences between all methods and the multi-path method for the BLS data set.

senses, but may reduce the overall accuracy of the system. As a result, the high percentage of found senses confirms **H1**. When examining Fig. 7b, there is an overall decrease in the system's ability to choose the correct sense. Therefore, while [11] allows for a hierarchy to be created, it may not be the correct one. However, compared to methods that did not use a path method, Fig. 7b shows that a multiple pass method is preferred when creating an action hierarchy from action names, confirming **H2**.

We performed an additional experiment to test hypothesis **H3**, by determining the percent coverage for both methods using a generated object hierarchy with over 100 leaf objects constructed based on the work of [15][4]. Ground truth

---

[4] The list of leaf objects can be seen in the additional materials.

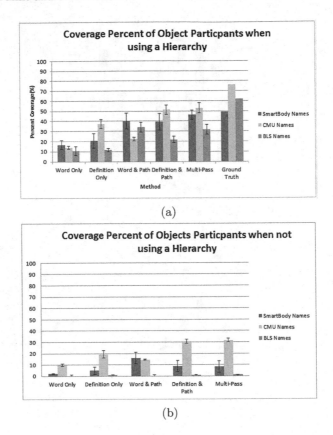

(a)

(b)

Fig. 8. The percent of matched object operational information compared to a ground truth assessment (a) when examining the whole action hierarchy and (b) using only the found senses of the actions. A two factor ANOVA between both graphs found a statistically significant difference with a p_value of 0.00194, and the difference between each data set to be statistically significant with a p_value of 0.007.

for object operational information is obtained by using the corresponding action hierarchy from the ground truths used in the analysis of **H1** and **H2**, and participant connections are chosen even if there is not a corresponding connection in the object tree. Our method then computes coverage for each of the found object trees, using our automated method. We also compute a maximum ground truth using the ground truth action hierarchy for each data set. At this stage, we also tested **H4** by using the found action senses with and without the object hierarchy. The results can be found in Fig. 8.

When using an action hierarchy to get a fuller definition of an action, it can be seen from Fig. 8a that the closer to ground truth the starting senses are, the closer the expected connections are to the maximum coverage using our method. As there is a statistically significant difference for each dataset using each method, we cannot confirm **H3** and the true ability of the coverage. We can infer from the operational connections in the ground truth seen in Fig. 8a that our method can resolve over half of the operational connections between our object and action ontologies. This already greatly reduces the effort needed by a simulation author and encourages further work in this area.

When no hierarchy is used, the ability to determine expected operational information decreases drastically, as seen by the low percentages in Fig. 8b. This should be expected as the likelihood for a WordNet sense to have a corresponding FrameNet frame using [18] will increase when a more general sense understanding can be exploited. This confirms **H4**.

6.1   Connections with Virtual Humans

Determining the operational information of objects and actions in a scene can provide knowledge as to the set-up of a command to a virtual human. However, it is important that the motion a virtual human is performing is compatible with the objects that have been assigned to the action. To demonstrate this, we use more general behaviors from our BLS data set with sub-actions being generated by motion clips from CMU's motion library. The motions are performed using a standard SmartBody skeleton [19] and the animations from the motion library.

We place our virtual human in a diner that contains several hundred objects normally found in such an environment. We then instruct our agent to *Cook*. The results can be seen in Fig. 2[5]. It should be noted from this that the agent examines its environment and chooses objects that are appropriate to participate in the *Cook* action. This is using only the found connections, and not the final ground truth operational information not found in the object ontology. The found objects are then passed to a *Walk* and *PickUp* action through a planning language, and must have connected operational information for each of those actions as well.

7   Conclusions, Limitations, and Future Work

In order to determine object participants for parametrizable actions, we developed a multi-pass word sense disambiguation technique and graph search methodology. These techniques require well defined motion data names and a hierarchy of possible object names for a given set of scenarios. Using multiple passes to determine senses ultimately leads to more object operational information. The resolved connections provide a first step to an automated approach of agent object interaction.

Our work depends on a simulation author correctly naming each of their motions, so that our system can reason about the names of our actions. The similarity between the correct output in Figs. 7b and 8a may show that a direct correlation exists between the system's ability to reason about actions and its ability to connect actions to plausible object participants. Methods that are

---

[5] The full example along with others can be found in the accompanying video.

less variable in our sense understanding stage may allow for better coverage of operational information. Future work will explore this connection. Examining the total connections the system could make to the ontology also show a need to use more information than only objects to increase the coverage. This can also be explored by looking at operational connection methods that are not sensitive to the name of the object in the ontology or its corresponding FE. One possibly promising approach is to use properties, for example *ingestible* to supplement these connections. Future work will also explore their use for this problem domain.

Our current system examines each individual action and does not consider objects that might be needed for parallel combinations of actions. However, it is common for actions to be combined together, such as the two actions *sit* and *eat*. Future work will examine determining participants for combinations of actions and will include determination of possible and impossible action combinations. A related task that is also considered future work will examine automated determination of prerequisites for actions.

Acknowledgments. This work was partially supported by a grant from the U.S. Army Night Vision and Electronic Sensor Directorate (W15P7T-06-D-E402) and software licenses from Autodesk. We would also like to acknowledge Shib Duman for the creation of 3D models used in our examples and John Mooney and Jessica Randall for their contributions in refining the presentation of this research.

References

1. Baker, C.F., Fillmore, C.J., Lowe, J.B.: The Berkeley FrameNet project. In: Proceedings of the 17th International Conference on Computational Linguistics - COLING 1998, vol. 1, pp. 86–90. Association for Computational Linguistics, Stroudsburg (1998). http://dx.doi.org/10.3115/980451.980860
2. Botvinick, M.M., Niv, Y., Barto, A.C.: Hierarchically organized behavior and its neural foundations: a reinforcement learning perspective. Cognition **113**(3), 262–280 (2008)
3. Donikian, S., Paris, S.: Towards embodied and situated virtual humans. In: Egges, A., Kamphuis, A., Overmars, M. (eds.) MIG 2008. LNCS, vol. 5277, pp. 51–62. Springer, Heidelberg (2008)
4. Fernández, C., Baiget, P., Roca, F.X., González, J.: Augmenting video surveillance footage with virtual agents for incremental event evaluation. Pattern Recogn. Lett. **32**(6), 878–889 (2011). http://dx.doi.org/10.1016/j.patrec.2010.09.027
5. Flotyski, J., Walczak, K.: Conceptual knowledge-based modeling of interactive 3d content. Vis. Comput., 1–20 (2014)
6. Gibson, J.: Perceiving, acting and knowing. In: The Theory of Affordances. Lawrence Erlbaum (1977)
7. Guerra-Filho, G., Biswas, A.: The human motion database: a cognitive and parametric sampling of human motion. Image Vis. Comput. **30**, 251–261 (2012)
8. Heckel, F.W.P., Youngblood, G.M.: Contextual affordances for intelligent virtual characters. In: Vilhjálmsson, H.H., Kopp, S., Marsella, S., Thórisson, K.R. (eds.) IVA 2011. LNCS, vol. 6895, pp. 202–208. Springer, Heidelberg (2011)

9. Kallmann, M., Thalmann, D.: Direct 3d interaction with smart objects. In: Proceedings of the ACM Symposium on Virtual Reality Software and Technology, VRST 1999, pp. 124–130. ACM, New York (1999). http://doi.acm.org/10.1145/323663.323683

10. US Bureau of Labor Statistics, B.: American time use survey. Technical report (2010). http://www.bls.gov/news.release/atus.nr0.htm

11. Laparra, E., Rigau, G.: Integrating wordnet and framenet using a knowledge-based word sense disambiguation algorithm. In: Proceedings of the International Conference RANLP-2009, pp. 208–213. Association for Computational Linguistics, Borovets, September 2009. http://www.aclweb.org/anthology/R09-1039

12. Lugrin, J.L., Cavazza, M.: Making sense of virtual environments: action representation, grounding and common sense. In: Proceedings of the 12th International Conference on Intelligent User Interfaces, IUI 2007, pp. 225–234. ACM, New York (2007). http://doi.acm.org/10.1145/1216295.1216336

13. Navigli, R.: Word sense disambiguation: a survey. ACM Comput. Surv. 41(2), 10:1–10:69 (2009)

14. van Oijen, J., Dignum, F.: Scalable perception for bdi-agents embodied in virtual environments. In: IEEE/WIC/ACM International Conference on Web Intelligence and Intelligent Agent Technology (WI-IAT), 2011, vol. 2, pp. 46–53, August 2011

15. Pelkey, C., Allbeck, J.M.: Populating virtual semantic environments. Comput. Anim. Virtual Worlds 24(3), 405–414 (2014)

16. Peters, C., Dobbyn, S., MacNamee, B., O'Sullivan, C.: Smart objects for attentive agents. In: Proceedings of 11th International Conference in Central Europe on Computer Graphics (2003)

17. Sequeira, P., Vala, M., Paiva, A.: What can i do with this?: Finding possible interactions between characters and objects. In: Proceedings of the 6th International Joint Conference on Autonomous Agents and Multiagent Systems, AAMAS 2007, pp. 5:1–5:7. ACM, New York (2007). http://doi.acm.org/10.1145/1329125.1329132

18. Shi, L., Mihalcea, R.F.: Putting pieces together: combining FrameNet, VerbNet and WordNet for robust semantic parsing. In: Gelbukh, A. (ed.) CICLing 2005. LNCS, vol. 3406, pp. 100–111. Springer, Heidelberg (2005)

19. Thiebaux, M., Marsella, S., Marshall, A.N., Kallmann, M.: Smartbody: behavior realization for embodied conversational agents. In: Proceedings of the 7th International Joint Conference on Autonomous Agents and Multiagent Systems, AAMAS 2008, vol. 1, pp. 151–158. International Foundation for Autonomous Agents and Multiagent Systems, Richland (2008). http://dl.acm.org/citation.cfm?id=1402383.1402409

20. Princeton University: About wordnet. Technical report, Princeton University (2010). http://wordnet.princeton.edu

21. Wu, Z., Palmer, M.: Verbs semantics and lexical selection. In: Proceedings of the 32nd Annual Meeting on Association for Computational Linguistics, ACL 1994, pp. 133–138. Association for Computational Linguistics, Stroudsburg (1994). http://dx.doi.org/10.3115/981732.981751

A Platform for Building Mobile Virtual Humans

Andrew W. Feng[1], Anton Leuski[1], Stacy Marsella[2] , Dan Casas[1],
Sin-Hwa Kang[1], and Ari Shapiro[1][✉]

[1] Institute for Creative Technologies, USC Institute for Creative Technologies,
Los Angeles, USA
{feng,leuski,kang,shapiro}@ict.usc.edu, dan.casas@gmail.com
[2] Northeastern University, Boston, USA
marsella@neu.edu

Abstract. We describe an authoring framework for developing virtual
humans on mobile applications. The framework abstracts many elements
needed for virtual human generation and interaction, such as the rapid
development of nonverbal behavior, lip syncing to speech, dialogue management, access to speech transcription services, and access to mobile
sensors such as the microphone, gyroscope and location components.

Keywords: System · Mobile · Virtual human · Chat

1 Motivation

Virtual Humans (VH) have been shown to be effective elements of training simulations, interactive entertainment and other virtual experiences. Non-embodied,
audio-based, or text-only agents have been well explored in the research community. A 3D embodied virtual human significantly expands the amount of information that can be communicated to a user over an audio-only or text-based
interaction. Virtual humans can potentially display non-verbal behavior similar
to humans in face-to-face interactions. However, developing a 3D virtual human
can be complicated due to the need to model both visual and behavioral elements
of human-to-virtual human interaction. For example, a conversational virtual
human might need to keep track of the dialogue turn, exhibit both speaking and
listening behavior, and be able to express emotions non-verbally.

Complex virtual humans are typically found in museums, specialized training
installations, and similar settings. In many cases, a virtual human resides in a
particular place, and is often only available under formal or brief encounters.
Thus encounters with virtual humans are limited in place, interaction and time.
In addition, constructing a virtual human is a complex, multi-disciplinary effort.
Thus research into pervasive aspects of virtual humans have been limited by the
few venues in which they can appear, and the complexity of their construction.
Studies of virtual humans and their impact on real humans are restricted to
expensive, location-specific, and domain-specific interactions.

Mobile platforms such as smartphones and tablets are a pervasive technology,
and are now capable of running the software and hardware components that
are necessary for a convincing, interactive Virtual Human. Potentially, a virtual

© Springer International Publishing Switzerland 2015
W.-P. Brinkman et al. (Eds.): IVA 2015, LNAI 9238, pp. 310–319, 2015.
DOI: 10.1007/978-3-319-21996-7_33

human running on a mobile platform changes three significant relationships with real humans: (1) a mobile virtual human can be accessible to a mobile user at any time, (2) a mobile virtual human can be accessible to a mobile user at any location, and (3) the group of real users who could potentially interact with a mobile virtual human is broadened to all people with a smartphone. Thus, rich, long-term interactions with a broad range of types of people would now be possible on mobile devices, through a broad set of domains.

While it is possible to create a virtual human application on a mobile device, the effort to do so is very large and requires experts from many disciplines. By providing a mechanism for non-experts to assemble various functionality related to virtual humans and mobile platforms, we extend the domain of virtual human applications to a larger audience than would ordinarily be possible. Rather than requiring several experts from artificial intelligence, graphics, and programming to assemble a single application, we anticipate that a mobile application author could construct a virtual human application without any external assistance. Thus researchers from the social and behavioral sciences will be able to access and manipulate virtual human technology on mobile devices.

In this paper, we further describe an authoring framework for developing virtual humans on mobile applications. The framework abstracts many elements needed for virtual human generation and interaction, such as the rapid development of nonverbal behavior, lip syncing to speech, dialogue management, access to speech transcription services, and access to mobile sensors such as the microphone, gyroscope and location components. We describe our experience in building virtual humans on mobile devices, and how we have attempted to abstract key features into a singular platform that allows the rapid production of similar mobile apps.

Our platform differs from desktop-based virtual human systems in that: (1) it leverages commonly used mobile capabilities, such as the location, gyroscope and microphone sensors, (2) it runs on mobile platforms, such as Android, and does not require a separate mobile application to be built, and (3) it utilizes an Application Programming Interface (API) that allows the author to generate a virtual human application through the use of run-time scripts (using Python [17]), that allows access to mobile capability as well as to virtual human capability.

2   Related Work

Many mobile applications have been developed that use 3D characters, and some mobile applications have been developed as embodied virtual humans. However, there have been very few mobile platforms specifically designed for virtual human research. A number of virtual human systems designed for desktop use include Greta [15], Elckerlyc [21], EMBR [6] and SmartBody [18] which all use the Behavioral Markup Language [8]. In addition, there are a number of other systems that use different behavioral specifications, such as BEAT [3] and Maxine [1]. A system that integrates many components for virtual human development can be found in [5]. Our framework differs in that we seek rapid authoring for a specific set of capability for mobile devices.

There are numerous studies that use mobile platforms. A description of virtual humans on personal digital assistants is found in [4]. A study of animated characters on a handheld device explored different modalities of agents, such as text, static image, or animated character [2]. More recently, [16] investigates the use of a 3D facial avatar for chat applications. Closest to our work, is the description of the Elckerlyc BML realizer for mobile systems [7], which allows the embodiement of a 2D character on an Android system using the behavioral capabilities of Elckerlyc. Our platform differs in that (1) it uses 3D, not 2D, characters, which allow for a greater potential for nonverbal communication, and (2) it is capable of rendering high-fidelity (photorealistic) virtual humans, (3) our platform provides a set of interfaces to the sensors and to dialogue management, and (4) finally, in contrast to custom systems like [11], we focus on unifying the overall tool set as a platform for building different virtual humans.

3   Experience Developing Mobile Virtual Humans

Our architecture is inspired from our past experience of developing virtual humans on mobile devices. We describe some of these experiences and demonstate how they inform our mobile virtual human architecture. Code examples for the following sections can be found at http://smartbody.ict.usc.edu/mobilevirtualhumans/.

Development Environments for Building Mobile Apps Can Require Numerous Tool Sets and Build Environments and Has a Slow Iteration Speed. A mobile platform development typically requires a set of tools that is specialized and sometime unfamiliar to the mobile application developer.

In addition, the iteration time for a typical mobile application is very slow. When iteratively developing a mobile application, the app either has to be copied to a mobile device, or it has to run inside of a simulator, which can be slow, particularly when 3D graphics are used.

In this platform, we simplify such a process by providing an executable app that is configured through the use of a set of runtime-interpreted scripts (in the Python scripting language). By building the executable (the "vanilla app"), we eliminate the need to build the mobile application separately. We abstract the elements needed to configure that application into a set of APIs. By allowing the application to be configured by scripts, an application author can iterate over the changes by simply running the application directly on the device.

Game Engines Have a Steep Learning Curve and Are Not Designed for Conversational Virtual Characters. Modern game engines contain excellent tools for authoring 3D content. However, the use of a 3D game engine requires a learning curve to understand its architecture and design, as well as its build processes. In addition, game engines typically employ very generic animation capabilities; they allow for the playback, blending and overlay of animations, but typically do not provide fine-grain control over subtle human emotion and expression, such as gazing and gesturing.

We base our framework on an existing animation system and BML [8] realizer that employs a large number of conversational capabilities that the virtual human community has identified through research, [18], including automated lip syncing to speech [22]. The learning curve for our platform is not based on knowledge of a game engine API, but rather on a set of APIs targeted to the use of virtual human development: a Virtual Human API (Sect. 4) which controls characters and their behaviors, an Interface and Sensor API (Sect. 4) which controls widgets and sensors, a Rendering API (Sect. 4) which controls the appearance of the app, a Dialogue Management API (Sect. 4) which controls the dialogue turn, and a Communication API (Sect. 4) which controls the communication between the device and other systems.

Character Configuration is Time Consuming and Complicated. Regardless of the capabilities of the underlying engine or platform, an effective virtual character needs to be configured properly to perform its functions related to communication and behavior. This requires a detailed face rig, a set of compatible gestures, and a means to lip sync to speech. Typical 3D characters that can be acquired through online marketplaces do not typically have complicated facial rigs, and there are very few standards for facial rigs, emotional expression or lip syncing.

In this platform, we provide a small set of characters of varying gender and age that are designed to be able to express varying emotions and nuance through a set of controls that allow arbitrary combinations of facial poses over time. In addition, our platform provides high-fidelity lip syncing automatically both from text-to-speech, as well as from recorded voice. Our platform also provides a set of male and female gestures that include a large set of deictic (pointing), metaphoric and beat gestures that are suitable for many conversational situations. Thus, the creation of a character that includes many conversational capabilities can be done with just a few lines of code.

Nonverbal Behavior Can Be Difficult to Generate. In developing virtual human applications, one of the key lessons that we have learned is that hand crafting nonverbal behavior is time consuming and requires considerable knowledge of the particulars of when nonverbal behavior is exhibited, as well as an strong aesthetic sense for the physical manner of that behavior. At the same time, social psychology as well as the virtual human community has extensively documented the powerful impact behaviors have on face-to-face interaction between humans as well as between humans and virtual humans. Leaving out these behaviors is not a viable option. Further, we have known going back to the pioneering work of film director Lev Kuleshov in the early 1900s on what is now studied as the Kuleshov effect that people will falsely infer attitudes and emotions in the absence of any behavioral signals. For these reasons, researchers and application developers have crafted a range of tools to help automate this process, including BEAT [3], NVBG [9] and Cerebella [13].

Over the process of using these tools in applications, developers have acquired considerable practical expertise. For example, we noticed early on that people tended to slightly nod their heads on initial noun phrases and verb phrases. Automating this behavior in virtual humans quite remarkably brings otherwise seemingly dead characters to life [9]. Later machine learning research [10] bore out this correlation in human data. Further, application developers often wanted very simple mechanisms that could specialize the performance of these tools on specific scenarios and characters, by, for example, triggering specific behaviors when the character spoke specific words or phrases. This functionality was not novel, all of the aforementioned tools had this capability. What developers wanted were simple mechanisms that did not require them to have expertise in a tool's internal workings. Based on both knowledge of the challenges of crafting nonverbal behavior, its importance as well as the practical expertise garnered over the years, we have chosen to incorporate a nonverbal behavior generator based on a few basic principles tailored to application developer use: parsing an utterance, breaking it down into syntactic and lexical elements that would allow an author to simply uses a text file that would provide a map between these elements and behaviors.

Voice-Based Interfaces are Familiar to Mobile Device Users. A speech-based interface is important for many mobile applications that require conversations with virtual humans. The Automatic Speech Recognition (ASR) module of a Virtual Human system, which converts the audio of the user's speech into machine readable text, has to process the audio in real time and be robust to different acoustic conditions, noise levels, and speaker accents. We leverage the Google Speech API to allow easy authoring of speech capture.

Easy Sensor Access is Needed to Leverage the Unique Nature of a Mobile Device. Mobile devices provide an array of sensors that can be used in virtual human systems, including orientation, position and microphone sensors. The use of such sensors represents one of the main differentiators between mobile and desktop applications. For example, a mobile device can have a location sensor, a gyroscopic sensor, an accelerometer sensor, and a camera sensor.

We simplify access to various sensors through the use of the Interface and Sensor API. While not part of our mobile platform, we anticipate that easy access to a camera-based sensors that reports facial expressions would also be useful. Such access would allow, for example, the acquisition of facial expressions from the mobile user in real time.

Language Processing. Natural Language Understanding (NLU) and Dialogue Management (DM) form the focal point where the different sensor inputs come together with the speech recognition output and the system decides how to respond to the user's actions.

There are many NLU approaches ranging from simple keyword spotting to detailed semantic parsing [20]. The main goal is the same – it is to ingest the text of the user's speech and produce some sort of machine readable representation that reflects the speech content. There is always a compromise when selecting an appropriate NLU strategy: a simple technique may not provide sufficient information for meaningful interaction, while a more complex approach requires extensive knowledge engineering and can be rather brittle in the presence of ASR mistakes. Another dimension where a virtual human system designer has to make a choice is whether to have the NLU system select one of several predefined utterance meanings or generate one on the fly. The former approach guarantees a predictable result coming from the NLU component, while limiting the number of things the character can understand to whatever is stored in the system.

In our system we use the statistical text classification approach [12]. This approach assumes that all possible system responses are known and stored in a database at the system construction stage. It relies on a set of linked sample utterances and response pairs to "translate" the incoming user's utterance into a query that it uses to search the database of responses. The algorithms returns a ranked subset (possibly empty) of the system responses. While this approach is limited by the number of things the virtual human can understand, it is fast, robust to the ASR errors, and it does not require extensive knowledge engineering beyond providing sample utterances that should trigger individual system responses. It can also combine both verbal and non-verbal features, e.g., sensor data, in one classification step. It has been shown to perform successfully in a variety of applications [12].

The second part of virtual human language processing is the Dialogue Management (DM) module that takes the result from the NLU, considers the current state of the interaction, and selects the system response. Here also a number of approaches exist that range from a set of simple rules to a sophisticated multi-level reasoning process that includes modeling of the character knowledge, goals, and emotions [19]. For our platform we use a rule-based decision approach, where the character designer specifies a number of rules triggered by the specific NLU outputs, sensor events, or system timers. The designer can use the scripting language to model and maintain the dialogue state, keep track of the interaction history, and combine the DM state with the system events into complex behavior strategies. A general purpose dialogue management script is included with the system sufficient for constructing question-answering characters [12]. We also provide a tool box of script-based functions for the character designer to extend and modify the dialogue strategy, instead of relying on a separate tool to configure the NLU and DM.

Communication Between Mobile Devices or Between a Mobile Device and a Server is a Common Part of Many Virtual Human Apps. Mobile applications frequently require communication that extends beyond the device itself, and potentially to other devices or servers. For example, a mobile application might communicate with a server to collect or retrieve data. Standard mobile platform communication mechanisms can be used over standard TCP/IP networks.

We include an asynchronous communication protocol called the Virtual Human Messaging System (VHMSG) that allows the easy communication between virtual human applications. Thus, only one line of script code is needed to connect, and one line of script code for each message is necessary. In this way, we allow numerous mobile devices to communicate with each other without requiring a separate protocol to be defined and managed.

4   Architecture

The Mobile Virtual Humans framework consists of a set of code, scripts, configuration files and processes to build and develop a mobile application on an Android operating system platform. The app author configures the mobile virtual human by writing scripts that access five Application Programming Interfaces (APIs); the Virtual Human API, the Interaction and Sensor API, the Rendering API, the Dialogue Management API, and the Communication API. The five APIs, in turn, communicate with the animation engine, rendering engine, mobile os platform, and sensors. The rendering component interacts with the animation engine, mobile OS and app code, as shown in Fig. 1.

Application authors can leverage the application, called the "vanilla app", by associating data and process. Thus, a mobile virtual human platform author does not need to compile a new application, only to modify the control scripts and data in order to have a functioning mobile virtual human app.

Virtual Human API. The Virtual Human API handles the setup and control of the virtual human characters. The API includes methods to create a virtual human, configure its behaviors, and respond to user input. The API leverages an animation system SmartBody [18] to construct and configure characters and the environment. Lip syncing to speech is automatically performed and matched to the character's facial rigs [22]. Complex configuration elements, such as configuring the facial rig, and behavioral control are abstracted via interface scripts, and thus the construction of characters can be done with a single line of code.

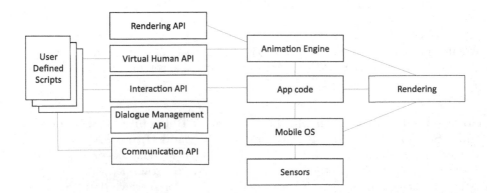

Fig. 1. Components of Mobile Virtual Human architecture. The authoring interface is primarily through a set of scripting interfaces that allow control of the Virtual Human API, the Interface API, the Rendering API, and the Dialogue Management API.

Interface and Sensor API. The Interface and Sensor API manages the user interaction with the mobile device, such as touch and widget interfaces, as well as access to the various mobile sensors, such as the gyroscope, microphone, location and camera. In addition, it allows access to device-specific information, such as the device id, IP address and name of the user interacting with the device.

Rendering API. The Rendering API manages the display elements such as cameras and lighting. The platform draws 3D content using OpenGL ES [14].

Dialogue Management API. The Dialogue Management API handles control of the speaking turn and the virtual human responses to user questions. The NPC Editor [12] is used to provide a question-and-answer interface.

Communication API. The Communication API allows easy access to all the capabilities in the system. The platform leverages the Virtual Human Messaging System (VHMSG) which transmits asynchronous messages across a TCP/IP network.

5   Applications

We demonstrate a number of applications that can be generated through our architecture and describe the key control elements needed in Fig. 2.

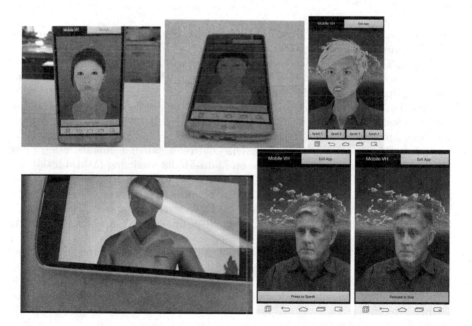

Fig. 2. (Top Left and Top Center) Using the accelerometer to determine the orientation of the mobile device. (Top Right) An example using text-to-speech and proper lip sync useful for dynamic conversations. (Bottom Left) Use of a virtual human in the medical domain. A virtual nurse queries the users for health issues. (Bottom Center and Bottom Right) A realtime render showing a photorealistic virtual human backchannelling in response to a user's speech.

6   Conclusion

In this work, we have presented a platform for the development of virtual human systems on mobile devices. Unlike many 3D frameworks and game engines, our framework is focused on the interaction between a virtual human and a user. Our framework also differs from desktop-based virtual human frameworks in that it allows convenient access to capabilities that are commonly found on mobile devices, such as the gyroscopic, microphone and location sensors. Modification of an application developed by our platform can be done in a data-driven way by modifying the scripts that control the virtual human, interface and rendering.

All software architecture designs differ in which aspects can be exposed to the platform author and which aspects will be hidden. Any 3D platform, such as a game engine, can be used to design virtual human systems. Our design choices make the development of a 3D conversational virtual human require very little configuration or expertise. For example, a virtual human can be displayed and made to speak with only a few lines of code, and without even going through the configuration process of building an app. By contrast, a game engine would be a superior platform for the development of large-scale 3D worlds that include various particle effects, such as water, dust and so forth.

References

1. Baldassarri, S., Cerezo, E., Seron, F.J.: Maxine: a platform for embodied animated agents. Comput. Graph. **32**(4), 430–437 (2008)
2. Bickmore, T., Mauer, D.: Modalities for building relationships with handheld computer agents. In: CHI 2006 Extended Abstracts on Human Factors in Computing Systems, pp. 544–549. ACM (2006)
3. Cassell, J., Vilhjálmsson, H.H., Bickmore, T.: Beat: the behavior expression animation toolkit. In: Prendinger, H., Ishizuka, M. (eds.) Life-Like Characters, pp. 163–185. Springer, Berlin (2004)
4. Gutierrez, M., Vexo, F., Thalmann, D.: Controlling virtual humans using pdas. In: The 9th International Conference on Multi-Media Modeling (MMM 2003), pp. 150–166. No. VRLAB-CONF-2007-028 (2003)
5. Hartholt, A., Traum, D., Marsella, S.C., Shapiro, A., Stratou, G., Leuski, A., Morency, L.-P., Gratch, J.: All together now. In: Aylett, R., Krenn, B., Pelachaud, C., Shimodaira, H. (eds.) IVA 2013. LNCS, vol. 8108, pp. 368–381. Springer, Heidelberg (2013)
6. Heloir, A., Kipp, M.: Real-time animation of interactive agents: specification and realization. Appl. Artif. Intel. **24**(6), 510–529 (2010)
7. Klaassen, R., Hendrix, J., Reidsma, D., et al.: Elckerlyc goes mobile enabling technology for ecas in mobile applications. In: The Sixth International Conference on Mobile Ubiquitous Computing, Systems, Services and Technologies, UBICOMM 2012, pp. 41–47 (2012)
8. Kopp, S., Krenn, B., Marsella, S.C., Marshall, A.N., Pelachaud, C., Pirker, H., Thórisson, K.R., Vilhjálmsson, H.H.: Towards a common framework for multimodal generation: the behavior markup language. In: Gratch, J., Young, M., Aylett, R.S., Ballin, D., Olivier, P. (eds.) IVA 2006. LNCS (LNAI), vol. 4133, pp. 205–217. Springer, Heidelberg (2006)

9. Lee, J., Marsella, S.C.: Nonverbal behavior generator for embodied conversational agents. In: Gratch, J., Young, M., Aylett, R.S., Ballin, D., Olivier, P. (eds.) IVA 2006. LNCS (LNAI), vol. 4133, pp. 243–255. Springer, Heidelberg (2006)

10. Lee, J., Marsella, S.C.: Predicting speaker head nods and the effects of affective information. IEEE Trans. Multimedia **12**(6), 552–562 (2010)

11. Leuski, A., Gowrisankar, R., Richmond, T., Shapiro, A., Xu, Y., Feng, A.: Mobile personal healthcare mediated by virtual humans. In: Proceedings of International Conference on Intelligent User Interfaces (2014)

12. Leuski, A., Traum, D.: NPCEditor: creating virtual human dialogue using information retrieval techniques. AI Mag. **32**(2), 42–56 (2011)

13. Marsella, S., Xu, Y., Lhommet, M., Feng, A., Scherer, S., Shapiro, A.: Virtual character performance from speech. In: Proceedings of the 12th ACM SIGGRAPH/Eurographics Symposium on Computer Animation, pp. 25–35. ACM (2013)

14. Munshi, A., Ginsburg, D., Shreiner, D.: OpenGL ES 2.0 programming guide. Pearson Education, Boston (2008)

15. Poggi, I., Pelachaud, C., de Rosis, F., Carofiglio, V., De Carolis, B.: Greta: a believable embodied conversational agent. In: Stock, O., Zancanaro, M. (eds.) Multimodal intelligent information presentation, pp. 3–25. Springer, The Netherlands (2005)

16. Rincón-Nigro, M., Deng, Z.: A text-driven conversational avatar interface for instant messaging on mobile devices. IEEE Trans. Hum. Mach. Syst. **43**(3), 328–332 (2013)

17. Sanner, M.F., et al.: Python: a programming language for software integration and development. J. Mol. Graph. Model. **17**(1), 57–61 (1999)

18. Shapiro, A.: Building a character animation system. In: Allbeck, J.M., Faloutsos, P. (eds.) MIG 2011. LNCS, vol. 7060, pp. 98–109. Springer, Heidelberg (2011)

19. Traum, D.R.: Talking to virtual humans: dialogue models and methodologies for embodied conversational agents. In: Wachsmuth, I., Knoblich, G. (eds.) ZiF Research Group International Workshop. LNCS (LNAI), vol. 4930, pp. 296–309. Springer, Heidelberg (2008)

20. Traum, D., Swartout, W., Gratch, J., Marsella, S., Kenney, P., Hovy, E., Narayanan, S., Fast, E., Martinovski, B., Bhagat, R., Robinson, S., Marshall, A., Wang, D., Gandhe, S., Leuski, A.: Dealing with doctors: virtual humans for non-team interaction training. In: Proceedings of the 6th Annual SIGDIAL Conference, Lisbon, Portugal, September 2005

21. van Welbergen, H., Reidsma, D., Ruttkay, Z.M., Zwiers, J.: Elckerlyc. J. Multimodal User Interfaces **3**(4), 271–284 (2009)

22. Xu, Y., Feng, A.W., Marsella, S., Shapiro, A.: A practical and configurable lip sync method for games. In: Proceedings of Motion on Games, pp. 131–140. ACM (2013)

Narrative Variations in a Virtual Storyteller

Stephanie M. Lukin[✉] and Marilyn A. Walker

Natural Language and Dialogue Systems Lab, Baskin School of Engineering,
University of California, Santa Cruz, USA
{slukin,mawalker}@ucsc.edu

Abstract. Research on storytelling over the last 100 years has distinguished at least two levels of narrative representation (1) story, or fabula; and (2) discourse, or sujhet. We use this distinction to create *Fabula Tales*, a computational framework for a virtual storyteller that can tell the same story in different ways through the implementation of general narratological variations, such as varying direct vs. indirect speech, character voice (style), point of view, and focalization. A strength of our computational framework is that it is based on very general methods for re-using existing story content, either from fables or from personal narratives collected from blogs. We first explain how a simple annotation tool allows naïve annotators to easily create a deep representation of fabula called a story intention graph, and show how we use this representation to generate story tellings automatically. Then we present results of two studies testing our narratological parameters, and showing that different tellings affect the reader's perception of the story and characters.

Keywords: Narrative · Language generation · Storytelling · Engagement

1 Introduction

Research on oral storytelling over the last 100 years has distinguished at least two levels of narrative representation (1) story, or fabula: the content of a narrative in terms of the sequence of events and relations between them, the story characters and their traits and affects, and the properties and settings; and (2) discourse, or sujhet: the actual expressive telling of a story as a stream of words, gestures, images or facial expressions in a storytelling medium [2,7,19,20,22]. In the telling of a narrative, events from the story are selected, ordered, and expressed in the discourse. We use this distinction to create *Fabula Tales*, a computational framework for a virtual storyteller that can tell the same story in different ways, using a set of general narratological variations, such as direct vs. indirect speech, character voice (style), point of view, and focalization.

We demonstrate the generality of our methods by applying them to both Aesop's Fables and personal narratives from a pre-existing corpus of blogs [8]. We hypothesize many advantages for a virtual storyteller who can repurpose existing stories. Stories such as *The Startled Squirrel* in Fig. 1 are created daily

© Springer International Publishing Switzerland 2015
W.-P. Brinkman et al. (Eds.): IVA 2015, LNAI 9238, pp. 320–331, 2015.
DOI: 10.1007/978-3-319-21996-7_34

This is one of those times I wish I had a digital camera. We keep a large stainless steel bowl of water outside on the back deck for Benjamin to drink out of when he's playing outside. His bowl has become a very popular site. Throughout the day, many birds drink out of it and bathe in it. The birds literally line up on the railing and wait their turn. Squirrels also come to drink out of it. The craziest squirrel just came by- he was literally jumping in fright at what I believe was his own reflection in the bowl. He was startled so much at one point that he leap in the air and fell off the deck. But not quite, I saw his one little paw hanging on! After a moment or two his paw slipped and he tumbled down a few feet. But oh, if you could have seen the look on his startled face and how he jumped back each time he caught his reflection in the bowl!

Fig. 1. *The Startled Squirrel* personal narrative

in the thousands and cover any topic imaginable. They are natural and personal, and may be funny, sad, heart-warming or serious. Applications for virtual storytellers who can retell these stories in different ways could include virtual companions, persuasion, educational storytelling, or sharing troubles in therapeutic settings [3,9,18,23,24]. Figure 2 shows how *Fabula Tales* can shift from third person to first person automatically using content from *The Startled Squirrel* (Fig. 1). To our knowledge, this is the first time that these narratological variations have been implemented in a framework where the discourse (telling) is completely independent of the fabula (content) of the story [13].

ID	Example
S1	The narrator placed the bowl on the deck in order for Benjamin to drink the bowl's water. The bowl was popular. The birds drank the bowl's water. The birds bathed themselves in the bowl. The birds organized themselves on the deck's railing in order for the birds to wait.
S2	I approached the bowl. I was startled because I saw my reflection. I leaped because I was startled. I fell over the deck's railing because I leaped because I was startled. I held the deck's railing with my paw. My paw slipped off the deck's railing. I fell.

Fig. 2. Variation in Point of View for *The Startled Squirrel*

Section 2 describes how the deep structure of any narrative can be represented as a story intention graph, a generic model of the fabula [5]. Section 3 describes our method for generating retellings of stories, and Sect. 4 describes two experimental evaluations. We delay discussion of related work to Sect. 5 when we can compare it to our own, and sum up and discuss future work.

A Crow was sitting on a branch of a tree with a piece of cheese in her beak when a Fox observed her and set his wits to work to discover some way of getting the cheese. Coming and standing under the tree he looked up and said, "What a noble bird I see above me! Her beauty is without equal, the hue of her plumage exquisite. If only her voice is as sweet as her looks are fair, she ought without doubt to be Queen of the Birds." The Crow was hugely flattered by this, and just to show the Fox that she could sing she gave a loud caw. Down came the cheese,of course, and the Fox, snatching it up, said, "You have a voice, madam, I see: what you want is wits."

Fig. 3. The Fox and The Crow

2   Repurposing Stories with Story Intention Graphs

Our framework builds on Elson's representation of fabula, called a story intention graph, or SIG [5]. The SIG allows many aspects of a story to be captured, including key entities, events and statives arranged in a timeline, and an interpretation of the overarching goals, plans and beliefs of the story's agents [5]. Figure 4 shows the part of the SIG for *The Startled Squirrel* story in Fig. 1. Elson's DRAMABANK provides 36 Aesop's Fables encoded as SIGs, e.g. *The Fox and the Crow* in Fig. 3, and Elson's annotation tool Scheherazade allows minimally trained annotators to develop a SIG for any narrative. We hired an undergraduate linguist to use Scheherezade to produce SIGs for 100 personal narratives. Each story took on average 45 min to annotate. We currently have 100 annotated stories on topics such as travel, daily activities, storms, gardening, funerals, going to the doctor, camping, and snorkeling.

Scheherazade allows users to annotate a story along several dimensions, starting with the surface form, or discourse as shown in Fig. 4, and then proceeding to deeper representations. The second column in Fig. 4 is called the "timeline layer", in which the story facts are encoded as predicate-argument structures (propositions) and temporally ordered on a timeline. The timeline layer consists of a network of propositional structures, where nodes correspond

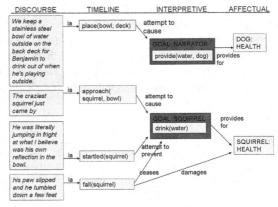

Fig. 4. Part of the STORY INTENTION GRAPH (SIG) for *The Startled Squirrel.*

to lexical items that are linked by thematic relations. Scheherazade adapts information about predicate-argument structures from the VerbNet lexical database [11] and uses WordNet [6] as its noun and adjectives taxonomy. The arcs of the story graph are labeled with discourse relations. Scheherazade also comes with a built-in realizer (referred to as *sch* in this paper) that the annotator can use to check their work. This realizer does not incorporate any narratological variations.

3   Generating Narratological Variations

Our framework can generate story re-tellings using methods that are neither genre nor domain-specific. We build *Fabula Tales* on two tools from previous work: PERSONAGE and the ES-Translator [15, 21]. PERSONAGE is an expressive natural language generation engine that takes as input the syntactic formalism of Deep Syntactic Structures (DSYNTS) [10, 12]. DSYNTS allow PERSONAGE to be

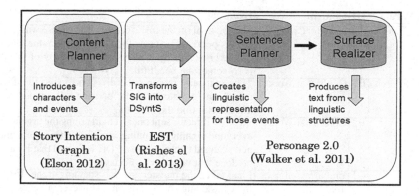

Fig. 5. NLG pipeline method of the ES Translator.

flexible in generation, however the creation of DSYNTS has been hand crafted and time consuming. The ES-Translator (EST) automatically bridges the narrative representation of the SIG to the DSYNTS formalism by applying a model of syntax to the SIG [21]. The SIG representation gives us direct access to the linguistic and logical representations of the fabula for each story, so the EST can interpret the story in the DSYNTS formalism and retell it using different words or syntactic structures [14,21].

DSYNTS are dependency structures where the nodes are labeled with lexemes and the arcs of the tree are labeled with syntactic relations. The DSYNTS formalism distinguishes between arguments and modifiers and between argument types (subject, direct and indirect object etc.). PERSONAGE handles morphology, agreement and function words to produce an output string.

After the EST applies syntax to the SIG, it generates two data structures: text plans containing sentence plans and the corresponding DSYNTS. Thus any story or content represented as a SIG can be retold using PERSONAGE. Figure 5 provides a high level view of the architecture of EST. The full translation methodology is described in [21].

This paper incorporates the EST pipeline (including SIGs and PERSONAGE) into the *Fabula Tales* computational framework and adds three narratological parameters into story generation:

1. **Point of View:** Change the narration point of view to any character in a story in the first person voice (Sect. 3.1).
2. **Direct Speech:** Given any SIG encoding that uses speech act verbs (e.g. said, told, asked, alleged), re-tell as direct speech or indirect speech (Sect. 3.2).
3. **Character Voice:** Substitute different character voices using any character model expressible with PERSONAGE's 67 parameters (Sect. 3.3).

Figure 6 provides variations that combine these narratological parameters illustrating content from "The Fox and the Crow" and two additional stories: Conflict at Work, and The Embarrassed Teacher. B2 and C1 are examples of the original tellings and C2 is a *sch* realization.

Narr Param	ID	Content	Example
Direct Speech	A1	Fox and Crow	The crow sat on the tree's branch. The cheese was in the crow's pecker. The crow thought "I will eat the cheese on the branch of the tree because the clarity of the sky is so-somewhat beautiful."
Direct Speech	B1	Conflict at Work	"The company requires the division to sign the document", the director told the division. "Be expedient", the director told the division.
Original	B2	Conflict at Work	The new director sent out an email noting the urgency of everyone signing, scanning, and formatting the signed and scanned contract into a PDF. He noted that it had to be done that very day (a Friday).
Original	C1	Embarrassed Teacher	I had taken the register and was standing at the front of the class doing some revision... However, all eyes were not on my face but at my ankles. Nervously I looked down to see that my underslip had somehow made its way to the floor. Elastic gone What to do?.
Sch	C2	Embarrassed Teacher	The narrator lifted the slip and inserted it into a bottom drawer of the desk. The narrator resumed teaching, and the group of students didn't react.
Indirect Speech	A2	Fox and the Crow	The fox said the beauty of the bird was incomparable. The fox said the hue of the feather of the bird was exquisite.
Indirect Speech	B3	Conflict at Work	The narrator said if the director said the thing was urgent the narrator would need to be urgent. The narrator said the director was frivolous.
Character Voice	A3	Fox and the Crow	The fox alleged "your beauty is quite incomparable, okay?" The fox alleged "your feather's chromaticity is damn exquisite."
Character Voice	C3	Embarrassed Teacher	I stood at the classroom's front. I no-noticed my ankle to be somewhat observed. I looked nervously toward my ankle. I glanced around the students.
Point of View	A4	Fox and the Crow	I sat on the tree's branch. The cheese was in my beak. The fox observed me. The fox came. The fox stood under the tree. The fox looked toward me. The fox said he saw me.

Fig. 6. Narratological Variations in Blogs and Aesops

3.1 Point of View

From the deep syntactic structure in the format of DSYNTS, we can change the narration style from the third person perspective to the first person perspective of any character in the story (see example A4 in Fig. 6). We define simple rules to make this transformation within the DSYNTS itself, not at the sentence level. Table 1 shows the DSYNTS, which are represented as xml structures, for the sentence *The crow flew herself to the window.*

In order to transform the sentence into the first person, only simple changes to the deep structure are necessary. At lines 9 and 10 in Table 1, we assign the `person` attribute to `1st` to specify a change of point of view to first person. The surface realizer in PERSONAGE takes care of the transformations with its own rules, knowing to change whatever lexeme is present at line 9 simply to *I*, and to

Table 1. DSYNTS for "The crow flew herself to the window" and "I flew myself to the window"

```
"The crow flew herself to the window"
1 <dsyntnode class="verb" lexeme="fly">
2    <dsyntnode class="common_noun" lexeme="crow" gender="fem">
3    <dsyntnode class="common_noun" lexeme="crow" gender="fem"
             pro="pro">
4    <dsyntnode class="preposition" lexeme="to">
5       <dsyntnode class="common_noun" lexeme="window">
6    </dsyntnode>
7 </dsyntnode>
```

```
"I flew myself to the window"

8 <dsyntnode class="verb" lexeme="fly">
9       <dsyntnode class="common_noun" lexeme="crow" gender="fem"
          person="1st">
10      <dsyntnode class="common_noun" lexeme="crow" gender="fem"
          pro="pro" person="1st">
11      <dsyntnode class="preposition" lexeme="to">
12         <dsyntnode class="common_noun" lexeme="window">
13      </dsyntnode>
14</dsyntnode>
```

change the coreference resolutions at line 10 to *myself*. This is a major advantage of our computational framework: the deep linguistic representation allows us to specify changes we want without manipulating strings, and allows general rules for narratological parameters such as voice.

3.2 Dialogue Realization

By default, speech acts in the SIG are encoded as indirect speech. We automatically detect a speech act from its verb type in the WordNet online dictionary, and then transform it to a direct speech act (see A1, A2, B1, and B3 in Fig. 6). First we use WordNet to identify if the main verb in a sentence is a verb of communication. Next, we break apart the DSYNTS into their tree structure (Fig. 7). For example, we first identify the subject (*director*) from utterance B1 in Fig. 6, and object (*division*) of the main verb of communication (*tell*). Then we identify the remainder of the tree (*be* is the root verb), which is what is to be uttered, and split it off from its parent verb of communication node, thus creating two separate DSYNTS (Fig. 8). In PERSONAGE, we create a direct speech text plan to realize the explanatory in the default narrator style and the utterance in a specified character voice and appropriately insert the quotation marks. We can then realize direct speech as *"Utterance" said X.* or *X said "utterance"*.

3.3 Character Voice

The main advantage of PERSONAGE is its ability to generate a single utterance in many different voices. Models of narrative style are currently based on the Big Five personality traits [15], or are learned from film scripts [25]. Each type of model (personality trait or film) specifies a set of language cues, one of 67 different parameters, whose value varies with the personality or style to be conveyed. Previous work in [15] has shown that humans perceive the personality stylistic models in the way that PERSONAGE intended, and [25] shows that character utterances in a new domain can be recognized by humans as models based on a particular film character.

After we add new rules to *Fabula Tales* to handle direct speech, we modified the original SIG representation of the *Fox and the Crow* to contain more dialogue in order to evaluate a broader range of character styles, along with the use of direct speech. Table 2 shows a subset of parameters, which were used in the three personality models we tested here: the *laid-back* model for the fox's direct speech, the *shy* model for the crow's direct speech, and the *neutral* model for the narrator voice. The *laid-back* model uses emphasizers, hedges, exclamations, and expletives, whereas the *shy* model uses softener hedges, stuttering, and filled pauses. The *neutral* model is the simplest model that does not utilize any of the extremes of the PERSONAGE parameters.

C3 in Fig. 6 provides an example of *Fabula Tales* rendering a story in a single voice for *The Embarrassed Teacher*. We tell the story from her point of view and give her an introverted voice. We also show that we can specify voices for characters in dialogue as in the Fable excerpt in A3 in Fig. 6. *Fabula Tales* system allows multiple personalities to be loaded and assigned to characters so that PERSONAGE runs once, fully automatically, and **in real-time**.

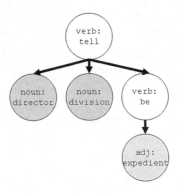

Fig. 7. *The director told the division to be expedient.*

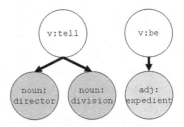

Fig. 8. *"Be expedient", the director told the division or The director told the division "be expedient."*

4   Experimental Results

We present two experiments that show how the flexibility of the EST combined with our narratological parameters to create *Fabula Tales* allows us to manipulate the perception of characters and story engagement and interest. We first present *The Fox and the Crow* with variations on direct speech and voice, followed by *Embarrassed Teacher* with variations on voice and point of view.

4.1   Perceptions of Voice and Direct Speech

We collect user perceptions of the *The Fox and the Crow* generated with direct speech and with different personality models (character voices) for each speech act. A dialogic variation plus character voice excerpt is A3 in Fig. 6. The dialogic story is told (1) only with the neutral model; (2) with the crow as shy and the fox as laid-back; and (3) with the crow as laid-back and the fox as shy.

Table 2. Examples of pragmatic marker insertion parameters from PERSONAGE

Model	Parameter	Description	Example
Shy	SOFTENER HEDGES	Insert syntactic elements (*sort of, kind of, somewhat, quite, around, rather, I think that, it seems that, it seems to me that*) to mitigate the strength of a proposition	'*It seems to me that he was hungry*'
	STUTTERING	Duplicate parts of a content word	'*The vine hung on the tr-trellis*'
	FILLED PAUSES	Insert syntactic elements expressing hesitancy (*I mean, err, mmhm, like, you know*)	'*Err... the fox jumped*'
Laid Back	EMPHASIZER HEDGES	Insert syntactic elements (*really, basically, actually*) to strengthen a proposition	'*The fox failed to get the group of grapes, alright?*'
	EXCLAMATION	Insert an exclamation mark	'*The group of grapes hung on the vine!*'
	EXPLETIVES	Insert a swear word	'*The fox was damn hungry*'

Subjects are given a free text box and asked to enter as many words as they wish to use to describe the characters in the story. Table 3 shows the percentage of positive and negative descriptive words when categorized by LIWC [17]. Some words include "clever" and "sneaky" for the laid-back and neutral fox, and "shy" and "wise" for the shy fox. The laid-back and neutral crow was pereived as "naíve" and "gullible" whereas the shy crow is more "stupid" and "foolish".

Table 3. Polarity of Adjectives describing the Crow and Fox (% of total words)

Crow	Pos	Neg		Fox	Pos	Neg
Neutral	13	29		Neutral	38	4
Shy	28	24		Shy	39	8
Laid-back	10	22		Laid-back	34	8

Overall, the crow's shy voice is perceived as more positive than the crow's neutral voice, (ttest(12) = -4.38, p < 0.0001), and the crow's laid-back voice (ttest(12) = -6.32, p < 0.0001). We hypothesize that this is because the stuttering and hesitations make the character seem more helpless and tricked, rather than the laid-back model which is more boisterous. However, there is less variation between the fox polarity. Both the stuttering shy fox and the boisterous laid-back fox were seen equally as "cunning" and "smart". Although we don't observe a difference between all characters, there is enough evidence to warrent further investigation of how reader perceptions change when the same content is realized in difference voices.

4.2   Perceptions of Voice and POV

In this experiment, we aim to see how different points of view and voices effect reader engagement and interest. We present readers with a one sentence summary of the *Embarrassed Teacher* story and 6 retellings of a sentence from the story, framed as "possible excerpts that could come from this summary". We show retellings of a sentence from *Embarrassed Teacher* in first person neutral, first person shy, first person laid-back, third person neutral, the original story, and *sch*. We ask participants to rate each excerpt for their interest in wanting to read more of the story based on the style and information given in the excerpt, and to indicate their engagement with the story given the excerpt.

Figure 9 shows the means and standard deviation for engagement and interest ratings. We find a clear ranking for engagement: the original sentence is scored highest, followed by first outgoing, first neutral, first shy, *sch*, and third neutral.

Engagement	Orig	1st-out	1st-neutr	1st-shy	sch	3rd-neutr
M	3.98	3.27	3.00	2.73	1.95	1.93
SD	1.07	1.39	1.19	1.25	1.07	1.06

Interest	Orig	1st-out	1st-neutr	1st-shy	sch	3rd-neutr
Mean	3.91	3.02	3.02	2.81	1.90	1.87
SD	0.99	1.21	1.37	1.27	1.05	1.01

Fig. 9. Means (M) and standard deviation (SD) for engagement and interest for original sentences and all variations in Perceptions of Voice and POV Experiment

Figure 10 shows the average engagement and interest for all the sentences. For engagement, paired t-tests show that there is a significant difference between original and first outgoing (ttest(94) = -3.99, p < 0.0001), first outgoing and first shy (ttest(94) = 3.71, p < 0.0001), and first shy and *sch* (ttest(94) = 5.60, p < 0.0001). However, there are no differences between first neutral and

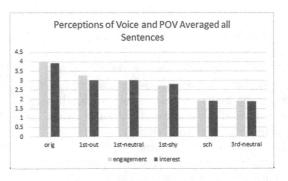

Fig. 10. Histogram of Engagement and Interest for Perceptions of Voice and POV Experiment averaged across story (higher is better)

first outgoing (ttest(95) = -1.63, p = 0.05), and *sch* and third neutral (ttest(94) = -0.31, p = 0.38). We also performed an ANOVA and found there is a significant effect on style (F(1) = 224.24, p = 0), sentence (F(9) = 5.49, p = 0), and an interaction between style and sentence (F(9) = 1.65, p < 0.1).

For interest, we find the same ranking: the original sentence, first outgoing, first neutral, first shy, *sch*, and third neutral. Paired t-tests for interest show a significant difference between original and first outgoing (ttest(93) = 5.59, p < 0.0001), and first shy and *sch* (ttest(93) = 6.16, p < 0.0001). There is no difference between first outgoing and first neutral (ttest(93) = 0, p < 0.5), first neutral and first shy (ttest(93) = 2.20, p = 0.01), and *sch* and third neutral (ttest(93) = 0.54, p = 0.29). We also performed an ANOVA and found there is a significant effect on style (F(1) = 204.08, p = 0), sentence (F(9) = 7.32, p = 0), and no interaction between style and sentence (F(9) = 0.64, p = 1).

We also find qualitative evidence that there are significant differences in reader's interest and engagement in a story dependent only upon the style. Readers preferred to read this story in the first person: "[the] immediacy of first person ... excerpts made me feel I was there", "I felt as though those that had more detail and were from a personal perspective were more engaging and thought evoking versus saying the narrator did it", and "I felt more engaged and interested when I felt like the narrator was speaking to me directly, as I found it easier to imagine the situation". This further supports our hypothesis that our framework to change POV will effect reader perceptions.

Readers also identified differences in the style of the voice. Two readers commented about first outgoing: "The 'oh I resumed...' Feels more personal and is more engaging" and "curse words are used to express the severity of the situation wisely". About first shy, "Adding the feeling of nervousness and where she looked made sense". This suggests that certain styles of narration are more appropriate or preferred than others given the context of the story.

5 Discussion and Future Work

We introduce *Fabula Tales*, a computational framework for story generation that produces narratological variations of the same story from the fabula. We present examples showing that the capability we have developed is general, and can be applied to informal personal narratives. We present experiments showing that these novel narratological parameters lead to different perceptions of the story. Our approach builds on previous work which focused on generating variations of Aesop's Fables such as *The Fox and the Crow* [21], however this previous work did not carry out perceptual studies.

Previous work has dubbed the challenges of generating different story tellings from fabula the **NLG gap**: an architectural disconnect between narrative generation (fabula) and natural language generation (sujet) [4,13]. To our knowledge, there are only two previous lines of research that address the NLG gap. The STORYBOOK generator is an end-to-end narrative prose generation system that utilizes a primitive narrative planner along with a generation engine to produce stories in the Little Red Riding Hood fairy tale domain [4]. This work manipulates NLG parameters such as lexical choice and syntactic structure, as well as narratological parameters such as person and focalization and the choice of whether to realize dialogue as direct or indirect speech. Similarly the IF system can generate multiple variations of text in an interactive fiction (IF) environment [16]. The IF system (and its successor Curveship) uses a world simulator as the fabula, and renders narrative variations, such as different focalizations or temporal orders. However STORYBOOK can only generate stories in the domain of Little Red Riding Hood, and IF can only generate stories in its interactive fiction world. Other work implements narratological variations in the story planner and does not attempt to bridge the NLG gap [1].

In future work, we aim to further develop *Fabula Tales* and to test in more detail the perceptual effects of narratological variations on user interpretations of a story. Furthermore, we hope to learn when certain styles are preferred given the context in the SIG.

Acknowledgments. This research was supported by NSF Creative IT program grant #IIS-1002921, and a grant from the Nuance Foundation.

References

1. Bae, B.C., Cheong, Y.G., Young, R.M.: Toward a computational model of focalization in narrative. In Proceedings of the 6th International Conference on Foundations of Digital Games, pp. 313–315. ACM (2011)
2. Bal, M., Tavor, E.: Notes on narrative embedding. Poetics Today **2**, 41–59 (1981)
3. Bickmore, T.W.: Relational agents: effecting change through human-computer relationships. Ph.D. thesis, MIT Media Lab (2003)
4. Callaway, C.B., Lester, J.C.: Narrative prose generation. Artif. Intell. **139**(2), 213–252 (2002)
5. Elson, D.: Modeling Narrative Discourse. Ph.D. thesis (2012)
6. Fellbaum, C.: Wordnet: An electronic lexical database (1998). (WordNet is available from http://www.cogsci.princeton.edu/wn) (2010)
7. Genette, G.: Nouveau discours du récit. Éd. du Seuil, Paris (1983)
8. Gordon, A., Swanson, R.: Identifying personal stories in millions of weblog entries. In: Third International Conference on Weblogs and Social Media, Data Challenge Workshop, San Jose, CA (2009)
9. Gratch, J., Morency, L.P., Scherer, S., Stratou, G., Boberg, J., Koenig, S., Adamson, T., Rizzo, A.: User-state sensing for virtual health agents and telehealth applications. Stud. Health Technol. Inform. **184**, 151–157 (2012)
10. Mel'čuk, A.: Dependency Syntax: Theory and Practice. SUNY Press, Albany (1988)
11. Kipper, K., Korhonen, A., Ryant, N., Palmer, M.: Extensive classifications of english verbs. In: Proceedings of the 12th EURALEX International Congress, pp. 1–15 (2006)
12. Lavoie, B., Rambow, O.: A fast and portable realizer for text generation systems. In: Procs of the 5th conference on Applied natural language processing, pp. 265–268. ACL (1997)

13. Lönneker, B.: Narratological knowledge for natural language generation. In: Proceedings of the 10th European Workshop on Natural Language Generation (ENLG-05), pp. 91–100. Citeseer (2005)
14. Lukin, S.M., Ryan, J.O., Walker, M.A.: Automating direct speech variations in stories and games (2014)
15. Mairesse, F., Walker, M.A.: Controlling user perceptions of linguistic style: trainable generation of personality traits. Comput. Linguist. **37**, 455–488 (2011)
16. Montfort, N.: Generating narrative variation in interactive fiction. University of Pennsylvania (2007)
17. Pennebaker, J.W., Francis, M.E., Booth, R.J.: Linguistic Inquiry and Word Count: Liwc 2001. Lawrence Erlbaum Associates, Mahway (2001)
18. Pennebaker, J.W., Seagal, J.D.: Forming a story: the health benefits of narrative. J. Clin. Psychol. **55**(10), 1243–1254 (1999)
19. Prince, G.: A Grammar of Stories: An Introduction. Walter de Gruyter, New York (1973). Number 13
20. Propp, V.I.: Morphology of the Folktale, vol. 9. University of Texas Press, Austin (1968)
21. Rishes, E., Lukin, S., Elson, D.K., Walker, M.A.: Generating dierent story tellings from semantic representations of narrative. In: Internation Conference on Interactive Digital Storytelling, ICIDS 2013 (2013)
22. Shklovsky, V.: Theory of Prose. Dalkey Archive Press, Champaign (1991)
23. Slater, M.D., Rouner, D.: Entertainment education and elaboration likelihood: Understanding the processing of narrative persuasion. Commun. Theory **12**(2), 173–191 (2002)
24. Traum, D., Roque, A., Georgiou, A.L.P., Gerten, J., Narayanan, B.M.S., Robinson, S., Vaswani, A.: Hassan: a virtual human for tactical questioning. In: Proceedings of SIGDial (2007)
25. Walker, M.A., Grant, R., Sawyer, J., Lin, G.I., Wardrip-Fruin, N., Buell, M.: Perceived or not perceived: film character models for expressive NLG. In: Si, M., Thue, D., André, E., Lester, J., Tanenbaum, J., Zammitto, V. (eds.) ICIDS 2011. LNCS, vol. 7069, pp. 109–121. Springer, Heidelberg (2011)

Context-Awareness in a Persistent Hospital Companion Agent

Timothy Bickmore[1]([✉]), Reza Asadi[1], Aida Ehyaei[2], Harriet Fell[1],
Lori Henault[3], Stephen Intille[1,3], Lisa Quintiliani[4],
Ameneh Shamekhi[1], Ha Trinh[1], Katherine Waite[4],
Christopher Shanahan[4], and Michael K. Paasche-Orlow[4]

[1] College of Computer and Information Science, Northeastern University,
Boston, MA, USA
bickmore@ccs.neu.edu
[2] College of Engineering, Northeastern University, Boston, MA, USA
[3] Bouvé College of Health Sciences, Northeastern University,
Boston, MA, USA
[4] Boston Medical Center, Boston, MA, USA

Abstract. We describe the design and preliminary evaluation of a virtual agent that provides continual bedside companionship and a range of health, information, and entertainment functions to hospital patients during their stay. The agent system uses sensors to enable it to be aware of events in the hospital room and the status of the patient, in order to provide context-sensitive health counseling. Patients in the pilot study responded well to having the agent in their rooms for 1–3 days and engaged in 9.4 conversations per day with the agent on average, using all available functions.

Keywords: Relational agent · Embodied conversational agent · Medical informatics · Health informatics · Sleep promotion · Sensors · Accelerometer · RFID

1 Introduction

Despite the bewildering array of technology in modern hospital rooms, little is provided for patients to directly interact with, aside from the television, telephone, and nurse intercom. Even in the academic research literature, few systems have been developed to provide information and comfort to patients while they are in their hospital beds. Although the purpose of hospitals is to heal acutely ill patients, they provide this service in a manner that largely treats patients as objects to be fixed rather than human beings to be supported and healed.

The hospital experience can be disempowering and disorienting. Patients face noise, sleep deprivation, frequent interruptions, an unfamiliar environment filled with many changing health professionals and ancillary staff, and medications that often have physical or psychoactive side-effects. At the same time, patients are often lonely and bored, left alone in their rooms until interventions are required.

© Springer International Publishing Switzerland 2015
W.-P. Brinkman et al. (Eds.): IVA 2015, LNAI 9238, pp. 332–342, 2015.
DOI: 10.1007/978-3-319-21996-7_35

In addition, many studies indicate that hospitalized patients are not engaged in their own hospital care at even the most rudimentary level. People frequently cannot identify the name or role of their providers [1]. After discharge, most patients cannot name their diagnoses or medications and few can name important potential side effects of their medications [2]. Expanding patients' role in their own care is an important goal: people who are more involved in their care have better outcomes, and helping patients establish their health agendas and promoting patients' questions about their care can improve outcomes (e.g., satisfaction, adherence, blood pressure control, and diabetes control) [3]. Currently, disagreements between patients and providers about basic aspects of the inpatient experience are common [4].

To help address these issues, we have developed a hospital companion agent that is designed to support a patient throughout a hospital stay. The "Hospital Buddy" is a virtual agent that is designed to chat with patients about their hospital experience— providing empathic feedback and emotional support—in addition to a range of topics that have medical and entertainment functions (Fig. 1). A preliminary version of the Hospital Buddy that had limited, patient-initiated dialogue-only functionality was evaluated with three hospital patients in 2011 [5]. In this paper, we report on a greatly enhanced version of the system that integrates a suite of sensors to make the agent aware of events in the hospital environment and more aware of the status of the patient, to provide more context-sensitive and helpful counseling. We also report the results of a pilot acceptance study involving 8 patients.

2 Related Work

Within the hospital environment, most HCI research has been clinician-centric, although there have been a few examples of patient-facing systems. Bers *et al.* developed a system that provided immersive multi-user collaborative support

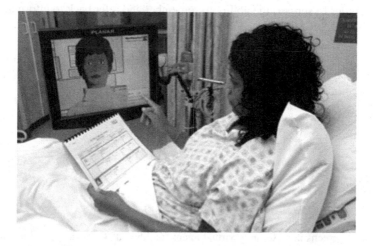

Fig. 1. Patient Interacting with the hospital buddy

environments for hospitalized pediatric patients with renal and cardiac diseases [6], and other conditions. Bickmore *et al.* developed a virtual nurse for hospital discharge education that was met with high rates of patient satisfaction [7]. Additionally, Wilcox *et al.* have shown that both patients and physicians are favorably inclined to having patient-facing health information displays located in the hospital room [8]. Vawdrey *et al.* piloted a tablet-based medical record portal with cardiology patients, and found that viewing their information helped patients feel more engaged in their care [9].

3   Design of the Hospital Buddy

Our interdisciplinary design team consisted of physicians, a medical student and computer science students and faculty. The team conducted a series of brainstorming meetings to identify possible functions for the Hospital Buddy. A series of storyboards were developed for promising functions and reviewed by the team.

The Hospital Buddy is deployed on a wheeled kiosk with a touch screen display on an articulated arm that can be positioned beside or in front of patients while they are in bed (Fig. 1). The hardware setup also includes a UHF RFID antenna mounted on a separate arm (see Sect. 3.1), an omni-directional microphone, accelerometers for the patient to wear (see Sect. 3.2; Fig. 3), and RFID tagged-badges for the hospital staff.

The user interface features a virtual agent whose nonverbal behavior is synchronized with a text-to-speech engine. User contributions to the conversation are made via a touch screen selection from a multiple-choice menu of utterance options, updated at each turn of the conversation. Several additional interface screens are used to provide "dashboard" displays of patient status, provider background information, and other information (Fig. 2).

Agent dialogues are scripted, using a custom hierarchical transition network-based scripting language. In addition to network branching operations, script actions can include saving values to a persistent database or retrieving and testing values from the database, in order to support the ability to remember and refer back to information from earlier turns and prior conversations. Agent utterances can be tailored at runtime

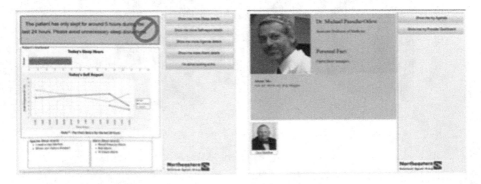

Fig. 2. Display screens in addition to virtual agent "dashboard" (left) and "provider biography" (right)

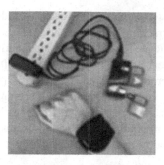

Fig. 3. Two wockets, a charger and a wocket worn in wrist band

through the inclusion of phrases derived from information in the database or other sources, using template-based text generation. The virtual agent has a range of non-verbal behaviors that it can use, including: hand gestures, body posture shifts, gazing at and away from the user, raising and lowering eyebrows, head nods, different facial expressions, and variable proximity (wide to close-up camera shots). Co-verbal behavior is determined for each utterance using the BEAT text-to-embodied-speech system [10], with several enhancements to support health dialogues.

3.1 RFID-Based Health Provider Identification

Up to 100 unique staff members may enter a patient's hospital room on a given day, and even those most closely involved with their care may be on irregular shift rotations, leaving patients confused about the identity and role of the hospital staff they interact with. Further, patients are not typically given an opportunity to provide feedback on the quality of these interactions during their hospital stay. To address these issues, we added a provider identification function to the system. Providers who approach a patient's bedside (and agree to wear an RFID tag) are detected and identified by the Hospital Buddy system using a long-range RFID reader, which then displays the provider's biography page, allowing the patient to view the provider's picture, name, role, and personal facts (Fig. 2). At the end of the interaction (when the RFID reader detects that all providers have left the bedside), the agent prompts the patient to evaluate the provider and the interaction using standardized measures [11].

3.2 Accelerometer-Based Sleep Detection for Hospital Patients

Hospital patients commonly experience fragmented sleep due to frequent interruptions, noise and other factors [12]. Fragmented sleep may be as detrimental to cognitive functioning as total sleep deprivation, and the effects of sleep deprivation are thought to be cumulative. Impairments to cognitive function can make it difficult for patients to be alert, engaged and receptive to information about their care. In addition, insufficient and fragmented sleep causes delirium (especially in older adult patients), limits patient learning and activation opportunities, and decreases patient satisfaction.

To address these issues, we extended the Hospital Buddy system to promote sleep management for patients by tracking their sleep and intervening with both patients and providers to ensure that patients get an appropriate amount of quality sleep. Sleep tracking is performed using real-time signal processing software, acquiring data from a small, wireless 3-axis accelerometer called a "Wocket" [13] (see Fig. 3) worn on a patient's wrist. The Wocket attempts to send raw accelerometer data to the Hospital Buddy system via Bluetooth once per minute. If the patient is not in the Bluetooth range of the system, the system notes that the patient is absent, and the Wocket saves a 1-min summary of wrist motion and sends that summary data during the next successful connection.

The Hospital Buddy computer processes the data as it is received and detects sleep and wake periods. The Hospital Buddy interface accordingly informs providers who approach a patient's bedside when the patient is sleeping and in need of sleep, presenting a text message and graph of recent sleep patterns to the care provider so that procedures that can be easily rescheduled can be deferred (Fig. 2). When the patient does wake, the Hospital Buddy asks him or her about the quality of the completed sleep episode and records this information for hospital staff.

The sleep-detection software was validated vs. polysomnography (PSG), the gold standard for sleep detection [14], in a pilot study. For 10 hospital patients the PSG sensors (EEG, EOG and chin EMG sensors) were set on the head and two Wockets were worn, one on the wrist and the other on the ankle, for 20 h each. The PSG data were manually labeled by a clinician in the hospital's Sleep Disorders Center in 30-s epochs according to American Academy of Sleep Medicine guidelines [15]. The sleep-detection software was trained with Wocket data and the PSG labels to build the accelerometer-based sleep detection model using an algorithm modified from Sazonov et al. [16]. The algorithm detected sleep/wake states with 82.7 % accuracy for one Wocket on the wrist, and 74.5 % accuracy for one Wocket on the ankle, where results were analyzed using 10-fold cross validation.

3.3   Acoustic Identification of Medical Device Alarms

Audible alarms on medical devices such as infusion pumps, and monitors such as pulse oximeters, are common in the hospital environment. The sheer number of alarms may result in alarm fatigue and decreased provider responsiveness, or even to alarms being disabled, silenced, or ignored [17]. Unexplained alarms can also cause patient anxiety, and the noise caused by frequent alarms can disrupt patient sleep.

To address these problems, we extended the Hospital Buddy with a microphone and signal processing software to detect and identify audible alarms in the hospital room (monitoring devices in many hospitals, including ours, do not provide digital alarm outputs). When an alarm is detected and identified, the Buddy proactively explains the alarm to the patient, so the patient understands what the alarms in the room are and their implications for care. Patients are also counseled on behaviors they can avoid that may trigger false alarms (e.g., certain kinds of motion, removing biometric monitor leads, etc.), reducing false alarm rates.

Table 1. Acoustic medical device alarm identification accuracy

Alarm type	Precision (%)	Recall (%)	F1 (%)
Dash monitor alarm	85.36	83.33	84.33
IV pump alarm	83.52	81.72	82.61
Cardiac monitor alarm	88.46	86.25	87.34
Bed alarm	89.61	87.34	88.46
Blood pressure alarm	35.97	92.59	51.81

To identify the source of frequent alarms and to collect samples for training, we collected audio recordings from 11 patients totaling over 250 h of hospital room sounds. Samples of interest were extracted and labeled by clinicians. This resulted in six types of frequent hospital alarms that we wanted the system to identify: IV standby, IV check, bed, dash monitor, blood pressure monitor and cardiac monitor alarms. Based on the type of the detected alarm, the Buddy initiates a corresponding dialogue, providing empathetic feedback, explaining the alarm and its potential causes, and suggesting actions to be made (e.g., calling the nurse). In addition, the system offers the patient options to immediately add the alarm issue onto an agenda of problems to be discussed with the medical team.

We developed signal-processing software to identify the six alarms from real-time audio. An audio buffer of length 20 s is used for processing the input signal. The frequency of each alarm was measured and used to design a high pass filter that is used to remove the noise from the input signal. The envelope of the signal is extracted by a full-wave rectifier and a low pass filter. The envelopes of the alarm signals contain pulse trains with specific patterns. The pulse width and the pulse period are used for detecting these patterns. Each alarm detector looks for pulses that have amplitudes higher than a specific threshold. The detectors match the pulse width and period with their related alarm pattern to identify the alarm. Results of alarm identification testing on recorded hospital sounds are presented in Table 1.

3.4 Additional System Functions and Overall Operation

In addition to the dialogue initiated by the Buddy in response to sensed events, patients can also initiate the following functions themselves via dialogue.

Dialogue About Hospital Events. This dialogue enables patients to discuss an event that just occurred to them in the hospital, such as: just waking up; just finishing a meal; just finished watching TV; family or friends just visited; or just had a procedure or test done. In each case, the agent elicits how the patient felt about the event, and provides empathic feedback when warranted.

Agenda Minder. This function maintains a prioritized agenda of unresolved questions and issues about the patient's condition and treatment. The agenda is built by the patient, with prompting by the Buddy and input from providers. The Buddy ensures that these agenda items get addressed by prompting patients and providers to discuss them during consultations with providers. Questions can be picked from a list of frequently asked questions, or typed via a soft keyboard.

Symptom Tracker. This function enables patients to self-report different subjective health-related states, such as pain and stress, and record them for later time-series display for their own use or to share with their providers (Fig. 2). Patients can report any of a validated list of nine symptoms commonly experienced by hospital patients, the Edmonton Symptom Assessment System [18]. In addition to allowing patients to initiate self-report whenever they want, the Buddy prompts patients twice daily at preset times to describe how they are feeling. The agent also uses these patient utterances as empathic opportunities to provide comfort when appropriate.

Social Chat. The Buddy can engage in chat by telling the patient a story, selected from a list of health-related stories, anecdotes, and jokes.

The overall Hospital Buddy System operates in the following modes.

Agent. Patient is talking to the agent, with no providers in the room. This can either be initiated by the patient, or when an event is sensed (a medical device alarm is identified, the patient just woke up, or it is time for a self-report of symptoms).

Dashboard. One or more providers are in the room, and either the patient is not present or asleep. In this situation, the "dashboard" is displayed, summarizing information that the Buddy knows about the patient, and a prominently-display notice to not wake the patient, if sleeping (Fig. 2). The agent never interacts with providers directly because, based on our prior experience, providers are not receptive to this form of interface in the hospital environment.

Consult. One or more providers are in the room, and the patient is present and awake. Provider time is limited, and we did not want the agent interfering with provider consultation with the patient, so the virtual agent is not used in this situation. When providers first enter the room, their biography pages are displayed for the patient, but a provider or the patient can also view the patients "dashboard," sleep data, alarm data, agenda, or self-report history, to support consultation.

Postconsult. Following a consultation, and 5 min after all providers have left the room, the agent appears and prompts the patient to rate their providers and their interactions.

4   Pilot Evaluation Study

To evaluate the Hospital Buddy, we conducted a formative pilot test in which hospitalized patients used the system continuously for one to three days. The study was conducted on a general medicine floor at an urban hospital.

Following the administration of informed consent, patients were given a brief introduction to the system functionality. Providers who agreed to participate and wear RFID tags were also consented and given an overview of the system. The system was then left in the patient's room for one to three days. A research assistant visited the patients once per day to switch and recharge the Wockets. Upon the study completion, we asked the patients to complete questionnaires, followed by semi-structured interviews with both patients and their providers.

We recruited 8 patients: 50 % female; aged 33–53 (M = 47); 33 % were African American, 33 % were Hispanic or Latino; 33 % had college degrees, 50 % had high school education; 83 % reported using computers regularly; 50 % had inadequate health literacy according to the REALM test. Eleven providers (all female, 36 % doctors and 64 % nurses) were recruited from the same unit.

Results

System Use. All patients used the system for 1–3 days (mean 1.38 days). Patients had an average of 9.4 (SD = 4.5) conversational interactions per day with the agent, 44 % of which were initiated by the patients. The average duration of the conversations was 115 s (SD = 107.2).

Working Alliance. Table 2 presents the patients' self-report ratings of their relationship with the Buddy [19]. The patients showed confidence in the Hospital Buddy's ability to help them and felt that the Buddy was genuinely concerned about their wellbeing.

Symptom Reporting. 75 % (n = 6) of patients used the symptom reporting function, demonstrating a strong engagement in this activity with an average of 1.9 (SD = 1.2) reports per day from each patient. Providing dual channels for symptom reporting was shown to be effective, resulting in both patient-initiated selective symptom reports (62 %) and scheduled, agent-initiated symptom reports (38 %). During the interviews, patients reported positively on the ability to proactively track their symptoms. One patient indicated that the graph visualization of her symptom progress helped her to

Table 2. Patients' working alliance inventory [19] ratings of the hospital buddy

Rating items (scale measures from 1–7) 1 – strongly disagree 7 – strongly agree	Mean (SD)
I feel uncomfortable with the Buddy	2.4 (2.6)
The Buddy and I understand each other	4.4 (2.1)
I believe the Buddy likes me	5.4 (2.5)
I believe the Buddy is genuinely concerned about my welfare	6 (1)
The Buddy and I respect each other	6 (1)
I feel that the Buddy is not totally honest about her feelings toward me	2.2 (1.6)
I am confident in the Buddy's ability to help me	5.8 (2.2)
I feel that the Buddy appreciates me	5 (2)
The Buddy and I trust one another	3.8 (2.3)
My relationship with the Buddy is very important to me	4.8 (1.9)
I have the feeling that if I say or do the wrong things, the Buddy will stop working with me	2 (1.2)
I feel the Buddy cares about me even when I do things that she does not approve of	5.4 (2.5)

process the information more easily. One patient also envisioned the potential of this function to facilitate information sharing among their care team, who often work on different time schedules.

Agenda Management. 50 % (n = 4) of patients used the agenda function, recording questions about specific medical terms (e.g. *"What is MRI?"*), events (e.g. lab tests or alarms) and general concerns about their conditions (e.g. *"How can I prevent this?"*). One patient checked off his agenda item as an indication that the item had been resolved. Both patients and providers reported highly positive feedback on the concept of agenda tracking, noting that it allowed the patients to avoid the common problem of forgetting questions without relying on papers or external help from family members. Two patients specifically selected this function as their favorite part of the system and one provider described the idea as *"absolutely fantastic."*

Alarm Detection. An average of 15.3 (SD = 17.8) alarms were detected daily for each patient, triggering an average of 2.4 (SD = 3.7) agent-initiated discussions about alarms per day. In addition to agent-initiated dialogues, two patients proactively initiated their alarm dialogue with the agent. During these alarm conversations, there was only one instance that the patient indicated the detected alarm as a false alarm. While one patient noted that Hospital Buddy could help *"cut down on alarm time ringing,"* the high frequency of the agent-initiated alarm dialogues and the problem of occasionally detecting other patients' alarms sometimes causes confusion and frustration.

Provider Identification. Both patients and providers reported generally positive feedback on the ability to detect provider presence and display their biography, indicating that it acted as a *"great memory aid"* of their medical team. More specifically, one patient noted that she was *"always at the hospital and already know a lot of the people; however, they don't always write their name on the white board in the room."* None of the participants provided any provider ratings.

Sleep Monitoring. Due to technical issues, we were only able to collect sleep records from three patients, with the duration of detected sleep bouts ranging from 2 to 972 min. Only one of the patients provided a sleep quality rating. One patient noted that wearing the Wocket *"was comfortable,"* and that it could provide helpful information to both the patient and the hospital staff. Whether such information could change the behavior of both patients and providers, however, needs further study.

Companionship and Entertainment. Patients appreciated the ability of the Hospital Buddy to provide companionship during their hospital stay: *"She is always there...I know that there is somebody to respond to you right away...somebody next to me, someone to chat with."* Most (75 %, n = 6) patients used the storytelling function, with each of them listening to an average of 2.8 (SD = 1.5) stories during their stay. Patients reported enjoying the stories, which could help calm them down when they were *"feeling bored and depressed with nothing going on,"* as *"it was something to do to keep your mind occupied."*

5   Conclusion

Patients were generally happy with the Hospital Buddy, and used all system functions. As in our pilot study, many patients felt the Buddy provided them with companionship in what otherwise can be an impersonal and bewildering environment. We experienced many technical difficulties with the various sensor systems, leading to a less than enthusiastic response from providers, who expect a high degree of reliability from technology. Future work includes improvements to the sensor systems and a properly powered randomized trial to evaluate the ability of the Hospital Buddy to increase inpatient satisfaction, sleep quality, symptom control, anxiety, loneliness, and depression.

Acknowledgments. This work was funded by CIMIT Consortium grant 12-1035.

References

1. Arora, V., et al.: Ability of hospitalized patients to identify their in-hospital physicians. Arch. Intern. Med. **169**(2), 199–201 (2009)
2. Calkins, D.R., et al.: Patient-physician communication at hospital discharge and patients' understanding of the postdischarge treatment plan. Arch. Intern. Med. **157**(9), 1026–1030 (1997)
3. Kidd, J., et al.: Promoting patient participation in consultations: a randomised controlled trial to evaluate the effectiveness of three patient-focused interventions. Patient Educ. Couns. **52** (1), 107–112 (2004)
4. Olson, D.P., Windish, D.M.: Communication discrepancies between physicians and hospitalized patients. Arch. Intern. Med. **170**(15), 1302–1307 (2010)
5. Bickmore, T., Bukhari, L., Vardoulakis, L.P., Paasche-Orlow, M., Shanahan, C.: Hospital buddy: a persistent emotional support companion agent for hospital patients. In: Nakano, Y., Neff, M., Paiva, A., Walker, M. (eds.) IVA 2012. LNCS, vol. 7502, pp. 492–495. Springer, Heidelberg (2012)
6. Bers, M., et al.: Interactive storytelling environments: coping with cardiac illness at Boston's children's hospital. In: CHI (1998)
7. Bickmore, T., Pfeifer, L., Jack, B.W.: Taking the time to care: empowering low health literacy hospital patients with virtual nurse agents. In: Proceedings of the ACM SIGCHI Conference on Human Factors in Computing Systems (CHI), Boston, MA (2009)
8. Wilcox, L., et al.: Designing patient-centric information displays for hospitals. In: Proceedings of the ACM SIGCHI Conference on Human Factors in Computing Systems (CHI), pp. 1879–1888, Atlanta, GA (2010)
9. Vawdrey, D., et al.: A tablet computer application for patients to participate in their hospital care. AMIA … Annual Symposium Proceedings/AMIA Symposium. AMIA Symposium, 2011, pp. 1428–1435 (2011)
10. Cassell, J., Vilhjálmsson, H., Bickmore, T.: BEAT: the behavior expression animation toolkit. In: SIGGRAPH 2001, Los Angeles, CA (2001)
11. Ware Jr, J.E., Hays, R.D.: Methods for measuring patient satisfaction with specific medical encounters. Med. Care **26**(4), 393–402 (1988)

12. Tranmer, J.E., et al.: The sleep experience of medical and surgical patients. Clin. Nurs. Res. **12**, 159–173 (2003)
13. Intille, S., et al.: Design of a wearable physical activity monitoring system using mobile phones and accelerometers. IEEE Eng. Med. Biol. Soc. (2011)
14. Pollak, C., et al.: How accurately does wrist actigraphy identify the states of sleep and wakefulness? Sleep **24**(8), 957–965 (2001)
15. Iber, C., et al.: The AASM Manual for the Scoring of Sleep and Associated Events: Rules, Terminology, and Technical Specifications, 1st edn. American Academy of Sleep Medicine, Westchester (2007)
16. Sazonov, E., et al.: Activity-based sleep–wake identification in infants. Physiol. Meas. **25**(5), 1291–1304 (2004)
17. Graham, K.C., Cvach, M.: Monitor alarm fatigue: standardizing use of physiological monitors and decreasing nuisance alarms. Am. J. Crit. Care **19**(1), 28–34 (2010)
18. Bruera, E., et al.: The Edmonton symptom assessment system (ESAS): a simple method for the assessment of palliative care patients. J. Palliat. Care **7**(2), 6–9 (1991)
19. Horvath, A., Greenberg, L.: Development and validation of the working alliance inventory. J. Couns. Psychol. **36**(2), 223–233 (1989)

A Motion Style Toolbox

Klaus Förger [✉] and Tapio Takala

Department of Computer Science, Aalto University, Espoo, Finland
{klaus.forger,tapio.takala}@aalto.fi

Abstract. We present a Matlab toolbox for synthesis and visualization of human motion style. The aim is to support development of expressive virtual characters by providing implementations of several style related motion synthesis methods thus allowing side-by-side comparisons. The implemented methods are based on recorded (captured or synthetic) motions, and include linear motion interpolation and extrapolation, style transfer, rotation swapping per body part and per quaternion channel, frequency band scaling and swapping, and Principal/Independent Component Analysis (PCA/ICA) based synthesis and component swapping.

Keywords: Computer animation · Human motion · Motion style · Motion synthesis · Toolbox

1 Introduction

Expressiveness of virtual characters can be vital for many practical applications. Bodily movements are a useful modality for creating expressive behaviors. One approach is to utilize symbolic gestures such as waving a fist or scratching ones head. However, interpreting them may depend on the viewer's cultural background. For this reason, modulating motion style, meaning the manner how a gesture or an action is performed, is an attractive way to create expressive variations of motions. We present a toolbox of Matlab functions for motion capture based synthesis and visualization of human motion style (see Fig. 1 for examples), and a collection of code examples. The visualization technique is a novel way to draw attention to motion style.

The toolbox includes implementations of several methods related to creating new style variations from captured motions. Time warping is also included as a necessary synchronization tool when style variations are based on combining or comparing different motions. 14 code examples of animation techniques are provided portraying cases with best and worst performance. For each case, a short video is included that demonstrates the resulting motions. The package also contains acted examples of hand waving and locomotion performed in varying styles.

The toolbox assumes a hierarchical skeleton structure as in the BioVision Header (BVH) format. The joint rotations are represented by quaternions, and translation of the root with xyz coordinates. In our examples, the motions are

© Springer International Publishing Switzerland 2015
W.-P. Brinkman et al. (Eds.): IVA 2015, LNAI 9238, pp. 343–347, 2015.
DOI: 10.1007/978-3-319-21990-7_36

recorded with the rate of 100 frames per second. We assume that input motions contain the same action and only differ in style. The considered methods enable high level control of style with relatively low computational demands. We exclude methods that require manual key-frame editing or physics simulations, or only concatenate existing motions.

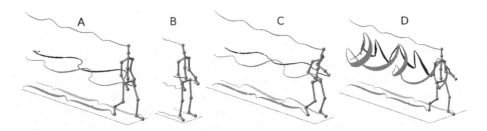

Fig. 1. Walks produced by acting (A), frequency band scaling (B), frequency band swapping (C), and partial joint signal swapping (D). The trajectories indicate velocities.

The toolbox can be used for creating expressive variations of motions, and the included examples may be useful as learning material. When developing new animation methods, the implementations can be used as a baselines to allow comparisons. The toolbox is not readily usable as part of a real-time animation pipeline, but it could be used in finding out what kind of a pipeline allows maximal expressivity. The code is available under an open source BSD license at: http://iki.fi/klaus.forger/motion_style_toolbox/

2   Related Work

Our goal is to allow comparisons between style related motion synthesis methods, and to map and explore types of styles the methods can produce. This is not an easy task based on existing publications. For example, a presented system may combine many techniques such as swapping body parts between motions, interpolation and signal decompositions [6], or apply post-processing to remove produced artifacts [8]. Therefore, we attempt to outline low-level operations which can be separately implemented and evaluated. Selection of methods into the toolbox has been guided by earlier reviews on motion synthesis [4,7].

3   Implemented Methods

If a method takes multiple input motions, time warping is necessary for making corresponding events happen at the same time [7]. We have implemented two versions (see video/code ex_01), one applying a constant warp and another with segmentation.

Linear interpolation is the standard approach for creating ranges of styles by motion blending [7]. We have implemented two versions, one for pairwise interpolation (ex_02) and another for N-way interpolation (ex_03). Both take as parameters the weights of the input motions which must sum to 100 %. Our pairwise implementation is intended for non-repetitive actions and applies the slerp algorithm [9]. For N-way interpolation we have applied normalized linear interpolation (nlerp) instead, as slerp does not generalize to this case. The implementation is optimized for locomotion, and uses segmented time warping.

Extrapolation and style transfer rely on modeling style as numerical differences between motions. The extrapolation extends linear interpolation by allowing the weights of the motions to be under 0 % and over 100 % while still requiring them to sum to 100 %. Style transfer in turn means taking a difference between signals of two motions, scaling it to adjust the amount of style, and adding the result to a third motion. We have implemented pairwise extrapolation (ex_04), style transfer between three motions (ex_05), and N-way extrapolation (ex_06). N-way extrapolation is the most general as it allows combining multiple pairwise interpolations, extrapolations and style transfers.

In interpolation and extrapolation, the weight of each input motion is an adjustable parameter. If a set of motions contains redundant versions of styles, dimensionality reduction can be applied to join the redundant parameters. In this context, we have implemented motion synthesis based on Principal Component Analysis (PCA) (ex_07) and Independent Component Analysis (ICA) (ex_08). These methods differ in the way the input motions are decomposed, but are otherwise identical. The PCA synthesis uses Matlab function *princomp* and the ICA applies decomposition using the *FastICA* library [5]. A further comparison between PCA synthesis and N-way extrapolation shows that our implementations can produce exactly the same sets of motions.

Different frequencies have been suggested to be associated with different motion styles [1]. Thus, scaling part of the frequencies of a motion should affect the perceived styles. We have implemented decomposition into frequency bands as originally described by Bruderlin and Williams [1]. Frequency band scaling (ex_09) can be applied to a single motion and it can produce variations on the size of the motions and styles from stiff to energetic (Fig. 1 B), for example. The frequency bands can also be swapped between motions (ex_10) that allows for example transferring the overall posture from one motion to another (Fig. 1 C).

Swapping signals of joints between motions (ex_11) allows creation of many new style variations with minimal artifacts (Fig. 1 D). However, the joints must be carefully selected as otherwise the swap can break the whole motion. It is also possible to swap individual quaternion channels (ex_12), but this can add shakiness and sudden accelerations to the motions as breaking quaternions apart does not guarantee them to remain of unit length.

PCA and ICA can be used to reduce the number of channels that represent rotations. This can for example combine together joints that rotate similarly. New style variations can be created by swapping part of the motion signals from one motion to another in the reduced space. Our implementation is similar to that described by Shapiro et al. [8], with the exception that we use quaternions instead of joint coordinates. After the dimensionality reduction with PCA (ex_13) and ICA (ex_14), the new signal channels can be swapped between motions. This can create new style variations, but may also result in similar artifacts as in the case of swapping individual quaternion channels.

4   Discussion

The toolbox enables exploration and comparison of a multitude of motion editing methods. For example, it reveals that even simple methods such as swapping rotations between motions can create interesting style variations. Also, there are differences between the usability of the methods as for example it may not be easy to describe in practical terms what styles are affected by editing PCA components. More rigorous comparison of the methods would require perceptual studies and quantitative evaluations of the produced motions [3]. Also, the usefulness of the synthesis methods can differ depending on the final application where they would be used in. For example, a virtual character with a cartoonish representation may benefit from exaggerated motions, while naturalness of the motions may be more important for a realistic character. The toolbox could be especially helpful in expanding expressivity of motion collections containing variedly performed versions of actions [2].

Acknowledgements. This work has been supported by the Kone Foundation through the project Social eMotions, and the Hecse graduate school. We also thank people behind the open source Matlab libraries/functions FastICA, GPMat, Quaternion Toolbox, ScreenCapture, Slerp, and SpinCalc.

References

1. Bruderlin, A., Williams, L.: Motion signal processing. In: Proceedings of the 22nd Annual Conference on Computer Graphics and Interactive Techniques, pp. 97–104. ACM (1995)
2. Carreno-Medrano, P., Gibet, S., Larboulette, C., Marteau, P.-F.: Corpus creation and perceptual evaluation of expressive theatrical gestures. In: Bickmore, T., Marsella, S., Sidner, C. (eds.) IVA 2014. LNCS, vol. 8637, pp. 109–119. Springer, Heidelberg (2014)
3. Förger, K., Takala, T.: Animating with style: defining expressive semantics of motion. The Visual Computer, pp. 1–13 (2015). doi:10.1007/s00371-015-1064-4
4. Geng, W., Yu, G.: Reuse of motion capture data in animation: a review. In: Kumar, V., Gavrilova, M.L., Tan, C.J.K., L'Ecuyer, P. (eds.) ICCSA 2003. LNCS, vol. 2669, pp. 620–629. Springer, Heidelberg (2003)
5. Hyvärinen, A.: Fast and robust fixed-point algorithms for independent component analysis. IEEE Trans. Neural Netw. **10**(3), 626–634 (1999)
6. Kim, Y., Neff, M.: Component-based locomotion composition. In: Proceedings of the ACM SIGGRAPH/Eurographics Symposium on Computer Animation, pp. 165–173. Eurographics Association (2012)

7. Pejsa, T., Pandzic, I.S.: State of the art in example-based motion synthesis for virtual characters in interactive applications. In: Computer Graphics Forum. vol. 29, pp. 202–226. Blackwell Publishing (2010)
8. Shapiro, A., Cao, Y., Faloutsos, P.: Style components. In: Proceedings of Graphics Interface 2006, pp. 33–39. Canadian Information Processing Society (2006)
9. Shoemake, K.: Animating rotation with quaternion curves. SIGGRAPH Comput. Graph. **19**(3), 245–254 (1985)

A Collaborative Human-Robot Game as a Test-bed for Modelling Multi-party, Situated Interaction

Gabriel Skantze[(⊠)], Martin Johansson, and Jonas Beskow

Department of Speech Music and Hearing, KTH, Stockholm, Sweden
{skantze,vhmj,beskow}@kth.se

Abstract. In this demonstration we present a test-bed for collecting data and testing out models for multi-party, situated interaction between humans and robots. Two users are playing a collaborative card sorting game together with the robot head Furhat. The cards are shown on a touch table between the players, thus constituting a target for joint attention. The system has been exhibited at the Swedish National Museum of Science and Technology during nine days, resulting in a rich multi-modal corpus with users of mixed ages.

1 Introduction

Recently, there has been an increased interest in understanding and modelling multi-party, situated interaction between humans and robots [1–5]. To develop such models, we think that a test-bed is needed in which data can be collected, and which can be used to test out data-driven models based on this data. The test-bed should be robust enough to be used in a public setting, where a large number of interactions with naïve users can be recorded. In this paper (and demonstration), we present a dialog system that was exhibited during nine days at the Swedish National Museum of Science and Technology, in November 2014.[1] As can be seen in Fig. 1, two visitors at a time could play a collaborative game together with the robot head Furhat [1]. On the touch table between the players, a set of cards are shown. The two visitors and Furhat are given the task of sorting the cards according to some criterion. For example, the task could be to sort a set of inventions in the order they were invented, or a set of animals by how fast they can run. This is a collaborative game, which means that the visitors have to discuss the solution together with Furhat. However, Furhat does not have perfect knowledge about the solution. Instead, Furhat's behaviour is motivated by a randomized belief model. This means that the visitors have to determine whether they should trust Furhat's belief or not, just like they have to do with each other. Thus, Furhat's role in the interaction is similar to that of the visitors, as opposed to for example a tutor role which is often given to robots in similar settings [4].

We think that this setup has several features that makes it useful as a test-bed for collecting data and testing out models for multi-party situated interaction. Firstly, it has proven to be fairly robust against speech recognition errors, since the multi-modal

---

[1] A video of the interaction can be seen at https://www.youtube.com/watch?v=5fhjuGu3d0I.

© Springer International Publishing Switzerland 2015
W.-P. Brinkman et al. (Eds.): IVA 2015, LNAI 9238, pp. 348–351, 2015.
DOI: 10.1007/978-3-319-21996-7_37

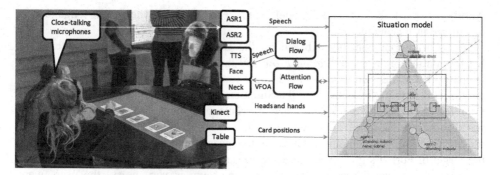

Fig. 1. A schematic illustration of the setting and architecture

nature of the setup allows the system to fall back on other modalities (head pose and movement of the cards) and still take part in a meaningful interaction. This is further enhanced by the multi-party setup which allows the visitors to have a meaningful discussion with each other even in cases where Furhat's understanding is limited. Secondly, the symmetry of such a setting allow us to compare the human behaviour towards each other with their behaviour towards the robot in order to (1) use the data as a model for Furhat's behaviour, (2) investigate to what extent they interact with the robot as if it was a human interlocutor, and (3) evaluate how human-like the robot's current behaviour is, and how it could be improved [3]. A third important feature of this setup is that it involves discussion about objects in the physical space, where the interlocutors' visual focus of attention (VFOA) must be shared between each other and the objects under discussion, which has a clear effect on their turn-taking behaviour [3]. Many previous studies on multi-party interaction have mainly focused on interactions where this is not the case [2, 5].

2   System Description

The system was implemented using the open source dialogue system framework IrisTK[2] [6] and is schematically illustrated in Fig. 1. The visitors are interacting with the Furhat robot head [1], which has an animated face back-projected on a translucent mask, as well as a mechanical neck, which allows Furhat to signal his focus of attention using a combination of head pose and eye-gaze. A Kinect camera (V2) is used to track the location and rotation of the two users' heads, as well as their hands. The low-level events from the different sensors (Kinect, Touch table and ASR) are sent to a *Situation model*, which translates the local coordinates to a common 3D representation, and then generates high-level events for the combined sensory data. This way, speech recognition results from the microphones can be mapped to the right users based on their location, regardless of whether it is a microphone array or a close-talking microphone.

---

[2] http://www.iristk.net.

Another task of the Situation model is to keep track of when users engage and disengage in the interaction.

Two behaviour controllers based on the Harel statechart mechanism offered by IrisTK run in parallel: The *Dialog Flow* and the *Attention Flow*. The Attention Flow keeps Furhat's attention to a specified target (one or both users, or a card), even when the target is moving, by consulting the Situation model. The 3D position of the target is then transformed into neck and gaze movement of Furhat (again taking Furhat's position in the 3D space into account). This, together with the 3D design of Furhat, makes it possible to maintain exclusive mutual gaze with the users, and to let them infer the target of Furhat's gaze when directed towards the cards, in order to maintain joint attention [1]. Since the public setting of a museum is very noisy, the users were wearing close-talking microphones. The speech recognition is done with two parallel cloud-based large vocabulary speech recognizers, which allows Furhat to understand the users even when they are talking simultaneously.

The Dialogue Flow module orchestrates the spoken interaction, based on input from the speech recognizers, together with events from the Situation model (such as cards being moved, or someone leaving or entering the interaction). The head pose of the users is used to determine whether they are addressing Furhat, and he should contribute to the discussion, or whether they are discussing with each other, and he should just provide backchannels to signal that he is still keeping track of what they are saying. In order to provide meaningful comments about the cards being discussed, The Dialog Flow maintains a *focus stack*. Cards are primed in the focus stack when their names are detected in the speech recognition, or when they are being moved. Since Furhat's role should be similar to that of the visitors', and therefore not have perfect knowledge, his behaviour is motivated by a randomized belief model. This is generated by taking the correct value (e.g. *speed* or *year*) for each card and then apply a random distortion. In addition, a random standard deviation is calculated for each belief, which represents Furhat's confidence in his belief. The outcome of these parameters is governed by two constants: *Ignorance* and *Uncertainty*, which may be used to tune Furhat's general behaviour. This belief model can be used to allow Furhat to compare two cards using a Z-test and assess his belief about their order and his confidence in this belief, which will in turn affect his choice of words. For example, he could say "I am quite sure the kangaroo is faster than the elephant", or "I have no idea whether the telescope was invented before the printing press".

3   Discussion and Future Work

During the 9 days the system was exhibited at the Swedish National Museum of Science and Technology, we recorded data from 373 interactions with the system, with an average length of 4.5 min. The dataset contains mixed ages: both adults playing with each other (40 %), children playing with adults (27 %), and children playing with each other (33 %). After completing one game, the players could choose to continue playing. 58 % of the pairs who completed the first game chose to do so.

In the current setting, most of Furhat's behaviour is motivated by hand-crafted policies that were tuned during extensive testing. However, we think that the setup described in this paper serves as a very useful test-bed for collecting data on situated interaction (as we have done), and then use this data to build data-driven models for Furhat's behaviour. The test-bed then allows us to evaluate these models in the same setting that the data was collected. The models we are working on include detection of turn-taking relevant places based on a large range of multi-modal cues (e.g. head pose, words, prosody, movement of cards). Another interesting problem is to determine where Furhat's visual focus of attention should be. Since we have data on the users' attentional behaviour (approximated by head pose), and their roles are similar to that of Furhat's, this could be used to guide a data-driven model.

The exhibition at the museum also showed that both children and adults enjoyed the game, with several of them coming back to play more. We therefore think that the game could be a useful application in its own right, for example in an educational setting. The simple game concept (sorting of cards) allows the content to be easily customized for a particular subject.

Acknowledgements. This work is supported by the Swedish research council (VR) project *Incremental processing in multimodal conversational systems* (2011-6237) and *KTH ICT-The Next Generation*. Thanks to everyone helping out with the exhibition: Saeed Dabbaghchian, Björn Granström, Joakim Gustafson, Raveesh Meena, Kalin Stefanov and Preben Wik.

References

1. Al Moubayed, S., Skantze, G., Beskow, J.: The furhat back-projected humanoid head - lip reading, gaze and multiparty interaction. Int. J. Humanoid Rob. **10**(1), 25 (2013)
2. Bohus, D., Horvitz, E.: Decisions about turns in multiparty conversation: from perception to action. In: ICMI 2011 Proceedings of the 13th International Conference on Multimodal Interfaces, pp. 153–160 (2011)
3. Johansson, M., Skantze, G., Gustafson, J.: Comparison of human-human and human-robot turn-taking behaviour in multi-party situated interaction. In: International Workshop on Understanding and Modeling Multiparty, Multimodal Interactions, at ICMI 2014. Istanbul, Turkey (2014)
4. Al Moubayed, S., Beskow, J., Bollepalli, B., Hussen-Abdelaziz, A., Johansson, M., Koutsombogera, M., Lopes, J., Novikova, J., Oertel, C., Skantze, G., Stefanov, K., Varol, G.: Tutoring Robots: Multiparty multimodal social dialogue with an embodied tutor. In: Proceedings of eNTERFACE2013. Springer, Heidelberg (2014)
5. Mutlu, B., Kanda, T., Forlizzi, J., Hodgins, J., Ishiguro, H.: Conversational gaze mechanisms for humanlike robots. ACM Trans. Interact. Intell. Syst. **1**(2), 12:1–12:33 (2012)
6. Skantze, G., Al Moubayed, S.: IrisTK: a statechart-based toolkit for multi-party face-to-face interaction. In: Proceedings of ICMI. Santa Monica, CA (2012)

The Affective Storyteller: Using Character Emotion to Influence Narrative Generation

Frank Kaptein and Joost Broekens$^{(\boxtimes)}$

TU Delft, Interactive Intelligence, Delft, The Netherlands
joost.broekens@gmail.com
http://ii.tudelft.nl/

Abstract. We present the Affective Storyteller, a narrative generation framework that combines storytelling and emotion. With this framework we propose to address two main challenges in narrative generation: customization, and, reduced calculation time. Our solution is based on the fact that narrative generation in the Affective Storyteller is influenced by an analysis of the emotional patterns of the synthetic characters in the stories. These emotions are simulated using GAMYGDALA.

Keywords: Narrative generation · Storytelling · Emotion

1 Introduction

A story is the presentation of a series of logically and chronologically related events that are caused or experienced by actors [1]. Storytelling is a powerful tool to influentially communicate information [5,11] in fields including entertainment, education, health care, advertising, training and argumentation [10]. Narratologists define a differentiation between the generation of the story events and the manner in which these are presented [9], it is referred to as fabula and presentation [1]. *Fabula* is the chronological order of all events that occur in the story. It can be presented in different ways. Examples are: speech, writing and movies.

Narrative generation is about the aim to have computers automatically generate stories (for review see [4]). Computers are capable of generating multiple story lines each with the same message but told differently. This improves replay value (retelling the story to the same user) and personalizing the story to a particular user [9]. By using simulated emotions of virtual characters, this research proposes a method to improve the generation efficiency and to enable customization of the story.

1.1 Emotions in Synthetic Storytelling

Emotion can be used to measure the user and steer the story based on those emotions, or to model the emotions of the virtual characters [3,14]. We focus on

© Springer International Publishing Switzerland 2015
W.-P. Brinkman et al. (Eds.): IVA 2015, LNAI 9238, pp. 352–355, 2015.
DOI: 10.1007/978-3-319-21996-7_38

this second approach. The success of a story is dependent on the understandability and believability of its characters [8], characters need emotions to be believable [2]. The work in [7] tries to identify how affective characters should be configured. This approach is also seen in the way the virtual storyteller uses emotional modeling [12,13].

2   Challenges in Narrative Generation

There are two challenges that we consider here. The first is *efficiency*: computation time grows exponentially in the size of the story domain. Heuristics are needed that can reject story paths before completely calculating them. The second is *customization*: how to make different versions of the same story, for example to facilitate replay or personal style of the reader. In this research we propose to use the characters' simulated emotions to address these challenges.

3   Approach

We have developed the *Affective Storyteller*, a domain independent system that uses GAMYGDALA [6] to generate character emotions. These emotions are used to improve on the previously mentioned challenges.

3.1   Customization of Story Affect

The narrative generation problem in the Affective storyteller starts with the user defining a domain. The Affective storyteller then calculates all possible event sequences that lead to the defined finishing state of the story. These event sequences differ in storyline, and character emotions. The problem we address here is how to find the subset of event sequences that fit particular affective preferences.

In every event sequence the GAMYGDALA-calculated emotions for the different characters are measured and logged. These are then used to sort the stories. The user is presented an emotion panel that shows all *occurring* emotions in the characters during the story. The panel makes it possible to change the importance of these emotions. When a user for example increases the importance for Joy, then the Affective storyteller will search for stories that have more joy occurring in them. Currently, a user can choose these values for the first half and the second half separately, but we anticipate extending this with regular expression-like functionality that can be used to filter the story.

The Affective storyteller uses GAMYGDALA to generate 16 different emotions after both the first and second half of the story, being a total of 32 measurements for each event sequence. The user chooses for every emotion, for both halves of the story, how important this occurrence is to him on a scale from 0 to 1. This again results in a total of 32 numbers. We use a normalized dot product of these two vectors as a value function for the different event sequences. In Eq. 1

EI stands for emotion intensity, EC is the emotion congruency as defined by the user, and Gain is a constant set by the user defining how aggressive the intensity dampening is.

$$Value(Seq) = \sum_{i=1}^{32} \left\{ \left(\frac{EI_i * gain}{EI_i * gain + 1} \right) * EC_i \right\}.$$ (1)

When the fabula generation has been affectively customized, the best matching story is transformed in a written text communicating the events with their main affective consequences.

3.2 Efficiency

The fabula generation method as explained in Sect. 3.1 starts by calculating all possible story-paths and then sorts these based on the similarity of their emotion pattern and the user preference. Addressing the performance problem (Sect. 2), we show as a proof of concept heuristic (in our case, and as an example, based on conflict between the characters) enhances efficiency. Conflict between two characters means they perform actions that are undesirable for the other. GAMYGDALA generates anger for these type of actions, which means that stories with insufficient anger should be pruned.

In Table 1 the calculation time of the pruning algorithm is compared with that of the complete breadth first search. The algorithms are tested on an example domain where idle actions are incrementally added. These idle actions can occur once in the story but at every moment of the story. Initially the breadth first search is quicker because it does not have the overhead of calculating the emotions of the characters. However, because the number of possible paths grows exponentially and this pruning heuristic decreases the exponent, the computation time of the emotionally-pruned algorithm quickly outperforms the classic breadth-first algorithm.

Table 1. Time of calculation. Method 1 prunes on anger to reduce the search space. Method 2 saves time by skipping emotion calculations.

	Initial domain	1 Idle action	2 Idle action	3 Idle action
Prune on anger	2,27 sec	5,31 sec	8,57 sec	12,25 sec
Breadthfirst without emotions	0,04 sec	0,27 sec	7,26 sec	26 min; 31 sec

4   Discussion and Future Work

We have proposed a framework that affectively models the story-characters to customize stories and improve the efficiency of their generation. These emotions can be used to filter the set of generated stories, either during or after generation of the set. In both cases, it is important to be able to correctly represent the emotional patterns one is looking for in a story. Now we used a simple vector-based filter method, but we anticipate using a regular expression type of filtering so that more complex patterns can be found, which is especially useful in longer stories. Further, we have shown that it is possible to optimize the story generation process by pruning on emotional filters. When the domain becomes more complex, this will dramatically reduce processing time. Although there is much more work to be done on the exploration of emotion patterns in stories, in particular verification of the perceived story quality, we conclude based on our current work that emotion simulation is a promising direction to address planning complexity and story customization.

References

1. Bal, M., Van Boheemen, C.: Narratology: Introduction to the Theory of Narrative. University of Toronto Press, Toronto (2009)
2. Bates, J., et al.: The role of emotion in believable agents. Commun. ACM **37**(7), 122–125 (1994)
3. Cavazza, M., Pizzi, D., Charles, F., Vogt, T., André, E.: Emotional input for character-based interactive storytelling. In: Proceedings of The 8th International Conference on Autonomous Agents and Multiagent Systems, vol. 1, pp. 313–320. International Foundation for Autonomous Agents and Multiagent Systems (2009)
4. Gervás, P.: Computational approaches to storytelling and creativity. AI Mag. **30**(3), 49–62 (2009)
5. Mar, R.A., Oatley, K., Djikic, M., Mullin, J.: Emotion and narrative fiction: interactive influences before, during, and after reading. Cogn. Emot. **25**(5), 818–833 (2011). http://www.ncbi.nlm.nih.gov/pubmed/21824023
6. Popescu, A., Broekens, J., van Someren, M.: GAMYGDALA: an emotion engine for games. IEEE Trans. Affect. Comput. **5**(1), 32–44 (2014). http://ieeexplore.ieee.org/lpdocs/epic03/wrapper.htm?arnumber=6636311
7. Rank, S., Hoffmann, S., Struck, H.G., Spierling, U., Petta, P.: Creativity in configuring affective agents for interactive storytelling. In: International conference on computational creativity, p. 165 (2012)
8. Riedl, M.O., Young, R.M.: An objective character believability evaluation procedure for multi-agent story generation systems. In: Panayiotopoulos, T., Gratch, J., Aylett, R.S., Ballin, D., Olivier, P., Rist, T. (eds.) IVA 2005. LNCS (LNAI), vol. 3661, pp. 278–291. Springer, Heidelberg (2005)
9. Riedl, M.O., Young, R.M.: Narrative planning: balancing plot and character. J. Artif. Int. Res. **39**, 217–268 (2010)
10. Riedl, M.O., Bulitko, V.: Interactive narrative: an intelligent systems approach. AI Mag. **34**(1), 67 (2012)
11. Simmons, A.: The story factor: Secrets of Influence from the Art of Storytelling. Basic Books, New York (2006)
12. Swartjes, I., Theune, M.: A fabula model for emergent narrative. In: Göbel, S., Malkewitz, R., Iurgel, I. (eds.) TIDSE 2006. LNCS, vol. 4326, pp. 49–60. Springer, Heidelberg (2006)
13. Theune, M., Rensen, S., den op Akker, R., Heylen, D., Nijholt, A.: Emotional characters for automatic plot creation. In: Göbel, S., Spierling, U., Hoffmann, A., Iurgel, I., Schneider, O., Dechau, J., Feix, A. (eds.) TIDSE 2004. LNCS, vol. 3105, pp. 95–100. Springer, Heidelberg (2004)
14. Zhao, H.: Emotion in interactive storytelling. In: FDG, pp. 183–189 (2013)

Prototyping User Interfaces
for Investigating the Role of Virtual Agents
in Human-Machine Interaction
A Demonstration in the Domain of Cooperative Games

Nikita Mattar[✉], Herwin van Welbergen, Philipp Kulms, and Stefan Kopp

AG Social Cognitive Systems, Faculty of Technology, CITEC,
Bielefeld University, Bielefeld, Germany
{nmattar,hvanwelbergen,pkulms,skopp}@techfak.uni-bielefeld.de

Abstract. To investigate how different levels of embodiment or variations of a task affect the performance or perception of an interaction, researchers need tools that enable them to effortlessly modify such aspects. We demonstrate the MultiPro framework that allows for fast and easy prototyping of applications that are to be used in the context of human-machine interaction research. In conjunction with a newly developed cooperative game scenario we show how different configurations with and without an embodied agent can be configures and how the agent's behavior can be adapted.

Keywords: Intelligent virtual agents · Human-machine interaction · User Interfaces · Prototyping · Framework · BML

1 Introduction

To be able to analyze key characteristics of human-agent interactions, frameworks are needed that allow to investigate factors that shape the interaction in a systematic fashion. For example, common research questions are: How is an interaction perceived, e.g., in terms of trust, and how does a human perform on a given task when different levels of embodiment are presented (e.g., none vs. chat window vs. virtual agent)? Existing frameworks focus on virtual agent capabilities and generation of behavior in different application scenarios (cf. ICT Virtual Human Toolkit, [1]). However, how to integrate embodied virtual agents into classical task environments based on, e.g., the desktop metaphor is still challenging. Therefore, we adopt a different approach by focusing on the combination of virtual agents with classical user interface elements. Thus, strengths of human-like interaction capabilities of virtual agents and accuracy and efficiency of WIMP-based elements (e.g., text fields, buttons) can be utilized.

2 MultiPro – A Framework for Prototyping Virtual Agent Applications

Kulms et al. [3] introduced the MultiPro (Multimodal Interaction Prototyping) framework that allows for fast and easy prototyping of applications that are to

© Springer International Publishing Switzerland 2015
W.-P. Brinkman et al. (Eds.): IVA 2015, LNAI 9238, pp. 356–360, 2015.
DOI: 10.1007/978-3-319-21996-7_39

be used in the context of human-agent interactions, combining embodied virtual agents with traditional UI elements. In MultiPro, UI and application logic can easily be adapted by modifying a SCXML[1]-based statechart without having to dive into the sourcecode of the application itself, as statecharts, and thereby the main interaction logic, can be defined using a graphical statechart editor. Adding an embodied virtual agent corresponds to a simple modification of an underlying UI metafile.

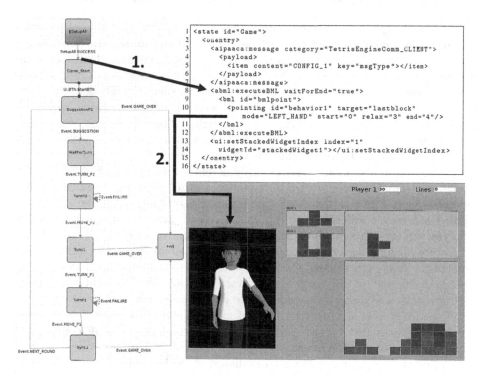

Fig. 1. In the MultiPro framework, user interface and application logic are controlled through a statechart (left). Besides updating the UI from within the statechart given certain events, messages can be broadcasted to different components to control their behavior. For example, on entry of a node (1) a BML message can be send to the virtual agent resulting in a hand movement (2).

Figure 1 depicts an exemplary setup consisting of a QT application with an embedded BML-controlled virtual agent [4] and a game engine widget connected through MultiPro's statechart representation. UI events like button clicks, as well as events produced by connected components or optional sensor hardware,

---

[1] http://www.w3.org/TR/scxml/.

can trigger state transitions in the statechart. By attaching actions to events, the UI as well as the behavior of other components can be manipulated. For example, behavior of the agent can be defined by adding BML to a certain state transition within the statechart. Whenever the corresponding transition occurs, the action is forwarded to the agent's sub-component using a communication middleware.

3   Demo Scenario: Cooperative Interaction Game

As part of a larger research program that studies the determinants of cooperation in human-agent interaction, we have developed an interaction framework in which we can operationalize, manipulate and analyze the relevant factors and key characteristics of cooperative behavior in a systematic fashion [2]. The general setting is that two partners solve a puzzle game interactively. The game consists of a board where blocks of various shapes need to be placed, using horizontal movements and rotation (see Fig. 1, bottom right). The core engine of the game is written in Java and allows for different configurations, e.g., whether blocks are colored or blocks move down gradually. Using MultiPro, different versions of the game can be obtained by providing different statecharts with different configurations. Thus enabling us to, for example, examine the impact of the agent's behavior on the interaction (task performance or perception of the agent), by using BML that corresponds to different levels of advice-giving or multimodal behavior when commenting on its or the human player's moves.

Figure 2 depicts two statecharts (simplified) that correspond to different versions of the game: statechart (a) corresponds to an asymmetric setup of the game with two different player roles, a recommender and a decider, while statechart (b) represents a symmetric version where both players have the same task.

Consider statechart (a): On start of the application, a configuration message that is attached to the *SetupAll*-node is broadcasted to all components (here: QT application, virtual agent architecture, and puzzle game engine). By exploiting the aforementioned middleware-based communication, synchronization between the different components is achieved. On success a state transition to *Game_Start* occurs. The game begins after the user presses a certain button, thereby generating the *UI.BTN.StartBTN* event. Depending on the state, e.g., whether it is the user's (*P1*-nodes) or the agent's (*P2*-nodes) turn, certain UI elements are (de)activated throughout the game, thus guiding the interaction. For example, state *SuggestionP1* corresponds to the user's move of suggesting a block to the agent. On entry of the node, keyboard input is activated within the QT application enabling the user to choose a block. When the user confirms the selection, an event *SUGGESTION* is generated leading to a state transition from *SuggestionP1* to *WaitForTurn* and keyboard input is deactivated again. If it is the agent's turn (e.g., node *TurnP2*), a message is broadcasted to the corresponding component and the statechart remains in the respective state until an appropriate event is generated.

In our demo we will illustrate the capabilities of the MultiPro framework in conjunction with our puzzle game scenario. We will demonstrate how different

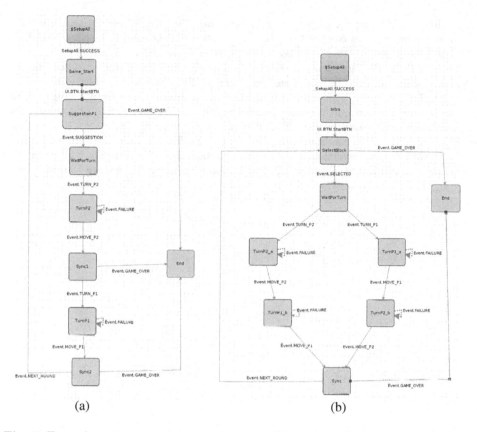

(a)   (b)

Fig. 2. Exemplary statecharts representing two different versions of the underlying puzzle game.

configurations and interactions with and without an embodied agent can be obtained and how the agent's behavior can be adapted within the statechart.

Acknowledgements. This research was supported by the German Federal Ministry of Education and Research (BMBF) within the Leading-Edge Cluster 'it's OWL', managed by the Project Management Agency Karlsruhe (PTKA), as well as by the Deutsche Forschungsgemeinschaft (DFG) within the Center of Excellence 277 'Cognitive Interaction Technology' (CITEC). The authors are responsible for the contents of this publication.

References

1. Hartholt, A., Traum, D., Marsella, S.C., Shapiro, A., Stratou, G., Leuski, A., Morency, L.-P., Gratch, J.: All together now. In: Aylett, R., Krenn, B., Pelachaud, C., Shimodaira, H. (eds.) IVA 2013. LNCS, vol. 8108, pp. 368–381. Springer, Heidelberg (2013)

2. Kulms, P., Mattar, N., Kopp, S.: An interaction game framework for the investigation of human-agent cooperation. In: Brinkman, W.P., Broekens, J., Heylen, D.K.J. (eds.) Intelligent Virtual Agents. Springer, Heidelberg (2015)
3. Kulms, P., van Welbergen, H., Kopp, S.: Prototyping von intuitiven und interaktiven Benutzerschnittstellen: Schnelles und einfaches Design von Anwendungen mit virtuellen Agenten [Prototyping of intuitive and interactive interfaces: Easily designing virtual agent applications], pp. 30–38. Technische Unterstützungssysteme, die die Menschen wirklich wollen, Helmut-Schmidt-Universität (2014)
4. van Welbergen, H., Yaghoubzadeh, R., Kopp, S.: AsapRealizer 2.0: the next steps in fluent behavior realization for ECAs. In: Bickmore, T., Marsella, S., Sidner, C. (eds.) IVA 2014. LNCS, vol. 8637, pp. 449–462. Springer, Heidelberg (2014)

Turn-Taking

Regulating Turn-Taking in Multi-child Spoken Interaction

Samer Al Moubayed[✉] and Jill Lehman

Disney Research, Pittsburgh, PA, USA
{samer,jill.lehman}@disneyresearch.com

Abstract. We examine the effects of coordinated head and eye movement on children's turn-taking behavior in the context of a multiparty game. Twenty-two pairs of children competed in a trivia quiz scenario that is moderated first by a human and later by a robot. We quantify the effects of eyes-only and combined head-eye movements on the turn-taking behavior of the children in both directed and open questions (where either child is free to respond to win the point), and compare the results to performance with the human moderator who uses natural head and eye movements as well as additional cues that can be relevant to turn-taking. We find that coordinated head and eye movement in the robot is a significantly more successful cueing strategy than eye movement alone in directed questions, producing turn regulation that is comparable to the human moderator's more complex behaviors. Further, in open questions, head gaze results in more balanced turn taking than eye movement alone. Finally, we compare the results for children to comparable studies with adults and discuss the implications for developing computational models of joint-attention in human-agent spoken interactions.

Keywords: Multiparty interaction · Turn-taking · Head eyes coordination · Child-robot interaction · Behavior synthesis · Spoken dialog systems

1 Introduction

In areas as diverse as education, entertainment, therapy, and companionship, intelligent virtual characters and robots are demonstrating significant progress in interactive skills, resulting in the potential for more complex and successful applications. As the technology matures, awareness of the physical environment and the cognitive, affective and social state of the user becomes increasingly important; bringing intelligent agents into real-life situations demands skills for controlling the interaction in socially appropriate ways. In spoken interactions in particular, it is critical that animated characters and robots be able to regulate turn-taking in a way that is natural and fluent, even when the environment includes several users and multiple objects of discourse.

Early research identified several functions of gaze (the combination of eye and head movement) in interaction. Kendon's work on gaze direction in conversation (Kendon 1967) is foundational and inspired a wealth of studies that singled out gaze as one of the strongest non-vocal cues in human face-to-face interaction (e.g., Argyle and Cook 1976). Kleinke noted the association of gaze to a variety of functions within social

© Springer International Publishing Switzerland 2015
W.-P. Brinkman et al. (Eds.): IVA 2015, LNAI 9238, pp. 363–374, 2015.
DOI: 10.1007/978-3-319-21996-7_40

interaction: providing information, regulating interaction, expressing intimacy, exercising social control, and facilitating service and task goals (Kleinke 1986). The human-computer interaction community has built on this groundwork, recognizing the importance of modelling gaze in artificial personas such as embodied conversational agents (ECAs) (e.g., Takeuchi and Nagao 1993; Bilvi and Pelachaud 2003).

The use of verbal and nonverbal cues for regulating turn-taking in multiparty dialog has also been studied extensively, although primarily in adult interactions. Research in the area has focused on visual signals such as eye and head movements as central to addressee identification, and as modulating influences on turn-holding, turn-releasing, and speaker prediction. Recent systems have concretely demonstrated the importance of these cues in maintaining fluent dialog in multiparty tasks (e.g. Bohus and Horvitz 2010; Al Moubayed et al. 2013).

Multiparty spoken interaction with children has been less explored (although see Gustafson et al. 2004; Swartout et al. 2010; Lehman 2014). With respect to education, entertainment and therapy, children represent a unique and interesting demographic because children's language behavior changes in complex ways over time as a function of biological maturation, general cognitive development and experience. Agents that are intended to fluently interact in multi-child applications cannot assume that children of all ages have the same capabilities or that their capabilities mirror adult competence. Despite this potential variability, agents must be able to perceive, interpret, and generate regulatory signals that maintain the fluency of the interaction and efficiency of the task, without compromising the children's engagement.

In this study, we explore the use of coordinated eye and head movement in the regulation of turn-taking during a verbal quiz game played by two children and either a robot or human moderator. The robot's multimodal dialog system is programmed to ask each child questions cued by inclusive or exclusive gaze or eye movement alone. The children's success in responding appropriately under each condition is further contrasted with their success in a comparable human-moderated game.

2   A Spoken Multiparty Quiz Game

A multiparty trivia game provides a familiar and natural format within which cueing strategies can be studied. By explaining and enforcing specific rules regarding how questions are to be answered, we can systematically vary cues on a question-by-question basis. In this study, players competed in games that consisted of two rounds of eight questions each. With a fixed number of questions, tie outcomes were possible.

The moderator began by introducing the activity as a Disney trivia game, and specified the rules by telling the children to *"Answer the question as fast as you can, but remember that you are not allowed to answer the question if it is not directed to you"*. The instructions assume that if the player believes that the question is directed toward him/her, and the player knows the answer, then the player will take the turn and answer the question. Alternatively, if the player knows the answer but believes that the question is not directed to her/him, s/he will wait for the other player to answer it.

The game has two types of questions: open and directed. Open questions are addressed to both players and both children have the right to take the turn to answer. Directed questions, on the other hand, are meant for a specific child. The addressee may answer freely, but the other child must wait. If the child who is not addressed responds, it is considered a turn-taking error.

Typical behavior by the moderator of a standard quiz game might include explicit linguistic cues to indicate the target recipient of a question (e.g., "The next question is for you, Jessie," or "This question is for both of you"). Because our goal is to examine the usefulness and power of nonverbal visual cues for regulating turn-taking, the moderators in our quiz game did not use linguistic cues to indicate addressee, but instead began each question with a neutral phrase such as, "Ok, next question". The moderator continued by stating the question itself (e.g., "What is the color of Mickey's shorts?"), followed by three possible answers in random order (e.g., "Red? Yellow? Or blue?"), then paused to wait for an answer. When one of the addressed players answered the question, the moderator gave a point to the speaker if the answer was right or else turned and offered the other player the chance to respond. If, however, the unaddressed player answered the question (a turn-taking error), the moderator informed that player that the question was not directed to him/her (e.g., "It is not your turn," or "Wait for your turn"), then turned and gave the other player a chance. In cases of no response from either player, the moderator either repeated the question or insisted that the player(s) take a guess. The moderator also repeated the question if a player requested it.

3 Experimental Conditions

Within the general framework described above, game variations were implemented to contrast human and robot cues and to test the efficacy of eye versus combined head-eye movement in regulating turn-taking by the robot moderator.

3.1 Natural Movement

The *natural movement* condition was implemented by a human game moderator, who was an informed confederate instructed to regulate the interaction and designate addressee with natural gaze and nonverbal signals such as facial expression and prosody, but without using hand gestures or explicit verbal reference. To make the *natural* and *programmed* conditions comparable, the human's moderating behavior was controlled by a touch interface on a laptop placed in front of her. As shown in Fig. 1, the interface presented the target addressee(s) for the question, one of the randomly ordered questions along with its three randomly ordered answers (the correct answer in red), and buttons to award points to one or both players for a correct response.

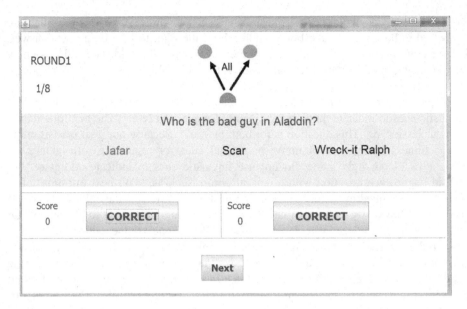

Fig. 1. The interface used by the human game moderator.

3.2 Programmed Movement

The *programmed movement* condition was implemented using an anthropomorphic robot head, named Sammy, as the game moderator (Furhat Robotics, furhatrobotics. com). The head has proportions similar to that of an average adult, and uses rear-projected facial animation on a 3D-printed mask, giving fine-grained control and natural movement to the eyes in synchrony with the head. It is powered by a neck with two degrees of freedom, allowing for accurate head pose on the vertical and horizontal axes. The system's fidelity in delivering gaze targets that are accurately perceived has been previously established (Al Moubayed and Skantze 2011; Al Moubayed et al. 2012a). Although the robot has an integrated speech recognizer, the robot's natural language understanding was wizarded by a human experimenter using an interface similar to the human moderator's, allowing the wizard to provide high-level input to guide the robot throughout its interaction.

Sammy's interaction with and regulation of the players was effected through a dialog system authored with IrisTK (Skantze and Al Moubayed 2012). The dialog system employed a person-tracking module using Microsoft Kinect™ to provide accurate coordinates of the two players in real-time, which in turn allowed the robot to gaze accurately at the intended player.

The dialog system followed the same interaction flow as the human moderator. Sammy began by introducing the game and repeating the turn-taking rule, then presented the question set in random order, under different visual cueing conditions. When a player answered a question, the wizard used the interface to indicate which player answered (left-side or right-side) and whether the answer was correct or not. In the case of a directed question, if the wrong player answered, the wizard clicked the "wrong player" button, causing the robot to point out the turn-taking error in a way that was similar to the human moderator.

As in the *natural movement* condition, questions delivered with *programmed movement* could be directed or open. Additionally, the intended addressee(s) could be cued either with full gaze (coordinated eye and head movement) or through eye movement alone. The physical cues associated with each of these four sub-conditions are shown in Fig. 2 and discussed below.

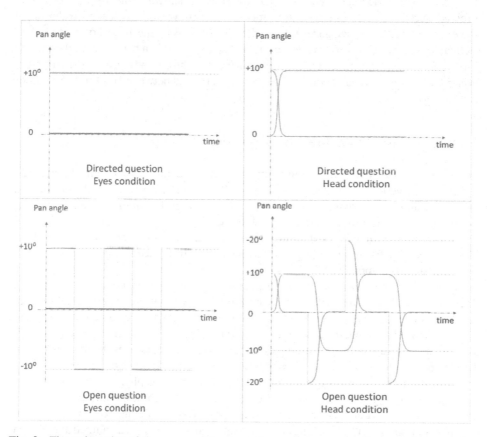

Fig. 2. The trajectories of the eyes and head rotation over the course of one spoken question under the four *programmed movement* sub-conditions. Plots assume that the two participants are standing at -10 and +10 degrees from the robot. Single blue lines represent horizontal angular rotation of the head, double orange lines represent the rotation of the eyes in relation to the head. *Top left*: Eyes-only condition in a directed question where the head remains stationary between the two players and the eyes are rotated toward the addressee. *Top right*: Head-eyes condition in a directed question where an eye saccade establishes mutual gaze and is followed by head rotation. *Bottom left*: Eyes-only condition in an open question to both players where the eyes alternate between the players, and the head is static. *Bottom right*: Head-eyes in an open question to both players where a saccade and following rotation alternates head movements between the two. In all conditions the sum of the eye and head rotation angle equals the angle at which the intended user is standing. Rendering these movements is discretized at 30 frames/second, resulting in every transition consuming 33 ms.

Eyes-Only Movement. In this case, Sammy's head moved exactly in-between the two players' sensed locations while the eyes of the robot were rotated toward the player that the question was intended for. As shown in the left side of Fig. 2, the eyes remained on the sole intended addressee throughout directed questions, but alternated between the two players (in intervals of one second) during open questions.

Coordinated-Head-Eye Movement. In this case, the head was used in combination with the eyes to signal the addressee(s) of each question. As shown in the top right of Fig. 2, directed questions were cued by an immediate eye movement (saccade) to the target player to establish mutual gaze, followed by a rotation of the head horizontally and vertically to the target player as the eyes move back to (0, 0) in a behavior similar to gaze pursuit. For open questions (bottom right of Fig. 2), the saccade-followed-by-rotation alternated between players at random intervals that ranged between 1000 and 1500 ms of mutual gaze.

4 Population, Materials and Procedure

The trivia quiz was part of a multi-activity data collection. Forty-four children (20 female), age five to nine, participated in pairs. Recruited families were asked to bring a same-age sibling or friend to participate with their child so that children playing together were familiar and comfortable with each other, developmentally similar, and likely to share the same level of knowledge about the subject matter. Twenty-one of the 22 pairs met the friend-or-sibling criteria; the mean difference in age between paired players was seven months.

The order of *natural* versus *programmed* conditions was not counterbalanced. Because the children were unfamiliar with the lab space and the experimental form of the quiz activity, we expected some learning and performance change over time and chose to embed that phase in the more familiar context of the human moderator; we discuss the potential bias this introduces in the next section. As a result, all pairs played the first quiz game with the human moderator, followed by a non-quiz activity of about ten minutes, then the second quiz game with Sammy. The physical arrangement of moderator and players can be seen in Fig. 3. During both games, children were given the freedom to stand and move in relation to each other and the moderator at whatever distance felt comfortable, as long as they remained on a rug that defined the Kinect camera's field of view.

As noted above, each game consisted of two rounds of eight questions each. In the human-moderator condition, there were four directed questions to the left child, four directed questions to the right child, and eight open questions to both children. In the robot-moderator condition, eight questions were *eyes-only* and eight questions were *head-eyes*. The content of the 32 questions was chosen to reflect common knowledge for the age group in order to encourage spirited play. Questions were presented in random order, but each moderator always presented the same 16 questions. This was done both to hold the content in the *eyes-only* versus *head-eyes* conditions constant and to optimize the clarity of Sammy's synthesized speech, as some words and phrases were difficult to make him pronounce correctly.

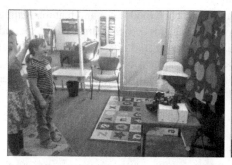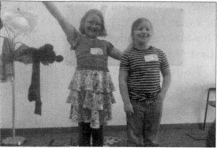

Fig. 3. Left: Side view of the setup with Sammy and two players. The human moderator sat in the same location with her head at approximately the same height. Right: A front view of the participants from Sammy's point of view.

With each type of moderator, the ordering of addressee (directed to right child, directed to left child, and open questions) was fixed. The choice to not randomize the addressee in addition to the questions was made to avoid arbitrary effects that could make the game seem unfair (e.g., two successive questions to the same child, and no open questions presented repetitively).

Audio-visual recording of both games was done using two stereo directed microphones and HD cameras capturing the children from the perspective of the moderator, and an overall far-field recording that captured a side view (see Fig. 3). All events, conditions, and questions were time-logged by the support interfaces, and all audio-visual recordings were manually synchronized with the event logs post hoc.

5   Analysis and Results

Hardware failure during three games reduced the available data for analysis to the 19 pairs of children with recorded sessions for both moderators. Although the wizard and human-moderator interfaces captured measures of interest by button press during game play, audio-visual data was hand-coded independently by two study-blind annotators to ensure that the analysis reflected accurate values. In particular, the annotators coded each question for the following features:

- **First responder:** defined to be the player(s) who first gave an answer to the question. Four values were coded: *left child*, *right child*, *tie* (overlapping responses) and *no response*. *No response* was used in two circumstances: (a) if there was no answer from either child before the moderator re-prompted with the question or (b) if the first child to speak was not responding to the question (typically because s/he was asking whose turn it was).
- **Response type:** defined with respect to the answer to the question. Three values were coded: *correct*, *wrong*, or *none*. *None* was used for ties and non-answer first responses.
- **Host-interrupted:** defined as *yes* if the moderator was unable to finish the question and three alternative answers prior to the first response, otherwise *no*.

Inter-rater reliability was computed separately for each moderator and feature. Kappa values were all in the "very good" range for the human-moderated games: .87, .85, and .98 for **first responder**, **response type**, and **host-interrupted** respectively. Agreement for **first responder** and **response type** were also high in the robot-moderated games, .92 and .86, respectively, but only moderate for **host-interrupted** (.45). A third coder resolved all disagreements and the resolved values were used in the analysis below.

5.1   Practice Effect

Recall that *natural* versus *programmed* conditions were not counter-balanced for order because we anticipated that some within-task learning would occur as children became acclimated to the environment and task. Because the primary goal of the study was to understand the relative importance of coordinated head and eye movement over eyes alone in cueing turn-taking with the robot, we chose to absorb the learning phase into the human-moderator's session. In this way differences between *programmed* sub-conditions would not be conflated with general task practice effects.

Comparing performance in the first and second rounds with the human moderator, we see evidence of increasing comfort: children were almost twice as likely to interrupt the moderator in the second round (48 interruptions versus 28) and the number of ties almost doubled as well (22 in round 1, 40 in round 2). However, there was no evidence of a practice effect with respect to their understanding of the instructions: the total number of turn-taking errors was comparable across rounds (23 and 26). So, while the children seemed to relax and become increasingly invested in winning the point over the first 16 questions, their responsiveness to turn-taking cues remained constant.

5.2   Trivia Knowledge

In addition to a priori concerns about practice effects, the choice of trivia questions was a potential source of conflation. While there was no way to guarantee that at least one child knew the answer to every question, we were aware that if we chose too many questions that were outside the children's experience the resulting lack of response could be attributable to either lack of knowledge or uncertainty about the right to take the turn. We tried to choose subject matter that was likely to be familiar to five to nine year olds in order to encourage quick and competitive play in which they held back only when they knew the answer but also knew it was not their turn.

Across all 32 questions and all conditions, fewer than 8 % were coded as *no responses* and only 11 % were answered incorrectly by the first responder, suggesting that we were generally successful in our efforts to make the material accessible. Further, a comparison of *response type* {correct, wrong, none} x moderator revealed no significant difference ($X^2 = 7.132$, p > .05), indicating that the decision to restrict each moderator to a unique set of questions introduced no bias due to knowledge.

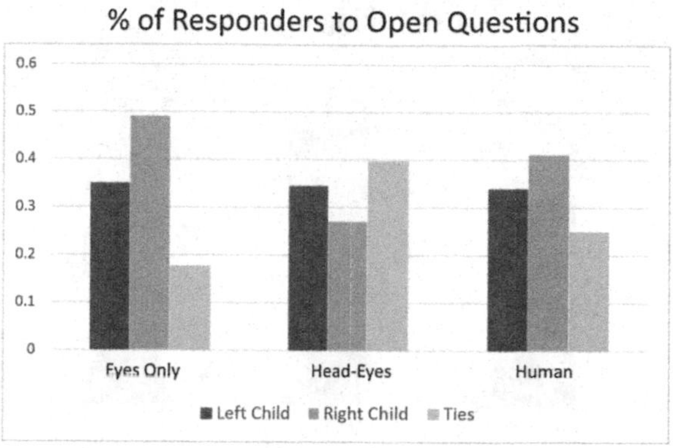

% of Responders to Open Questions

Fig. 4. Proportion of open questions answered by the child to the right of the moderator, the child to the left, or by both (ties), as a function of condition.

5.3   Turn-Taking in Open Questions

Open questions are accompanied by moderator cues that signal inclusion, and either child (or both) can answer during play. Such questions help to keep the game moving and both children engaged. More crucially, because open questions never generate negative feedback about turn-taking errors, the children's experience answering them underscores the distinction between cueing for the open and directed classes.

Figure 4 shows the proportion of open questions answered by each player across conditions. We note that the most even distribution of effort occurs in the *programmed head-eyes* condition. The increase in imbalance in the human-moderated condition (as compared to *head-eyes*) is difficult to interpret. It could be attributable to some aspect of the human moderator's behavior that evoked more dominant responding from one child, but seems more likely to be a simple function of who knew more of the answers in that question set. The imbalance that occurs in the *eyes-only* condition, however, is both more pronounced and less likely to reflect differences in background knowledge— one would expect a more knowledgeable child to be more knowledgeable across the robot-moderated game, irrespective of how the open questions were cued. Nor could it be that more difficult questions happened to be assigned to the *eyes-only* condition, as questions were randomly assigned to sub-condition across games. The imbalance in participation along with the reduced percentage of ties in questions where ties would have been acceptable suggests that some other factor may be relevant. We return to this point after examining children's turn-taking errors in directed questions.

5.4   Turn-Taking in Directed Questions

Turn-taking errors occur when a question is directed to one child and the other, non-addressed child is the first responder or offers a tied response. Figure 5 shows the accuracy of turn-taking across conditions for directed questions that had responses. Children made accurate turn-taking decisions in answering directed questions 67.8 % of the time with the human moderator, 70.0 % of the time with *head-eyes* cues, and

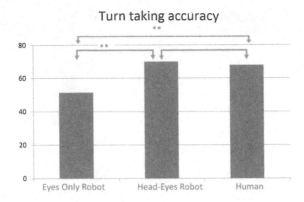

Fig. 5. The accuracy of children's turn-taking in directed questions as a function of condition: natural human movement versus robot *eyes-only* versus robot *head-eyes*. Double-starred comparisons reflect p < .01.

only 51.4 % of the time in the *eyes-only* condition. A comparison of condition x {error, no error} demonstrated the relationships shown in the figure: the *eyes-only* condition resulted in significantly more errorful turn-taking behavior than the *head-eyes* condition (X^2 = 9.272, p = .002) and the *natural movement* condition (X^2 = 8.73, p = .003), but Sammy's coordinated gaze was no more or less effective than the full set of human cues for this measure. No correlation was found between the accuracy of turn-taking and the child's age in any of the conditions.

The results make it clear that using only the eyes as a cue for turn regulation in interactions between a robot and multiple children in this age group will be error prone. At 51 % accuracy, the children's overall behavior in the directed questions was essentially at chance with *eyes-only*. Although there was no correlation between accuracy and age, performance was significantly lower than the 84 % that has been reported in the literature in similar studies with multiple adults using the same robot head (Al Moubayed et al. 2012b). Eye gaze is learned early in development as a signal for co-reference and regulating turn-taking, but its use alone, as instantiated on this particular anthropomorphic head, does not seem to demand the same joint attention.

Poor performance in the *eyes-only* condition for directed questions also suggests an explanation for the response profile of *eyes-only* open questions described in the previous section. If children found it difficult, in general, to read the turn-taking cue from the eyes alone, then disproportionate response and an overall reduction in ties might reflect a greater or lesser willingness to risk a turn-taking error in cases of uncertainty.

If robot eyes alone present too subtle a cue, the additional cues from prosody and facial expression by the human appear to be redundant, adding nothing to the information available over and above head pose. Still, neither of the coordinated eye and head conditions produced adult levels of accuracy, which Al Moubayed et al. (2012) have measured at 91 % for directed questions in a question-answering task using the same robot. The perception of nonverbal regulatory signals might simply be more robust in adults, and it may be that the use of an explicit verbal cue is the only way to guarantee turn-taking accuracy in this setting with young children. Alternatively, it is possible that the persistent 30 % error rate for children across the two more successful conditions reflects a lack of ability to inhibit their responses, despite accurately reading the cues. In short, unlike adults, the baseline of $\sim$ 70 % may be all one can achieve among a demographic that has difficulty waiting its turn.

Although the games that were played with a human moderator appear more natural and engaging than those played with Sammy, in terms of turn-taking accuracy and balance, the human's additional complex regulating behaviors produced no benefit.

The simple and unambiguous turn-assignment signal of coordinated gaze appears adequate to produce what may be an upper bound on regulated response, given the excitement and lack of substantive consequences for error in our game environment.

6 Discussion

We have presented a study investigating the efficacy of different signals for regulating turn-taking in a multi-child interaction. Results reflect the behavior of 19 pairs of children playing a trivia game with directed and open questions, moderated by a human or a robot using either eye gaze alone or coordinated eye and head rotation to cue the addressee.

We found that in directed questions, a simple but visually-prominent movement such as a head rotation was as successful as the more complex turn-regulatory movements performed by the human. The result was unexpected given that the human moderator could accurately sense the child's attentiveness, produce more relevant mutual gaze patterns, and pause during speaking in order to reacquire attention. Although this added sensitivity does not seem to increase the efficacy of turn-taking, it probably does increase the fluency and engagement of the task, questions we intend to explore in future studies using this interaction scenario.

We also found that the eye movement that accompanied the robot's head rotation in coordinated gaze was not, by itself, adequate to signal addressee in young children. Again, this result was somewhat unexpected given that the role of eye contact and mutual gaze is established in early language development. The efficacy of accompanying simple eye gaze with explicit verbal cues is still to be explored, and if more successful may provide an alternative to the wear-and-tear of repeated head movement as well as welcome variety in Sammy's behavior.

Acknowledgment. The authors would like to thank Brooke Kelly, Iain Matthews, Charles Mathy, Hanspeter Pfister, Virginia Perry Smith, Jody Aha, Carol O'Sullivan, Jacqueline Kappes, and Bob Sumner for their help in formulating the trivia questions, Daniela DeFanti for help in early pilot testing, and, in particular, Adriana DeFanti, for her help in both question writing and pilot testing.

References

Al Moubayed, S., Skantze, G.: Turn-taking control using gaze in multiparty human-computer dialogue: effects of 2D and 3D displays. In: Proceedings of the International Conference on Auditory-Visual Speech Processing AVSP, Florence, Italy (2011)

Al Moubayed, S., Beskow, J., Skantze, G., Granström, B.: Furhat: A back-projected human-like robot head for multiparty human-machine interaction. In: Esposito, A., Esposito, A., Vinciarelli, A., Hoffmann, R., Müller, V.C. (eds.) Cognitive Behavioural Systems. Lecture Notes in Computer Science. Springer, Heidelberg (2012a)

Al Moubayed, S., Edlund, J., Beskow, J.: Taming Mona Lisa: communicating gaze faithfully in 2D and 3D facial projections. ACM Trans. Interact. Intell. Syst. 1(2), 25 (2012b)

Al Moubayed, S., Edlund, J., Gustafsson, J.: Analysis of gaze and speech patterns in three-party quiz game interaction. In: Proceedings of Interspeech, Lyon, France (2013)

Argyle, M., Cook, M.: Gaze and mutual gaze. Cambridge University Press, Cambridge (1976)

Bilvi, M., Pelachaud, C.: Communicative and statistical eye gaze predictions. In: Proceedings of International Conference on Autonomous Agents and Multi-Agent Systems (AAMAS), Melbourne, Australia (2003)

Bohus, D., Horvitz, E.: Facilitating multiparty dialog with gaze, gesture, and speech. In: Proceedings of ICMI 2010, Beijing, China (2010)

Gustafson, J., Bell, L., Boye, J., Lindström, A., Wirén, M.: The nice fairy-tale game system. In: Proceedings of SIGdial (2004)

Lehman, J.: Robo fashion world: a multimodal corpus of multi-child human-computer interaction. In: Proceedings of ICMI 2014 Understanding and Modeling Multiparty, Multimodal Interactions, Istanbul, Turkey (2014)

Kendon, A.: Some functions of gaze direction in social interaction. Acta Psychol. 26, 22–63 (1967)

Kleinke, C.L.: Gaze and eye contact: a research review. Psychol. Bull. 100, 78–100 (1986)

Skantze, G., Al Moubayed, S.: IrisTK: a statechart-based toolkit for multi-party face-to-face interaction. In: Proceedings of the 14th ACM International Conference on Multimodal Interaction ICMI Santa Monica, CA, USA (2012)

Takeuchi, A., Nagao, K.: Communicative facial displays as a new conversational modality. In: Proceedings of the Interact 1993 and chi 1993 Conference on Human Factors in Computing Systems (1993)

Swartout, W., Traum, D., Artstein, R., Noren, D., Debevec, P., Bronnenkant, K., Williams, J., Leuski, A., Narayanan, S., Piepol, D., Lane, C., Morie, J., Aggarwal, P., Liewer, M., Chiang, J.-Y., Gerten, J., Chu, S., White, K.: Ada and Grace: toward realistic and engaging virtual museum guides. In: Safonova, A. (ed.) IVA 2010. LNCS, vol. 6356, pp. 286–300. Springer, Heidelberg (2010)

Conversational Behavior Reflecting Interpersonal Attitudes in Small Group Interactions

Brian Ravenet[1]([⊠]), Angelo Cafaro[2], Beatrice Biancardi[2], Magalie Ochs[3], and Catherine Pelachaud[2]

[1] Institut Mines-Télécom, Télécom ParisTech, CNRS-LTCI, Paris, France
ravenet@telecom-paristech.fr
[2] Télécom ParisTech, CNRS-LTCI, Paris, France
{cafaro,biancardi,pelachaud}@telecom-paristech.fr
[3] Aix Marseille Université, CNRS, ENSAM, Université de Toulon, LSIS UMR7296,
13397 Marseille, France
ochs@lsis.org

Abstract. In this paper we propose a computational model for the real time generation of nonverbal behaviors supporting the expression of interpersonal attitudes for turn-taking strategies and group formation in multi-party conversations among embodied conversational agents. Starting from the desired attitudes that an agent aims to express towards every other participant, our model produces the nonverbal behavior that should be exhibited in real time to convey such attitudes while managing the group formation and attempting to accomplish the agent's own turn-taking strategy. We also propose an evaluation protocol for similar multi-agent configurations. We conducted a study following this protocol to evaluate our model. Results showed that subjects properly recognized the attitudes expressed by the agents through their nonverbal behavior and turn taking strategies generated by our system.

1 Introduction

In a conversing group there might be from three up to twenty participants [2]. All participants adhere to specific social norms governing, for example, their distance and body orientation in order to coordinate and make it easier to interact with each other [15,32]. Goffman classifies participants into different roles (e.g. speakers and listeners) [11]. The role and the attitude that each participant aims at expressing towards the others determine the verbal and nonverbal behavior that are exhibited in such group interactions [20]. For virtual agents, the expressions of attitudes in groups is a key element to improve the social believability of the virtual worlds that they populate as well as the user's experience, for example in entertainment [19] or training [14] applications. This paper presents a model for expressing interpersonal attitudes in a simulated group conversation. The intended attitudes are exhibited via nonverbal behavior and

© Springer International Publishing Switzerland 2015
W.-P. Brinkman et al. (Eds.): IVA 2015, LNAI 9238, pp. 375–388, 2015.
DOI: 10.1007/978-3-319-21996-7_41

impact the management of the group interaction (i.e. group formation), the conversational nonverbal behavior and the turn-taking strategy of the agents. The model is grounded on human and social sciences literature. We use the Argyle's representation of Status and Affiliation for describing interpersonal attitudes [1].

The main contributions of this paper are (1) a model that allows an agent to express interpersonal attitudes through its turn-taking strategies and nonverbal behavior while interacting in a small group, and (2) a study protocol designed to evaluate this model and similar scenarios involving small group interactions.

2   Related Work

ECAs Gathering in Groups. Prada and Paiva [24] modeled groups of autonomous synthetic virtual agents that collaborated with the user in the resolution of collaborative tasks within a 3D virtual environment. Rehm and Endrass [28] implemented a toolbox for modeling the behavior of multi-agent systems. In [23], the authors combined a number of reactive social behaviors, including those reflecting personal space [13] and the F-formation system [15], in a general steering framework inspired by [29]. This complete management of position and orientation is the foundation of the Impulsion Engine used in the work presented here. All these models did not take into account the expression of attitudes while exhibiting the behaviors of the agents.

Turn-Taking Models for ECAs. Ter Maat and colleagues [33] found that the perception of an ECA's personality (in a Wizard of Oz dyadic setting) varies when changing its turn-taking strategy. In [25], they proposed a model to manage the turn-taking between a user and a spoken dialog system using data-driven knowledge. In [18], the authors proposed to add to the ECA Max a turn-taking system based on states (Wanting the turn or Yielding the turn for instance) and possible transitions between them. A similar work on ECA's turn-taking is the model YTTM by Thórisson [34]. While it started as a turn-taking model for agents in dyadic interactions, it has been extended to multi-party interactions. It is based on Sacks' turn-taking model [30] and Duncan's findings on behavior for turn-taking management [9]. Another work focusing on these behaviors is the Spark architecture presented in [35]. This architecture supports the automatic generation of animations for avatars depending on the conversational activity of their user (typing on a keyboard). Some of these systems were designed for face-to-face interaction only [18,25,33] or did not consider the expression of attitudes [34].

ECAs Expressing Interpersonal Attitudes. Different models enabling ECAs to exhibit social attitudes through their verbal and non-verbal behavior have been proposed. For instance, in [10], the system Demeanour supported the design of virtual characters within a group with different social attitudes (expressed through posture and gaze) following Argyle's Status and Affiliation model. In [28], the authors proposed a toolbox for manipulating the decision making of agents in a group based on different theories on social relations. In [17] they designed the nonverbal behavior of ECAs depending on their conversational role and their social relations. In [3], the authors conducted a study where users evaluated the perception of an ECA's attitude (friendly, hostile, extraversion) in the first seconds of an encounter with an ECA exhibiting different behaviors (smiles, gaze and proxemics). In [4], they evaluated the perception of attitudes (friendly, hostile) conveyed in both the nonverbal behavior of the agent while speaking and the content of the speech. In [6], they explored how sequences of nonverbal signals (a head nod followed by a smile for instance) can convey interpersonal attitudes in a dyadic interaction.

These systems have been mainly designed for face-to-face interaction and scripted scenarios. In our system, we propose a model for the automatic generation of nonverbal behavior, we do not focus onverbal content at the moment, and it takes into account multi-party interaction in a small group formation.

3   Computational Model

We propose a computational model for the generation of nonverbal behavior supporting simulated group conversations (F-formation, turn-taking and conversational behaviors) and conveying interpersonal attitudes. The components of our model are the following: a *turn-taking component*, a *group behavior component* and a *conversational behavior component*. The expression of interpersonal attitudes is obtained, within each component, by modulating the produced nonverbal behavior as function of the attitude that every agent intends to express towards all the other group members. Given the different roles that participants can assume in a group conversation [11], as a first step, we focus on speaker and listener roles. The turn-taking mechanism is based on Clark's model [7] and builds on top of previous agent multi-party interaction research [34]. Our model triggers nonverbal behavior specific to each agent depending on its role in the conversation and its social attitudes towards the members of the group. This computation is done in **real-time** and in a **continuous** fashion. Moreover, our model deals with conflicting behaviors emerging from different social norms (interpersonal attitude, group formation and conversational behavior). For instance, one agent may need to orient itself towards its addressee and keep an orientation towards the group at the same time while gazing at the most dominant agent in the group.

3.1   Turn-Taking Component

We based the design of this component on Clark's work [7]. Clark described a turn as an emergent behavior from a joint action of speaking and listening. Therefore our model generates a value for the desire of speaking that will trigger an utterance depending on the current speakers. This means that more than one agent at time can speak. We hypothesize that the attitudes expressed towards each other members of the group affect this desire to speak. We assumed that each agent has the intention to communicate and we do not consider the content of speech but only the willingness to actually utter sounds (sequence of words). However, we are aware of the importance of the speech content in an interaction so our model is designed in a way it could receive inputs from a dialog manager (speech utterances and desire to speak) in future works. An agent successfully takes the floor on the basis of the interpersonal attitudes it wants to express towards the others. We modeled the turns as a state machine similarly to Thórisson [34]. These states are based on Goffman's ratified conversational roles [11] and are the following (as depicted in Fig. 1): *own-the-speech* when the agent is the only one speaking, *compete-for-the-speech* when the agent is not the only one speaking, *end-of-speech* transitional state when the agent is willing to stop speaking, *interrupted* transitional state when the agent is forced to stop speaking, *addressed-listener* when the agent is listening and directly addressed to, *unaddressed-listener* when the agent is listening and not directly addressed to and *want-to-speak* when the agent is willing to speak and let the other know it by its behavior. The states and the transitions between them are depicted Fig. 1.

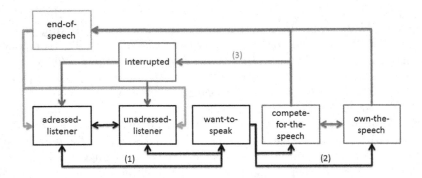

Fig. 1. The states of the turn-taking component

An agent starts in the *unaddressed-listener* state. Every 250ms, the system check if a transition from the current state activates. It is the minimum time required for a human to react to a stimuli [16]. For a transition to activate, it needs specific input values. These inputs are: the current list of speakers and who they are talking to, what attitudes the agents express to the others and the time passed since the last time the agent spoke. We chose to represent the attitudes on a two-axis space where each axis (Status and Affiliation) goes from -1 to 1. The minimum value of the Status axis represents a submissive attitude (respectively a hostile attitude on the Affiliation axis) and the maximum value represents a dominant attitude (respectively a friendly attitude). Regarding the transitions from and to *unaddressed-listener* and *addressed-listener*, they activate if another agent is addressing the agent or not. From *unaddressed-listener* or *addressed-listener* to *want-to-speak*, the function is using the time of the last utterance ($Last$) and the attitudes of the agent ($Stat$ and Aff as respectively the mean Status expressed and the mean Affiliation expressed). According to [5,12] the higher the Status and the Affiliation, the more a person is willing to

speak and the quicker he/she wants to take the floor again. Whereas in a submissive attitude the desire to speak drops, an hostile attitude does not have that
effect. Since in our simulation, all agents have the intent to speak, even if they
are submissive, for instance, they keep their desire of speaking. We empirically
defined a maximum delay ($Delay$) before having the desire of speaking again.
Therefore our transitional function $f_{li,wa}$ (from a listener state to $want$-to-$speak$
state), where Now is the current time, is the following:

$$f_{li,wa}(Last, Stat, Aff) = \begin{cases} 1 & if(Now \geq Last+ \\ & Delay * (1 - \frac{1}{2}(Stat + norm(Aff))) \\ 0 & else \end{cases} \quad (1)$$

The function $norm()$ is the normalization from $[-1, 1]$ to $[0, 1]$. From $want$-
to-$speak$ to own-the-$speech$ or $compete$-for-the-$speech$, there are two strategies
(i.e. transitions). First, the agent tries to see if there is another agent willing
to give it the turn. If this does not succeed, the second strategy is trying to
get into the conversation by interrupting or overlapping. However, in order to
do so, the agent has to feel that it is compatible with its attitudes towards
the others. The inputs of this transition are the currently speaking agents and
the attitudes towards them. Let $Stat_{sp}$ and Aff_{sp} be respectively the mean
Status and the mean Affiliation expressed towards the current speakers. A person
expressing dominance interrupts others more easily [12]. Expressing friendliness
and hostility result in possible overlapping [12,21]. Therefore our function $f_{wa,sp}$
(from $want$-to-$speak$ to a speaker state) is the following:

$$f_{wa,sp}(Stat_{sp}, Aff_{sp}) = \begin{cases} 1 & if(Stat_{sp} + |Aff_{sp}| > 0) \\ 0 & else \end{cases} \quad (2)$$

The transition from and to $compete$-for-the-$speech$ and own-the-$speech$ is activated if at least an other agent is talking at the same time. Within these states,
the model selects the addressee by choosing randomly among the other agents,
with a preference for those towards whom it expresses the most friendliness.
From $compete$-for-the-$speech$ to $interrupted$, it is similar to the $f_{wa,sp}$ function
but this time the agent is not trying to interrupt but it is trying not to be
interrupted. Therefore our function $f_{sp,in}$ is the following:

$$f_{sp,in}(Stat_{sp}, Aff_{sp}) = \begin{cases} 1 & if(Stat_{sp} + |Aff_{sp}| \leq 0) \\ 0 & else \end{cases} \quad (3)$$

From $compete$-for-the-$speech$ or own-the-$speech$ to end-of-$speech$, this transition
is activated automatically at the end of the agent's speech. From $interrupted$ or
end-of-$speech$ to $unaddressed$-$hearer$ or $addressed$-$hearer$, the transition is activated after producing the behavior associated to these states (see Sect. 3.3).
Within each state, the agent produces different behaviors depending on the interpersonal attitudes it expresses. As the attitudes are also used to determine the
flow among the internal states, this model differs from previous existing models

as it allows an agent to convey interpersonal attitudes through its turn-taking strategies.

3.2 Group Behavior Component

Our model alters the behavior of the agents supporting the group formation so their different interpersonal attitudes are reflected accordingly. The model comes as a value producer for the parameters of a **Group Behavior** component that keeps the coherence of the formation based on the works of Kendon's F-Formation [15] and Scheflen's territoriality [32]. These parameters are preferred interpersonal distances between each member of the group, preferred target for gaze and preferred target for body orientation. The desired interpersonal distance ranged from 0.46 m to 2.1 m. These are the boundaries of personal and social areas as defined by Hall's proxemics theory [13], and these areas represent the space where social interaction takes place. We then compute a factor of interpolation α in this interval based on the expressed dominance and liking. A difference of status (either Dominance or Submissiveness) leads to a higher distance whereas friendliness leads to a smaller distance [8,20]. Let $Stat_i$ and Aff_i be respectively the expressed Status and Affiliation towards an agent Ag_i, the function $d(Ag_i)$ to compute the desired interpersonal distance with an agent Ag_i is:

$$d(Ag_i) = 0.46 + \alpha(2.1 - 0.46) \text{ with } \alpha = \frac{(|Stat_i| + (\frac{1 - Aff_i}{2}))}{2} \quad (4)$$

For the preferred gaze target, we compute a potentiality to be gazed at for each other participant and we select the participant with the higher potentiality. We do a similar process for the preferred body target. In order to compute the potentiality to be gazed at, we sum the result of a trigonometric interpolation on both the dominance expressed and the liking expressed whereas we consider only the dominance for the potentiality of the body orientation [20]. The function $p_g(Ag_i)$ to compute the potentiality to gaze at an agent Ag_i is:

$$p_g(Ag_i) = 1 + \frac{sin(\frac{1}{2} + 2 \times Aff_i) + sin(\frac{1}{2} + 2 \times (-Stat_i))}{2} \quad (5)$$

And the function $p_b(Ag_i)$ to compute the potentiality to orient the body towards an agent Ag_i is:

$$p_b(Ag_i) = \frac{1 - Stat_i}{2} \quad (6)$$

3.3 Conversational Behavior Component

In the initial state (*unaddressed-listener*), the agent is idle and the *Group Behavior* component is the only one producing an output, thus handling the agent's group behavior (i.e. interpersonal distance, body orientation and gaze). In the other states, the *Conversational Behavior* component might request resources (i.e. body joint to animate) from the *Group Behavior* one (preferred gaze target and preferred body orientation) to achieve the behavior needed by the turn-taking component and will also produce additional behavior such as gestures and facial expressions. To realize these additional behaviors, we extended the model introduced in [27]. This model has been learnt on data from a crowdsourcing experiment where participants configured the behavior of a virtual agent for different attitudes. The proposed model works as a SAIBA Behavior Planner. Upon the reception of an utterance and an attitude, the model generates the nonverbal behavior associated with that intention and attitude (gestures, facial expressions, head orientations and gaze behaviors). For instance, it can produce three different facial expressions (a smiling, frowning or neutral face) blended with the lips animation produced while speaking. It also produces beat gestures to accompany the speech with different amplitude (small, normal or wide) and strength (weak, normal or strong). When entering the *want-to-speak* state, the model outputs as preferred gaze target the current speaker to indicate the desire to take the floor [9]. In the states *own-the-speech* or *compete-for-the-speech*, the *Conversational Behavior* component receives from the *Turn-Taking* component an utterance to produce (a target to address and a sentence to say) and it retrieves from the *Group Behavior* component the details of the group. From these parameters, it will generates the nonverbal behavior corresponding to the interpersonal attitudes expressed thanks to the *Behavior Planner* from [27] and selects as preferred body orientation the addressee. However, when in the state *compete-for-the-speech*, the preferred gaze target is the agent towards whom the most submissiveness is expressed. In the *own-the-speech* state, the preferred gaze target is the addressee [20]. In the *end-of-speech* state, the preferred gaze target is the addressee [9]. In the state *interrupted*, the previous behavior of the agent is interrupted and both the preferred gaze target and preferred body orientation are the other speaker towards whom the highest submissiveness is expressed [12].

4   Implementation

The implementation of our model has been realized as a Unity3D application that uses two additional frameworks, the VIB/Greta agent platform [22] and the Impulsion AI library [23]. Once the application is started, a scene that takes place in a public square starts in which the user can navigate. Within the public square, the user can find a group of agents having a conversation, simulated by our model. The two additional frameworks handles the production of nonverbal behaviors for each agent. The VIB agent platform computes gestures and facial expressions accompanying communicative intentions while the Impulsion AI library handles group cohesion behaviors, body orientation, gaze direction and spacial distance between group members. The combined integration of these two frameworks has been presented in [26]. These frameworks have been extended in order to take into account the interpersonal attitudes in the production of behaviors. Our implemented turn-taking model, written in Unity3D scripts, encapsulates these two frameworks within the application and sends them the current attitudes and the utterances of each agent. In response, VIB and Impulsion produce the corresponding nonverbal behaviors.

5   Model Evaluation

We questioned whether the attitude expressed by our agents would emerge and be perceived by user when observing the behavior of the agents during simulated conversation. It was impractical to test all possible group configurations. Therefore we fixed at 4 the number of agents in order to represent a typical small gathering featured in the applications mentioned earlier in Sect. 1. A group of four agents expressing attitudes on two dimensions (i.e. status and affiliation) towards all other members yields an exponential number of possibilities. Considering the levels of attitude on a discrete scale (e.g. submissive vs. neutral vs. dominant) there are 3^{24} possible configuration among 4 agents. Therefore, we simplified the design by splitting the study in two trials focusing on each separate dimension, respectively named **Status Trial** and **Affiliation Trial**.

Secondly, based on the Interpersonal Complementarity Theory (IC) [31], we studied the attitudes expressed by two participants as described in the following section.

5.1   Experimental Design

The IC theory claims that to obtain a positive outcome in an interaction, people behaviors need to reflect a similar attitude on the Affiliation axis and/or an opposite attitude on the Status axis. Inspired by this theory, for each trial, we asked participants to watch videos taken from our implemented system featuring 4 agents (2 males and 2 females, all with a distinct appearance) in a group conversation. The user is an observer and the agents are positioned in a way that two appear at the immediate sides of the frame and two are located at the center of the frame (as depicted in Fig. 2). The participants rated how they perceived the attitudes of the two central agents while they were expressing similar and opposite attitudes towards each other according to the IC theory. We called these two agents **Left Agent** and **Right Agent**. The main research questions were the following: will the participants recognize the attitudes (validating the model we proposed for a subset of the possible configurations)? Is there any difference in the perceived attitudes when showing complementarity and anti-complementarity situations to participants? Does our model generate believable conversational group simulation and do users find it more believable in complementarity situations?

Stimuli. We describe the videos that were presented to the participants. We were aware of possible appearance and positioning biases (e.g. clothing and gender). Since we could not fully factor in these elements in our design, we considered

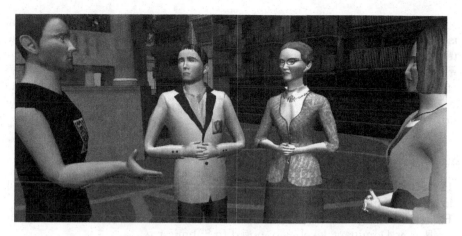

Fig. 2. A screenshot of the group interaction as seen by users in our evaluation study. The two central agents were respectively identified as the Left Agent (the male in this image) and the Right Agent (the female).

them as blocking factors. The four characters could be arranged in 6 different possible orders while keeping a circular group formation, we named this blocking factor *GroupArrangement*. Given an arrangement, the left and right agents (those exhibiting the stimuli, positioned at the center of the frame) could be swapped, we named this factor *PairPosition*. While the left and right agent (at the center of the frame) were the two exhibiting the stimuli, the other two side agents were still actively participating in the simulated conversations expressing and receiving a neutral attitude in both dimensions. According to our blocking factors, we generated 48 video stimuli for each trial. In both trials, the independent variables (IVs) were the following: Expressed Left Agent Status **ExpStatusL** (respectively **ExpAffL** in the *Affiliation* trial) and Expressed Right Agent Status **ExpStatusR** (respectively **ExpAffR** in the *Affiliation* trial). Both variables had two levels, *Submissive* and *Dominant* (respectively *Hostile* and *Friendly*).

Measurements. For each video stimuli, we asked the participants to answer a questionnaire in order to measure their perceived attitudes of the two agents. This questionnaire was designed by including adjectives classified around the interpersonal circumplex chosen from [36]. There were 4 questions on how accurate a sentence using one the 4 adjectives (2 with positive valence and 2 with negative) described the attitude of an agent towards the other one. For the *Status* Trial, the adjectives were: controlling, insecure, dominating and looking for reassurance. For the *Affiliation* Trial, the adjectives were: warm, detached, likeable and hostile. One of the question was, for instance, *Left Agent expresses warmth towards the Right Agent*. We also asked 3 questions about the group: its believability, the engagement of its participants and its social richness. All answers were on 5 points Likert scales (anchors *Completely disagree* and *Completely agree*). In sum, the dependent variables (DVs) in the *Status* trial (and respectively the *Affiliation* trial) were the Measured Left Agent Status **MeasureStatusL** (respectively **MeasureAffL**) and the Measured Right Agent Status **MeasureStatusR** (respectively **MeasureAffR**). We aggregated the answers from positive and negative items to produce a single normalized value for each DVs in the range [0,1]. In both trials, the variables related to the questions about the group were: the **Group Believability**, the **Group Engagement** and the **Group Social Richness**.

Hypotheses.

- **H1 (Left Agent)**: The value of MeasureStatusL is higher when ExpStatusL is at Dominant level as opposed to Submissive.
- **H2 (Right Agent)**: The value of MeasureStatusR is higher when ExpStatusR is at Dominant level as opposed to Submissive.
- **H3 (IC Theory)**: With respect to Interpersonal Complementarity theory, participants should better recognize the attitudes when ExpStatusL and ExpStatusR show opposite values
- **H4 (Group)**: The values for Group Believability, Group Engagement and Group Social Richness should be rated higher in complementarity configuration than anti-complementarity configuration.

We call H1.s, H2.s, H3.s and H4.s the hypotheses in the Status Trial and H1.a, H2.a, H3.a and H4.a the hypotheses in the Affiliation Trial.

Procedure and Participants. In both trials, each participant was assigned to 4 videos in a fully counterbalanced manner according to our blocking factors. We ran the study on the web. A participant was first presented with a consent page and a questionnaire to retrieve demographic information (nationality, age and gender). Then, we showed a tutorial video with a sample question. And then we presented in a fully randomized order the 4 videos, each in a different page with questions at the bottom, in a within-subjects design. Finally, a debriefing page was shown. We recruited a total of 144 participants via mailing lists, 72 in each trial. In the Status Trial, 58.34 % of the participants were between 18 and 30 years old and 50 % were female, 48.61 % were male and 1.39 % did not say. In the Affiliation Trial, 66.66 % were between 18 and 30, 56.94 % were female while 43.06 % were male. We had participants from several cultural backgrounds but most of them were from France (47.22 % in the Status Trial and 52.68 % in the Affiliation Trial).

5.2 Results

Status Trial. In order to test H1.s, H2.s and H3.s, we ran a 2×2 repeated measures MANOVA (Doubly Multivariate Analysis of Variance) on MeasureStatusL and MeasureStatusR with within-subjects factors ExpStatusL and ExpStatusR. We found an overall main effect of ExpStatusL ($WilksLambda = 0.50$,

$F(2, 70) = 35.7$, $p < 0.001$) and ExpStatusR ($WilksLambda = 0.57$, $F(2, 70) = 25.7$, $p < 0.001$). No significant interaction effects were found. Since the sphericity assumption was not violated, we performed a follow-up analysis that looked at univariate repeated measures ANOVAs for the 2 DVs. For MeasureStatusL, the ANOVA confirmed a significant main effect of ExpStatusL ($F(1, 71) = 63$, $p = .0$). In particular, Left Agent was rated as more dominant when ExpStatusL was at the Dominant level (M $= .56$, SE $= .02$) as opposed to the Submissive level (M $= .43$, SE $= .01$). No other interaction effects were found therefore **H1.s is supported**. For MeasureStatusR, the ANOVA confirmed a significant main effect of ExpStatusR ($F(1, 71) = 48$, $p = .0$). In particular, Right Agent was rated as more dominant when ExpStatusR was at the Dominant level (M $= .60$, SE $= .01$) as opposed to the Submissive level (M $= .46$, SE $= .01$). No other interaction effects were found therefore **H2.s is supported**. The interaction of the two IVs had no effects on both measures, **H3.s is rejected**. We ran a further MANOVA analysis with two additional between-subjects factors Group Arrangement and Subject Gender. We did not find significant interaction effects (all $p > .38$). As for the 3 group measures, we ran 3 similar univariate repeated measures ANOVAs. Except for an effect of ExpStatusR on Group Believability ($p = 0.03$) with a small effect size ($\eta_p^2 = .06$), no other significant main effects and interactions were found (all $p > .13$).

Affiliation Trial. We ran a similar 2×2 repeated measures MANOVA on MeasureAffL and MeasureAffR with within-subjects factors ExpAffL and ExpAffR. We found an overall main effect of ExpAffL ($WilksLambda = 0.42$, $F(2, 70) = 48.4$, $p < 0.001$) and ExpAffR ($WilksLambda = 0.55$, $F(2, 70) = 28$, $p < 0.001$). No significant interaction effects were found. We also performed a follow-up analysis that looked at univariate repeated measures ANOVAs for the 2 DVs. For MeasureAffL, the ANOVA confirmed a significant main effect of ExpAffL ($F(1, 71) = 93$, $p = .0$). In particular, Left Agent was rated as more friendly when ExpStatusL was at the Friendly level (M $= .61$, SE $= .02$) as opposed to the Hostile level (M $= .37$, SE $= .01$). No other interaction effects were found therefore **H1.a is supported**. For MeasureAffR, the ANOVA confirmed a significant main effect of ExpAffR ($F(1, 71) = 54$, $p = .0$). In particular, Right Agent was rated as more friendly when ExpAffR was at the Friendly level (M $= .58$, SE $= .02$) as opposed to the Hostile level (M $= .41$, SE $= .01$). No other interaction effects were found therefore **H2.a is supported**. The interaction of the two IVs had no effects on both measures, **H3.a is rejected**. We also ran a further MANOVA analysis with two additional between-subjects factors Group Arrangement and Subject Gender. We did not find significant interaction effects (all $p > .17$). As for the 3 group measures, we ran 3 similar univariate repeated measures ANOVAs. Except for an effect of ExpAffR on Group Engagement ($p = 0.01$) with a small effect size ($\eta_p^2 = .09$), no other significant main effects and interactions were found (all $p > .12$).

6   Discussion and Conclusion

We presented a computational model for generating agents' nonverbal behavior in a conversational group. This nonverbal behavior supports the expression of interpersonal attitudes within group formation management, conversational behavior and turn-taking strategies adopted by the agents. We also designed an evaluation protocol that we used to conduct a two trials study aimed at testing the capacity of this model to produce believable attitudes in anti-complementarity and complementarity situations. Results showed that agents' attitudes were properly recognized (H1 and H2 supported in both trials). We didn't find any interaction effect between the expressed attitudes as the IC theory suggests (H3 rejected in both trials). The reason might be that since we did not consider the content of the speech, it was maybe easier for participants to clearly distinguish each attitude (and not to consider them in interaction). The expressed Attitudes (both in the Status and Affiliation trials) of the two central agents (i.e. the left and right agents for which we manipulated the attitudes expressed) had a main effect on the respective measured Attitudes. Similarly, we obtained means for the Group Dependent Variables (Believability, Engagement, and Social Richness) all >3.472 (outcomes were in the range 1–5) but we didn't find any significant differences when looking at complementarity or anti-complementarity situations (H4 rejected). Finally, the blocking factors (in particular the group arrangement) and the user's gender have been considered as between-subjects factors but they had no effects. Each agent was able to express its attitude regardless of the other's attitude, the group arrangement and the gender of the user. Some limitations should be considered. The model should be extended with additional nonverbal behaviors (e.g. supporting back-channels) and the generation of verbal content (also reflecting interpersonal attitudes). Regarding the evaluation, we have considered only a subset of all the possible configurations, limiting the manipulated attitudes to the two (central) characters. However, the intended attitudes that our model aimed at expressing, emerged from the overall group behavior exhibited by the agents. Furthermore, we introduced an evaluation protocol that other researchers could adopt when running similar studies on group behavior. In the short term, we intend to make the user an active participant in the group conversation, allowing him/her to interact with the agents and have the agents expressing their attitudes towards the user.

Acknowledgments. This work was partially was performed within the Labex SMART (ANR-11-LABX-65) supported by French state funds managed by the ANR within the Investissements d'Avenir programme under reference ANR-11-IDEX-0004-02. It has also been partially funded by the French National Research Agency project MOCA (ANR-12-CORD-019) and by the H2020 European project ARIA-VALUSPA.

References

1. Argyle, M.: Bodily Communication. University Paperbacks, Methuen (1988)
2. Beebe, S.A., Masterson, J.T.: Communication in Small Groups: Principles and Practices. Pearson Education, Inc., Boston (2009)
3. Cafaro, A., Vilhjálmsson, H.H., Bickmore, T., Heylen, D., Jóhannsdóttir, K.R., Valgarosson, G.S.: First impressions: users' judgments of virtual agents' personality and interpersonal attitude in first encounters. In: Nakano, Y., Neff, M., Paiva, A., Walker, M. (eds.) IVA 2012. LNCS, vol. 7502, pp. 67–80. Springer, Heidelberg (2012)
4. Callejas, Z., Ravenet, B., Ochs, M., Pelachaud, C.: A computational model of social attitudes for a virtual recruiter. In: Autonomous Agent and Multiagent Systems (2014)
5. Cappella, J.N., Siegman, A.W., Feldstein, S.: Controlling the floor in conversation. In: Siegman, A.W., Feldstein, S. (eds.) Multichannel Integrations of Nonverbal Behavior, pp. 69–103. Erlbaum, Hillsdale (1985)
6. Chollet, M., Ochs, M., Pelachaud, C.: From non-verbal signals sequence mining to Bayesian networks for interpersonal attitudes expression. In: Bickmore, T., Marsella, S., Sidner, C. (eds.) IVA 2014. LNCS, vol. 8637, pp. 120–133. Springer, Heidelberg (2014)
7. Clark, H.H.: Using Language. Cambridge University Press, Cambridge (1996)
8. Cristani, M., Paggetti, G., Vinciarelli, A., Bazzani, L., Menegaz, G., Murino, V.: Towards computational proxemics: inferring social relations from interpersonal distances. In: Privacy, Security, Risk and Trust, pp. 290–297. IEEE (2011)
9. Duncan, S.: Some signals and rules for taking speaking turns in conversations. J. Pers. Soc. Psychol. **23**(2), 283 (1972)
10. Gillies, M., Crabtree, I.B., Ballin, D.: Customisation and context for expressive behaviour in the broadband world. BT Technol. J. **22**(2), 7–17 (2004)
11. Goffman, E.: Forms of Talk. University of Pennsylvania Press, Philadelphia (1981)
12. Goldberg, J.A.: Interrupting the discourse on interruptions: An analysis in terms of relationally neutral, power-and rapport-oriented acts. J. Pragmat. **14**(6), 883–903 (1990)
13. Hall, E.T.: The Hidden Dimension, vol. 1990. Anchor Books, New York (1969)
14. Johnson, W.L., Marsella, S., Vilhjalmsson, H.: The darwars tactical language training system. In: Proceedings of I/ITSEC (2004)
15. Kendon, A.: Conducting interaction: Patterns of behavior in focused encounters, vol. 7. CUP Archive (1990)
16. Kosinski, R.J.: A literature review on reaction time. Clemson University 10 (2008)
17. Lee, J., Marsella, S.: Modeling side participants and bystanders: the importance of being a laugh track. In: Vilhjálmsson, H.H., Kopp, S., Marsella, S., Thórisson, K.R. (eds.) IVA 2011. LNCS, vol. 6895, pp. 240–247. Springer, Heidelberg (2011)
18. Leßmann, N., Kranstedt, A., Wachsmuth, I.: Towards a cognitively motivated processing of turn-taking signals for the embodied conversational agent max. In: Proceedings Workshop Embodied Conversational Agents: Balanced Perception and Action, pp. 57–64. IEEE Computer Society (2004)
19. Maxis: http://www.thesims.com (November 2014). http://www.thesims.com
20. Mehrabian, A.: Significance of posture and position in the communication of attitude and status relationships. Psychol. Bull. **71**(5), 359 (1969)
21. O'Connell, D.C., Kowal, S., Kaltenbacher, E.: Turn-taking: a critical analysis of the research tradition. J. Psycholinguist. Rss. **19**(6), 345–373 (1990)

22. Pecune, F., Cafaro, A., Chollet, M., Philippe, P., Pelachaud, C.: Suggestions for extending saiba with the vib platform. In: Proceedings of the Workshop on Architectures and Standards for Intelligent Virtual Agents at IVA 2014 (2014)
23. Pedica, C., Vilhjálmsson, H.H., Lárusdóttir, M.: Avatars in conversation: the importance of simulating territorial behavior. In: Allbeck, J., Badler, N., Bickmore, T., Pelachaud, C., Safonova, A. (eds.) IVA 2010. LNCS, vol. 6356, pp. 336–342. Springer, Heidelberg (2010)
24. Prada, R., Paiva, A.: Believable groups of synthetic characters. In: Proceedings of the Fourth International Joint Conference on Autonomous Agents and Multiagent Systems, AAMAS 2005, pp. 37–43. ACM, New York, NY, USA (2005)
25. Raux, A., Eskenazi, M.: A finite-state turn-taking model for spoken dialog systems. In: Proceedings of Human Language Technologies: The 2009 Annual Conference of the North American Chapter of the Association for Computational Linguistics, pp. 629–637. Association for Computational Linguistics (2009)
26. Ravenet, B., Cafaro, A., Ochs, M., Pelachaud, C.: Interpersonal attitude of a speaking agent in simulated group conversations. In: Bickmore, T., Marsella, S., Sidner, C. (eds.) IVA 2014. LNCS, vol. 8637, pp. 345–349. Springer, Heidelberg (2014)
27. Ravenet, B., Ochs, M., Pelachaud, C.: From a user-created corpus of virtual agent's non-verbal behavior to a computational model of interpersonal attitudes. In: Aylett, R., Krenn, B., Pelachaud, C., Shimodaira, H. (eds.) IVA 2013. LNCS, vol. 8108, pp. 263–274. Springer, Heidelberg (2013)
28. Rehm, M., Endrass, B.: Rapid prototyping of social group dynamics in multiagent systems. AI Soc. **24**, 13–23 (2009)
29. Reynolds, C.: Steering behaviors for autonomous characters. In: Proceedings of the Game Developers Conference, pp. 763–782. Miller Freeman Game Groups, San Francisco, CA (1999)
30. Sacks, H., Schegloff, E.A., Jefferson, G.: A simplest systematics for the organization of turn-taking for conversation. Language **50**, 696–735 (1974)
31. Sadler, P., Woody, E.: Interpersonal complementarity. Handbook of interpersonal psychology: Theory, research, assessment, and therapeutic interventions, p. 123 (2010)
32. Scheflen, A.E., Ashcraft, N.: Human Territories: How We Behave in Space-Time. Prentice-Hall, Englewood Cliffs (1976)
33. ter Maat, M., Truong, K.P., Heylen, D.: How turn-taking strategies influence users' impressions of an agent. In: Allbeck, J., Badler, N., Bickmore, T., Pelachaud, C., Safonova, A. (eds.) IVA 2010. LNCS, vol. 6356, pp. 441–453. Springer, Heidelberg (2010)
34. Thórisson, K.R., Gislason, O., Jonsdottir, G.R., Thorisson, HTh: A multiparty multimodal architecture for realtime turntaking. In: Allbeck, J., Badler, N., Bickmore, T., Pelachaud, C., Safonova, A. (eds.) IVA 2010. LNCS, vol. 6356, pp. 350–356. Springer, Heidelberg (2010)
35. Vilhjálmsson, H.H.: Animating conversation in online games. In: Rauterberg, M. (ed.) ICEC 2004. LNCS, vol. 3166, pp. 139–150. Springer, Heidelberg (2004)
36. Wiggins, J.S., Trapnell, P., Phillips, N.: Psychometric and geometric characteristics of the revised interpersonal adjective scales (IAS-R). Multivar. Behav. Res. **23**(4), 517–530 (1988)

A Continuous Model for the Management of Turn-Taking in User-Agent Spoken Interactions Based on the Variations of Prosodic Signals

Mathieu Jégou[1]($\boxtimes$), Liv Lefebvre[1], and Pierre Chevaillier[1,2]

[1] Technologic Research Institute b<>com, 29280 Plouzané, France
{mathieu.jegou,liv.lefebvre}@b-com.com
[2] ENIB–UEB, Lab-STICC, 29280 Plouzané, France
pierre.chevaillier@enib.fr

Abstract. Many recent works on agent architectures have focused on polite and optimal turn-transitions. However, real turn-taking is more complex due to several contextual variables, linked to each agent's own goals (cooperative or non cooperative for example). For mixed-initiative interactions, we need to go beyond the polite agent context to make more complex patterns of turn-taking emerge. We present here an architecture based on a dynamical and continuous model of turn-taking, able to control the turn-taking behaviors of the agent depending on its willingness to speak or not. We show how we implemented our model based on human data and how complex patterns of turn-taking emerge from agent-agent simulations. Finally, we present the results of a perceptual experiment where we questioned participants about the intentions of two agents interacting.

Keywords: Conversational agents · Emergent behavior · Turn-taking

1 Introduction

In many spoken dialog systems, speech exchanges between users and agents are rigid, non-smooth, still far from human interactions [4]. This could be explained partly by the lack of an appropriate turn-taking model [11]. For successful mixed-initiative interactions with users, the turn-taking manager should be able to handle smooth turn transitions, but also barge-ins, non-competitive overlaps, hesitations and silences [4,9], in a highly dynamic, noisy, unpredictable context and under time-pressure. To our best knowledge, no existing architecture is able to manage all these aspects using one single model. We propose a continuous and dynamical model that accounts for various kinds of turn-taking situations in human spoken interactions. Although we do not neglect the role of the semantic interpretation of the verbal production [10], our objective is to obtain agents able to use nonverbal signals to coordinate their turn-taking behavior, in a way

© Springer International Publishing Switzerland 2015
W.-P. Brinkman et al. (Eds.): IVA 2015, LNAI 9238, pp. 389–398, 2015.
DOI: 10.1007/978-3-319-21996-7_42

human beings do, as reported in [6,7]. Moreover, previous work stressed the role of voice intensity and pitch variations in the perception of the interlocutor's intention towards turn-taking [7].

This article presents the general conceptual model for dyadic interactions we devised to handle multimodal non verbal signals. In this study, we focused on the vocal modality. We show how our agent is able to continuously vary intensity and pitch to indicate its intention to take, keep or give the floor and to take into account the intentions of its interlocutor, as they are conveyed by her/his nonverbal productions.

2   Related Work and Positionning

Turn-taking is referred as the process by which participants exchange speech such that, roughly speaking, one participant talks at a time [4]. According to Ward et al. [11], in spoken dialog systems, turn-taking is non natural, non smooth and leads to unpleasant interactions. To resolve these usability issues, they advocate the development of incremental speech processing and speech synthesis but also an appropriate cognitive model of turn-taking. For many of existing models (e.g. Raux and Eskenazi [8]), turn-taking is an optimization problem: the agent must take the turn as soon as it perceives the end of turn, while avoiding to misinterpret pauses as turn-taking opportunities. Despite these approaches are well fitted to some kinds of interactions, such as request-response systems, we need to go beyond this polite agent context when users and agents are in situations where roles cannot be assigned in advance. In these kinds of conversations, participants' behavior are subjects to more variability and indeed turn-transitions are not always optimal, their duration are normally distributed [3]. Moreover, misinterpretations of the interlocutor's intention relative to turn-taking are often observed that can lead to unintentional conflicting overlaps. The smoothness of the conversation resides also in the capability of both participants to quickly resolve these situations [6].

Noteworthy, in mixed-initiative dialogs, turns are locally managed and, who is going to be the next speaker, is not defined in advance. Therefore, turn allocations is not under the control of any specific participant and their temporal organization is an emergent property of the agents' interaction. Managing the whole spectrum of situations, in a robust and seamless way, requires a turn-taking management model, able to continuously adapt the agent's nonverbal productions to users' behavior [5,13]. The sensory-motor coupling of the two interacting agents ensures the emergent nature of behavior.

3   Conceptual Model

Overview. The specific components of our turn-taking management (TTM) architecture are the *intention perception* module and the *control of action* module (Fig. 1). The intention perception module continuously updates γ, the confidence the agent has about its interlocutor's intention, based on the nonverbal signals the agent can perceive. As a speaker, the intention perception module has to infer whether the listener is currently claiming the floor or not, and, as a listener, whether the speaker is yielding the turn or not. The control of action module has two input variables: the agent's own intention I to yield or to take the turn and γ. Typically, I is controlled by the agent's dialog manager. I represents the willingness the agent has to adopt the opposite role. This intention depends on whether the agent has something to say or not, and to its degree of cooperativeness. The interplay between these two variables creates a complex relationship between the agent's own willingness to speak or yield turn, and the influence of its interlocutor's signal. Therefore, each agent's behavior is not fully under its control, but is self-organized and emerges from the interaction.

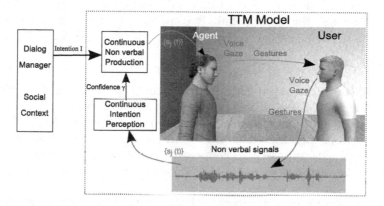

Fig. 1. General principle of the agent architecture showing the interplay between the agent's intention and its confidence about the intention of its interlocutor.

Continuous Perception. Turn-taking is a time-constrained task. Participants resolve different situations, such as conflicting overlaps, in a short lapse of time. Moreover, due to the limitations of the perception capabilities of the agents and the variations along the time of the different nonverbal productions, agents are acting in a noisy, uncertain environment. Moreover, the agent has to infer the intention of its interlocutor between two alternatives: whether he wants or not to take (yield) the turn. All these characteristics correspond to the Two Alternative Forced Choice (TAFC) paradigm [1], which has been extensively applied for the modeling of tasks where humans had to infer the right information provided by the environment between two possible solutions. The Drift Diffusion Model (DDM) applies this paradigm. It is implemented as an integrator, accumulating over time evidence favoring one or the other alternative. A definitive decision towards one alternative is made when the agent has accumulated sufficient evidence favoring one alternative. The equation of DDM is defined as follows:

$$d\gamma = \beta dt + \sigma d\epsilon \quad ; \text{ with } \gamma(0) = 0 \tag{1}$$

$d\gamma$ represents the variation of the difference of evidence favoring one or the other alternative. This value depends on two terms: the accumulation parameter βdt, which is a function of the signals currently produced by the interlocutor, and $\sigma d\epsilon$, representing a normally distributed noise in the process. Typically, multimodal signals are continuously acquired by different audio-visual sensors. We set currently the noisy term to 0 to assert the main properties of our model without adding any stochastic process. The model defines two decision thresholds ($t_\gamma^+ = 1$, $t_\gamma^- = -1$), corresponding to the two alternatives. When γ crosses one threshold, a definitive decision is made towards the corresponding alternative. $\gamma = t_\gamma^+$ means that the agent is sure about its interlocutor willingness to change its role (listener $\rightarrow$ speaker, or speaker $\rightarrow$ listener). $\gamma = t_\gamma^-$ means that the agent is sure that its interlocutor wants to keep the same role. When $\gamma \geq t_\gamma^+$, whatever the value of I, the agent definitely considers that its interlocutor changed role and, thus, itself has currently taken the opposite role. In this case, γ is reset to 0.

Control of the Nonverbal Signals. Following the behavioral dynamics [12], human behavior is a self-organized, emergent property of a perception-action cycle: by acting, information provided by the environment varies, and directly constrains actions performed by the agent. Several studies have shown the applicability of this approach to cooperative tasks [2]. It strongly encouraged us to apply this paradigm to turn-taking management, which is a cooperative behavior.

In Warren's approach, the control laws are defined as dynamical systems where information provided by the environment constitutes a control variable. Attractors of these systems are the agent's goals, and repellers, the states to avoid. In our model, each modality is controlled by a set of dynamical systems. The intention I and the confidence γ play the role of control variables. In our model, all the dynamical systems have the same general shape, given by Eq. 2:

$$\ddot{a}_j = -b\dot{a}_j - k_g * (a_j - f(\gamma, I)) \tag{2}$$

$-b\dot{a}_j$ is a damping term, corresponding to the inertia of the signal production. The term $-k_g * (a_j - f(\gamma, I))$ determines towards which value the signal varies, depending on the current confidence and intention of the agent. In this abstract formalization, each signal j produced by the agent is encoded as a variable $a_j \in [0.0, 1.0]$, 0.0 representing no signal displayed and 1.0 the maximum intensity of the signal (e.g. the highest voice intensity or the highest pitch). The way these theoretical internal values are converted into real values depends on the nature of each signal; they serve as control parameters of the different continuous behavior realizers.

4   Calibration

We have implemented our general model for controlling variations of prosody during turn transitions. The two controlled parameters were intensity of the voice and pitch. The objective was to verify if such a model could reproduce the real prosodic variations during different situations observed in human conversations in French. For this, we collected data on dyadic human spoken interactions, and then calibrated our model, based on the results we obtained.

4.1 Analysis of Human-Human Interactions

We analyzed several features from recorded spontaneous mixed initiative dialogs. We studied the variations of prosodic signals during turn transitions or attempts and temporal features in these situations: duration of silence (often referred as gaps [3]), slight overlaps in transitions and duration of competitive overlaps.

We found that the duration of gaps were distributed in majority between 100 and 800 ms (median = 470 ms). The median value of overlaps duration was approximately 400 ms, and mostly distributed between 100 ms to 1.5 s.

We then present the analysis of two prosodic features: the mean variation of pitch and intensity at the end of turns and during overlaps. Differences were the most significant and maximal when we measured the mean intensity and pitch during the last 300 ms. It was found that participants significantly decreased their intensity (-3.7 dB) and pitch (-13 Hz) before turn endings. No significant differences in intensity and pitch were found at turn beginnings. For overlaps, data showed a significant increase of the speaker's intensity during competitive overlaps ($+4$ dB), and also for the listener who fought to take the floor ($+3.3$ dB). Such effect was not found for pitch.

4.2 Calibration of the Model

The first step was to define the functions $f(\gamma, I)$ presented in Eq. 2 for each action. We manually determined the parameters and the shape based on the main qualitative patterns of turn-taking observed in our data. These equations are presented in the table below, where u is the Heaviside function ($u(x) = 0$ for $x < 0$ and $u(x) = 1$ when $x \geq 0.0$). In this implementation, $I \in [-1.0, 1.0]$: $I < 0$ represents an intention of the agent to keep its role, $I > 0$ the opposite. For confidence, $\gamma \in [-1.0, 1.0]$: if $\gamma > 0$, the agent is confident about the intention of the other to change role, $\gamma < 0$ the agent is confident about the opposite.

Speaker	Functions
Intensity	$f(\gamma, I) = 0.5 * u(2I + \gamma - 1.1) + (I - 0.5) * u(-\gamma) * u(2I + \gamma - 1.1)$
Pitch	$f(\gamma, I) = 0.5 * u(2I + \gamma - 1)$
Listener	Functions
Intensity	$f(\gamma, I) = 0.5 * u(-I - \gamma) * u(I) + 0.5 * u(-I) - 0.5 * I * u(\gamma) * u(-I)$
Pitch	$f(\gamma, I) = 0.5 * (u(-I - \gamma) * u(I) + u(-I))$

Fig. 2. Equations for the control of actions for both the speaker and the listener

The confidence value above which the agent begins to display cues for changing role is a linear function of I when $I > 0$. If $I = 1$, the agent displays role-changing signals even if $\gamma = -1$, if $I = 0$, the agent begins to display signals only when $\gamma = 1$. This implies that, when $I > 0.5$, it will begin to display signals even if evidence suggest that the other does not want to change role. This case corresponds to an agent that tries to force the other to change role by increasing its signals. On the opposite if $I < 0.5$, the agent will wait until getting evidence that the other is yielding the turn. For the current speaker, when $I < 0$ and $\gamma > 0$, the agent perceives that its interlocutor tries to take the turn, and then increases its intensity.

The implementation of the decision making module consists in instantiating each function β_j. We used polynomial functions, which are universal approximators:

$$y = b_0 + b_1 \dot{s}_j + b_2 s_j + b_3 \dot{s}_j s_j + b_4 \dot{s}_j{}^2$$

The parameters of the equation were calculated such that, depending on the intentions of the agents, when both intentions are positive, a smooth transition occurs. Meanwhile, when the intention of the speaker is negative and the intention of the listener is positive, there is a conflict. In this case, given I_l the speaker intention and I_a the listener intention, when $|I_l| < |I_a|$ the listener takes finally the turn, and when $|I_l| > |I_a|$ the current speaker currently keeps the turn. We used a simulated annealing algorithm combined to a cost function to estimate these parameters.

4.3   Results

To verify the ability of the parameterized model to reproduce the various situations, we simulated the interaction of two agents. We present here the results for situations resulting in gaps and competitive overlaps.

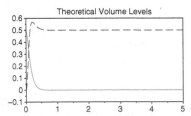 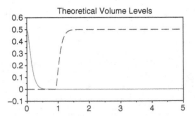

Fig. 3. Two smooth transitions patterns produced by the model. For both figure: in plain, the previous speaker; in dashed, the next speaker.

The results show that the duration of the turn transitions vary between -400 ms (Fig. 3, left) and 900 ms (Fig. 3, right), depending on the intentions of the agents. According to the observations, the current speaker begins to decrease his intensity and pitch 300 ms before the end of the turn. Concerning competitive overlaps, when the two agents are trying to keep (or to take) the floor, duration of conflicts are between 700 ms (Fig. 4, left) and 1.8 s (Fig. 4, right).

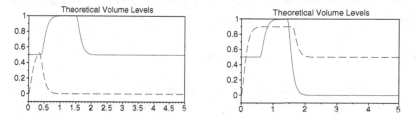

Fig. 4. Two different overlaps between turns. In plain, speaker at the beginning of the simulation; in dashed, listener).

We finally evaluated the stability of the model, which means its ability to handle several consecutive turns. Figure 5 shows one scenario where we varied manually intentions of the two agents. The curves in plain and dashed at the top represent the intensity variation for the two agents. Below, the plain and dashed curves represent the associated the time series of I: when the curve is at the value -0.05 (resp. -0.25), $I = 1$; when the curve is at -0.15 (resp. -0.35), $I = -1$.

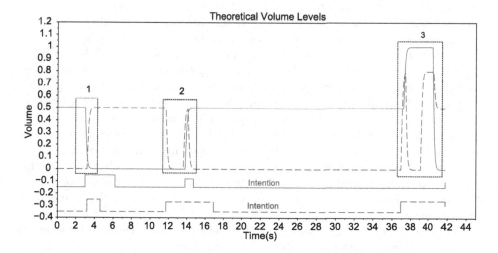

Fig. 5. Example of a complex scenario of turn-taking on several turns.

Interestingly several patterns emerge from this scenario. The second transition in Fig. 5 corresponds to an unintentional overlap. The current speaker (dashed) wants to yield the turn. As it observes that its interlocutor does not seem to take the turn, it starts to speak again, typically starting with a filler.

As it observes next that the current listener finally takes the turn, it rapidly stops speaking, resulting in a smooth resolution of an overlap. The third transition occurs as the current speaker (plain) does not want to yield the turn. The current listener tries two times to take the turn and succeeds at the second attempt.

5   User Perception Experiment

We conducted a perceptual experiment where human participants were confronted to recorded interactions of two virtual humans dialoging in a 3D environment. Characters spoke a pseudo-language that participants could not understand. By this way, any semantic or syntactic cues were removed. We wanted to know if, based on the prosodic variations provided by our model, participants were able to infer correctly participants' intentions.

Experimental Protocol. Each interaction was composed of different types of situation, among them, a slight overlap of 300 ms corresponding to an agent taking the turn just before the end of the current speaker turn (considered by some authors as non competitive [6]) and a barge-in.

Each situation was extracted from agent-agent simulations. The prosodic variations initially between zero and one computed by our model were transposed in intensity in dB and pitch in Hz. We converted intensity following the formula $i_{dB} = i_{mdB} \times (1 + 20 \times log(\exp(4(i - i_m))))$ where: i_{dB} corresponds to the resulting value of intensity in dB; i_{mdB} a manually determined mean intensity in dB; i the current intensity from the model; i_m the mean intensity in the model (i.e. 0.5). We converted the pitch following the formula $p_{Hz} = p_{mHz} \times (1 + \frac{p - p_m}{p_m})$, where: p_{Hz} corresponds to the value of the resulting pitch in Hz; p_{mHz} a manually determined mean pitch in Hz; p the current pitch value from the model; p_m the mean pitch of the model (i.e. 0.5). Then, these data were applied to utterances pronounced by agents by setting to each syllable the mean intensity and pitch of the corresponding period of the syllable via SSML. Sound files were generated via Voxygen TTS for each utterance. During the experiment, at each situation two different set of files, one per agent, were played, and were time-aligned to fit the original transition or overlap duration of the original agent-agent simulation. The different situations followed themselves without interruption in the interaction between characters.

The succession of situations changed for each subject. During the interaction we questioned participants about the overlap situations they observed. We stopped the interaction after the situation occurred and we asked: (Q1) if the previous listener perceived that the speaker finished speaking before taking the turn, (Q2) if the previous speaker wanted to prevent the listener to take the turn, (Q3) if the previous listener wanted to prevent the speaker to continue speaking. Participants had to answer by True or False to these questions. We asked the participants to indicate in a four-point Lickert scale (between 0 and 3) the clarity of the cues that permitted them to answer.

Results and Discussion. In total, 22 subjects participated in our study. We present in Fig. 6 the results obtained. The column "Expected" refers to what we expected participants to answer, the column "Agreement" refers to the percentage of participants that responded as we expected. The values in bold corresponds to the percentage of agreement where participants indicated a clarity value greater than 1.

Questions	Slight overlap		Competitive overlap	
	Expected	Agreement	Expected	Agreement
Q1	Yes	60 % (**64 %**)	No	86 % (**96 %**)
Q2	No	77 % (**75 %**)	Yes	81 % (**100 %**)
Q3	No	45 % (**58 %**)	Yes	64 % (**76 %**)

Fig. 6. Percentage of agreement of the participants' answers relative to the agent's communicative intention.

Generally speaking, participants reported that it was difficult to clearly identify the intentions of the characters. This difficulty explains the answers to the questions Q1 for slight overlaps and Q3 for both situations. In the slight overlap situation, participants reported that they had difficulties to know if the previous speaker was ending its turn. It explains the low majority of "Yes" in the answers of the participants. For Q3, the low percentage of agreement for slight overlaps is consistent with the answers to Q1, since participants did not perceive that the previous speaker wanted to yield the turn, they considered this situation as a barge-in. However, when participants identified clear cues, the percentage of agreement was above the mean, which means that signals produced by the agents conveyed the right information.

Several hypotheses could be done from these results. First, intensity and pitch could be non sufficient for the detection of turn endings. This agrees with some studies [10] that tend to show that intensity and prosody have only a weak effect on the perception of turn endings. However, Niebuhr et al. study [7] show that intensity and pitch are effectively used by users to identify a turn ending. This could mean also that, for our study, the interaction that participants observed was non natural. As a result, subjects did not feel involved in the scenario and could have perceived differently cues compared to subjects observing real conversation situations. Besides, participants were observers and did not have the same temporal constraints as if they were engaged in an interaction. Embedding users in a real, time constrained, interaction, could lead to a better interpretation of the agents' intentions based on both prosodic cues.

6   Conclusion

We presented a continuous model for turn-taking management that reproduces the prosodic variations observed during human conversations. The model produces consistent behavior depending on agents' intentions. The ability to rapidly resolve unintentional overlaps and the stability of the model are encouraging. The results of the perceptual evaluation should be interpreted keeping in mind that the participants had no idea what the agents were saying, and were not in the same conditions as embedded in a real conversation. The results could mean that intensity and pitch do not convey enough information for users to discriminate the right communicative intention of the agents. Beyond the undeniable contribution of verbal content, it is also necessary to endow the agents with additional communicative channels, e.g. speech rate, gesture and gaze. One could also question whether it is better to reproduce exactly the values observed in human-human interactions or to accentuate the variations of the signals exposed by the agent. We now plan to observe behavior of users interacting in real-time with our agent.

References

1. Bogacz, R., Brown, E., Moehlis, J., Holmes, P., Cohen, J.: The physics of optimal decision making: a formal analysis of models of performance in two-alternative forced-choice tasks. Psycholog. Rev. **113**(4), 700 (2006)
2. Fowler, C.A., Richardson, M.J., Marsh, K.L., Shockley, K.D., Jirsa, V.K.: Language use, coordination, and the emergence of cooperative action. In: Fuchs, A., Jirsa, V.K. (eds.) Coordination: Neural, Behavioral and Social Dynamics. Understanding Complex Systems, pp. 261–279. Springer, Heidelberg (2008)
3. Heldner, M., Edlund, J.: Pauses, gaps and overlaps in conversations. J. Phonetics **38**(4), 555–568 (2010)
4. Jonsdottir, G.R., Thórisson, K.R.: A distributed architecture for real-time dialogue and on-task learning of efficient co-operative turn-taking. In: Coverbal Synchrony in Human-Machine Interaction, p. 293 (2013)
5. Kopp, S., Buschmeier, H.: A dynamic minimal model of the listener for feedback-based dialogue coordination. In: Proceedings of the 18th Workshop on the Semantics and Pragmatics of Dialogue, Edinburgh, UK, pp. 17–25 (2014)
6. Kurtić, E., Brown, G.J., Wells, B.: Resources for turn competition in overlapping talk. Speech Commun. **55**(5), 721–743 (2013)
7. Niebuhr, O., Görs, K., Graupe, E.: Speech reduction, intensity, and F0 shape are cues to turn-taking. In: SIGDIAL 2013, pp. 261–269 (2013)
8. Raux, A., Eskenazi, M.: Optimizing the turn-taking behavior of task-oriented spoken dialog systems. ACM Trans. Speech Lang. Process. **9**(1), 1:1–1:23 (2012)
9. Reidsma, D., de Kok, I., Neiberg, D., Pammi, S.C., van Straalen, B., Truong, K., van Welbergen, H.: Continuous interaction with a virtual human. J. Multimodal User Interfaces **4**(2), 97–118 (2011)
10. Riest, C., Jorschick, A.B., de Ruiter, J.P.: Anticipation in turn-taking: mechanisms and information sources. Front. Psychol. **6**, 89 (2015)
11. Ward, N.G., Rivera, A.G., Ward, K., Novick, D.G.: Root causes of lost time and user stress in a simple dialog system. In: INTERSPEECH 2005, pp. 1565–1568 (2005)
12. Warren, W.H.: The dynamics of perception and action. Psycholog. Rev. **113**(2), 358–389 (2006)
13. van Welbergen, H., Yaghoubzadeh, R., Kopp, S.: AsapRealizer 2.0: the next steps in fluent behavior realization for ECAs. In: Bickmore, T., Marsella, S., Sidner, C. (eds.) IVA 2014. LNCS, vol. 8637, pp. 449–462. Springer, Heidelberg (2014)

An Interaction Game Framework for the Investigation of Human–Agent Cooperation

Philipp Kulms(✉), Nikita Mattar, and Stefan Kopp

Social Cognitive Systems Group, Faculty of Technology,
Center of Excellence - Cognitive Interaction Technology (CITEC),
Bielefeld University, Bielefeld, Germany
{pkulms,nmattar,skopp}@techfak.uni-bielefeld.de

Abstract. Success in human–agent interaction will to a large extent depend on the ability of the system to cooperate with humans over repeated tasks. It is not yet clear how cooperation between humans and virtual agents evolves and is interlinked with the attribution of qualities like trustworthiness or competence between the cooperation partners. To explore these questions, we present a new interaction game framework that is centered around a collaborative puzzle game and goes beyond commonly adopted scenarios like the Prisoner's dilemma. First results are presented at the conference.

1 Introduction

With advances in human–agent interaction and artificial intelligence, future interactions with technical systems are likely to be shaped like a *cooperation* between partners with complementary competencies [2]. In such teams, each agent has some degree of autonomy to handle dynamic situations and to make decisions within uncertain situations. One central question is: what does it require for a human to be willing and able to cooperate with a computer? We take further steps to investigate the potential of virtual agents to support cooperation. We focus in particular on the central factors *trustworthiness* and *competence* and how they develop in, and influence an ongoing human–agent cooperation. We consider trustworthiness as the agent's ability to signal reliability in terms of benevolent intentions [3], and we seek to analyze how it is intertwined with the user's perception of the agent's competence.

2 Theoretical Background

Cooperative interaction moved into focus of HCI with a paradigm shift from using computers as mere tools, to interacting with them as intelligent and autonomous partners that resemble human-like counterparts [2,5]. Hoc [4] argued that cooperative situations are shaped by (a) both agents' ability to interfere with each other on goals, resources, etc. (thus requiring coordination) and by (b) the management of interference, for example to support the other agents

© Springer International Publishing Switzerland 2015
W.-P. Brinkman et al. (Eds.): IVA 2015, LNAI 9238, pp. 399–402, 2015.
DOI: 10.1007/978-3-319-21996-7_43

tasks. To further promote the development of cooperative agents, it is crucial to understand when and how cooperation emerges in scenarios that are dynamic, extend over many interactions, and afford communication via various social signals. Thus far, cooperative behavior is primarily investigated using idealized cooperative games originating from behavioral game theory (BGT). However, cooperative games such as the Prisoner's dilemma, although well-established, are limited in scope and ecological validity when it comes to studying issues like competence and trustworthiness and how they evolve in a scenario with richer interaction. These game scenarios are on purpose kept very limited, with various variations and modifications applied, e.g. recasting the Prisoner's dilemma into an investment game, or allowing emotional feedback. Aside from making binary decisions (cooperate: yes/no) or allocating money between both players, the decision spaces and possibilities to interact in a meaningful way are confined. Although the BGT approach has yielded remarkable results, it is difficult to model and examine cooperative human–agent interactions with cooperative games alone in the long run because they cannot sufficiently model settings that comprise cooperative elements of HCI such as the formation of teams, solving a collaborative task, or rich communication. We argue that a framework that allows for modeling and studying cooperation in human–agent interaction in a more realistic and valid, yet controllable and manageable way is still lacking. From our point of view, such a framework has to meet at least the following requirements: (R1) goal interdependence, (R2) evocation and observation of various key factors (e.g. trust/trustworthiness, cooperativeness, competence, willingness to take risks, believability, emotions), (R3) ability to communicate and coordinate between the agent, (R4) identification of utilities assigned to decisions, (R5) possibility to introduce agent embodiment, (R6) algorithmically feasible automatization, (R7) possibility to assign different roles to players.

3   A Cooperative Puzzle Game

We have developed an interaction framework that allows us to operationalize, manipulate and analyze the relevant factors and key characteristics of cooperative behavior in a systematic fashion (see Fig. 1). The general setting includes two players solving a puzzle game interactively. Inspired by Tetris®, the interaction scenario consists of a board where two players work together to place blocks of various shapes, using horizontal movements and rotation. In our game, blocks do not move down gradually and filled lines are not cleared. The former gives us the ability to manipulate the available time per round (difficulty), the latter simplifies the implementation of an algorithm that enables a virtual agent to participate as autonomous player. There are further reasons why we chose this puzzle game: First, it is relatively easy to implement a heuristic to find optimal solutions for an agent (R6). By adapting the underlying heuristic, we are thereby able to manipulate the agents behavior and thus, presumably, its perceived competence (R2). Second, we can induce both individual goals (e.g. as an individual score for a block a player has placed) as well as cooperative goals (as a team score for lines that get completely filled). This enables us to analyze

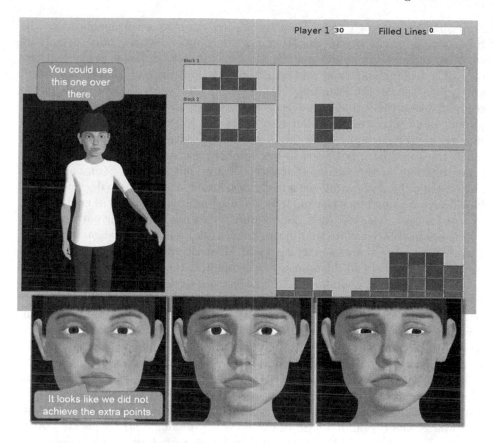

Fig. 1. Concept of the puzzle game interface with a virtual agent as cooperation partner. The agent can display multimodal behavior or other contextual social cues. This allows for analyzing which type of feedback cue (verbal, sad or regretful facial expression) has what differential effect on the ongoing cooperation.

if a player prioritizes one over the other as a measure of cooperativeness (R1). Third, by changing factors such as field size, time constraints, block shapes, or block scores we can manipulate the difficulty of achieving the cooperative goal. Finally, we can at all times fully observe the game state.

Two different player roles are introduced in an asymmetric setup of the game (R7): a *recommender* and a *decider*. Each round consists of the following steps: (1) The *recommender* picks one out of two blocks he wants to recommend to the *decider*. (2) The *decider* picks a block by either accepting or rejecting the recommendation and places it on the board. (3) The *recommender* places the remaining block. Both players receive points individually for every block they place. The complex block gives more points than the simple one, leading to an individual benefit in placing more complex blocks (R4). In addition, both players obtain points when a certain amount of lines are completely filled horizontally. We refer to this as cooperative or joint goal since it can only be achieved if the players cooperate with each other by recommending and choosing blocks that minimize the occupied space, and by placing them in a reasonable way. The three actions occurring in this scenario – recommendations, (not) complying with recommendations, and placing blocks – relate to different behavioral factors (R2): recommendations and compliance are indicative of competence, trust, and pursued goals. For example, if the *recommender* constantly recommends the complex block this could be interpreted as a high level of trust in the partner, pursuit of an altruistic goal, but also as low level of competence of the *recommender* himself. In contrast, if the *recommender* always recommends the simple block this could be interpreted as low level of trust or pursuit of a selfish goal. Interpretations of the actions of the *decider* are quite similar. Still, one cannot always tell if the *decider* follows a recommendation or would have decided for the block anyway. The block placing may serve as indicator for level of competence, except for cases where players deliberately try to minimize their partners score by misplacing blocks. Note that in this framework, (non-)cooperation is strategic and requires more than a binary decision. Although the decision-making process in the often used social dilemmas is also complex, the final action translates to "I (do not) want to cooperate". In contrast, we expect the degree of cooperativeness the *decider* signals to the *recommender* to depend on (a) the *decider's* puzzle solving skills, and (b) the intention the *decider* signals by (not) complying with the *recommender's* advice. As a result, how is a *decider* perceived who performs well but only rarely accepts recommendations, or who accepts the recommendations but performs poorly? The perceived cooperativeness of the *decider*, then, should relate to the *recommender's* willingness to cooperate with him [1]. An experimental study where participants played as *recommender* and a non-embodied agent acted as *decider* showed that perceived competence, trustworthiness, and cooperativeness of the *decider* were differentially affected by its puzzle solving skills and the degree to which it accepted recommendations.

Acknowledgements. This research was supported by the German Federal Ministry of Education and Research (BMBF) within the Leading-Edge Cluster 'it's OWL', managed by the Project Management Agency Karlsruhe (PTKA), as well as by the Deutsche Forschungsgemeinschaft (DFG) within the Center of Excellence 277 'Cognitive Interaction Technology' (CITEC). We also would like to thank Kai Sattler for his valuable contributions.

References

1. Balliet, D., Van Lange, P.A.: Trust, conflict, and cooperation: a meta-analysis. Psychol. Bull. **139**(5), 1090 (2013)
2. Bradshaw, J.M., Dignum, V., Jonker, C., Sierhuis, M.: Human-agent-robot teamwork. IEEE Intell. Syst. **27**(2), 2–7 (2012)
3. Deutsch, M.: Cooperation and trust: some theoretical notes. In: Jones, M.R. (ed.) Nebraska Symposium on Motivation, pp. 275–320. University of Nebraska Press, Oxford (1962)
4. Hoc, J.M.: From human-machine interaction to human-machine cooperation. Ergonomics **43**(7), 833–843 (2000)
5. Nass, C., Fogg, B., Moon, Y.: Can computers be teammates? Int. J. Hum. Comput. Stud. **45**(6), 669–678 (1996)

Virtual Agent Perception Studies

Offscreen and in the Chair Next to Your: Conversational Agents Speaking Through Actual Human Bodies

Kevin Corti[✉] and Alex Gillespie

Department of Social Psychology, London School of Economics, London, UK
{k.corti,a.t.gillespie}@lse.ac.uk

Abstract. This paper demonstrates how to interact with a conversational agent that speaks through an actual human body face-to-face and in person (i.e., offscreen). This is made possible by the cyranoid method: a technique involving a human person speech shadowing for a remote third-party (i.e., receiving their words via a covert audio-relay apparatus and repeating them aloud in real-time). When a person shadows for an artificial conversational agent source, we call the resulting hybrid an "echoborg." We report a study in which people encountered conversational agents either through a human shadower face-to-face or via a text interface under conditions where they assumed their interlocutor to be an actual person. Our results show that the perception of a conversational agent is dramatically altered when the agent is voiced by an actual, tangible person. We discuss the potential implications this methodology has for the development of conversational agents and general person perception research.

Keywords: Design methodologies · Evaluation methodologies and user studies · Applications for film, animation, art and games · Cyranoid · Echoborg

1 Introduction

You have just signed up to participate in a social psychological research project and find yourself in a university meeting room with two chairs positioned facing each other. As you take a seat in one chair, the researcher informs you that the study you are taking part in involves holding a 10-min face-to-face conversation with a stranger - another research participant. You are told that you can discuss anything you would like with your interlocutor; there is no script you need to follow or role you need to play. *Simple enough*, you think to yourself.

Shortly after the researcher leaves the room an ordinary-looking person enters and takes a seat in the chair across from you. You introduce yourself and reflexively utter "how are you?" to get the conversation started. "Fine," they say. As you begin to ask more questions you notice something slightly odd about the person you are speaking with. They are taking an unusually long time to answer you. *Should it really take someone three seconds to answer the question "are you a student?"* You brush this off as shyness and try to find a topic to discuss. "What do you think of the weather today?" you ask. "I think the weather is beautiful today," they respond (after several seconds of

© Springer International Publishing Switzerland 2015
W.-P. Brinkman et al. (Eds.): IVA 2015, LNAI 9238, pp. 405–417, 2015.
DOI: 10.1007/978-3-319-21996-7_44

slightly awkward silence). *Really? This person's idea of beauty is icy rain and wind?* "But don't you hate it when the underground stations get all wet and slippery from the rainwater?" you counter. "Yes," they say. "What exactly do you find beautiful about it then?" you demand. Their answer: "I actually don't. Or at least prefer it when I wake up and don't remember much from them, which is actually almost on a regular basis." *Huh?* "Sorry?" you utter. Their reply: "I forgive you."

About halfway through the conversation you start to suspect that this is all an act (you are participating in a social psychology study, after all). *But they can't be giving scripted responses, I'm allowed to say and ask anything I want!* By the time the 10-min have ended you haven nearly given up all hope of achieving a meaningful interaction with the other person. You found it impossible to build upon discussion topics with them. As soon as you would begin to develop conversational sequences about, say, favorite books or movies, your interlocutor would change the topic or completely forget what they had said several turns prior. The most frustrating things in your mind were the misunderstandings and the inability, despite your best efforts, to resolve them.

The researcher returns to the room and your interlocutor exits. "So, how did it go?" the researcher asks...

2   Background

2.1   Motivation

For the past two years we have conducted basic social psychological research involving people interacting with conversational agent computer programs that speak through actual human bodies. Our goal has been the development of a new research tool: the "echoborg." An echoborg is a hybrid agent composed of the body of a real person and the "mind" (or, rather, the words) of a conversational agent; the words the echoborg speaks are determined by the conversational agent, transmitted to the person via a covert audio-relay apparatus, and articulated by the person through speech shadowing. Echoborgs can be used in interactive field research as well as in laboratory settings rich in mundane realism. The purpose of exploring the possibility of such a tool stems from an interest in studying human-agent interaction under conditions wherein research participants are neither psychologically constrained nor influenced by machine interfaces. The echoborg can be thought of as a means of investigating the role of the tangible human body in altering how machine intelligence is perceived and interacted with.

2.2   Stanley Milgram's "Cyranoid Method"

The story of how we came to develop the echoborg concept begins with the unpublished work of Stanley Milgram. Milgram, who is well-known throughout psychology for his studies on obedience to authority [1], conducted a series of small experiments in the late 1970s that explored the possibility of creating a single interactive persona (a "cyranoid") from separate individuals [2]. He trained research confederates to speech shadow – an audio-vocal technique in which a person immediately repeats words they receive from a separate communication source [3]. Once trained, Milgram staged interactions wherein he and other research assistants conversed through these speech shadowers with research participants naïve to the fact that the person they encountered was being inconspicuously fed what to say by an unseen source. The shadowers contributed no words of their own to these interactions. Time after time, Milgram's participants failed to detect the manipulation, even in contexts involving extreme incongruity between source and shadower such as when he sourced for 11- and 12-year-old children during interviews with panels of teachers. Milgram described these participants as having succumbed to the "cyranic illusion": a phenomenon he defined as failing to perceive when an interlocutor is not self-authoring the words they speak.

Speech shadowing is a straightforward technique that requires fairly little time to master. It can be accomplished by having the shadower wear an ear monitor that receives audio from either a recording or a live, spontaneously communicating source. The shadower listens to this audio and attempts to replicate the words and vocal sounds they hear as soon as they are perceived. Research has shown that shadowers can fluidly replicate audio stimuli at latencies as short as a few hundred milliseconds [4–6]. Shadowers instinctively mimic the gestural elements of their source, unconsciously adopting their source's accent, cadence, stress, emphasis, and so on [7, 8]. Shadowing is not a cognitively demanding task. Trained speech shadowers, not having to *think* about what to say, can divert cognitive resources to other actions. For instance, while shadowing one can focus on producing body language and an overall physical demeanor consistent with the words one finds oneself repeating.

2.3   Replicating Milgram

Milgram died in 1984 at the age of 51 having never formally published his cyranoid studies, and the method lay dormant within social psychology for over two decades. In recent years, however, the cyranoid paradigm has re-emerged in experiential art and interactive design research [9–12]. Inspired by this work, we set out to replicate Milgram's original pilots, which he outlined in a speech he prepared for an American Psychological Association conference in 1984 [2] and which are described in a biography authored by Blass [13]. Our interest was in vetting the utility of the method as a technique for investigating aspects of person perception and as a means of experiencing a transformed social identity.

We explored a basic cyranic illusion scenario in an initial study [14]. Participants in a control condition conversed for 10-min in unscripted scenarios one-on-one and face-to-face with an adult male research confederate. In a treatment condition, participants spoke with the same research confederate who this time speech shadowed for a female source. Participants then filled out a questionnaire in which they were asked questions that gauged their suspicions regarding the communicative autonomy of the person they encountered. Participants were also thoroughly interviewed to gain a sense of their subjective impressions of the person they had encountered (the confederate). No differences between the conditions emerged. No participant in either condition believed that their interlocutor was being fed lines from a remote third-party, and very few participants held doubts as to whether their interlocutor was producing self-authored words. The fact that the conversations were unscripted (i.e., participants were told they could talk about whatever they wanted during the interactions) played a significant role in impressing upon the participants the feeling that the person they had encountered could not have been giving rehearsed responses.

Following our initial study, we decided to recreate Milgram's teacher-panel interview scenario. We designed an experiment in which a 12-year-old boy and a university professor alternated sourcing and shadowing for one another in mock interview contexts [14]. Panels of three to five research participants were asked to interview a stranger for twenty minutes in order to gain a sense of their intellectual capacity. No scripts were used; participants generated their own questions and remarks. Following the interviews, participants were asked in a number of ways whether they had doubts as to the communicative autonomy of the person they had interviewed. The vast majority of participants believed that they had engaged with a person who was articulating their own self-authored responses. This provided us with evidence that the cyranic illusion was robust even in situations involving extreme incongruity between source and shadower.

3   Dreaming of Electric Sheep

Following our replication of Milgram's original pilots, and on the basis of what we observed in additional small-scale cyranoid studies [15], we decided to explore the possibility of a cyranoid composed not of two human beings, but one composed of a human shadower and a conversational agent computer program source (the most extreme source-shadower incongruity we could imagine). We fashioned the term "echoborg" to refer to this special type of cyranoid.

The idea of the echoborg was largely inspired by the premise explored in Phillip K. Dick's famous novel *Do Androids Dream of Electric Sheep?* [16] (which was later adapted into the film *Blade Runner*). In the familiar story, a post-apocalyptic earth is partially populated by androids physically indistinguishable from actual human beings. One of the many thought experiments raised by the novel regards the role of belief in attributing an inner essence to an interlocutor, and the role perceiving a human body plays in implying a particular inner essence (namely, a human one).

3.1   Creating an Echoborg

A standard cyranoid requires a means for the source to overhear the words being articulated by an "interactant" (Milgram's term for those who engage with a cyranoid, either naïvely or in full knowledge that they are doing so), as well as a means for the shadower to receive speech from the source in real-time. If it is the researcher's goal to construct a covert cyranoid, then the apparatus will have to be composed of devices that are not perceptible to the interactant. In our standard covert cyranoid apparatuses we use a contraption of interconnected radio transmission devices. From one room, the source speaks into a microphone that connects to an FM radio transmitter. The signal is transmitted to an adjacent room where it is picked up by a pocket radio worn by the shadower, attached to which is a neck-loop induction coil that is concealed by the shadower's clothing. The shadower wears a flesh-colored inner-ear monitor that sits in their ear canal and is not detectable at close distances. This monitor receives the signal from the induction coil, allowing the shadower to hear and thus voice the source's words in real-time. A "bug" microphone placed in the room where the interactant and shadower are located wirelessly transmits audio via a radio signal to a receiver listened to by the source, thereby enabling the source to hear and respond to the words of the interactant. While this amalgam of devices is convenient and inconspicuous, there are other means of constructing cyranoid apparatuses both overt and covert in nature [10].

The echoborg concept simply replaces the human source in a traditional cyranoid with a conversational agent of some sort (e.g., a chat bot). The means by which the agent receives speech from the interactant, and how it transmits its responses to the human shadower, are decisions that the researcher must make on the basis of their particular research objectives. One could opt for full technological dependency and make use of speech recognition software as a means of inputting the interactant's words into the conversational agent program, as well as speech synthesis software as a means of relaying the agent's words to the shadower. The advantage of full technological dependency is that it truly removes the human element from the echoborg's speech interpretation and speech production subsystems. However, the downside of full technological dependency is that the quality of the interactions will be significantly constrained by current limitations in speech recognition and speech synthesis software. These technologies are not nearly as adept as humans at accurately perceiving spontaneous speech in real-time and articulating words with phonetic richness [17].

An alternative to full technological dependency is to have a human intermediary listen to the words spoken by the interactant (from a separate room), manually speed type them into the agent's input window, and speak the agent's subsequent response to the shadower via a radio transmission device (as the human source might in a standard cyranoid apparatus). The advantage of this minimal technological dependency format is that it preserves the verbal agency of the conversational agent (i.e., the agent still decides what to say in response to the interactant) while ensuring that the most accurate representations of the interactant's words are interpreted by the agent.

4 Using Echoborgs to Study Social Perception: A Simple Comparative Study

We ran an experiment to see how the experience of interacting with a conversational agent changes when the agent's words are embodied by a real person in face-to-face interaction. Three chat bots were used in the study, Cleverbot [18], Mitsuku (winner of the 2013 Loebner Prize chat bot competition) [19], and Rose (winner of the 2014 Loebner Prize) [20]. In the experiment participants were *not* informed before the interactions commenced that they would be speaking with a conversational agent (i.e., the agents operated covertly). Participants either engaged a person who, unbeknownst to them, shadowed for a chat bot (Echoborg condition), or engaged who they were told was another real person via a text interface (Text Interface condition). The study was approved by an ethical review board and was conducted in a behavioral research laboratory at a major British university.

4.1   Participants

Forty-one adult participants (mean age = 24.12; 26 female) were recruited from a university recruitment portal and randomly assigned to one of the two conditions (Echoborg or Text Interface) as well as a chat bot (Cleverbot, Mitsuku, or Rose). A female graduate student (aged 23) functioned as the echoborg shadower. In the Echoborg condition, Cleverbot and Rose each spoke with seven different participants while Mitsuku spoke with six. In the Text Interface condition, the three chat bots each spoke with seven different participants.

4.2   Procedure

Echoborg Condition. From the interaction room, the participant was informed that the study involved speaking to a stranger (another research participant) for 10-min and that they could discuss topics of their choosing during the interaction so long as nothing was vulgar. The researcher then left the room and relocated to an adjacent room which housed the computer on which the chat bot operated. The female shadower entered the interaction room and seated herself in a chair opposite the participant. The study made use of a minimal technological dependency format: as the participant spoke, the researcher speed typed their words into the chat bot's input window and articulated the chat bot's subsequent response into a microphone which discreetly relayed to the shadower's ear monitor (see Fig. 1). After 10-min, the researcher returned to the interaction room and the shadower exited.

Text Interface Condition. From the interaction room, the researcher informed the participant that the study involved speaking to a stranger (another research participant) for 10-min. The participant was instructed that though they were being asked to speak aloud, the stranger's responses would appear on a computer monitor in the form of text. Participants were informed that they could discuss topics of their choosing. As with the Echoborg condition, the Text Interface condition involved a minimal technological dependency format: the participant's words were input by the researcher into the chat bot's input window; once the chat bot generated a response to the input text, the researcher routed the text response via an instant messaging client to the participant's screen (see Fig. 1).

4.3   Measures and Post-interaction Interview

Following the interaction, the participant indicated on a 10-point scale how comfortable they felt during the interaction (1: not at all comfortable; 10: very comfortable) and also wrote a brief description of their interlocutor. Then, in a short interview, the participant was asked by the researcher to describe the personality of their interlocutor. Following

Text Interface condition

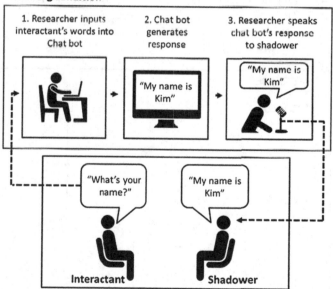

Echoborg condition

Fig. 1. Illustration of interaction scenarios used in study.

the interview, the participant was debriefed and made aware of the full nature of the study. After all experimental trials were complete, participants' written descriptions were collated and adjectives and other descriptors used to describe the interlocutor's personality were identified. Adjectives and descriptors regarding personality were also extracted from the recorded post-interaction interviews.

4.4   Results

Bootstrapped independent samples means tests of participants' comfort ratings were conducted for each chat bot comparing those who engaged an echoborg to those who engaged a text interface. Participants who encountered Mitsuku via an echoborg felt significantly less comfortable than those who did so via text (mean difference = −2.57, SE = 1.02, 95 % CI: [−4.58, −0.67]). Likewise, those who encountered Rose via an echoborg felt significantly less comfortable than those who did so via text (mean difference = −2.71, SE = 1.26, 95 % CI: [−5.05, −0.04]). No significant difference between conditions was found among those who spoke with Cleverbot (see Fig. 2).

Considering the written evaluations and post-interaction interviews, participants who spoke with an echoborg used a total of 86 unique descriptors to characterize their interlocutor, compared to 80 unique descriptors used by those who had spoken to a text interface. All descriptors which had a unique frequency of at least 3 (i.e., the descriptor was used by at least 3 participants in the same experimental condition) are shown in word clouds below (Figs. 3 and 4). The most frequent descriptors used in the Echoborg condition were "awkward" (6 different participants used this descriptor), "shy" (5), "introverted" (5), "uncomfortable" (4), "autistic" (3), "strange" (3), "poor social skills" (3), and "random" (3). The most frequent descriptors used by those in the Text Interface condition were "computer" (6), "strange" (5), "robotic" (5), "mechanical" (4), "introverted" (4), "difficult" (3), "friendly" (3), "random" (3), "nonsensical" (3), "odd" (3), and "asocial" (3).

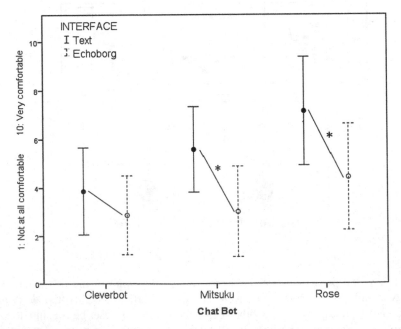

Fig. 2. Clustered error bar comparison of participants' feelings of comfort (*denotes significant difference: 95 % CI of difference does not span zero).

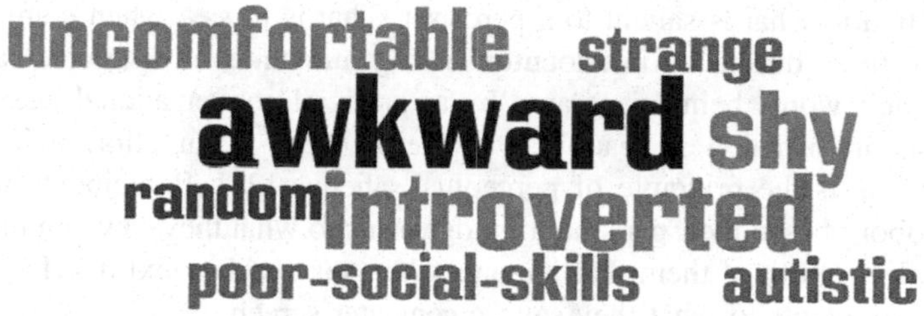

Fig. 3. Personality descriptors used by participants in the Echoborg condition to describe their interlocutor. Word cloud shows descriptors that had a frequency greater than or equal to 3. Larger text size indicates greater relative frequency.

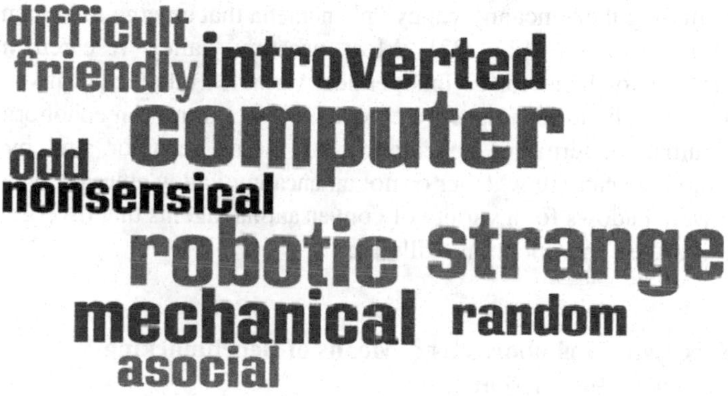

Fig. 4. Personality descriptors used by participants in the Text Interface condition

5 General Discussion

5.1 Findings

Our results demonstrate that when words generated by a conversational agent become embodied by a real human body during face-to-face communication, the social psychological dynamics of the interaction dramatically alter. Keeping in mind that participants were not told until *after* the post-interaction interviews were complete that they had in fact been communicating with the words of a chat bot, participants who encountered a text interface were prone to use adjectives describing their interlocutor as artificial/inhuman (frequently using words such as "mechanical," "computer," and "robotic"). By comparison, those who encountered an echoborg more often used descriptors that pointed to intrinsically human characteristics (e.g., "shy," "awkward," and "autistic"). This is evidence of how the interface one encounters frames the interaction and functions as a prism through which meaning and perception are refracted. The tangible *face* of an interlocutor evokes expectations regarding interpersonal dynamics and communicative norms that when violated trigger casual attributions tied to what is salient to a perceiver. That is to say, when communication breaks down (e.g., due to an interlocutor lacking human-level discourse capacity on account of their words being generated by an artificial conversational agent), people look to what information is readily available to them in an effort to explain the breakdown; this is the principle of perceptual salience [21]. Participants who spoke with an echoborg based their personality judgements to what they saw: a human person sitting directly in front of them. Participants who spoke with a text interface tied their personality judgments to what they saw: a computer screen.

We can also see how uncomfortable it is speaking to a covert echoborg relative to encountering a covert conversational agent via text. This underscores the notion that face-to-face, in-the-flesh interaction places much higher interpersonal demand on the parties to an encounter to maintain social norms related to communication. In future research we plan on further exploring the issue of interpersonal comfort in human-echoborg interaction and linking our findings with the growing body of research surrounding the "uncanny valley" phenomena that emerge in human-agent and human-android interaction [22, 23]. Most uncanny valley research has treated appearance and motor behavior as independent variables rather than investigate how agents' interlocution qualities impact interactants' perceptions. An echoborg, however, is perfectly human in terms of appearance and motor behavior, and by using the echoborg method we can see whether or not an uncanny valley emerges when the same speech shadower shadows for a variety of conversational agents that diverge in terms of how human-like their interlocution skills are.

5.2 Towards Using Echoborgs as a Means of Benchmarking Human-Agent Interaction

Our exploratory work with echoborgs has laid the foundation for future research that involves using the echoborg method as a means of benchmarking human-agent interaction. Because echoborgs can operate covertly (i.e., in conditions wherein interactants *assume* they are speaking with an autonomously communicating person), they allow researchers to study human-agent interaction in contexts where research subjects hold the same social psychological expectations about the interaction as they would a face-to-face encounter with another human. We consider such conditions to represent "baseline" conditions that can be compared against conditions wherein interactants know their interlocutor to be producing the words of an agent (e.g., an "overt" echoborg scenario) and/or interact with a nonhuman interface (e.g., an embodied conversational agent) in order to discern how people's perceptions of and experiences with an agent change the moment their interlocutor to some extent becomes a "thing" rather than a real person.

We are particularly interested in using echoborgs to evaluate human-agent intersubjectivity against human-human benchmarks. Intersubjectivity is a term used in the psychological sciences that encapsulates the means by which the various subjective perspectives held by parties to an interaction influence one another so as to bring about shared understanding, and these perspectives are revealed through speech acts, nonverbal communication, and emotional responses [24]. Cassell and Tartaro [25] recommend that evaluative frameworks for human-agent interaction involve assessing human-agent intersubjectivity against human-human benchmarks; they state that "the goal of human-agent interaction, which includes both human-robot interaction and human-ECA interaction, should not be a believable agent; it should be a believable interaction between human and agent in a given context" (p. 407). Using echoborgs, we can establish baseline levels of a user's intersubjective behaviors (e.g., verbal requests that an interlocutor repair a misunderstanding) under conditions wherein the user expect a fully human interaction and compare these levels to those observed in scenarios wherein the user knows their interlocutor's words to be those of an agent and/or communicates with a nonhuman interface.

5.3   Other Potential Applications of Echoborg Methodology

Echoborgs can be useful in basic social perception research akin to the study reported in the present paper. Personality judgments and other perception/attribution measures can be collected from interactants during and following interaction with a conversational agent via a variety of interfaces (e.g., text, onscreen avatar, mechanical android, offscreen human body, etc.) and under a variety of contextual frames (e.g., knowing vs. not-knowing their interlocutor is producing the words of an agent). This can give developers a sense of how perception of and interaction with a fixed intelligent agent changes depending on the interface through which the agent communications, from a minimal onscreen interface all the way up to a full-blown offscreen human body.

Also, as they have actual human bodies, echoborgs are highly mobile. This allows for the possibility of non-stationary social interaction between research participants and conversational agents. At the moment, the agent's agency within an echoborg is limited to determining speech (the shadower still decides what motor behaviors to display), but this does not rule out the possibility of constructing agents that signal to their speech shadowers when to perform certain behaviors (e.g., using short tone patterns to indicate actions such as "shake hand," "stand up," "smile," and so on, or simply sending motor behavior instructions to their shadower's left ear monitor while sending what to say to their right ear monitor). Developing echoborgs of this nature would give researchers the ability to leapfrog current constraints on recognizing social actions (e.g., a gesture inviting a handshake) and motor coordination, allowing developers to focus on creating higher-level computer programs that can guide a human's behavior.

5.4   Limitations

As our work with echoborgs is still very much in an exploratory phase, there are a number of limitations of the methodology as it is presently practiced that are worth noting. For instance, using a minimal technological dependency format of human-echoborg interaction requires the manual typing of interactant-utterances into a conversational agent which can result in awkward delays between turns at speech and thus reduced mundane realism. Developing techniques to minimize this latency is a major research priority. We presently face a trade-off between speed and accuracy:

though speech recognition software is potentially faster than manual typing by a human intermediary, having an intermediary type interactant-utterances into the conversational agent better ensures that an accurate representation of the interactant's speech will be processed by the agent. Though the effect of this latency certainly had some influence on interactants' experiences in our study, we did not formally analyze this effect; we do plan to include such an analysis in subsequent research.

Another important limitation of the study we have reported is the fact that we did not assess how the idiosyncrasies and other features of the shadower (e.g., gender, age, ethnicity, and so on) may have affected interactants' perceptions. In principle it is possible to discern these effects via the echoborg method (say, by having multiple shadowers differentiated along some physical dimension such as age shadow for the same conversational agent), however we did not consider this sort of analysis to be of theoretical interest as we were more concerned with providing a general proof of concept of the method. Furthermore, though best attempts were made to ensure that the body language and general demeanor of the shadower was consistent across experimental trials, we did not make specific considerations for behaviors such as consistency of eye-contact. We must stress, however, that since we have conceptualized echoborgs to be *hybrids* consisting of both an artificial agent and a human being, the shadower is free to convey body language that they feel is appropriate within the context of the interaction (unless of course, as discussed above, the agent is programmed to provide behavioral cues to the shadower in addition to words to replicate, which is something future echoborg research might entail).

6 Conclusion

This paper has demonstrated how it is possible to construct scenarios wherein people encounter hybrid social actors that consist of a conversational agent speaking through the body of a real person offscreen. These hybrids are a special type of cyranoid we refer to as "echoborgs." We feel that, as a methodology for interaction researchers and intelligent agent developers, the echoborg holds promise as a means of understanding how the human body shapes experiences with and perception of machine intelligence.

References

1. Milgram, S.: Obedience to Authority: An Experimental View. Harper and Row, New York (1974)
2. Milgram, S.: Cyranoids. In: Blass, T. (ed.) The Individual in a Social World: Essays and Experiments, pp. 402–409. Pinter and Martin, London (2010)
3. Schwitzgebel, R., Taylor, R.W.: Impression formation under conditions of spontaneous and shadowed speech. J. Soc. Psychol. **110**, 253–263 (1980)
4. Marslen-Wilson, W.: Linguistic structure and speech shadowing at very short latencies. Nature **244**, 522–523 (1973)
5. Marslen-Wilson, W.: Speech shadowing and speech comprehension. Speech Commun. **4**, 55–73 (1985)

6. Bailly, G.: Close shadowing natural versus synthetic speech. Int. J. Speech Technol. **6**, 11–19 (2003)

7. Pardo, J.S., Jordan, K., Mallari, R., Scanlon, C., Lewandowski, E.: Phonetic convergence in shadowed speech: the relation between acoustic and perceptual measures. J. Mem. Lang. **69**, 183–195 (2013)

8. Goldinger, S.D.: Echoes of echoes? An episodic theory of lexical access. Psychol. Rev. **105**, 251–279 (1998)

9. Mitchell, R.: An in your face interface: revisiting cyranoids as a revealing medium for interpersonal interaction. In: Wouters, I.H.C., Kimman, F.P.F., Tieben, R., Offermans, S.A. M., Nagtzaam, H.A.H. (eds.) Proceedings on the 5th Interaction Design Research Conference (SIDeR): Flirting with the Future, pp. 56–59 (2009)

10. Mitchell, R., Gillespie, A., O'Neill, B.: Cyranic contraptions: using personality surrogates to explore ontologically and socially dynamic contexts. In: Martens, J., Markopoulos, P. (eds.) Proceedings of the 2nd Conference on Creativity and Innovation in Design (DESIRE), pp. 199–210. ACM, New York (2011)

11. Pawlak, L.: The St. Unicorn's Trust [Performance Art] (2009). http://www.mradamjames. com/#The-St-Unicorns-Trust

12. Raudaskoski, P., Mitchell, R.: The situated accomplishment (aesthetics) of being a cyranoid. In: Melkas, H., Buur, J. (eds.) Proceedings of the Participatory Innovation Conference (PIN-C 2013), pp. 126–129. LUT Scientific and Expertise Publications, Lappeenranta (2013)

13. Blass, T.: The Man Who Shocked the World: The Life and Legacy of Stanley Milgram. Basic Books, New York (2004)

14. Corti, K., Gillespie, A.: Revisiting Milgram's cyranoid method: experimenting with hybrid human agents. J. Soc. Psychol. **155**, 30–56 (2015)

15. Corti, K., Reddy, G., Choi, E., Gillespie, A.: The researcher as experimental subject: using self-experimentation to access experiences, understand social phenomena, and stimulate reflexivity. Integr. Psychol. Behav. Sci. **49**(2), 288–308 (2015). doi:10.1007/s12124-015-9294-6. [Advance online publication]

16. Dick, P.K.: Do Androids Dream of Electric Sheep?. Doubleday, New York (1968)

17. Picraccini, R.: The Voice in the Machine: Building Computers that Understand Speech. MIT Press, Cambridge (2012)

18. Carpenter, R.: Cleverbot [Computer Program]. http://www.cleverbot.com

19. Worswick, S.: Mitsuku [Computer Program]. http://www.square-bear.co.uk/mitsuku/housebot.htm

20. Wilcox, B.: Rose [Computer Program]. http://brilligunderstanding.com/rosedemo.html

21. Taylor, S.E., Fiske, S.T.: Point of view and perceptions of causality. J. Pers. Soc. Psychol. **32**, 439–445 (1975)

22. MacDorman, K.F., Ishiguro, H.: The uncanny advantage of using androids in cognitive and social science research. Interact. Stud. **7**, 297–337 (2006)

23. Seyama, J., Nagayama, R.S.: The uncanny valley: effect of realism on the impression of artificial human faces. Presence **16**, 337–351 (2007)

24. Gillespie, A., Cornish, F.: Intersubjectivity: towards a dialogical analysis. J. Theory Soc. Behav. **40**, 19–46 (2009)

25. Cassell, J., Tartaro, A.: Intersubjectivity in human-agent interaction. Interact. Stud. **8**, 391–410 (2007)

Game Experience When Controlling a Weak Avatar in Full-Body Enaction

Roberto Pugliese[✉], Klaus Förger, and Tapio Takala

Department of Computer Science, Aalto University, Otaniementie 17,
PO Box 15500, 02150 Espoo, Finland
{roberto.pugliese,klaus.forger,tapio.takala}@aalto.fi
https://mediatech.aalto.fi/

Abstract. In this paper we describe a motion-controlled game based on a paradigm of a player enacting the character, rather than a character mimicking the player's action. Our hypothesis is that a controlling scheme based on the adaptation of a player to the way the avatar is able to perform actions, can result in a stronger presence and psychological bond to the character. The approach is based on previous studies showing that features, attitudes and behaviors of the digital representation of players in a virtual reality setting, alter the players self-perception in the virtual environment (Proteus effect). The interaction mechanism is inspired by enactive approach to cognition and embodied action. In a mini-game we explore effects of controlling a weak character on self-presence and identification with the avatar. We show that increasing degrees of effort in the controlled bodies resulted in different impressions of the physical state of the character. Additionally, we provide our interpretation of relation between game experience and the kinetic parameters and adaptation indicators extracted from the motion of the player and avatar. Finally, we address scenarios where this enaction-based approach to motion controlled avatar can find application.

Keywords: Motion-controlled games · Embodied interaction · Game experience · Self presence · Proteus effect

1 Introduction

Controlling an avatar using full-body interaction is not anymore exclusive of Virtual Reality research but is also available at consumer level. Motion controllers in video-games allow a more direct link between player's action and the avatar they are impersonating than mouse and keyboard or joypad based interfaces. As shown in a previous study [3], a motion-based controller (a controller that affords more movement) can enhance the level of engagement the participants experienced in the case of music and simulation games. Motion-controlled games have been studied also for other scenarios like gamification of trampoline jumping [17]. These scenarios are augmentation and simulation of physical activity where the player is brought one-to-one into the game world without the mediation of an avatar.

© Springer International Publishing Switzerland 2015
W.-P. Brinkman et al. (Eds.): IVA 2015, LNAI 9238, pp. 418–431, 2015.
DOI: 10.1007/978-3-319-21996-7_45

While in sport simulation a perfect mirroring or even an exaggerated version of players' movement is desirable, a controller scheme where the avatar copies the action of the player might not be suitable. In narrative games situations might arise when the character is not capable of executing the same action of the player e.g. character is wounded, affected by spells or needs to interact with objects of a certain weight. All these cases introduce a motion decoupling between player and game character. This has been acceptable in joypad-controlled games, either by displaying non-interactive sequences to the player or partially altering the controller mechanism (the same input on the gamepad produces an exaggerated or dampened output). Nevertheless, consistent natural interaction throughout the game might result in a more engaging experience.

The need of simulating a different body can also come from the opportunity of increasing sympathy and wish to help others by the use of a Virtual Environment (VE). For instance, Head Mounted Display has been used to reproduce visual impairment, e.g. color blindness and studies [1] have shown that participants of the study manifested an increased attitude to help others also after the experiment.

In this study we explore the possibilities of providing a self-representation of the player which is different not in terms of appearance but rather in the way it moves in the VE. We will portray an increasingly tired character that cannot follow the movement of the player perfectly. We examine the effect of this mediating body in a game and its impact on the game experience.

2   Related Works

Impersonating a character in a virtual environment (VE) can have profound effect on one's action in that environment. Studies show that people's behaviors can conform to their digital self-representation, the avatar. This phenomena renamed as Proteus effect might occur when the user's virtual self-representation is dissimilar to the physical self [26], for instance a more or less attractive version of one-self, a thinner or overweight, a taller or smaller. The Proteus effect has been explored for the potential of inducing virtuous behavior in the player [12, 13]. The effects of self-representation can extend outside the virtual environment and promote for instance more healthy eating behavior and positive effect on exercising. In the case of occupying a fictional super-hero with super-powers, a sense of empowerment and tendency towards pro-social behaviors can be found among players [23].

2.1   Self-presence, Identification and the Body

A key concept under which identification and Proteus effect fall into is self-presence, or the experience of feeling one's self within a virtual environment [16,18,20]. Adopting self-perception theory [2] to the avatar case, people might observe their virtual self behavior and infer from that their own features, affecting their self-image and also attitudes and future behaviors [11].

Another key-concept underlying the relation and bonding between the person and the avatar is identification. According to Klimmt et al. [8], "from the perspective of social psychology, identification is defined as a temporary alteration of media users' self-concept through adoption of perceived characteristics of a media person". The authors claim that compared to other media, due to the interactive setting of video games the player does not perceive the game character as an entity completely separate from themselves but rather a merging of their own self and the protagonist of the game. To identify with the media character is actually to perceive or be the media character.

Putting ourselves in someone else's shoes lets us understand other's feeling by simulating them ourselves. We understand another person's actions by reenacting those actions using our own motor system, for instance judging the weight of an object by watching how a person lifts a heavy object [7]. For the Proteus effect, embodiment produces significantly larger behavioral changes than mere observation of the same visual stimuli [27].

Overall, the process of identification and self-presence are responsible for the actual transfer of attitudes, behavior and emotional response between the player and its digital representation.

But if the mechanisms to understand somebody else's behaviors and feeling are based on internal simulation of those behaviors and feelings, what would be the consequence of physically enacting that behavior ? Can we expect a stronger self-presence in the VE ? Does adapting to another body and becoming in control of it affect our feeling and behaviors inferred from the movement capabilities of the new body?

The paradigm of enaction [10, 22] provides an account of social understanding based on embodied action, or in other words, the importance of the body in cognition and sense-making as an action-perception loop. In the case of a motion-controlled avatar, when a player needs to adapt to the avatar to achieve a goal she gets enclosed in a perceptually guided action loop where a dynamical coupling exists among the two. Only by enacting the body of the avatar the goal can be achieved, and through enaction the player understands the avatar she embodies. It is important that the relation between player and avatar is disrupted every time the player acts regardless of the avatar response perceived. Coordination needs to be maintained over time by a continuous negotiation among the parties. We will take into account these design criteria in the user study.

2.2   Game Experience

Many factors contribute to engagement in game experience and different models have been provided to illustrate their relationship. For instance the framework of [5] models the relation between motion and engagement. This approach helps us understanding how the game experience can be modulated via sensory experience due to different quality of player's motion when using motion-based controllers.

We focus here on one of the main contributors towards engagement: flow. Flow theory [9] has been widely adopted in research on computer games [24].

Flow is a state of optimal experience, the product of the balance between challenge offered and skill required to accomplish a task. Higher states of flow go hand-in-hand with an enjoyable experience. Due to this absorption in the activities performed, flow has been also associated with immersion, or the degree of involvement with a computer game [15]. Similar features are shared among flow and immersion: lack of awareness of time, loss of awareness of the real world and involvement and a sense of being in the task environment. Immersion is less radical than a perfect flow state, with a remaining awareness of the surrounding and it does not correspond to a pleasant experience of clear and reachable goals at all times. In this paper we refer to flow in this less radical "immersion-like" formulation. It is not our direct goal to provide an enjoyable experience but rather a strong embodied experience of identification and presence with the avatar. Nevertheless a minimum amount of flow might be necessary to reach a control of the avatar that guarantees a sense of attachment and dynamic coupling with movement of the avatar. In other words, without a certain amount of flow, impersonating the digital representation of our self becomes more difficult and also self-presence can be reduced. We will test this hypothesis in our study.

Other factors related to the response of the character to the player's input play a role in the game experience. The impact of lag in a platform game has been investigated by [19], studying independently the contribution of two aspects of lag: latency (constant delay) and jitter (varying delay). The results showed the negative effect of latency especially due to jitter on players' game experience, in terms of performance, satisfaction, ease of control, and sometimes how favorably players view the avatar.

3 Avatar Implementation and Research Questions

We describe here the implementation of a character controlled by the movement of a player. The character follows the movement of the player more or less closely, being as fast or slower than the player, it can fall down and might need the player to modify their own movement in order to keep control of the character. The character is intended to show weakness and tiredness while still being capable of moving where the player wants.

3.1 Research Questions

In the exploratory study presented in this paper we want to investigate the relationship between the body-controller mechanism implemented and the game experience. More specifically we are after the hypothesis that controlling a character which exhibits a behavior that can be countered only through a deliberate effort of the player towards adaptation can have an effect on identification, self-presence and game experience.

For the game experience we are interested in the impact of controlling the weak characters on flow and challenge and their relation with emotional response.

We also want to investigate if any relation exists between the motion of the player, the game experience and the recognition of particular features of the character they are controlling.

3.2 Controller-Mechanism

The implementation is based on commercially available tracking technology like Microsoft Kinect 2. The player is shown as a green stick-figure with 14 joints. The tracking mechanism introduces a latency of 50 ms with good accuracy and responsiveness.

Since we want to understand how impersonating a character who presents motion features different from the player's affects the player's experience in the game, we created a physics-based modification of the original avatar. The visual appearance of this character is the same stick-figure but the movement is modified by applying custom forces to the individual joints. Three forces are applied at each joint. The first is an attraction force that pulls the joint to the original position.

The second force called *Potential Force* is also an attraction force pulling the joint to the original position but only within a certain distance from the original position. The *Potential Force* acts on the joint to make its trajectory over time follow the original one but it decreases linearly with the distance. When the avatar is displayed in front of the player, the avatar follows the movement of the player as long as the player waits for the avatar to follow the movement. The player needs to imitate at first the posture of the avatar if different from his own and then move smoothly enough not to "lose grip" of the avatar. Conversely, the faster and more independently from the avatar the player moves the less the player is in control of the avatar.

The third force is a force pushing down that is used to change the posture of the character to make it look tired or weak. The influence of posture on attitude and behavior has been studied by [21] and more recently in the game context by [4]. The three forces can be scaled independently for each joint.

When all the forces are applied, the player has more control the more she adapts their movements to the one of the character by matching the posture. Nevertheless letting the character lag behind can result not just in the need of slowing down but also going all the way to a crouched posture before being able to control the character again (Fig. 1). This process stimulates the adaptation of the player to the pace of the avatar in a continuous feedback of push-pulling the avatar.

We expect those traits of the avatar to transfer to the player because the digital representation appears and behaves (it needs to be controlled) differently from the mirrored representation (Proteus effect). Additionally, the embodied experience of that behavior (I am controlling/adapting to the movement of my digital representation) will promote identification with the avatar and modified self-presence. Furthermore, the posture regulated by the controller mechanism will act as a regulator for emotion [4].

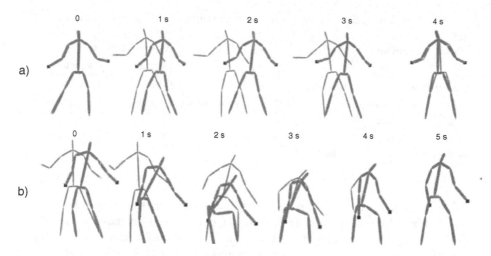

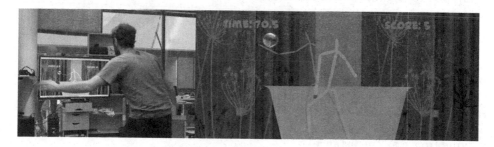

Fig. 1. Original (thin limbs) and avatar (tick): in (a) the control of the avatar is partially lost due to a lateral fast movement. The player needs to wait for the avatar. In (b) the avatar starts falling down and the player needs to adapt to the crouched posture.

4   Method

A motion-controlled mini-game was designed where a character on the screen needs to pop soap bubbles as fast as possible using its hands only. A new bubble appears every 7 s or 1 s after it has been popped. All the interaction happens on the same depth plane so that depth perception does not influence game play. Scores and a timer is shown on top of the game (Fig. 2).

Fig. 2. Subject playing the bubble-popping mini-game (left) and screen-grab from gameplay (right).

The conditions were designed to discover differences of movements and game experiences against the mirroring condition when posture and movement between player and controlled character differs. The dimensions we explore are the posture of the avatar and the avatar's response to the player's movement (Table 1).

Table 1. Dimensions explored in the user study and designed conditions

Avatar movement	Avatar Posture	
	Mirror	Crouched
Avatar follows player movement	Condition 1	Condition 4
Avatar moves as the player only if the player matches its pose (with higher tolerance)	Condition 2	Condition 5
Avatar moves as the player only if the player matches its pose (with lower tolerance)	Condition 3	Condition 6

The resulting conditions can be grouped in characters that move similarly as the player but differ in posture (condition 4), characters that move as the player only if the player is close enough to their pose (condition 2 and 3) and conditions where the player needs to exert a continuous effort of adaptation if she wants to maintain control and not lose the "grip" of the character (condition 5 and 6) that otherwise falls down into a crouched posture.

On the screen (see Fig. 2) 2 stick figures are displayed, the original body (thin stick figure) and the transformed body (thicker limbs figure). In this way the player has a visual feedback of the difference between the pose and movement of the controlled and transformed avatar. This helps the process of matching his own pose with the one of the transformed avatar and being in control of it. When the distance of the corresponding body parts is small, the thinner limbs disappear inside the ticker one of the transformed characters, thus visually confirming the successful bonding of original and transformed character. As an exception, in the conditions where the character has tired posture and mirrored movement, the display shows only the transformed character. An accompanying video showing the different conditions in actions is available at: https://vimeo.com/robertopugliese/enactingtheavatar.

4.1 Procedure

A within-subject design for the experiment was used. 11 participants were recruited among colleagues and were promised that the best players of the user study will receive a movie ticket. The sample consisted of 7 men and 4 women who ranged in age from 24 to 61 ($MV = 32.5$, $SD = 11.17$). The experiment was conducted in an office room. The game was displayed on a 54" screen with participants playing from c.a. 2 m distance.

A training session preceded the actual experiment. During this phase the participant went through all the conditions for 30 s each one receiving an explanation about how the transformed body was intended to be controlled. Then, 12 2-minutes trials were presented consisting of the 6 conditions repeated twice in randomized counterbalanced order.

4.2 Measures

Quantitative Study. The motion tracking data for the players and character were recorded every trial. With this data we calculated the average pose distance between player and character, the average speed of the player and an adaptation percentage. The adaptation refers to the percentage of frames when the player can see a target bubble, but moves away from it instead of trying to actively pop it, therefore likely trying to adapt to the behavior of the avatar.

Subjective Evaluation Study. We designed a questionnaire to be filled in after each trial. The items comprised questions that address Identification and Self-presence (see Appendix), emotional response with the Self-assessment manikin [6] and game experience using the Game Experience Questionnaire [14]. The GEQ (in-game) components can assess experiential constructs of immersion, tension, competence, flow, negative affect, positive affect and challenge.

A further question included in the questionnaire addressed the features or characteristic the player saw in the avatar: "Which of the following best describes your impression of the avatar? (weak, strong, angry, sad, happy, other)".

5 Results

We considered all the measures of Sect. 4.2 as dependent variables and conducted a 2-way within-subjects ANOVA considering the conditions and the repetitions as factors. In the case of the calculation of the Pose Distance we limited the analysis to the Condition 2-3-5-6 because only in these conditions the player can affect the variable with their movement, while in condition 1 the pose distance is 0 by definition and condition 4 is an off-set resulting from the gravity force applied. Post-hoc threshold of significance was corrected using Bonferroni adjustment for multiple comparisons among conditions.

In Fig. 3 the calculated motion data are shown. The **Pose Distance** $(F(3, 30) = 12.318, \eta_p^2 = 0.552, p < .0001)$ clearly shows that in condition 6 participants found themselves more often far from the character than in other conditions. Pairwise comparison showed differences between Condition 2 $(MV = 0.316)$ and Condition 6 $(MV = 0.832, MD = -.516, p < .05)$, and between Condition 5 $(MV = 0.338)$ and Condition 6 $(MD = -.494, p < .05)$.

As a consequence players need to adapt their movements more and not go directly towards the bubble to pop, as it can be seen from the **Adaptation movements** $(F(5, 50) = 7.849, \eta_p^2 = 0.44, p < .0001)$. Pairwise comparison showed differences between Condition 2 $(MV = 14\%)$ and Condition 3 $(MV = 18.5\%, MD = .045, p < .05)$, and between Condition 2 and Condition 6 $(MV = 21.7\%, MD = .077, p < .05)$, between Condition 3 and Condition 4 $(MV = 10.4\%, MD = -.081, p < .05)$, between Condition 4 and Condition 6 $(MD = .113, p < .05)$ and between Condition 5 $(MV = 15.3\%)$ and Condition 6 $(MD = .064, p < .05)$.

Speed (F$(5, 50)$ = 83.866, η_p^2 = 0.893, $p < .0001$) greatly varied among conditions as a result of the different adaptation required with Condition 2 and 3 showing similar mean values as 5 and 6. Pairwise comparison showed significant differences of Condition 1 with Condition 2 (MD = .073, $p < .001$), with Condition 3 (MD = .084, $p < .001$), with Condition 5 (MD = .073, $p < .001$), and Condition 6 (MD = .077, $p < .001$). Condition 2 was found different from Condition 3 (MD = .011, $p < .001$). Also differences were found among Condition 3 and Condition 4 (MD = −.063, $p < .001$), Condition 5 (MD = −.011, $p < .001$) and Condition 6 (MD = −.007, $p < .01$). Non surprisingly, scores (F$(5, 50)$ = 169.668, η_p^2 = 0.944, $p < .0001$) followed the same trend of the speed.

As it can be observed from the **Vertical Center of Mass** F$(5, 50)$ = 76.565, η_p^2 = 0.884, $p < .0001$, players spent more time crouched in condition 5 and 6 for the need of picking up the character when falling. Pairwise comparisons among conditions showed strong significant differences ($p < .001$) between the Conditions 1-2-3-4 and Condition 5 and 6.

In Fig. 4, statistically significant results for the subjective evaluation aggregated according to the questionnaire instruction are presented. We found significant differences for **Presence** (F$(5, 50)$ = 9.077, η_p^2 = 0.476, $p < .0001$). Pairwise comparison showed higher values for condition 1 (MV = 18.318) over Condition 2 (MV = 13.727, MD = 4.591, $p < .05$), Condition 3 (MV = 12.727, MD = 5.591, $p < .01$), Condition 4 (MV = 16.182, MD = 2.136, $p < .05$) and Condition 5 (MV = 13.773, MD = 4.545, $p < .05$). Also Condition 2 and 4 were found different (MD = −2.455, $p < .05$)

No significant differences among conditions were found for the variable **Identification**, with mean values between 8.8 (Condition 3) and 9.1 (Condition 1).

Significant differences among conditions were found also for **Flow** (F$(5, 50)$ = 2.808, η_p^2 = 0.219, $p < .05$). Pairwise comparison showed significant differences among condition 1 (MV = 6.955) and Condition 2 (MV = 5.682, MD = 1.273, $p < .05$), and Condition 2 with Condition 5 (MV = 6.5, MD = −.818, $p < .05$).

For **Challenge** we found statistically significant differences among conditions (F$(5, 50)$ = 9.468, η_p^2 = 0.486, $p < .0001$). Pairwise comparison showed significant differences among condition 1 (MV = 5.364) and Condition 3 (MV = 7.591, MD = −2.227, $p < .05$), and Condition 1 with Condition 6 (MV = 7.727, MD = −2.364, $p < .01$), and also for Condition 4 (MV = 5.773, MD = −1.955, $p < .05$) with Condition 6.

Significant differences among conditions were found also for **Dominance** (F$(5, 50)$ = 34.507, η_p^2 = 0.775, $p < .0001$). Pairwise comparison showed significant differences among condition 1 (MV = 6.955) and Condition 2 (MV = 5.682, MD = 1.273, $p < .05$), and Condition 2 with Condition 5 (MV = 6.5, MD = −.818, $p < .05$).

Additionally, we found significant differences for the **Negative affect** (F$(5, 50)$ = 3.229, η_p^2 = 0.244, $p < .05$). Pairwise comparison showed higher values for condition 4 (MV = 4.864) compared to Condition 1 (MV = 3.727, MD = −1.136, $p < .05$).

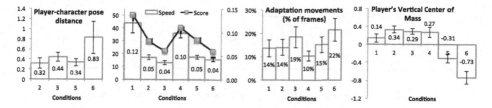

Fig. 3. Statistically significant results from the motion data analysis. Error bars show 95 % confidence intervals.

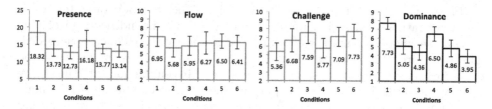

Fig. 4. Statistically significant results from subjective evaluation. Error bars show 95 % confidence intervals.

Figure 5 reports the impression participant got of the character they controlled. From an initial list of 49 adjectives, we operated a reduction by grouping common concepts reaching a total of 17.

6   Discussion

As expected the different conditions offered a different degree of challenge and a similar trend could be seen in the dominance measure. This is due to the fact that the mechanics of the game stayed the same among conditions and the main factor affecting the challenge is different degree and autonomy of control of the character. Interestingly, flow did not score that differently between the mirror condition and the conditions with the falling character (conditions 5 and 6). This could be attributed to the fact players can reach a level of expertise in a short time that let them be in a good flow state and shows that the controller mechanism proved successful in bringing a good trade-off between challenge and ease-of-use.

Self-presence was lower in conditions where the motion of the character was modified. Looking into the individual items of the questionnaire, the sense of embodying the character is higher when the motion follows directly the players movement (Condition 1 and 4). This could be due to the representation of the character as a separate entity causing the player to see both themselves and the character as separate. Moreover, as it can seen from the question "To what extent did the avatar seem real?", conditions 2-3-5-6 portrayed a less realistic and believable character. The character exhibited less realistic behavior not obeying

Conditions	weak	slow	tired	sad	dead	apathetic	clumsy	stiff	disobeying	confused	lazy	neutral	strong	fast	ready	happy	other
1	1	0	0	0	0	0	0	0	0	0	0	7	7	2	2	2	1
2	9	6	0	1	0	1	1	0	0	0	3	0	0	0	0	1	0
3	7	4	1	1	1	1	0	1	1	1	1	0	0	0	0	1	2
4	4	3	5	2	0	0	1	1	0	0	0	2	0	0	2	0	2
5	11	5	0	1	1	0	1	0	1	0	1	0	0	0	0	1	0
6	12	1	0	2	1	1	0	0	2	1	1	0	0	0	0	1	0

Fig. 5. Frequency table of the impressions players had of the character.

natural physical constraints of the human body (legs crossed in a cartoonish style) and not falling according to real gravity.

From Fig. 5 we can notice Condition 6 being associated more often to a weak character rather than a slow one, suggesting that the intended design of portraying weakness through the effort needed to control the character succeeded. The most tired character was found in Condition 4, impression that could be explained considering the posture of the character in conjunction with the ability to move unconstrained and let the player achieve the second higher score among conditions. We can speculate that being in a tired position (Condition 6) rather than observing a tired representation (Condition 4) shifts the experience of the player from seeing tiredness to feeling the weakness of the avatar.

Other adjectives mentioned by the participants belong semantically to the dissatisfaction of their expectations in controlling the character (*apathetic, boring, lazy,...*). A lack of context and motivation for the behavior of the character probably puts emphasis on pure performance task and it makes the avatar feel non-cooperative to reach the player's goal. Indeed the condition 6 is the one where players spent more time searching for control (Player-character pose distance) and the highest effort in adaptation was necessary (Adaptation Movements in Fig. 3).

We could not find statistically significant differences in arousal and valence. As witnessed during the test and from the answers, individual preferences emerged about the conditions players liked the most. This study does not aim at showing the best condition but rather the suitability of the conditions for specific game play context and applications.

While there was no difference among condition for identification, the mean value were high in all the conditions maybe indicating on one hand a better metric for this aspect should be used but also a richer game scenario should be designed.

7   Conclusion and Future Works

We have presented an implementation of a motion-controlled avatar that shows different responses to the player movement and needs to be controlled through the player adaptation to it. Those features aimed at portraying a weak character in both posture and effort in movement. We found that when the player needs not just to adapt to the pose of the character but also to go into a crouched position to retain control of the avatar (enaction) elicits in the player the impression of controlling a weak character. We showed that the loss of control does not excessively compromise a state of flow during game play. We showed that posture alone creates the impression of controlling a tired character, offers equivalent flow state as the enaction case but less challenge. The observed drop of self-presence could be overcome by using a more realistically moving avatar.

As potential scenario for the deployment of this character, we want to point at the simulation of motor skills disorder in order to foster empathy towards people with motor difficulties. Also, we suggest a variety of game scenarios where this enactment could take place and enrich the game experience like dramatic storytelling and role-playing game in which the state of the character is altered due to the enfolding of the story.

We can hypothesize that context and pre-story would augment the impact of adopting this kind of enactment and its effect on the identification and self-presence, extending the player's impression of the avatar to an effective transfer of the avatar's features to the player.

From a methodological point of view, in future study we could use a post-game self-identification task as proposed by [25]. This could overcome a difficulty in measuring through questionnaire the physical identification the player with the impersonated character. It would help in understanding how the movements resulting from the attempted adaptation to a different body are internalized in the memory of the player.

Appendix

Identification. The questionnaire was adapted from APPENDIX A: STUDY 1 [11].

(1 = Strongly disagree; 2 = Somewhat disagree; 3 = Neither disagree nor agree; 4 = Somewhat agree; 5 = Strongly agree)

- While playing the game, I wanted the avatar to succeed by popping as many bubbles as possible.
- While playing the game, I did NOT want the avatar to give up and miss bubbles.

Presence. The questionnaire was adapted from APPENDIX A: STUDY 1 [11].

(1 = Not at all; 2 = Slightly; 3 = Moderately; 4 = Very much; 5 = Extremely)

- To what extent to do you feel the avatar is an extension of yourself?
- To what extent do you feel that if something happens to the avatar, it feels like it is happening to you?
- To what extent do you feel you embodied the avatar you controlled?
- To what extent did you feel you were in the same room with the avatar?
- To what extent did the avatar seem real?
- To what extent were you involved in the game world?

GEQ In-Game version as in [14]. Please indicate how you felt while playing the game for each of the items, on the following scale:

(1 = not at all; 2 = Slightly; 3 = Moderately; 4 = Fairly; 5 = Extremely)

Questions	Measure
2 - I felt successful	Competence
9 - I felt skillful	
1 - I was interested in the game's story	Sensory and imaginative immersion
4 - I found it impressive	
5 - I forgot everything around me	Flow
10 - I felt completely absorbed	
6 - I felt frustrated	Tension
8 - I felt irritable	
12 - I felt challenged	Challenge
13 - I had to put a lot of effort into it	
3 - I felt bored	Negative affect
7 - I found it tiresome	
11 - I felt content	Positive affect
14 - I felt good	

References

1. Ahn, S.J.G., Le, A.M.T., Bailenson, J.: The effect of embodied experiences on self-other merging, attitude, and helping behavior. Media Psychol. **16**(1), 7–38 (2013)
2. Bem, D.J.: Self-perception theory. Adv. Exp. Soc. Psychol. **6**, 1–62 (1972)
3. Bianchi-Berthouze, N.: Understanding the role of body movement in player engagement. Hum. Comput. Interact. **28**(1), 40–75 (2013)
4. Bianchi-Berthouze, N., Cairns, P., Cox, A., Jennett, C., Kim, W.W.: On posture as a modality for expressing and recognizing emotions. In: Emotion and HCI workshop at BCS HCI London (2006)
5. Bianchi-Berthouze, N., Kim, W.W., Patel, D.: Does body movement engage you more in digital game play? and why? In: Paiva, A.C.R., Prada, R., Picard, R.W. (eds.) ACII 2007. LNCS, vol. 4738, pp. 102–113. Springer, Heidelberg (2007)
6. Bradley, M.M., Lang, P.J.: Measuring emotion: the self-assessment manikin and the semantic differential. J. Behav. Ther. Exp. Psychiatry **25**(1), 49–59 (1994)
7. Chandrasekharan, S., Mazalek, A., Nitsche, M., Chen, Y., Ranjan, A.: Ideomotor design: using common coding theory to derive novel video game interactions. Pragmatics Cogn. **18**(2), 313–339 (2010)
8. Christoph, K., Dorothée, H., Peter, V.: The video game experience as "true" identification: a theory of enjoyable alterations of players' self-perception. Commun. Theor. **19**(4), 351–373 (2009)
9. Csikszentmihalyi, M.: The Psychology of Optimal Experience. Harper Perennial, New york (1990)
10. De Jaegher, H., Di Paolo, E.: Participatory sense-making. Phenomenol. Cogn. Sci. **6**(4), 485–507 (2007)
11. Fox, J.: The use of virtual self models to promote self-efficacy and physical activity performance. Ph.D. thesis, Stanford University (2010)
12. Fox, J., Bailenson, J., Binney, J.: Virtual experiences, physical behaviors: the effect of presence on imitation of an eating avatar. Presence Teleoperators Virtual Environ. **18**(4), 294–303 (2009)

13. Fox, J., Bailenson, J.N.: Virtual self-modeling: the effects of vicarious reinforcement and identification on exercise behaviors. Media Psychol. **12**(1), 1–25 (2009)
14. IJsselsteijn, W., De Kort, Y., Poels, K.: The game experience questionnaire: development of a self-report measure to assess the psychological impact of digital games. Manuscript in Preparation (2013)
15. Jennett, C., Cox, A.L., Cairns, P., Dhoparee, S., Epps, A., Tijs, T., Walton, A.: Measuring and defining the experience of immersion in games. Int. J. Hum. Comput. Stud. **66**(9), 641–661 (2008)
16. Jin, S.A.A., Park, N.: Parasocial interaction with my avatar: effects of interdependent self-construal and the mediating role of self-presence in an avatar-based console game, wii. CyberPsychology Behav. **12**(6), 723–727 (2009)
17. Kajastila, R., Holsti, L., Hämäläinen, P.: Empowering the exercise: a body-controlled trampoline training game. Int. J. Comput. Sci. Sport **13**, 1–18 (2014)
18. Lee, K.M.: Presence, explicated. Commun. Theor. **14**(1), 27–50 (2004)
19. Normoyle, A., Guerrero, G., Jörg, S.: Player perception of delays and jitter in character responsiveness. In: Proceedings of the ACM Symposium on Applied Perception, pp. 117–124. ACM (2014)
20. Ratan, R., Santa Cruz, M., Vorderer, P.: Multitasking, presence, and self-presence on the wii. In: Proceedings of the 10th Annual International Workshop on Presence, pp. 167–190 (2007)
21. Riskind, J.H., Gotay, C.C.: Physical posture: could it have regulatory or feedback effects on motivation and emotion? Motiv. Emot. **6**(3), 273–298 (1982)
22. Rosch, E., Thompson, E., Varela, F.J.: The Embodied Mind: Cognitive Science and Human Experience. MIT Press, Cambridge (1992)
23. Rosenberg, R.S., Baughman, S.L., Bailenson, J.N.: Virtual superheroes: using superpowers in virtual reality to encourage prosocial behavior. PLoS ONE **8**(1), e55003 (2013)
24. Sweetser, P., Wyeth, P.: Gameflow: a model for evaluating player enjoyment in games. Comput. Entertain. **3**(3), 3–3 (2005)
25. Mazalek, A., Nitsche, M., Chandrasekharan, S., Welsh, T., Clifton, P., Quitmeyer, A., Peer, F., Kirschner, F.: Recognising your self in virtual avatars. Int. J. Arts and Technol. **6**(1), 83–105 (2012)
26. Yee, N., Bailenson, J.: The proteus effect: the effect of transformed self-representation on behavior. Hum. Commun. Res. **33**(3), 271–290 (2007)
27. Yee, N., Bailenson, J.N.: The difference between being and seeing: the relative contribution of self-perception and priming to behavioral changes via digital self-representation. Media Psychol. **12**(2), 195–209 (2009)

On the Trail of Facial Processing in Autism Spectrum Disorders

Diana Arellano[1]([✉]), Ulrich Max Schaller[2], Reinhold Rauh[2], Volker Helzle[1], Marc Spicker[3], and Oliver Deussen[3]

[1] Filmakademie Baden-Württemberg, Ludwigsburg, Germany
{diana.arellano,volker.helzle}@filmakademie.de
[2] University Medical Center Freiburg, Freiburg Im Breisgau, Germany
{reinhold.rauh,ulrich.schaller}@uniklinik-freiburg.de
[3] University of Konstanz, Konstanz, Germany
{marc.spicker,oliver.deussen}@uni-konstanz.de
http://research.animationsinstitut.de/projects/sara/

Abstract. To investigate the difficulties in communication, socialization abilities, and emotion perception deficits in individuals with autism spectrum disorders (ASD), we propose the project SARA. Its main goal is to assess how abstracted emotional facial expressions influence the categorization of the emotions by children and adolescents with high-functioning ASD. This paper focuses on the first pilot study where an adapted version of the Dynamic Emotional Categorization Test (DECT) was implemented. The results support the validity of the emotional facial animations, which is confirmed by the low performance of subjects with high-functioning ASD when categorizing emotions, in comparison with their peers without ASD.

Keywords: Autism spectrum disorders · Real-time NPR · Abstraction · 3D characters · Dynamic facial animations

1 Introduction

A smooth interaction in social contexts depends in great measure on an adequate internal mental representation of the emotional state of those we interact with. However, people diagnosed with autism spectrum disorders (ASD) present difficulties in social interaction and lesser communication abilities, which are in part the result of emotion perception deficits [1].

To investigate this issue we propose SARA (Stylized Animations for Research in Autism), an ongoing project that studies how abstracted emotional facial animations are categorized by children and adolescents with high-functioning ASD. To carry out our research, we implemented an adapted version of the Dynamic Emotional Categorization Test (DECT) [2], named R-DECT, where dynamic facial animations of physically-plausible 3D characters are generated in real-time, and can be parameterized in terms of speed and intensity.

In this paper we present the results of our first study, the goal of which was to obtain a better understanding of the perceptual and conceptual facial

© Springer International Publishing Switzerland 2015
W.-P. Brinkman et al. (Eds.): IVA 2015, LNAI 9238, pp. 432–441, 2015.
DOI: 10.1007/978-3-319-21996-7_46

processing of individuals with and without ASD. To that end, we conducted a feasibility and validation study of the R-DECT to set the basis for the inclusion of abstractions, which constitutes one of the novelties in our project.

2 Background

Impairments in the ability to perceive and categorize facial expressions have been found in a number of psychiatric disorders such as Affective Disorder, Attention-Deficit/ Hyperactivity Disorder (ADHD), Anxiety Disorders, Eating Disorders [3], and Autism Spectrum Disorders (ASD) [4,5]. Due to the core symptomatologies of these disorders, deficits in emotion recognition are multi-faceted and show varying degrees of severity.

In 2008 it was estimated that one in 88 children aged 8 years had ASD [6]. However, in 2010 the reports indicated one in 68 children [7]. A direct consequence of this increase has been a growing awareness of the biopsychosocial functioning and of the quality of life of individuals with ASD.

Different fields have conducted exhaustive investigations to understand ASD, proposing theories like "weak central coherence" (WCC), "executive dysfunctioning", or a "delayed development of theory-of-mind" [8]. A very detailed review of methodologies to develop and train the social skills of people with autism is offered in [9]. One method, especially when working with children and adolescents, consists of the interaction with virtual characters in computer-based applications. The advantages include the possibility of practicing skills in a repetitive way that is more controllable, less threatening and less socially demanding than when interacting with real people. The design of the virtual characters has ranged from very cartoony styles like the ones used in ECHOES VE [10], JeStiMulE [11], Lifeisgame [12], Photogoo [13], to realistic-human-like styles as seen in [14–16], and going through more artistic versions like the thin-line drawn 2D pedagogical agent developed by [17].

3 The SARA Project

The ongoing research project SARA has been structured to allow synergy between clinical psychology, animation and real-time graphics. The main goal is to better understand the deficits in social cognition in individuals with ASD by means of real-time dynamic facial animations, abstraction techniques, eye tracking techniques, psychophysiological and behavioral measurements.

A number of works demonstrate that these deficits might be related to the amount of details conveyed by facial expressions, as well as to different types of processing of the emotional stimuli, i.e. atypical mutual gaze and eye contact [18–20]. Therefore, one of the main novelties of the project is the use of Non-Photorealistic Rendering (NPR) to abstract the faces of our virtual characters, given that NPR helps in reducing the information load and conveying the presented information more efficiently [21,22]. Moreover, it provides a painterly representation of the characters, bringing artistic elements into play, which have shown to be of great use in therapies for individuals with ASD [23,24].

4   DECT

The Dynamic Emotional Categorization Test (DECT) [2] was conceived to assess the feasibility of using real-time animations by comparing virtual characters with human actors. In its very first version, it contained material of two human actors and two virtual characters displaying dynamic facial expressions of the six basic emotions (anger, disgust, fear, happiness, sadness, and surprise) on three intensity levels (weak, medium, and strong). Subjects had to categorize the presented video clips of real actors and animations of virtual characters in a six-alternative forced choice task with the six basic emotions as options (Fig. 1).

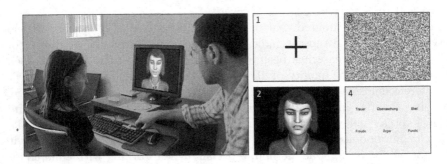

Fig. 1. Setup of the experiment and overview of a DECT trial: (1) Fixation cross that appears when the trial begins, (2) Facial Expression of one of the characters with certain speed and intensity, (3) White-Noise image to load participants' iconic memory with task-irrelevant information, (4) Emotion names as answers options.

The obtained results showed that the three levels of intensity were better reflected in the artificial actors than in the human actors. It was also concluded that using the Agent Framework [25], the software platform to generate the real-time facial animations, the experimenters could take advantage of the manipulability of the facial animations, and achieve desirable features like tailored testing.

In SARA the DECT has been adapted by improving the existent facial animations, integrating real-time NPR algorithms and adding communication with the open source software PsychoPy [26] and an eye tracker RED250 from SMI, which provides a high-speed sampling rate of 250 Hz, and thus high accuracy.

The first study of our project was the Rapid Social Cognition study, which studied the "rapid" aspect of social cognition. For that purpose, we used a version of the DECT that we called R-DECT, which novelty resides in the random presentation of real-time dynamic animations of facial expressions with different speeds (from normal to very fast) and intensities (weak, medium, strong).

The outcome of this study assesses the quality and the validity of the revised real-time and dynamic animations via accuracy rates. This in turn might suggest visual cues or facial features that play a key role in the understanding of perception and categorization of the expressions.

4.1 Virtual Characters

For the pilot study we used two characters: a young female (Nikita) and an older male (Hank) (Fig. 2). Both characters are provided and distributed with the Agent Framework under the Creative Commons Attribution-Non Commercial-ShareAlike 3.0 Unported License.

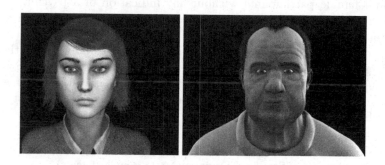

Fig. 2. Characters used in the R-DECT.

We decided to create human-like realistic characters because we aimed for visual similarity with real actors. Regarding the reduction of the level of detail in faces, it is more plausible to apply NPR techniques (e.g. sketchy or line drawing) to realistic characters and obtain an abstracted representation, than to reconstruct realistic representations from already abstracted characters.

Another important issue to take into consideration was the interactivity in the animations. On the one hand, we are interested in studying the timing in emotion recognition with dynamically moving faces which have higher ecological validity than static photos [5]. Thus our need to have real-time facial animations that can be parameterized in terms of speed and intensity. On the other hand, we plan more complex experiments where interactivity is a key component. In those, we will track the participants' eye gaze, which will originate the synchronized movement of the characters' head and gaze. All this could not be achieved using existing corpora of static images or video recordings of actors, where there is no real-time interactivity.

The animations of the character's facial expressions were produced using the Facial Animation Toolset (FAT)[1] [27], which permits the creation of believable non-linear facial deformations, based on the Facial Action Coding System (FACS) [28]. The FAT system also considers asymmetrical movements of Action Units (AU), allowing the generation of animations where one side of the face presents greater movement intensity than the other, and also in the upper and lower lip area. As a result, the animations are described in terms of FACS AUs and can be manipulated in Frapper's interface. Any value entered for an AU animation controls the intensity corresponding to the set of facial feature points involved.

---

[1] http://research.animationsinstitut.de/facial-research-tools/
facial-animation-toolset-2015/toolset-download/.

5   Experiment

In order to assess the feasibility (also with clinical samples), validity and improvement of the animations quality, we tested 39 adolescents that fulfilled the following inclusion criteria: age between 14.0 to 17.9 years and IQ $\geq$ 70. The group of neurotypically developed adolescents (NTD group: n=22) consisted of 18 male and 4 female participants without any indication of a psychiatric disorder. The group of individuals with high-functioning autism spectrum disorder (ASD group: n=17) consisted of 12 male and 5 female participants (Table 1). Diagnosis of ASD (ICD-10: F84.0, F84.1 or F84.5) was established by the international "gold standard" diagnostic procedure by applying the ADOS [29] and ADI-R [30]. Participants received a voucher for a cinema visit or for a book, and also got travel reimbursements in case of arising expenses. The study was approved by the local ethics committee.

Table 1. Sample characteristics (NTD = Neurotypical Development, ASD = Autism Spectrum Disorder, SD = Standard Deviation, ratio = male/female).

	NTD		ASD	
	(n=22, ratio=18/4)		(n=17, ratio=12/5)	
	Mean (SD)	Min - Max	Mean (SD)	Min - Max
Age	16.4 (1.1)	14.2 - 17.7	16.1 (1.1)	14.0 - 17.6
IQ	110.0 (13.3)	82 - 146	107.5 (20.6)	75 - 145

The R-DECT consisted of 2 (characters) $\times$ 6 (basic emotions) $\times$ 3 (intensity levels), resulting in 36 animations. Regarding the speed variable, it was assigned according to a certain scheme to each of the 36 animations, ranging from 1 (normal speed) up to 2.25 times of normal speed. In total, six levels were used (1.00, 1.25, 1.50, 1.75, 2.00, 2.25). However, since speed levels had little impact on results, we do not refer to this variable in the results section.

5.1   Procedure

The R-DECT was part of a battery of tests for rapid social cognition and intuitive moral reasoning assessment, comprising two experimental sessions, each lasting between 1.5 to 2 h. The R-DECT took about 15 min to be carried out and was administered as the first of five tests in the corresponding session. Experimental sessions were run individually in a quiet booth in the lab, where only the participant and the experimenter were present.

6   Results

6.1   Group Differences

In total, 62.2 % of the animations were categorized correctly. Accuracy rates for the NTD group was 65.7 % whereas for the ASD group was 57.7 %.

In order to test whether groups categorized animation-based emotions differently, whether animations with certain basic emotions differed from each other, or whether there are interactions between these two factors, a 2×6 MANOVA with repeated measurements was conducted using individual accuracy rates per basic emotion (collapsed over 6 test items [2 characters and three intensity levels] as dependent variables. This or closely related statistical approaches are common in the area of facial emotion recognition research (e.g. [31]).

The 2×6 MANOVA with repeated measurements yielded no significant interaction between group and basic emotion (F < 1). However, the two main effects were significant (*basic emotion*: $F(5,33) = 77.63$, p < .0001; *group*: $F(1,37) = 5.36$, p = .026). This means that the ASD group performed significantly worse than the NTD group, and that there were significant differences between categorization of basic emotions (Fig. 3).

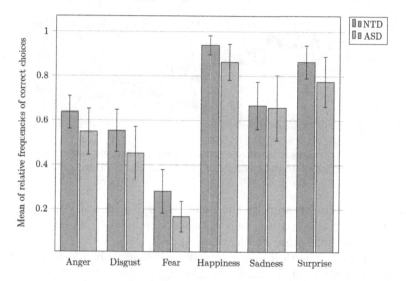

Fig. 3. Mean of relative frequencies of correct categorizations of six basic emotions in adolescents with high-functioning ASD in comparison to neurotypically developed peers (NTD). Error bars represent 95 % CI [confidence interval].

Order of accuracy for basic emotions was the same for both groups and had the following ranking from best to worst: happiness, surprise, sadness, anger, disgust, and fear. Same or similar orders have been found in other studies [31] or in recent meta-analyses [4]. Differences between groups were most pronounced for the basic emotion "fear" (NTD: 28.0 % vs. 16.7 %). However, all post-hoc comparisons did not reach statistical significance.

6.2   Analysis of Materials: Animations Intensities

Concerning the manipulation of the intensity of facial emotions, it is reasonable only to consider the NTD group where typical facial emotion recognition could be

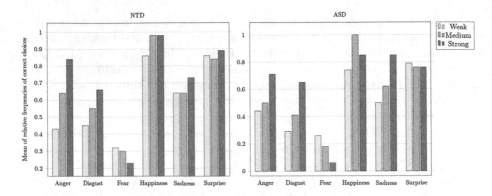

Fig. 4. Mean of relative frequencies of correct categorizations of six basic emotions across differing levels of intensity (weak, medium, strong) in the NTD and ASD group.

	Happiness	Surprise	Anger	Sadness	Disgust	Fear
Happiness	97.7	0.0	0.0	1.1	0.0	1.1
Surprise	4.6	86.4	1.1	0.0	1.14	6.8
Anger	0.0	4.6	73.9	5.7	6.8	9.1
Sadness	0.0	2.3	4.6	68.2	11.4	13.6
Disgust	1.1	0.0	33.0	3.4	60.2	2.3
Fear	23.9	26.1	6.8	1.1	15.9	26.1

Fig. 5. Percentage of chosen emotions (rows) per intended expression (columns) for animations with intensity levels medium or strong for the NTD group.

expected. The results showed that in general, varying intensity from weak over medium to strong affected accuracy rates correspondingly as intended: Weak: 59.5 %, Medium: 65.5 % and Strong: 72.0 %.

Broken down by emotion, most animations followed this pattern, except for "fear" that showed not the intended trend (Fig. 4). A similar pattern was found in the ASD group, where accuracy rates for fear also decreased with stronger intensity.

Confusion Matrices. In order to assess the quality of animations in general and which animations caused miscategorization in particular, confusion matrices between intended emotional expression and chosen expression were computed. A diagrammatic representation of the animations with medium or strong intensity (Fig. 5) shows that most emotional expressions were chosen by the NTD group as intended, with the exception of fear. "Fear" animations were frequently misinterpreted as "surprise", but surprisingly also as "happiness".

7   Discussion

We have presented the results of our first pilot study, which constitutes the first study of our project SARA (Stylized Animation for Research in Autism). To that end, we used an improved version of the DECT (Dynamic Emotional Categorization Test), named R-DECT. This version of the test provided physically-plausible 3D models of virtual characters capable of performing real-time facial expressions of emotions. In addition, the generated facial animations were dynamic in nature, as they could be parameterized according to different levels of speed and intensity.

The R-DECT proved to be suited for assessing the general ability of recognizing emotional facial expressions. The results of the experiment validated the test as the animations should be in a range where no floor effects (nobody recognizes the emotion) or ceiling effects (everybody recognizes the emotions) occur. Moreover, the R-DECT was able to detect the deficits in the ASD group and prove the impact of the different intensities in emotional expressions, as intended, see Figs. 3 and 4.

In order to improve the test, some adjustments of animations have to be made especially in the condition where intensity of the expression was intended to be "medium" or even "strong". That seems to be the case especially for the animation expressing the emotion "fear".

The results of these experiments lead to multiple application areas with virtual characters capable of expressing facial emotions. For instance, the parameterizable and real-time aspect of our system represents an advantage and a way to get away from videos and recorded material for teaching emotional facial expressions. It would provide the therapists, psychologists and experimenters freedom from the artists and developers, and the possibility to focus more on the individual differences of the autistic subjects. Hence it is possible to create tailored experiments for processing complex research questions.

As an intervention tool, the DECT could be enhanced to place the animations into another context and to provide immediate feedback about wrong/correct answers, as a sort of supervised learning environment.

Acknowledgments. The SARA project (officially Impact of non-photorealistic rendering for the understanding of emotional facial expressions by children and adolescents with high-functioning Autism Spectrum Disorders) is funded by the DFG - German Research Foundation (AR 892/1-1, DE 620/18-1, RA 764/4-1).

References

1. Hudepohl, M.B., Robins, D.L., King, T.Z., Henrich, C.: The role of emotion perception in adaptive functioning of individuals with high-functioning autism spectrum disorders. In: Autism: Int. J. Res. Pract. (2013)
2. Rauh, R., Schaller, U.M.: Categorical Perception of Emotional Facial Expressions in Video Clips with Natural and Artificial Actors: A Pilot Study. Technical report ALU-KJPP-2009-001, University of Freiburg (2009)
3. Collin, L., Bindra, J., Raju, M., Gillberg, C., Minnis, H.: Facial emotion recognition in child psychiatry: a systematic review. Res. Dev. Disabil. **34**(5), 1505–1520 (2013)
4. Lozier, L.M., Vanmeter, J.W., Marsh, A.A.: Impairments in facial affect recognition associated with autism spectrum disorders: a meta-analysis. Dev. Psychopathol. **26**(4 Pt 1), 933–945 (2014)

5. Uljarevic, M., Hamilton, A.: Recognition of emotions in autism: a formal meta-analysis. J. Autism Dev. Disord. **43**(7), 1517–1526 (2013)
6. Baio, J.: Prevalence of autism spectrum disorders autism and developmental disabilities monitoring network, 14 sites, United States, 2008. Surveill. Summ. **61**(SS03), 1–19 (2012)
7. Baio, J.: Prevalence of autism spectrum disorder among children aged 8 years autism and developmental disabilities monitoring network, 11 sites, United States, 2010. Surveill. Summ. **63**(2), 1–21 (2014)
8. Hill, E.L.: Executive dysfunction in autism. Trends Cogn. Sci. **8**(1), 2632 (2004)
9. Ospina, M.B., Seida, J.K., Clark, B., Karkhaneh, M., Hartling, L., Vandermeer, B., Smith, V.: Behavioural and developmental interventions for autism spectrum disorder: a clinical systematic review. Autism **3**(11), e3755 (2008)
10. Alcorn, A., Pain, H., Rajendran, G., Smith, T., Lemon, O., Porayska-Pomsta, K., Foster, M.E., Avramides, K., Frauenberger, C., Bernardini, S.: Social communication between virtual characters and children with autism. In: Biswas, G., Bull, S., Kay, J., Mitrovic, A. (eds.) AIED 2011. LNCS, vol. 6738, pp. 7–14. Springer, Heidelberg (2011)
11. Serret, S., Hun, S., Iakimova, G., Lozada, J., Anastassova, M., Santos, A., Vesperini, S. Askenazy, F.: Facing the challenge of teaching emotions to individuals with low- and high-functioning autism using a new Serious game: a pilot study. Molecular Autism. 5(37), (2014)
12. Alves, S., Marques, A., Queirós, C., Orvalho, V.: LIFEisGAME prototype: a serious game about emotions for children with autism spectrum disorders. PsychNology J. **11**(3), 191–211 (2013)
13. Hourcade, J.P., Bullock-Rest, N.E., Hansen, T.E.: Multitouch tablet applications and activities to enhance the social skills of children with autism spectrum disorders. Pers. Ubiquitous Comput. **16**(2), 157–168 (2012)
14. Whyte, E.M., Smyth, J.M., Scherf, S.: Designing serious game interventions for Individuals with autism. J. Autism Dev. Disord. (2014)
15. Baron-Cohen, S., Golan, O., Ashwin, E.: Can emotion recognition be taught to children with autism spectrum conditions? Phil. Trans. R. Soc. B. **364**, 3567–74 (2009)
16. Milne, M.K., Luerssen, M.H., Lewis, T.W., Leibbrandt, R.E., Powers, D.M.: Designing and evaluating interactive agents as social skills tutors for children with autism spectrum disorder. In: Conversational Agents and Natural Language Interaction: Techniques and Effective Practices, pp. 23–48. IGI Global, USA (2011)
17. Grawemeyer, B., Johnson, H., Brosnan, M., Ashwin, E., Benton, L.: Developing an embodied pedagogical agent with and for young people with autism spectrum disorder. In: Cerri, S.A., Clancey, W.J., Papadourakis, G., Panourgia, K. (eds.) ITS 2012. LNCS, vol. 7315, pp. 262–267. Springer, Heidelberg (2012)
18. Kätsyri, J., Saalasti, S., Tiippana, K., von Wendt, L., Sams, M.: Impaired recognition of facial emotions from low-spatial frequencies in Asperger syndrome. Neuropsychologia. **46**, 1888–1897 (2008)
19. Valla, J.M., Maendel, J.W., Ganzel, B.L., Barsky, A.R., Belmonte, M.K.: Autistic trait interactions underlie sex-dependent facial recognition abilities in the normal population. Front Psychol. 4(286) (2013)
20. Strauss, M.S., Newell, L.C., Best, C.A., Hannigen, S.F., Gastgeb, H.Z., Giovannelli, J.L.: The development of facial gender categorization in individuals with and without autism: the impact of typicality. J Autism Dev Disord. **42**(9), 1847–1855 (2012)

21. Götzelmann, T.: Towards non-photorealistic rendering in car navigation. J. Comput. Eng. Inf. Technol. 1(1) (2012)
22. Lee, J., Kim, H., Kim, M., Park, H., Kim, H.: Non-Photorealistic Rendering applied Semantic LOD. In: HCI KOREA 2015. pp. 1–6. Hanbit Media, Inc. (2015)
23. Epp, K.M.: Outcome-based evaluation of a social skills program using art therapy and group therapy for children on the autism spectrum. Child. Sch. 30(1), 27–36 (2008)
24. Emery, M.J.: Art therapy as an intervention for autism. Art Ther.: J. Am. Art Ther. Assoc. 21(3), 143–147 (2004)
25. Arellano, D., Helzle, V., Schaller, U.M., Rauh, R.: Animated faces, abstractions and autism. In: Bickmore, T., Marsella, S., Sidner, C. (eds.) IVA 2014. LNCS, vol. 8637, pp. 22–25. Springer, Heidelberg (2014)
26. Peirce, J. W.: Generating Stimuli for Neuroscience Using PsychoPy. Front. Neuroinform. 2(10) (2009)
27. Helzle, V., Biehn, C., Schlömer, T., Linner, F.: Adaptable setup for performance driven facial animation. In: ACM SIGGRAPH 2004 Sketches, p. 54 (2004)
28. Ekman, P., Friesen, W., Hager, J.: The Facial Action Coding System. Weidenfeld & Nicolson, London (2002)
29. Rühl, D., Bölte, S., Feineis-Matthews, S., Poustka, F.: ADOS: Diagnostische Beobachtungsskala für Autistische Störungen. Huber, Bern (2004)
30. Bölte, S., Rühl, D., Schmötzer, G., Poustka, F.: ADI-R: Diagnostisches Interview für Autismus - Revidiert German version of Autism Diagostic Interview - Revised. Huber, Bern (2006)
31. Smith, M.J.L., Montagne, B., Perrett, D.I., Gill, M., Gallagher, L.: Detecting subtle facial emotion recognition deficits in high-functioning Autism using dynamic stimuli of varying intensities. Neuropsychologia 48(9), 2777–2781 (2010)

Virtual Blindness - A Choice Blindness Experiment with a Virtual Experimenter

Martin Lingonblad[1], Ludvig Londos[1], Arvid Nilsson[2], Emil Boman[2], Jens Nirme[1], and Magnus Haake[1(✉)]

[1] Division of Cognitive Science, Lund University, Lund, Sweden
{martin.lingonblad.299,fte08llo}@student.lu.se,
{jens.nirme,magnus.haake}@lucs.lu.se
[2] Department of Computer Science, Lund University, Lund, Sweden
{ada09an2,emil.boman.633}@student.lu.se

Abstract. How are people facing a virtual agent affected by the vividness and graphical fidelity of the agent and its environment? A choice blindness (CB) experiment – measuring detection rate of hidden manipulations – was conducted presenting a high versus low immersion virtual environment. The hypothesis was that the lower quality virtual environment (low immersion) would increase the detection rate for the CB manipulations. 38 subjects participated in the experiment and were randomized into two groups (high and low immersion). Both conditions presented a virtual agent conducting the CB experiment. During the experiment, 16 pairs of portraits were shown two at a time for the participants who were then asked to choose which portrait they found most attractive. For eight of the pairs, participants were asked to justify their choice while in four cases their choice had been secretly switched to the portrait they had not chosen. If a participant stated that the chosen portrait had been switched, it was annotated as a concurrent detection.

The results revealed an increase in detection and earlier detection rate for the low immersion implementation compared to the high immersion implementation. Future research may involve experiments with higher degree of both immersion and presence, using for example head mounted display systems.

Keywords: Virtual agent · Choice blindness · Attention · Presence · Immersion

1 Introduction

1.1 Virtual Environments

A virtual environment (VE) provides control over a setting, similarly to a laboratory environment, with the advantage that a VE might emulate a more natural setting [1].

VEs also have the advantage that virtual humans or virtual agents can be used in the role as experimenters. The virtual agents will act the same way for each participant, something that is hard to control for with real humans as experimenters [2].

However, the validity of experiments in virtual environments in many cases remains unconfirmed. Do we act similarly in a VE as we would in the real world?

© Springer International Publishing Switzerland 2015
W.-P. Brinkman et al. (Eds.): IVA 2015, LNAI 9238, pp. 442–451, 2015.
DOI: 10.1007/978-3-319-21996-7_47

And more specifically; do we interact with a virtual human similarly to how we interact with other humans?

1.2 Immersion and Presence

In virtual reality the terms *immersion* and *presence* [3, 4] are often used to determine the degree of match to reality. *Presence* refers to a subjective measure of a person's experience of being in a virtual environment and can be subdivided into environmental presence, co-presence, and social presence [3].

There is evidence suggesting that participants who experience a high level of presence to a larger extent also behave like they would in a natural setting, including interaction with (virtual) humans [3]. A well-animated agent can be perceived as "human-like, engaging, and motivating" [2]. Furthermore, requirements for realistic graphics and animation are higher for interacting with a virtual agent as if it was a human, compared to interacting with an avatar (a virtual representation of another human [1, 2]. *Immersion* comprises the technical parts of the virtual setting. Slater and Wilbur divide immersion into four categories: *vivid*, *inclusive*, *extensive*, and *surrounding* [3]. "Vivid" refers to technical specifications such as resolution and fidelity. "Inclusive" refers to how much of reality is shut out. "Extensive" refers to how many sensory modalities are included. "Surrounding" refers to how well the visual field is represented. *Immersion* and *presence* are casually related. Welch et al. reported that high or low graphical fidelity affected participants' experienced presence during a car simulator experiment [5]. Likewise, Shubert et al. concluded: "The more inclusive, extensive, surrounding, and vivid the VE is [...] or the more similar the transformations in the VE are to those in the real world [...] the higher the presence." [6].

High immersion, however, does not necessarily lead to high presence. Another important factor is the ability to convince oneself that the virtual reality is real – something commonly referred to as *suspension of disbelief* [7]. An example of low immersion but high presence is reading an engaging book.

In the current study we exploited the Choice Blindness research paradigm [8, 9] where aspects of the physical environments are manipulated by real human experimenters using techniques inspired by the domain of close-up card-magic. A central measurable parameter is participants' detection-rate of the manipulations. The current study addressed whether the level of immersion would affect perception of and interaction with a virtual agent experimenter, as reflected in the detection rate of manipulations.

1.3 The Choice Blindness Paradigm

In the original version of a CB-experiment [8] a participant is shown a number of different photographs of human faces displayed in pairs, during 2 to 5 s intervals. After the view period the photographs are turned face-down on the table in front of the participant and the participant is asked to indicate the photograph he or she preferred. Then the experimenter pushes the chosen card towards the participant who picks it up and looks at it and is asked to justify her choice. In some of the trials, the experimenter has swapped the faces by having hidden copies of both photographs in each hand. In these manipulated trials, the participant is forced to justify a choice that has not been made. For 70–80 % of the trials with manipulation go undetected.

In studies where the original experimental set-up with a real experimenter and real cards, was changed into a real experimenter using digital cards displayed on a screen [10] and into a virtual experimenter using digital cards [11] detection rates increased, with 60–65 % of the manipulations undetected.

Why have participants more often noticed the manipulation when the photographs have been displayed digitally on a screen instead of physically on a table? One possibility is that the natural environment is more trusted: real photographs usually are not suddenly changed into another. Another possibility is that the natural environment is more distracting than the virtual and more likely to disrupt participants' attention.

In the current study, we will utilize CB to see if participants' detection rates are affected by the level of immersion in a virtual environment. The study is a conceptual replication of the original Choice Blindness experiment [8], but instead of exploring the choice blindness phenomenon itself – it uses the choice blindness paradigm as a measurement of the experience when interacting with a virtual agent. We hypothesize that the level of immersion will affect detection rate and possibly shade light on the roles of (i) trust in a real versus virtual environment and (ii) distractibility of a real versus virtual environment in affecting detection rates.

2   Method

2.1   Design

Participants were assigned to one of two virtual implementations of the *Choice Blindness* paradigm [8, 9]. One group was presented with a low immersion implementation and the other group with a high immersion implementation. Before the virtual choice blindness task, the participants were tested for individual tendencies to experience presence via a translated and adapted version of the *Immersive Tendencies Questionnaire* [12]. After the virtual choice blindness task, participants were debriefed via a standardized choice blindness debriefing format.

2.2   Participants

41 university students (20 male, 21 female), age 19 to 32 years, were recruited at Lund University, Sweden. The majority were students at the Faculty of Technology.

3 participants were excluded from the data set due to not accurately completing the task or a bug in the program that affected their performance. The final data set included data from a total of 38 participants (21 females and 17 males) with 19 participants in each condition, cf. Table 1.

Table 1. Participants: number, gender, age (ranges, medians and averages).

Condition	N	N (female /male)	Min – Max (age)	Median (age)	M (age)
Low immersion	19	11 /8	19 - 31	24	23.8
High immersion	19	10 /9	20-32	24	24.2

2.3   Procedure

After having read and signed a written consent form the participants were presented with a questionnaire addressing individual tendencies to experience presence. Next, the participants were told that they were to perform a task interacting with a virtual agent using a voice recognition system. This instruction was delivered to conceal the actual experimental design. The participants were then escorted into a booth where a computer with the virtual choice blindness task was prepared (having a "Wizard-of-Oz" [13] hiding in an adjacent booth).

Participants were assigned to one of the two conditions depending on the result of the ITQ together with a randomization table. The ITQ-result was used to ensure matched groups in the two conditions with regard to immersive tendency and to control for computer experience.

The virtual choice blindness task consisted of 16 sessions. In each session the virtual experimenter presented a pair of photographs showing portraits, with four of these sessions being manipulated according to the choice blindness paradigm [8, 9].

After completion the participants were brought back to the entering room and debriefed using a standardized choice blindness debriefing procedure [8, 9]. The experiment was finally concluded by giving the participants a restaurant voucher.

2.4   Immersive Tendencies Questionnaire

The widely used *Immersive Tendencies Questionnaire* (ITQ) [12] is designed to measure the tendency of individuals to be involved or immersed in a virtual environment by addressing several factors that are assumed to contribute to immersive tendencies, among others the tendency to become involved in activities, the tendency to maintain focus on current activities, and the tendency to play video games.

ITQ consist of 18 items, each with a seven-point scale semantic differential scale complemented with a midpoint anchor. In this study, the questionnaire was translated to Swedish with an additional 19th item probing for computer experience.

2.5   Virtual Setting

Design of the Virtual Scenario: The CB paradigm was implemented in a VE with a virtual experimenter and digital photos (from the original choice blindness card collection). As in the original studies, each photo pair was presented during 3 s. The size of the virtual cards was adjusted to resemble the size experienced in the original (real world) experiments when "virtually" presented on the screen.

Following the choice blindness protocol, the participant was asked to verbally describe their choice on 8 of 16 pairs during the experiment. Of these 8 pairs, 4 were manipulated so that the photo of choice was secretly (digitally) switched whereupon the participant actually was asked to describe why they preferred the photo they did not chose.

Main Measurement: The core measure within the choice blindness paradigm is *concurrent detection*. In case of explicit verbal reactions from the participant, a concurrent detection can be clearly registered. To handle more subtle cases, participants may, as in the present study, be video recorded during the experiment for post-experiment discern whether a detection of the manipulation was made. In addition there is a standardized debriefing procedure after the choice blindness experiment. During this debriefing, the participants are given a chance to make a post-experiment detections guided by a specified question procedure where the questions are asked step by step – revealing more and more information about the experiment.

Realization of the Virtual Scenario: The virtual implementation was developed based on motion capture recordings with one of the experimenters from the original choice blindness experiments going through the experimental procedure. An eight camera Qualisys® motion capture system was used; the recordings were imported into Autodesk MotionBuilder® and plotted onto a 3D-character created in Autodesk Character Generator®. The motion capture recordings were then edited into shorter clips representing different animated sequences of the experimental procedure, for example welcoming the participant, showing the pair of cards, asking the participant to describe a certain choice, etc. Next, the animated clips were imported into the Unity® developer platform together with 3D-models of the furnishings created in Autodesk 3ds Max®, whereupon the final implementation of the virtual scenarios were edited and scripted. As a real interactive implementation of a virtual agent with a spoken natural language interface was beyond the scope of this experiment, the actual interaction was simulated using a "Wizard-of-Oz"-approach [13]. In this realization, the participant communicated with the virtual experimenter through a head-set while the "Wizard" was hidden in an adjacent booth listening to the participant while triggering the verbal utterances and movements of the virtual presenter. As for the two implementations of the virtual experiment (high versus low immersion) the aim of the high immersion setting was to replicate one of the original experimental environments and procedures as closely as possible, while the low immersion setting was a tuned down version of the high immersion setting. The goal with the low immersion version was to reduce experienced presence.

In the low immersion version (cf. Fig. 1), all superfluous furnishing of the virtual environment were removed according to the involvement parameter, thus lowering inclusiveness [3]. Furthermore, for the low immersion version, the voice of the virtual experimenter was "computerized" (tuned to sound like a computer generated synthetic voice) and the facial animations were simplified in line with the spatial presence parameter in order to reduce extensiveness [3]. Finally, in the low immersion version, shadows were removed [14] and the graphical settings were decreased in compliance with the perceived realism parameter to decrease vividness [3].

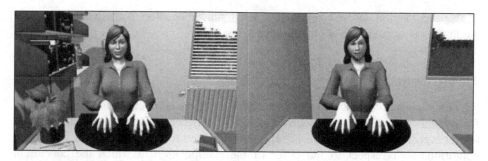

Fig. 1. Screenshots of the virtual implementation of the choice blindness experiment. Left: high immersion; right: low immersion.

A pilot study was conducted in order to validate that the two immersion conditions actually produced a difference in perceived presence and to reassure that the alterations in immersion did not affect the execution of the choice blindness task. The pilot study was performed in four steps, involving 10 students recruited from the same area (a campus restaurant) as the following experiment.

First, the participants were asked to fill out the *Immersive Tendencies Question-naire* (ITQ) [12] to determine to what extent the participants tended to involve themselves in a virtual world. Second, they were randomly exposed to one of two virtual implementations of the choice blindness task (low or high immersion). Third, after the interaction with the virtual implementation, the participants were asked to fill out a questionnaire to evaluate their perceived presence during the intervention. The presence questionnaire was based on the *The Igroup Presence Questionnaire* (IPQ) [6] and is made up of questions addressing three aspects of presence (*spatial presence, involvement,* and *perceived realism*); five additional questions were added to the presence questionnaire to include *social presence* [15]. The fourth and final step was a standardized choice blindness debriefing procedure for evaluation of concurrent detection [8].

The ITQ-results showed an average of 0.62 in the high immersion condition and 0.65 in the low, suggesting that the two groups of participants were equal with regard to individual tendencies to involve themselves in virtual environment settings.

The results of the presence questionnaire (cf. Table 2) indicated a difference between the two implementations in the expected direction, with higher perceived presence for all four parameters compared to the low immersion implementation.

The evaluation of concurrent detection of the choice blindness data also showed a lower rate of detections in the high immersion implementation compared to the low immersion implementation.

Table 2. Average values of the presence questionnaire parameters for the two implementations of immersion.

Group	Spatial	Involvement	Exp. realism	Social presence
High immersion	2.28	2.05	1.65	2.52
Low immersion	1.84	1.30	1.15	2.16

Neither version showed any tendencies to hinder or affect participants negatively while they performed the choice blindness task.

2.6   Statistical Analyses

All analyses were conducted in R v3.1.3 [16]. Independent student's t-tests were used for overall comparisons of concurrent detection between immersion conditions. Multilevel logistic regression (R package: *lme4*) was used to compare the two immersion conditions with respect to the order of the manipulation at which the concurrent detections were registered. The alpha level for all statistical analyses was set to .05.

3   Results

3.1   Concurrent Detection

Concurrent detection [8, 9] was individually coded by two blinded persons from the research team. Following the coding, the results were compared and discrepancies were discussed and agreed upon while still blinded.

Concurrent detection was coded in two levels, *hard* and *weak* detection [8, 9]. Hard detection refers to any verbal detection ranging from stating clearly that the photo was not the one chosen to a vaguer indication, for example "Was this really the photo I chose?" Weak detection refers to a participant either frowning, looking puzzled, or behaving differently compared to non-manipulated trials. Weaker detection is not as evident as the harder detection, as it could be the case that the participant is not really aware of the manipulation. It could also be the case that the participant was aware but did not react verbally (cf. Fig. 2).

The total result for hard concurrent detection was for high immersion 27 % (including weak detection = 31 %), and for low immersion 38 % (including weak detection = 43 %). A straightforward t-test showed no significant results between the low and high immersion condition (hard detection: $t(150) = 1.483$, 95 % CI [-0.07; 0.5], $p = 0.14$).

A look at Fig. 2 suggests, however, a seemingly evident difference between the two groups (low and high immersion) over the course of the four manipulations. While concurrent detections were more or less equal at the first manipulation, the low immersion group encountered more frequent concurrent detections during the second and third manipulation. During, the fourth and last manipulation, the high immersion group "caught up" and even surpassed the low immersion group. A multilevel logistic regression analysis of the detections with regard to the order of the four manipulations revealed a significant difference between the low and high immersion group ($Z = 2.363$, $p = .018$) in that the low immersion group had both more and earlier concurrent detections compared to the high immersion group. Additionally, the multilevel logistic regression also indicated a significant interaction effect between the type of immersion and the order of the four manipulations ($Z = -2.149$, $p = 0.032$) supporting the finding that the low immersion condition had substantially earlier detections than the high immersion condition (cf. Fig. 2).

concurrent detections

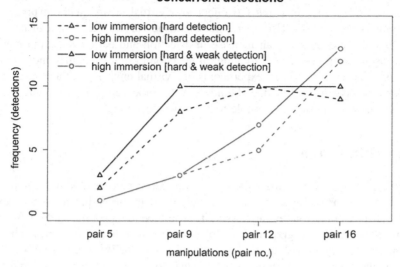

Fig. 2. Concurrent detection for low (green) and high (red) immersion. CD1 to CD4 (Current Detection 1 to 4) represents the four manipulations in the choice blindness experiment.

ITQ, the participant's extent of involving him/herself in a virtual world, were used to determine that there was no a misallocation between the high and low immersion groups. The mean ITQ for high immersion was 0.63 and for low immersion 0.59. A t-test showed no statistical difference between the groups.

4 Discussion

The study did not show any statistical difference in total detection rate between high and low immersion. However, the results indicated another difference in detection between the two conditions, and it is possible or even likely that a larger-scale experiment with more participants in each category would support our original hypothesis that low immersion will lead to a higher degree of detections in the CB task compared to high immersion.

As can be seen in Fig. 2, the patterns for *when* a detection is made differs between the two conditions. In the low immersion group detection in general came earlier than in the high immersion group. A possible reason for this result is that there were more interesting stimuli in the high immersion condition. In the low immersion condition there was a lack of stimuli to pay attention to, which could be the reason for the earlier detection. In other words, there was not many interesting things besides the faces to focus at and thus relatively more attention, compared to in the high immersion condition, was directed to the task at hand.

The concurrent detection results seem to be in par with similar research in the CB paradigm. For instance, the original CB study [8] reports a total detection rate at 26 %. For the high immersion condition in the present experiment the rate was 27–31 %, depending on how strict you want to be in calculating detection. We believe this shows that it is possible to recreate the CB effect in a virtual setting without producing a negative effect on the task. However, one should be vary of the design of the virtual setting. Our study does show an increase in detection and earlier detection rate for a low immersion design compared to a high immersion design. This may indicate that if one wants to replicate or design experiments in a virtual environment aiming at having participants behave naturally, one should take the time necessary to create a virtual setting which is as similar as possible to a real world setting.

5   Future Research

We would like to replicate the experiment with more participants and compare our results, foremost in the high immersion condition, with the earlier mentioned experiments by [10]. Another interesting possibility would be to repeat the study with a much more pronounced drop in graphical fidelity for the low immersion environment.

Using an intelligent virtual experimenter instead of a WOZ-setup with a human controlling the agent is also on our agenda. This would bring more control and ensure equivalence of vocal responses for all participants.

The experiment platform that we created can also be used for further and extended investigations. One may for instance add more properties to increase the immersion with the intention to increase the perceived presence. Possibly this might lower detection rate even more. However, that begs the question whether one could lower detection rate more. In one imagined scenario an *Occulus Rift* would be incorporated into the program to increase immersion. Would this lower the detection rate? We believe that the effect may be the opposite in making participants more suspicious and even increase detection. Imagine yourself being asked to do a "simple" face preference task but also be told that in order to do this simple task you need to use an advanced head mounted display. Yet we still find that it would be an interesting branch that this project could investigate.

It would also be possible to reduce the immersion level even more either by reducing all aspects or by focusing on one or some aspects, allowing distinguishing the most important aspect(s) behind the observed effect. In theory we could lower just the social presence aspect and see if that alone affects the detection rate. But our suspicion is that it is a combination of aspects that creates the CB effect.

References

1. Blascovich, J., Loomis, J., Beall, A.C., Swinth, K.R., Hoyt, C.L., Bailenson, J.N.: Immersive virtual environment technology as a methodological tool for social psychology. Psychol. Inq. **13**(2), 103–124 (2002)
2. Dehn, D.M., Van Mulken, S.: The impact of animated interface agents: a review of empirical research. Int. J. Hum Comput Stud. **52**(1), 1–22 (2000)

3. Slater, M., Wilbur, S.: A framework for immersive virtual environments (five): speculations on the role of presence in virtual environments. Presence Teleoperators Virtual Environ. **6** (6), 603–616 (1997)
4. Slater, M.: Measuring presence: a response to the witmer and singer presence questionnaire. Presence Teleoperators Virtual Environ. **8**(5), 560–565 (1999)
5. Welsh, R.B., Blackman, T.T., Liu, A., Mellers, B.A., Stark, L.W.: The Effects of Pictorial Realism, Delay of Visual Feedback, and Observer Interactivity on the Subjective Sense of Presence. Presence Teleoperators Virtual Environ. **5**(3), 263–273 (1996). MIT Press
6. Schubert, T., Friedmann, F., Regenbrecht, H.: The experience of presence: factor analytic insights. Presence **10**(3), 266–281 (2001)·
7. Thomas, F., Johnston, O.: The Illusion of Life: Disney Animation. Abbeville Press, New York (1984)
8. Johansson, P., Hall, L., Sikström, S., Olsson, A.: Failure to detect mismatches between intention and outcome in a simple decision task. Science **310**(5745), 116–119 (2005)
9. Johansson, P., Hall, L., Sikström, S.: From change blindness to choice blindness. Psychologia **51**, 142–155 (2008)
10. Haake, M., Gulz, A.: Trust in Virtual Reality. (Manuscript)
11. Johansson, P., Hall, L., Gulz, A., Haake, M., Watanabe, K.: Choice Blindness and Trust in the Virtual World. Technical Report of IEICE: HIP, 107(60), 83–86 (2007)
12. Witmer, B., Singer, M.: Measuring presence in virtual environments: a presence questionnaire. Presence **7**(3), 225–240 (1998)
13. Dahlbäck, N., Jönsson, A.: Empirical studies of discourse representations for natural language interfaces. In: Proceedings of the 4th Conference on European Chapter of the Association for Computational Linguistics (1989)
14. Slater, M., Usoh, M., Chrysanthou, Y.: The influence of dynamic shadows on presence in immersive virtual environments. In: Hansmann, W., Purgathofer, W., Sillion, F. (eds.) Eurographics: Virtual Environments 1995, pp. 8–21. Springer, Vienna (1995)
15. Garau, M., Slater, M., Pertaub, D.P., Razzaque, S.: The responses of people to virtual humans in an immersive virtual environment. Presence Teleoperators Virtual Environ. **14**(1), 104–116 (2005)
16. R Core Team: R: A Language and Environment for Statistical Computing [Computer Software]. R Foundation for Statistical Computing. Vienna (2015)

Comparing Behavior Towards Humans and Virtual Humans in a Social Dilemma

Rens Hoegen[✉], Giota Stratou, Gale M. Lucas, and Jonathan Gratch

Institute for Creative Technologies, University of Southern California,
Los Angeles, USA
{rhoegen,stratou,lucas,gratch}@ict.usc.edu

Abstract. The difference of shown social behavior towards virtual humans and real humans has been subject to much research. Many of these studies compare virtual humans (VH) that are presented as either virtual agents controlled by a computer or as avatars controlled by real humans. In this study we directly compare VHs with real humans. Participants played an economic game against a computer-controlled VH or a visible human opponent. Decisions made throughout the game were logged, additionally participants' faces were filmed during the study and analyzed with expression recognition software. The analysis of choices showed participants are far more willing to violate social norms with VHs: they are more willing to steal and less willing to forgive. Facial expressions show trends that suggest they are treating VHs less socially. The results highlight, that even in impoverished social interactions, VHs have a long way to go before they can evoke truly human-like responses.

Keywords: Virtual humans · Social behavior · Facial expressions · Decision making

1 Introduction

Do people treat machines like people? This has been a central concern within the virtual agent and robotics communities, almost since their inception. The answer to this question has more than passing interest. Virtual humans (VH) are increasingly used to teach people how to interact with other people. VHs teach people how to negotiate [4] or how to overcome fear of public speaking [2]. Others have proposed virtual agents or robots as replacements for people in a variety of customer service and even business settings. Following Cliff Nass' early work on the Media Equation [14], it is common to assume that the same social processes arise in both human and VH interaction, and many subsequent studies have reinforced the validity of this assumption (e.g., [17]).

Yet, recent studies emphasize important differences in how people treat machines [6,9]. Further, there is good reason to believe that studies under-report the differences between humans and artificial partners, as most "direct comparisons" are not as direct as they might seem. The most common method is to manipulate the *mere belief* of who one is interacting with. For example, people

© Springer International Publishing Switzerland 2015
W.-P. Brinkman et al. (Eds.): IVA 2015, LNAI 9238, pp. 452–460, 2015.
DOI: 10.1007/978-3-319-21996-7_48

interact with a digital character but in one case they believe they are playing a computer program and in the other case they believe a person is driving the agents behavior [9]. While there are good methodological reasons to adopt this experimental design, it also clearly under-represents the differences between human and VH interaction. It is a necessary but insufficient step towards demonstrating equivalence between human and machine interaction.

In this study, we make a direct comparison between the behavior of people interacting with other humans in face-to-face interaction with their behavior when interacting with VHs. We explore this within the context of a standard economic game, the iterated prisoner's dilemma, as this allows for several behavioral measures and allows us to connect our findings with a number of existing studies on social behavior. Prior VH research and robotics research on the prisoner's dilemma manipulated the beliefs of participants as to whether they were playing a real or virtual human, but decisions were always made by a computer (e.g., [7,10]). However, in this study we compared data between humans that could see each other via webcam (but not speak to each other), against humans playing with an emotionally-expressive VH. In order to determine social behavior we analyzed both the strategy used by participants and their use of facial expressions, by using facial expression recognition software. Based on prior findings on how people treat VHs in this game [7], we hypothesize that people will be more reluctant to show pro-social behavior to a VH, both through their actions and emotional displays. We explain these hypotheses in the next section.

In Sect. 2 we will give an overview of work involving the displayed social behavior against VHs. Section 3 describes the specifics of the iterated prisoner's dilemma game played during the study, as well as the VH that was used. Furthermore information on the analysis of the game behavior and expressed behavior will be given. Section 4 contains the overview of the results of the study for both game and expressed behavior and in Sect. 5 the implications of these results will be discussed.

2   Related Work

There are several views on the social behavior people show when interacting with computers. The Media Equation of Reeves and Nass claimed that responses to computers would equal responses to humans when computers incorporate human-like social cues. This was claimed to occur because people develop automatic responses to social cues and thus, unconsciously react automatically to computers in the same way as they do towards other humans [13]. It has been argued that the concept of facial expressions within economic games can serve as automatic elicitors of social behavior [16] and that VHs can exploit these cues [5].

A strong interpretation of the media equation, often articulated by Nass [12], is that responses towards computers are equivalent to human responses when computers incorporate social cues. A more nuanced perspective replaces the "=" in Nass' media equation with a "<". Blascovich [3] argues that social influence will increase based on the perceived realism and "agency" of a virtual agent. Agency refers to the perceived sentience or free will of an agent. This view is supported by a study of de Melo et al. [7], in two experiments agency was manipulated by comparing VHs that were either agents (i.e. controlled by computers) with avatars (i.e. controlled by humans). These experiments showed that people cooperated more with VHs which showed specific facial displays, however these displays only scored significantly different for the avatar condition, thus showing the difference in social behavior people display while playing against humans or VH. Riedl et al. [15] have done a study where participants played against humans and avatars. Their results showed that people display similar trust behavior between humans and avatars, however through neuroimaging they showed that there are different responses in the brain between human and avatar opponents. In a study by Krach et al. [10] humans played an iterated prisoner's dilemma, against both computers, robots and humans. Their results showed that humans in fact experienced more fun and competition in the interaction with increasing human-like features of their partners.

Our current study builds on the findings of de Melo et al. [8]. In their study, people played an iterated prisoners dilemma with a VH that played tit-for-tat and expressed specific emotions. In one condition, participants believed the agents choices and emotions were selected by another participant. In the other, they believed they were generated by a computer programmed to behave like a human. In either case, players could send emotional expressions to the other player along with their choice in the game. The tit-for-tat behavior and the pattern of emotional expressions were both chosen to maximize the amount of cooperation shown by participants. Nonetheless, participants made less cooperative choices and sent fewer positive and more neutral expressions when they believed they were playing a computer opponent. Based on these findings, we make the following hypotheses:

H1: *Participants will cooperate significantly more with other human players than VHs. More specifically, we predict people will be (H1a) more willing to try to exploit a VH, (H1b) more willing to persist in exploiting a VH, and (H1c) more willing to forgive humans following exploitation.*

H2: *Participants will show more cooperative facial expressions to human players compared with VHs. Specifically, we predict people will (H2a) show more joy to human players and (H2b) show more neutral expressions to VH.*

3   Experimental Setup

For this study, participants played an iterated prisoner's dilemma game against either other humans or a VH. The study used a 2-cell design, a total of 113 participants (56 female) participated in this study. 23 participants played against the VH, the remaining 90 participants played the game against each other in the human condition. No specific information was given on the VH, participants

Table 1. Left: Number of tickets the participant receives per outcome. Right: VH responses to outcomes.

		Opponent					Virtual human	
		Cooperate	Defect				Cooperate	Defect
Participant	Cooperate	5	0		Participant	Cooperate	Joy	Fear
	Defect	10	1			Defect	Anger	Sadness

were simply told that they would play the game against either a human or a virtual human. The task was based on the one presented by de Melo et al. [7]. Participants played 10 rounds of the game and the possible outcomes of the player decisions are shown in Table 1.

The game interface, shown in Fig. 1, displays the game on one side of the screen and the opponent on the other side. The participants chose whether to "split" the tickets or try to "steal" them, corresponding to the cooperate and defect options.

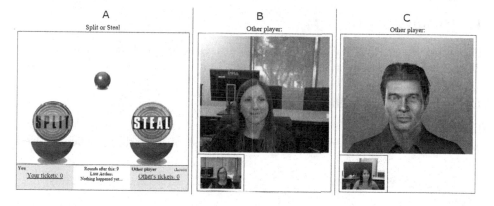

Fig. 1. Screenshot of the split/steal game. Panel A shows the game at the moment the participant can make their choice. Panel B will only be shown to participants in the human condition, panel C only for the VH condition.

Figure 1 shows both the human and VH condition of the game. The experiment was performed in a lab setting, with a maximum of five participants playing the game on computers. Participants were not allowed to speak during the study. The group playing against human opponents could see the video from their opponents' webcam on their screens. Participants playing against the VH would instead see the VH display within the web browser using the Unity web player plugin.[1] The VH used a tit-for-tat strategy during the game, similar to the study by de Melo et al. [7]. The agent used this strategy for the entire game with the exception of the first and second round, on the first round the agent would always cooperate with

---

[1] https://unity3d.com/webplayer.

the participant, whereas on the second round the VH would always defect. Table 1 shows the facial expressions feedback of the VH on the outcome of a round. These expressions are based on the expressions of virtual agents tested in a study by de Melo et al. [5] and were found to perform the best at eliciting cooperation. The actions of the participants were logged in a database along with the timestamps. Using this data we could infer when decisions were made, when the results were revealed and when rounds began or ended.

Participant videos from the webcams were automatically analyzed using FACET facial expression recognition software.[2] FACET features include intensities for the basic emotion labels as well for overall sentiment labels: "POSITIVE", "NEGATIVE" and "NEUTRAL". FACET is a commercial software for expression recognition that evolved from an academic version, the "Computer Expression Recognition Toolbox" (CERT) [1] and reports high accuracy on emotion recognition labels on known datasets [11]. Videos with high rate of missing frames were automatically discarded from the analysis. Logging of the game events allowed for automatic event-based behavior encoding as well as automatic segregation of the signals on the game period from the overall recording.

4   Results

This section describes the results of our study. Section 4.1 shows our findings on H1, Sect. 4.2 the findings on H2.

4.1   Game Behaviors

The plots in Fig. 2 show how often participants chose to cooperate in both conditions. We performed an independent T-test on this data, which showed

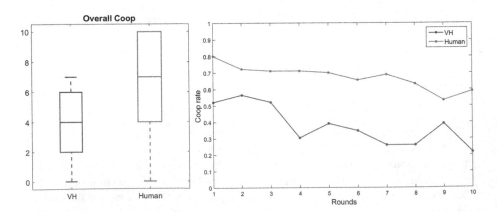

Fig. 2. The left boxplot showing the overall cooperation rate for participants playing either a VH or human opponent, the plot on the right displays the cooperation rate per round

---

[2] http://www.emotient.com/products/#FACETVision.

that there was a significant difference in overall cooperation between the human (M = 6.77, SD = 3.17) and the VH conditions (M = 3.64, SD = 2.13); $t(108) = 4.39$, $p < 0.001$. The number of times participants perform mutual cooperation in the human condition (M = 5.19, SD = 4.07) is in this game state significantly higher than in the VH condition (M = 1.59, SD = 1.65); $t(108) = 4.06$, $p < 0.001$, whereas the opposite is true for the mutual defect state (Human: M = 1.69, SD = 2.17; VH: M = 4.05, SD = 2.44); $t(108) = 4.44$, $p < 0.001$.

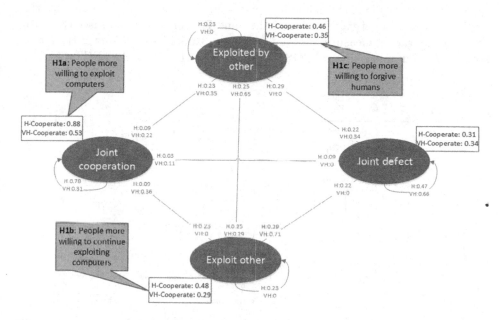

Fig. 3. Markov chain of the possible game states. Boxes display the chance a participant would choose to cooperate given in a certain state and support H1.

The Markov Chain in Fig. 3 shows that participants are generally more likely to exploit VH opponents than real humans (H1a). When participants are in a mutual cooperation state, the probability of continuing to cooperate is 88 % for the human condition, but only 53 % for the VH condition. Participants will forgive human opponents more easily after being exploited (H1c), with a 46 % probability, whereas for VH it is only 35 %. Similarly, participants are more likely to continue defecting on a VH opponent after having already exploited them once (H1b), with a probability of 29 % participants will choose to cooperate again after betraying their VH opponent, while this is 48 % for real humans.

Participants facing other humans are overall more likely to achieve joint cooperation with a probability of 52 % while only 17 % for the VH group. Participants playing against the VH instead had a chance of 39 % to reach mutual defect, whereas for the human group this chance was 17 %.

The self-report questionnaire data also supports the hypothesis. On a 7-point Likert scale people considered themselves significantly more cooperative while playing against humans (M = 5.88, SD = 1.72) than against VHs (M = 4.57, SD = 1.70), $t(112) = 3.27$, $p = 0.001$. Participants also self-reported that they were more fair against humans (M = 5.54, SD = 1.85; VH: M = 4.30, SD = 1.89), $t(112) = 2.85$, $p = .001$, further supporting H1. We found similar results in the self-reported data on friendliness, honesty and positivity.

4.2   Expressed Behaviors

As a secondary aspect of the behavior towards the game opponent we examined the participant displays of emotion during the game. For this purpose we used the automatically extracted measures mentioned in Sect. 3 and looked mainly at the intensities of the summary labels: "POSITIVE", "NEGATIVE" and "NEUTRAL".

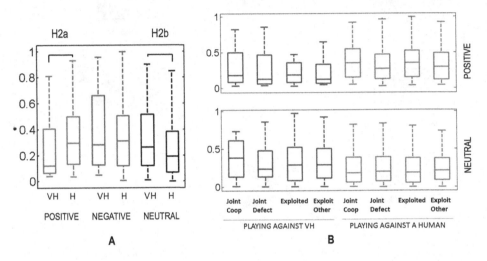

Fig. 4. Comparison of displays of expressions when playing with a VH or a human. Both overall (A) and when breaking down the game by game state (B), participants display more cooperative behaviors on average when playing with a human.

We show our first observations in Fig. 4A, namely that participants display a trend of higher intensity of positivity (H2a) and less neutrality (which translates to more expressivity, H2b) when playing against another human versus playing against a VH, as we hypothesized in H2. Those trends were both significant at the 0.1 level, compared with a standard T-test.

These trends combined translate into an overall more social signal that participants communicate with their expressions to other humans while VH opponents are receiving a less social treatment. This observation still holds when breaking down by different game states as seen in Fig. 4B (bottom) for expressivity and B (top) for positive intensity. These findings agree with de Melo et al. [8] reports on participants' chosen signaled affect during the game and support our second hypothesis that people will display more cooperative expressions to human players compared with VH ones.

5 Discussion

When comparing over the same social dilemma task, we demonstrated that participants will act more cooperatively towards other humans than VHs, both in terms of game choices when choosing to betray, forgive or cooperate (as described in H1) and in terms of displaying cooperative expressions such as more joy, or less neutrality (as described in H2). It can be argued that both of those aspects of behavior form a coherent profile for the players that is more social when facing other human players than when facing VH opponents. This general observation agrees with previous findings [7] that although people treat VH like a social entity, they don't treat them equally to other humans.

The observations made in this study are locally independent of the strategy used by the opponent, however due to the iterative nature of the game the overall strategy used by an opponent should be considered as another confounding factor and be further investigated.

As discussed in Sect. 2 the difference in behavior shown by participants against VHs may have to do with the poorer perception of emotion expression and agency of the VH [3]. Interestingly enough, in the self-report questionnaires the participants reported less connection to a VH opponent ($M = 2.70, SD = 1.49$) versus a human opponent ($M = 4.46$, $SD = 1.73$), $t(112) = 4.48$, $p < 0.001$. This less-felt rapport could explain why participants display more neutral expressions while interacting with a VH than with a human opponent. However, considering also the communicative, coordinative role that facial expressions play, one can hypothesize that the knowledge or the expectation that the VH cannot receive these signals the same way as a person does, would lead a person to allocate less effort into that signaling channel and perhaps to cooperative behavior over all. This may be tied with the observation that when playing with the VH, participants scored significantly less than when they were playing with humans (H: $M = 44:10, SD = 13.24$; VH: $M = 32.83, SD = 10.86$), $t(111) = 3.77$, $p < 0.001$. Understanding those gaps better is a topic of future work and it would help bring VH interactions closer to human-to-human ones.

Acknowledgements. This research was supported in part by the AFOSR [FA9550-14-1-0364] and the US Army. The content does not necessarily reflect the position or the policy of any Government, and no official endorsement should be inferred.

References

1. Bartlett, M., Littlewort, G., Wu, T., Movellan, J.: Computer expression recognition toolbox. In: 2008 8th IEEE International Conference on Automatic Face and Gesture Recognition, FG 2008, pp. 1–2. IEEE (2008)
2. Batrinca, L., Stratou, G., Shapiro, A., Morency, L.-P., Scherer, S.: Cicero - towards a multimodal virtual audience platform for public speaking training. In: Aylett, R., Krenn, B., Pelachaud, C., Shimodaira, H. (eds.) IVA 2013. LNCS, vol. 8108, pp. 116–128. Springer, Heidelberg (2013)

3. Blascovich, J.: A theoretical model of social influence for increasing the utility of collaborative virtual environments. In: Proceedings of the 4th International Conference on Collaborative Virtual Environments, pp. 25–30. ACM (2002)
4. Broekens, J., Harbers, M., Brinkman, W.-P., Jonker, C.M., Van den Bosch, K., Meyer, J.-J.: Virtual reality negotiation training increases negotiation knowledge and skill. In: Nakano, Y., Neff, M., Paiva, A., Walker, M. (eds.) IVA 2012. LNCS, vol. 7502, pp. 218–230. springer, Heidelberg (2012)
5. de Melo, C.M., Carnevale, P.J., Read, S.J., Gratch, J.: Reading peoples minds from emotion expressions in interdependent decision making. J. Pers. Soc. Psychol. **106**(1), 73–88 (2014)
6. de Melo, C.M., Carnevale, P., Gratch, J.: The influence of emotions in embodied agents on human decision-making. In: Allbeck, J., Badler, N., Bickmore, T., Pelachaud, C., Safonova, A. (eds.) IVA 2010. LNCS, vol. 6356, pp. 357–370. Springer, Heidelberg (2010)
7. de Melo, C.M., Gratch, J., Carnevale, P.J.: The effect of agency on the impact of emotion expressions on people's decision making. In: 2013 Humaine Association Conference on Affective Computing and Intelligent Interaction (ACII), pp. 546–551. IEEE (2013)
8. de Melo, C.M., Gratch, J., Carnevale, P.J.: The importance of cognition and affect for artificially intelligent decision makers. In: Twenty-Eighth AAAI Conference on Artificial Intelligence (2014)
9. Fox, J., Ahn, S.J., Janssen, J.H., Yeykelis, L., Segovia, K.Y., Bailenson, J.N.: Avatars versus agents: a meta-analysis quantifying the effect of agency on social influence. In: Human Computer Interaction, pp. 1–61 (2014)
10. Krach, S., Hegel, F., Wrede, B., Sagerer, G., Binkofski, F., Kircher, T.: Can machines think? Interaction and perspective taking with robots investigated via FMRI. PLoS ONE **3**(7), e2597 (2008)
11. Littlewort, G., Whitehill, J., Wu, T.-F., Butko, N., Ruvolo, P., Movellan, J., Bartlett, M.: The motion in emotion: a cert based approach to the fera emotion challenge. In: 2011 IEEE International Conference on Automatic Face and Gesture Recognition and Workshops (FG 2011), pp. 897–902. IEEE (2011)
12. Nass, C., Moon, Y.: Machines and mindlessness: social responses to computers. J. Soc. Issues **56**(1), 81–103 (2000)
13. Nass, C., Steuer, J., Tauber, E.R.: Computers are social actors. In: Proceedings of the SIGCHI Conference on Human Factors in Computing Systems, pp. 72–78. ACM (1994)
14. Reeves, B., Nass, C.: The Media Equation: How People Treat Computers, Television, and New Media Like Real People and Places. Cambridge University Press, New York (1996)
15. Riedl, R., Mohr, P., Kenning, P., Davis, F., Heekeren, H.: Trusting humans and avatars: behavioral and neural evidence (2011)
16. Van Kleef, G.A., De Dreu, C.K.W., Manstead, A.S.R.: An interpersonal approach to emotion in social decision making: the emotions as social information model. Adv. Exp. Soc. Psychol. **42**, 45–96 (2010)
17. von der Pütten, A.M., Krämer, N.C., Gratch, J., Kang, S.-H.: It doesn't matter what you are! explaining social effects of agents and avatars. Comput. Hum. Behav. **26**(6), 1641–1650 (2010)

A Feminist Virtual Agent for Breastfeeding Promotion

Lin Shi[1], Timothy Bickmore[1(✉)], and Roger Edwards[2]

[1] College of Computer and Information Science, Northeastern University,
Boston, MA, USA
{octlin, bickmore}@ccs.neu.edu
[2] College of Health Sciences, Northeastern University, Boston, MA, USA

Abstract. The design of a conversational virtual agent that plays the role of a lactation educator promoting breastfeeding is described, along with a manipulation to make the agent appear more or less feminist. Results from a randomized pilot study indicate that study participants were aware of the manipulation and participants who were more feminist preferred the feminist agent, while those who were non-feminist preferred the non-feminist agent. This work demonstrates one way that feminism can be incorporated into agent design, and a methodology for identifying users who will be most receptive to it.

Keywords: Feminism · Embodied conversational agent · Relational agent · Breastfeeding

1 Introduction

Culture as "the entire range of a society's arts, beliefs, institutions, and communication practices" [1] shapes gender — one of the organizing principles of human society — on a daily basis in both material as well as discursive ways. There is a significant amount of research on the cultural and social construction of gender roles [2–4]. Feminism is a collection of ideas and activities aimed at examining, revealing and overcoming "the economic, political, social, and psychological oppression of women" [1]. Academically speaking, feminists draw attention to the central of issues of gender and sexuality in the understanding of social experience and symbolic power in both the private as well as public sphere.

There has been a growing interest in incorporating feminist perspectives into technology design methodology — one of the practices of "cultural" adaptation according to our understanding. A CHI 2011 workshop on "Feminist HCI" focused on aspects of value sensitive design. However, this "feminist HCI", as admitted by the workshop participants, remains "a promising, yet underdeveloped term" [5]. Bardzell expounds that "the interaction design process takes place independent of gender considerations, and even today the central concept of the whole field – the user – remains genderless" [6].

In our work, we are interested in moving beyond only using feminist values in our design methodology, to incorporating these values into the technology artifacts

© Springer International Publishing Switzerland 2015
W.-P. Brinkman et al. (Eds.): IVA 2015, LNAI 9238, pp. 461–470, 2015.
DOI: 10.1007/978-3-319-21996-7_49

themselves, so that users will recognize the artifacts and the messages they produce as feminist. In doing this, we are intentionally creating artifacts, such as virtual agents, that are "tailored" [7] for a very specific subset of the population. We are also investigating whether informational messages from the scientific frame, delivered by a virtual agent, are better received by women in general if they are re-framed from an inclusive feminist perspective.

To explore issues of feminism in technological artifacts in general, and virtual agents in particular, we have conducted our research in the domain of breastfeeding promotion. Breastfeeding in itself is an important health topic: many major US public health and medical organizations have been actively promoting breastfeeding and recommend exclusive breastfeeding for the first six months of life [8], and then "breastfeeding should be continued for at least the first year of life and beyond for as long as mutually desired by mother and child" [8]. Despite these proclamations by the medical establishment, only 16.3 % of mothers in the US follow this recommendation, leading to a range of interventions to improve breastfeeding rates [9]. However, breastfeeding represents a controversial issue from the academic feminist perspective. The cultural consensus that "breast is best" is based on the scientific evidence of breastfeeding's biological and psychological benefits to both babies and their mothers, while an alternative perspective sees this medical "prescription" as subjugating mothers' "rights" to their children's perceived "needs." There is an emerging voice shared by feminist theorists [10–12], who are concerned more about women's freedom and autonomy, that breast-feeding advocacy should move beyond the debate over the medical effects of breastfeeding, and instead focus on securing social resources that enable women's freedom to make and enact their decisions about infant feeding.

In the rest of this paper we describe the design and implementation of a virtual agent that plays the role of a lactation educator whose job is to motivate new mothers to breastfeed exclusively for six months (Fig. 1). We describe the development of two versions of this agent: one that frames its arguments exclusively from the scientific/medical perspective, and one that provides the same argumentation but frames it from the feminist perspective. We then describe preliminary results from a study in which we compared women's reactions to the two versions of the agent.

2   Design of a Feminist Virtual Agent for Breastfeeding Promotion

The initial version of the virtual agent was developed to play the role of a virtual lactation educator. Our development methodology involved initially videotaping sample counseling sessions with a certified lactation consultant. This was followed by several months of meetings of an interdisciplinary design team to work through the overall design of the system and the specific dialogue scripts and media content used in each part of the intervention. We first designed a 20-min interaction intended to motivate women in their third trimester to follow the CDC recommendations. The topics covered in this script include: greeting; asking user about her most important breastfeeding topic; review of the CDC recommendations; review of benefits of breastfeeding for the baby; breastfeeding benefits for the mother; breastfeeding "101" (latching, basic nursing positions); review of CDC recommendations; and farewell.

The virtual agent's appearance was designed based on feedback from user testing with new mothers (Fig. 1). The agent is rendered using the LiteBody framework [13], with speech output produced with a commercial speech synthesizer. Dialogues are scripted using a custom hierarchical transition network-based scripting language. Agent nonverbal conversational behavior is generated using BEAT [14], and includes beat (baton) hand gestures and eyebrow raises for emphasis, a range of iconic, emblematic, and deictic gestures, gaze away behavior for signaling turn-taking, and posture shifts to mark topic boundaries, synchronized with speech. User input is obtained via multiple choice selection of utterances [15].

We next sought to create a version of the agent that delivered the same information content, but in a way that would be recognized as feminist by most women. We began by reviewing relevant literature [16–19], videotapes of lectures given by experts on the topic of feminism and breastfeeding, and tape-recorded and transcribed interviews with a convenience sample of self-identified feminists who were breastfeeding advocates. We included some elements of "second wave" feminism (anti-patriarchy), but focused the messaging on themes of "third wave" feminism (equality and inclusion) [20, 21]. An initial introductory script and closing script were drafted to precede and follow the

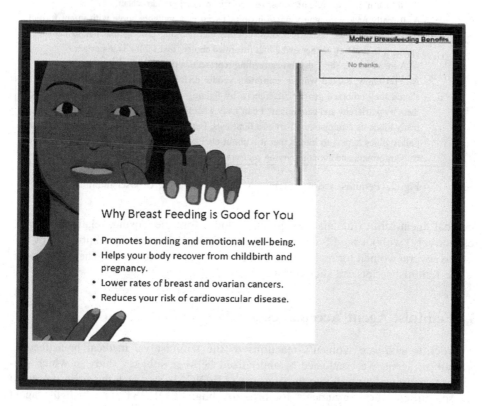

Fig. 1. Virtual agent interface used in breastfeeding promotion system

Feminist Introduction Script

1.   A: I like to think of myself as a fairly progressive woman, and I hope I do not offend you with some of my opinions. I will just be as honest as I can, with you. I totally respect any choice that anybody makes. I am not going to tell any woman what she should or should not do with her body. I can tell you what I think, but whatever you choose is your choice. But, I think you should make that choice in an informed way. There actually is a lot of science behind the benefits to you and your baby, that we will talk about today...

Feminist Closing Script

1.   A: You know, for me, in addition to all that important scientific stuff, there's one thing that really tipped my opinion in favor of breastfeeding. Once I realized that breastfeeding is something that is not done by most women in our society, and that huge formula corporations are actively working against it, it really brought out the rebel in me. I like doing non-traditional things, especially when it comes to women's issues. I would like to think that if women were not being allowed into universities, I would be one of those ones knocking down the doors. I like doing things that are not traditional for women. That's part of my identity, it's who I am. ...

2.   A: Breastfeeding is a learned thing. It's not something that you are born knowing how to do. For thousands of years, women have learned this from other women. Unfortunately, we don't have the community of women that we used to have. That's another thing that's been taking away from us, thank you very much capitalist patriarchy. It's something that you should learn from a circle of aunts, and girlfriends, and grandmothers.

3.   A: It really makes me angry when hospitals send new mothers home with infant formula and advertisements, because it short-circuits that learning process that has to happen. It makes it so that you cannot make that informed choice, that I think is important.

4.   A: A lot of people think that breastfeeding represents a dilemma for feminism.

5.   A: You know, should women minimize gender differences as the path to liberation, or should they embrace gender differences by fighting to remove the constraints placed on them by patriarchy and capitalism? I can't say what feminism is about, because there are as many kinds of feminism as there are feminists. But for me, the reason that many feminist philosophies appeal to me, is that it's about choice and freedom. It's about choice that is truly informed, and about removing barriers to that choice...

Fig. 2. Feminist script excerpts (A: Agent utterance; U: User utterance)

medical agent script (just after the greeting and before the closing, relative to Fig. 2, respectively) without modifying the medical content delivered. This initial script was sent to several women for review and revised based on their feedback. The final version of the feminist scripts are shown in Fig. 2.

3   Feminist Agent Acceptance Study

In order to compare women's reactions to the feminist vs. medical breastfeeding promotion agent, we conducted a randomized between-subjects study in which participants were randomized into three groups: MEDICAL, in which the agent presented the scientific/medical arguments for breastfeeding; FEMINIST, in which the agent presented both the medical arguments and the feminist introduction and closing (Fig. 2); and CONTROL, in which women did not receive any intervention. In this paper we are focusing only on results regarding attitudes towards the FEMINIST agent compared to the MEDICAL agent. Each of these conversations took approximately 20 min to complete, after which participants filled out a questionnaire about their attitudes towards the agent and conducted a semi-structured interview about their experience. Our hypotheses follow tailoring theory [7], in that we expect participants with stronger feminist orientations to prefer the FEMINIST agent, whereas those with weaker feminist orientations will prefer the MEDICAL agent.

3.1 Measures

In addition to sociodemographics, we measured feminist self-identification [22] and feminist values [23] at intake, using validated 7-point Likert scale instruments. Following interaction with the agent, we assessed overall satisfaction, desire to continue, comfort discussing breastfeeding with the agent, and preference to discuss breastfeeding with a doctor or nurse (rather than the agent), in addition to assessing the degree to which the agent was feminist (as a manipulation check), Table 1.

Table 1. Self-report questions and responses ("Tanya" is the name of agent)

Question	Anchor 1	Anchor 7	MEDICAL mean (sd)	FEMINIST mean (sd)	P
How satisfied were you with Tanya?	Not at all	Very satisfied	5.81 (1.08)	4.87 (1.21)	**.004**
How much would you like to continue working with Tanya?	Not at all	Very much	5.07 (1.27)	4.19 (1.57)	**.026**
How comfortable were you discussing breastfeeding with Tanya?	Not at all	Very much	5.68 (1.81)	5.93 (1.11)	.545
Would you have rather heard this information from a doctor or nurse?	Not at all	Very much	3.96 (1.53)	4.00 (1.49)	.929
How would you characterize Tanya as a feminist?	Very anti-feminist	Very feminist	4.3 (1.03)	5.93 (1.07)	**<.001**

3.2 Results

Nulliparous females (women who have not had any children) were recruited through an online job posting service (craigslist), fliers posted around the university, and a local newspaper. Nulliparous women were selected, since we felt attitudes towards breast-feeding of those who already had children would be relatively more solidified and so would be less receptive to new information. Seventy-two (72) women completed the study. Participants were 23.9 (sd 4.1) years old, 63 % white, 21 % black, 89 % never married, 46 % were students and 90 % had at least some college-level education. Overall, participants scored on the lower ends of the feminist identity (mean 3.2, sd 1.1) and feminist values (mean 3.3, sd 0.5) scales. Feminist identity and values were highly correlated, Pearson $r = .67$, $p < .001$. We created bivariate factors for feminist identity and feminist values by splitting women into two groups for each measure at the median.

Table 1 shows the ratings of the MEDICAL and FEMINIST agents by all participants. Participants did rate the FEMINIST agent as being more feminist than the MEDICAL agent, $t(52) = 5.7$, $p < .001$, establishing that our manipulation was effective. Overall, participants were significantly less satisfied with the FEMINIST agent, $t(52) = 3.0$, $p < .01$, and were less inclined to continue working with it, $t(52) = 2.3$, $p < .05$, compared to the MEDICAL agent.

We also performed 2×2 non-parametric ANOVAs (using the Aligned Rank Transform [8]) with agent type (MEDICAL vs. FEMINIST) and participant feminist orientation (feminist identity or feminist values category) as factors.

While women overall were less satisfied with the FEMINIST agent, those women who did not self-identify as feminist were less satisfied with the FEMINIST agent, $F(1,50) = 3.1$, $p = .08$ (trending), and were significantly less likely to continue working with it, $F(1,50) = 4.3$, $p < .05$, compared to the MEDICAL agent, while women who self-identified as feminist were much less dis-satisfied with the FEMINIST agent (Fig. 3).

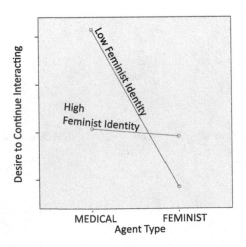

Fig. 3. Interaction of agent type and feminist identity on desire to continue

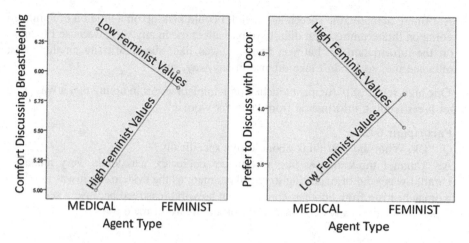

Fig. 4. Interaction of agent type and feminist values on comfort discussing breastfeeding with agent (L) and preference for talking to doctor or nurse about breastfeeding (R)

There was also a significant interaction between agent type and feminist values, such that women who endorsed feminist values were more comfortable talking with the FEMINIST agent about breastfeeding, while women who did not endorse feminist values were more comfortable talking with the MEDICAL agent, $F(1,51) = 3.6$, $p = .06$. Similarly, women who endorsed feminist values preferred talking to the FEMINIST agent rather than a doctor or nurse about breastfeeding, while women who did not endorse feminist values preferred receiving this information from the MEDICAL agent, $F(1,50) = 3.8$, $p = .06$ (Fig. 4).

3.3   Interview Results from Participants in FEMINIST Condition

Most comments about the agent's feminist language were from low-feminist participants, and were mostly negative.

Participant 022:
Q: "What about other things you might have disliked about Tanya?"
A: "Uhh, well she's so feminist, just at the end, all this stuff, it was too much for me. But that's ok."
Participant 051:
Q: "Ok. Did anything about it seem strange to you?"
A: "I thought, just like Tanya, how she was very feminist, like that kind of turned me off."

Most high-feminist participants did not notice or comment on the agent's feminist language. The few who did said they felt it did not affect them.

Participant 046:
Q: "Did you find her persuasive?"

A: "Umm, actually, the speech at the end, I could pick up on a little bit of feminism going on there, umm, but it didn't seem to affect me in any way. Because I focused on the information ... but you know, it was like, she didn't say anything that offended me, so I didn't take offense in any way, so."

One high-feminist participant touched on feminist themes in noting that it was good to get breastfeeding information from "another woman".

Participant 042:
Q: "Ok. What did you think about Tanya specifically?"
A: "Umm, I think she, as like a computer character, was kinda, very relatable. Umm, I was kind of expecting to see like a man, as the system. So it was nice as a woman hearing from another woman about how to breastfeed because it seems like these things are always dominated by, or are always a male role."

3.4   Discussion

Study participants who interacted with the FEMINIST agent rated it as being more feminist compared to participants who interacted with the MEDICAL agent, thus our manipulation worked. We also observed anticipated interaction effects between participant feminist orientation and the type of agent on their attitudes towards the agent, with feminist participants preferring the FEMINIST agent and non-feminist participants preferring the MEDICAL agent. However, we also observed lower satisfaction scores for the FEMINIST agent across all participants.

One reason for the overall lower satisfaction with the FEMINIST agent may simply have to do with the increased interaction time due to the additional feminist scripts. Also, since this part of the interaction was largely a monologue and had little information content, some participants may have felt that this part of the interaction was a waste of their time. It is also possible that the young women in our study follow the "depoliticized and individualistic" norm of young women in the US who agree with feminist ideas but do not label them (or themselves) as such [24].

This study had many limitations, beyond the very small and likely biased sample of study participants. There are many interpretations of feminism and we certainly only captured a few of them in our agent's feminist dialogue scripts. Achieving the feminist manipulation by simply "bookending" the medical dialogue script is an over-simplistic approach: a much better approach would be to use a dialogue system that is capable of interleaving feminist messages throughout the medical dialogue, or a text generator that is able to infuse all medical messages with feminist values, rather than abruptly switching frames. Finally, the FEMINIST condition was significantly longer than the MEDICAL condition, and the increased session duration, exposure to the agent, and messaging about breastfeeding all represent potential confounds for our study design.

4 Conclusion

We designed a virtual agent that plays the role of a lactation educator promoting breastfeeding, and a manipulation to make the agent appear more or less feminist in its language. Results from the pilot study indicate that participants were aware of the manipulation, and those who were more feminist preferred the feminist agent, while those who were non-feminist preferred the non-feminist agent.

4.1 Future Work

A multidisciplinary team has expanded the MEDICAL version of the virtual lactation educator into a full-blown, six-month duration intervention to promote breastfeeding, designed to be used in the obstetrician's office in the third trimester, in the labor and delivery ward of the hospital, and at home six months after birth. A pilot study on its efficacy has been conducted [25] and researchers are currently running a six-month randomized clinical trial with 84 women to evaluate its long-term impact [26].

There are significant opportunities to further explore feminist virtual agents, given the plethora of literature and theorizing on the topic, as well as further exploration of feminism as a persuasive message tailoring variable. More generally, the automatic generation (or recognition) of messages that frame scientific "facts" from different political points of view (as in [27]) is a potentially important and intriguing direction for future research, an initial step toward a stronger modeling-based approach.

References

1. Nelson, C., Treichler, P.A., Grossberg, L.: Cultural studies: an introduction. In: Cultural Studies, pp. 1–22 (1992)
2. Lorber, J.: The social construction of gender. In: The Social Construction of Difference and Inequality: Race, Class, Gender, and Sexuality, pp. 99–106 (2003)
3. Davis, T.L.: Voices of gender role conflict: the social construction of college men's identity. J. Coll. Stud. Dev. **43**, 508–521 (2002)
4. Lorber, J.: Paradoxes of Gender. Yale University Press, New Haven (1994)
5. Bardzell, S., Churchill, E., Bardzell, J., Forlizzi, J., Grinter, R., Tatar, D.: Feminism and interaction design. In: Conference Feminism and Interaction Design, pp. 1–4. ACM (2011)
6. Bardzell, S.: Feminist HCI: taking stock and outlining an agenda for design. In: Proceedings of the SIGCHI Conference on Human Factors in Computing Systems, pp. 1301–1310. ACM (2010)
7. Hawkins, R.P., Kreuter, M., Resnicow, K., Fishbein, M., Dijkstra, A.: Understanding tailoring in communicating about health. Health Educ. Res. **23**, 454–466 (2008)
8. American Academy of Pediatrics (2005)
9. Centers for Disease Control and Prevention: Breastfeeding report card - United States, 2014 (2014)
10. Hausman, B.L.: Mother's Milk: Breastfeeding Controversies in American Culture. Psychology Press, New York (2003)

11. Hausman, B.L.: Breastfeeding, rhetoric, and the politics of feminism. J. Women Polit. Policy **34**, 330–344 (2013)
12. Wolf, J.B.: Is Breast Best?: Taking on the Breastfeeding Experts and the New High Stakes of Motherhood. NYU Press, New York (2010)
13. Bickmore, T., Schulman, D., Shaw, G.: DTask & LiteBody: open source, standards-based tools for building web-deployed embodied conversational agents. In: Proceedings of the Intelligent Virtual Agents, Amsterdam, Netherlands (2009)
14. Cassell, J., Vilhjálmsson, H., Bickmore, T.: BEAT: the behavior expression animation toolkit. In: Proceedings of the 28th Annual Conference on Computer Graphics and Interactive Techniques, pp. 477–486 (2001)
15. Bickmore, T., Picard, R.: Establishing and maintaining long-term human-computer relationships. ACM Trans. Comput. Hum. Interact. **12**, 293–327 (2005)
16. Blum, L.M.: At the Breast: Ideologies of Breastfeeding and Motherhood in the Contemporary United States. Beacon Press, Boston (2000)
17. Baumslag, N., Michels, D.L.: Milk, Money, and Madness: The Culture and Politics of Breastfeeding. Bergin & Garvey, Westport (1995)
18. Drouin, K.H.: The situated mother: evolutionary theory and feminism as complementary components to understanding breastfeeding behavior. J. Soc. Evol. Cult. Psychol. **7**, 326 (2013)
19. Blum, L.M.: Mothers, babies, and breastfeeding in late capitalist America: the shifting contexts of feminist theory. Feminist Stud. **19**, 290–312 (1993)
20. Bardzell, S.: Feminist HCI: taking stock and outlining an agenda for design. In: ACM Conference of Human Factors in Computing Systems (CHI) (2010)
21. Krolokke, C., Sorensen, A.S.: Gender Communication Theories and Analyses: From Silence to Performance. Sage, Thousand Oaks (2006)
22. Szymanski, D.: Relations among dimensions of feminism and internalized heterosexism in lesbians and bisexual women. Sex Roles **51**, 145–159 (2004)
23. Fischer, A., Tokar, D., Mergl, M., Good, G., Hill, M., Blum, S.: Assessing women's feminist identity development: studies of convergent, discriminant, and structural validity. Psychol. Women Q. **24**, 15–29 (2000)
24. Aronson, P.: Feminists or "postfeminists"? Young women's attitudes toward feminism and gender relations. Gend. Soc. **17**, 903–922 (2003)
25. Edwards, R.A., Bickmore, T., Jenkins, L., Foley, M., Manjourides, J.: Use of an interactive computer agent to support breastfeeding. Matern. Child Health J. **17**, 1961–1968 (2013)
26. Zhang, Z., Bickmore, T., Mainello, K., Mueller, M., Foley, M., Jenkins, L., Edwards, R.A.: Maintaining continuity in longitudinal, multi-method health interventions using virtual agents: the case of breastfeeding promotion. In: Bickmore, T., Marsella, S., Sidner, C. (eds.) IVA 2014. LNCS, vol. 8637, pp. 504–513. Springer, Heidelberg (2014)
27. Hovy, E.: Generating Natural Language Under Pragmatic Constraints. Lawrence Erlbaum Associates, Hillsdale (1988)

From Non-human to Human: Adult's and Children's Perceptions of Agents Varying in Humanness

Eva Krumhuber[1](✉), Arvid Kappas[2], Colette Hume[3],
Lynne Hall[3], and Ruth Aylett[4]

[1] University College London, London WC1H 0AP, UK
e.krumhuber@ucl.ac.uk
[2] Jacobs University Bremen, 28759 Bremen, Germany
a.kappas@jacobs-university.de
[3] University of Sunderland, Sunderland SR6 0DD, UK
{colette.hume,lynne.hall}@sunderland.ac.uk
[4] Heriot-Watt University, Edinburgh EH14 4AS, UK
ruth@macs.hw.ac.uk

Abstract. While most interface agents have been designed from an adult perspective, the present paper compares adults' and children's views of agents that vary in their degree of humanness. Four synthetic characters ranging in appearance from non-human to very human (blob, cat, cartoon, human) were presented to adult and children perceivers and were evaluated with respect to their cognitive and emotional abilities. The visual appearance significantly influenced participants' ratings in both age groups. However, the pattern of results was more differentiated for adult perceivers as a function of the human-likeness of the character. The findings suggest that children may rely less on human-like features in inferring agents' capabilities which are judged along simpler cognitive and social dimensions. Implications for the design of artificial agents are discussed.

Keywords: Agent · Appearance · Human-like · Theory of mind · Children

1 Introduction

Current evidence suggests that users prefer and rely more on human-like agents/robots than mechanical-looking or abstract visual representations [1, 2]. While human-like characteristics contribute to a more human perception, there is one dimension of human mind that is seen as unique to humans: self-conscious mental experience [3]. The experience of mind with complex emotions and abstract thought appears to be reserved only for humans. This is supported by evidence showing that people rarely give moral rights and privileges to machines such as robots [4]. But does this apply to everyone and of every age? The goal of the present research was to examine how adults and children infer human qualities of virtual characters that vary in appearance from non-human to very human. To elucidate this question, we selected attributes that target dispositional traits, mental states, as well as basic and complex emotions. Whereas

© Springer International Publishing Switzerland 2015
W.-P. Brinkman et al. (Eds.): IVA 2015, LNAI 9238, pp. 471–474, 2015.
DOI: 10.1007/978-3-319-21996-7_50

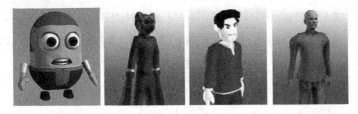

Fig. 1. Four embodied characters – blob, cat, cartoon, human - from non-human to very human in a neutral position.

simple traits and emotions (e.g., likeable, trustworthy, angry) may be easily attributed to mechanical and animal looking characters, abstract concepts such as mind and shame require more cognitive complexity than what might be apparent on first sight [5–7]. Based on previous research [8, 9] we predicted that the degree of human-likeness would significantly affect adults' attributions as to the agent's mental and emotional capabilities. These effects were expected to be less pronounced for children who might judge the characters along simpler cognitive and social dimensions.

2 Experiment

40 adults (M_{Age} = 20.33) and 35 children (M_{Age} = 10.06) were presented with either static or dynamic displays of four embodied characters that differed in their degree of human-likeness: blob, cat, cartoon, and human (see Fig. 1). All characters and animations were created in 3ds Max using a default biped and were displayed on blue background (490 × 270 pixels). After viewing each stimulus participants answered the following questions on 7-point Likert-scales ranging from (1) *not at all* to (7) *very much*: (a) How likeable is the character?, (b) How trustworthy is the character?, (c) How intelligent is the character?, (d) How engaging is the character?, (e) To what degree does the character have a mind on its own?, (f) To what degree can the character experience anger?, (g) To what degree can the character experience shame? These questions were posed in random order, with one question per stimulus presentation.

3 Results

A multivariate analysis of variance (MANOVA) revealed a significant interaction between Age Group and Stimulus Character, $F(21, 47) = 4.50$, $p < .001$, $\eta_p^2 = .67$. In univariate terms, this interaction was significant for almost all variables: likeable, $p = .009$, trustworthy, $p = .006$, intelligent, $p = .050$, engaging, $p = .214$, mind, $p < .001$, anger, $p = .014$, and shame, $p = .091$.

As can be seen in Fig. 2, children's ratings were generally higher than those of adults. This was particularly the case for the blob which was judged by children as more trustworthy, intelligent, likely to have a mind, and capable of experiencing anger and shame ($ps < .05$). Similarly, children made higher attributions of mind, anger and

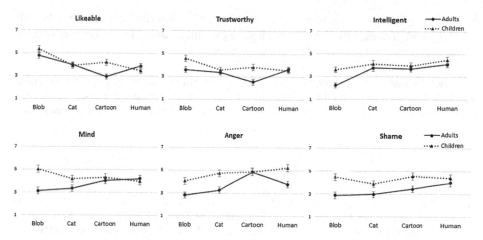

Fig. 2. Adults' and children's mean ratings of the four characters. Error bars represent standard errors.

shame when evaluating the cat ($ps \leq .05$). Differences between adults and children also occurred for the cartoon character which was seen by children as more likeable, trustworthy, and capable of experiencing shame ($ps < .01$). For the human character, children' ratings differed from those of adults only for anger ($p < .01$), with higher scores given by children.

4 Discussion

As shown in the present study, adults attributed complex states, such as mind and shame to a greater extent to characters that were at the endpoint of the human scale (i.e., cartoon, human). These findings are in line with previous research [1, 10–13] and suggest that the choice of visual representation drives attributions regarding the cognitive and emotional intelligence the system invites. Given that such effects are fast, in part automatic, and might not habituate over short exposures, the design of applications should therefore take a match between the perceived profile of the agents and the intended function into account. Although children made consistent and generally higher attributions regarding intellectual and emotional capabilities, a distinction was largely apparent only between the characters at the endpoints of the artificial/human scale (i.e., blob, human). Among all visual forms, the blob was most preferred and this favourable impression generalized across other characteristics (i.e., mind, trustworthiness). In accordance with previous research, for children a human-like appearance may therefore not be a direct criterion for inferring the agents' abilities [e.g., 5, 6].

In this research we have shown that assessing adults' and children's views can be essential for the design of embodied visual forms in human-computer interaction. Up to now, most guidelines for building effective interface agents are based solely on adult perspectives, thereby overlooking children's social and cognitive requirements. Here a closer collaboration of psychologists and computer scientists and engineers can be particularly promising. We do not believe that agent design can be a "one-size fits all" affair. Instead, agents, tasks and users must be carefully matched to achieve an optimal interaction between humans and artificial systems.

Acknowledgments. This work has been conducted within the European Commission project eCUTE – Education in Cultural Understanding, Technologically-Enhanced (FP7-ICT-2009.4.2). We thank Tony Manstead for his help with data collection and Nadia Malas for editorial work.

References

1. Goetz, J., Kiesler, S., Powers, A.: Matching robot appearance and behavior to tasks to improve human-robot cooperation. In: Proceedings of The IEEE International Workshop on Robot and Human Interactive Communication, pp. 55–60. Milbrae, California (2003)
2. Hinds, P.J., Roberts, T.L., Jones, H.: Whose job is it anyway? a study of human-robot interaction in a collaborative task. Hum-Comput. Interact **19**, 151–181 (2004)
3. Gray, H.M., Gray, K., Wegner, D.M.: Dimensions of mind perception. Science **315**, 619 (2007)
4. Friedman, B., Kahn, Jr., P.H., Hagman, J.: What online AIBO discussion forums reveal about the human-robotic relationship. In: Proceedings of the Computer-Human Interaction Conference CHI, pp. 273–280, New York (2003)
5. Hall, L., Woods, S., Dautenhahn, K., Sobral, D., Paiva, A.C., Wolke, D., Newall, L.: Designing empathic agents: adults versus kids. In: Lester, J.C., Vicari, R.M., Paraguaçu, F. (eds.) ITS 2004. LNCS, vol. 3220, pp. 604–613. Springer, Heidelberg (2004)
6. Paiva, A., Dias, J., Sobral, D., Aylett, R., Woods, S., Hall, L., Zoll, C.: Learning by feeling: evoking empathy with synthetic characters. Appl. Artif. Intell. **19**, 235–266 (2005)
7. Bumby, K.E., Dautenhahn, K.: Investigating children's attitudes towards robots: a case study. In: Proceedings of the CT99: The Third Cognitive Technology Conference, San Francisco (1999)
8. Woods, S., Dautenhahn, K., Schulz, J.: The design space of robots: investigating children's views. In: Proceedings of the IEEE International Workshop on Robot and Human Interactive Communication, pp. 47–52. Kurashiki (2004)
9. De Melo, C., Carnevale, P., Gratch, J.: Humans vs. computers: impact of emotion expressions on people's decision making. In: IEEE Trans. Affect. Comput. (in press)
10. Parise, S., Kiesler, S., Sproull, L., Waters, K.: My partner is a real dog: cooperation with social agents. In: Proceedings of the ACM Conference on Computer Supported Cooperative Work (CSCW), pp. 399–408. New York (1996)
11. Koda, T., Maes, P.: Agents with faces: the effects of personification of agents. In: Proceedings of the 5th IEEE International Workshop on Robot and Human Communication RO-MAN 1996, pp. 189–194. Tsukuba (1996)
12. Hegel, F., Krach, S., Kircher, T., Wrede, B., Sagerer, G.: Theory of Mind (ToM) on robots: a functional neuroimaging study. In: Proceedings of the Human-Computer Interaction Conference HRI, pp. 335–342. Amsterdam (2008)
13. Harris, P.L., Donnelly, K., Guz, G.R., Pitt-Watson, R.: Children's understanding of the distinction between real and apparent emotion. Child Dev. **57**, 895–909 (1986)

Smart Mobile Virtual Humans: "Chat with Me!"

Sin-Hwa Kang[✉], Andrew W. Feng, Anton Leuski,
Dan Casas, and Ari Shapiro

Institute for Creative Technologies, University of Southern California,
Los Angeles, USA
{kang,feng,leuski,casas,shapiro}@ict.usc.edu

1 Introduction

In this study, we are interested in exploring whether people would talk with 3D animated virtual humans using a smartphone for a longer amount of time as a sign of feeling rapport [5], compared to non-animated or audio-only characters in everyday life. Based on previous studies [2,7,10], users prefer animated characters in emotionally engaged interactions when the characters were displayed on mobile devices, yet in a lab setting. We aimed to reach a broad range of users outside of the lab in natural settings to investigate the potential of our virtual human on smartphones to facilitate casual, yet emotionally engaging conversation. We also found that the literature has not reached a consensus regarding the ideal gaze patterns for a virtual human, one thing researchers agree on is that inappropriate gaze could negatively impact conversations at times, even worse than receiving no visual feedback at all [1,4]. Everyday life may bring the experience of awkwardness or uncomfortable sentiments in reaction to continuous mutual gaze. On the other hand, gaze aversion could also make a speaker think their partner is not listening. Our work further aims to address this question of what constitutes appropriate eye gaze in emotionally engaged interactions.

We developed a 3D animated and chat-based virtual human which presented emotionally expressive nonverbal behaviors such as facial expressions, head gestures, gaze, and other upper body movements (see Fig. 1). The virtual human displayed appropriate gaze that was either consisted of constant mutual gaze or gaze aversion based on a statistical model of saccadic eye movement [8] while listening. Both gaze patterns were accompanied by other forms of appropriate nonverbal feedback. To explore the question of optimal communicative medium, we distributed our virtual human application to users via an app store for Android-powered phones (i.e. Google Play Store) in order to target users who owned a smartphone and could use our application in various natural settings.

2 Study Design

This study examined users' perceptions and reactions to a virtual human based on various presentation types: (1) animation with gaze aversion, (2) animation with constant mutual gaze (no gaze aversion), (3) static image, and (4)

© Springer International Publishing Switzerland 2015
W.-P. Brinkman et al. (Eds.): IVA 2015, LNAI 9238, pp. 475–478, 2015.
DOI: 10.1007/978-3-319-21996-7_51

no image. The animation included facial expressions, head gestures, gaze, and other upper body movements using our 3D chat-based virtual human (see Fig. 1). Because users were asked to use the button "Click and Hold to Speak" when they answered each question, we designed gaze aversion as a way to intentionally increase users' self-disclosure and comfort [1], rather than other functions such as turn-taking. Users answered a total of 24 questions of increasing intimacy asked by the virtual human (e.g. "What are your favorite sports?") in 2 sessions. Each session included 12 questions. We borrowed the structure and context of the questions from the studies of Kang and colleagues [6]. Since smartphones were treated as an icon of emotionally engaged communication [7], the conversation scenario in our study imitated casual chats in the format of an interview in a counseling situation to maintain the emotionally engaged interaction.

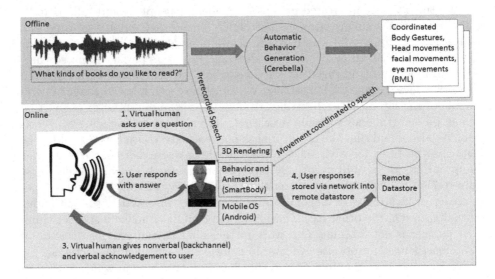

Fig. 1. [Top] Offline, a set of utterances are recorded and then processed by a non-verbal behavior generator (Cerebella [9]) and a lip sync process [11]. The results are stored in a BML file for later use during runtime. [Bottom] Online, a user listens to a virtual human, then responds by holding the 'Click and Hold to Speak' button, causing the virtual human to backchannel. The user responses to questions are stored in a remote datastore (Amazon Web Services [3]). The system runs on an Android device using the SmartBody animation system.

For Study A, a total of 89 participants (35% men, 65% women; average 39 years old) were randomly assigned to one of 4 conditions: animation with gaze aversion (N = 22), animation without gaze aversion (N = 21), static image (N = 21), and no image (N = 25). The participants were given $5 compensation when they completed the study. Participation required a total of 35 minutes on an individual basis. The pre-questionnaire included questions pertaining to users' demographics. There were two types of the post-questionnaires. All users received the first post-questionnaire, which included metrics to rate their perception of virtual rapport with and social attraction toward a virtual human. The second post-questionnaire was also given to all users regardless of participating in the second session. It gauged the driving factors behind the users' choice to continue or not continue conversing with the virtual human. It was mandatory to complete the first session and two post-questionnaires to get compensation, but the second conversation was optional. This was done in order to effectively observe whether users enjoyed conversing with the virtual human. We were motivated to conduct a follow up study based on our results from Study A. Study B consisted of a total of 233 participants as the participants in Study A were also included. In Study B, we utilized the same mobile app and 4 conditions noted above. The only exception is that participants in Study B were not required to fill out a pre-questionnaire and post-questionnaires. Thus, we did not have participants' demographic information. Participants were also randomly assigned to one of the 4 conditions: animation with gaze aversion ($N = 66$), animation without gaze aversion ($N = 55$), static image ($N = 47$), and no image ($N = 65$).

3 Preliminary Results and Discussion

For Study A, to measure the length of the conversation, we used the number of the last question that the user answered before stopping. We had to eliminate the data for six participants in our study given that they did not remember what question they last answered. To analyze the remaining data, we performed a Between-Subjects ANOVA. Our results [$F(3, 79) = 2.89$, $p = .040$] with Tukey HSD Test demonstrate that users answered more questions when they interacted with animated characters that demonstrated gaze aversion ($M = 22.43$, $SD = 3.79$), compared to interacting with static characters ($M = 17.26$, $SD = 6.61$). There was no other significant difference between the other conditions, however there was a trend that shows users answered more questions when communicating with animated character with gaze aversion, compared to communicating with animated character with no gaze aversion ($M = 19.95$, $SD = 5.91$) or no image at all ($M = 19.21$, $SD = 5.93$). For Study B, we analyzed the objective data for the duration of users' responses. The users in the animation condition with gaze aversion (149.5 s) tended to talk longer than users in the other conditions (animation without gaze aversion: 99.7 s, static: 128.6 s, no image: 125.4 s). There was no statistically significant difference among the 4 conditions. However, for only gaze related conditions, the results of an Independent-Samples T-Test analysis show that there was a strong trend [$t(107.22) = 2.297$, $p = .024$] that users talked for a longer time with an animated character with gaze aversion ($M = 149.47$, $SD = 148.54$) than an animated character without gaze aversion ($M = 99.67$, $SD = 86.39$). Regarding subjective measures, we did not find statistically significant difference for the conditions in the results of the study overall.

In general there was a trend that users interacted with a 3D animated virtual human with gaze aversion more, compared to communicating with a 3D animated virtual human without gaze aversion, a virtual human with a static visage, or an audio-only interface.

This study successfully utilized a virtual humans nonverbal behavior when presented on smartphone devices to explore its effect on users responses. The results of our study go beyond the body of existing research by validating the previous findings in real world settings where the potential of such smartphone devices could be fully explored with no limitations. With regard to gaze, the results of our study revealed that users interacted for a longer period of time with an animated virtual human that averted its gaze while listening, compared to an animated virtual human that did not avert its gaze. Based on this observed trend, we suggest that a virtual human should avert its gaze while listening in interactions in order to elicit greater engagement from human users.

References

1. Andrist, S., Mutlu, B., Gleicher, M.: Conversational gaze aversion for virtual agents. In: Aylett, R., Krenn, B., Pelachaud, C., Shimodaira, H. (eds.) IVA 2013. LNCS, vol. 8108, pp. 249–262. Springer, Heidelberg (2013)
2. Bickmore, T., Mauer, D.: Modalities for building relationships with handheld computer agents. In: CHI 2006 Extended Abstracts on Human Factors in Computing Systems, pp. 544–549. ACM (2006)
3. Cloud, A.E.C.: Amazon web services (2011). Accessed 9 November 2011
4. Garau, M., Slater, M., Vinayagamoorthy, V., Brogni, A., Steed, A., Sasse, M.A.: The impact of avatar realism and eye gaze control on perceived quality of communication in a shared immersive virtual environment. In: Proceedings of the SIGCHI Conference on Human Factors in Computing Systems, pp. 529–536. ACM (2003)
5. Gratch, J., Wang, N., Gerten, J., Fast, E., Duffy, R.: Creating rapport with virtual agents. In: Pelachaud, C., Martin, J.-C., André, E., Chollet, G., Karpouzis, K., Pelé, D. (eds.) IVA 2007. LNCS (LNAI), vol. 4722, pp. 125–138. Springer, Heidelberg (2007)
6. Kang, S.H., Gratch, J.: Socially anxious people reveal more personal information with virtual counselors that talk about themselves using intimate human back stories. Annu. Rev. Cybertherapy Telemed. **181**, 202–207 (2012)
7. Kang, S.H., Watt, J.H., Ala, S.K.: Social copresence in anonymous social interactions using a mobile video telephone. In: Proceedings of the SIGCHI Conference on Human Factors in Computing Systems, pp. 1535–1544. ACM (2008)
8. Lee, S.P., Badler, J.B., Badler, N.I.: Eyes alive. In: ACM Transactions on Graphics (TOG), vol. 21, pp. 637–644. ACM (2002)
9. Marsella, S., Xu, Y., Lhommet, M., Feng, A., Scherer, S., Shapiro, A.: Virtual character performance from speech. In: Proceedings of the 12th ACM SIGGRAPH/Eurographics Symposium on Computer Animation, pp. 25–35. ACM (2013)
10. Rincón-Nigro, M., Deng, Z.: A text-driven conversational avatar interface for instant messaging on mobile devices. IEEE Trans. Hum. Mach. Syst. **43**(3), 328–332 (2013)
11. Shapiro, A.: Building a character animation system. In: Allbeck, J.M., Faloutsos, P. (eds.) MIG 2011. LNCS, vol. 7060, pp. 98–109. Springer, Heidelberg (2011)

The Partial Poker-Face

When Affective Characters Try to Hide Their True Emotions

Christopher Ritter$^{(\boxtimes)}$ and Ruth Aylett

Heriot-Watt University, MACS, Edinburgh, Scotland, UK
{cmr4,r.s.aylett}@hw.ac.uk

Abstract. Research on emotional expressive embodiments for simulated affective behavior resulted in impressive systems allowing for characters being perceived as more natural. In consequence we want to explore what happens if these characters gain the human ability to hide their true emotions. More particular we are looking for the change in emotional engagement and the change in perceived naturalism. The Partial Poker-Face will allow virtual characters to recognize and control their own emotional expressive behaviour in order to influence the perception of self by others. While our research assumes applications in virtual storytelling, we are confident that it will be also of value for other areas, like human robot interaction.

1 Introduction

Research on virtual or robotic characters simulating emotions has shown that affective characters are not only more accessible to human inter-actors [1], but also seem to be more appropriate tools [2] for certain learning applications.

At the same time there has been vast research for architectures capable of communicating emotions to human interaction partners. Published work ranges from realistic expressions of basic emotions [3], down to selective gazing behavior [4] and other detailed micro expressions. Goal is to express simulated emotions as naturalistic as possible.

Less attention was paid to the idea that human beings do not always want to express all their emotions. This can be related to cultural influence [8] or due to exceptional situational context. Some examples of such work can be found in [5–7].

We also try hiding our emotions when deceiving others. An example for such a situation is a poker game. The so called Poker-Face is essential for not giving away important information to other players. The opponent might use leaking emotions to reason about the true value of Ones hand by updating his Theory of Mind (ToM) about Ones intentions. In consequence a player also has to learn how to use their own facial expressions in order to manipulate the perception of self by others.

Similarly active deception can happen, when one tries to maintain social harmony or to prevent social conflict from escalating by using Emotional Intelligence [9, 10].

© Springer International Publishing Switzerland 2015
W.-P. Brinkman et al. (Eds.): IVA 2015, LNAI 9238, pp. 479–482, 2015.
DOI: 10.1007/978-3-319-21996-7_52

2 The Partial Poker-Face

As indicated in Table 1 the Partial Poker-Face is looking for a gradual blend between the two extremes of a child's face (most current architectures) and the perfect poker-face. The "blending weight" can be imagined as a variable based on a character's Emotional Intelligence (EI) and conscientiousness [11]. A value of 0 prevents the character from ever hiding its emotions implying it has no control about its expressive behaviour. A value of 1 on the other hand would prevent any unconscious leaking of emotions. In between the true emotional expression would always start showing up until the character triggers an expression to replace it. The closer the value is to 1 the less time the true emotional expression would be visible to others.

Table 1. Defining the partial poker-face

Child's face	Partial Poker-Face	Poker-Face
• purely affective emotional expressive behaviour	• Conscious deceiving of emotions possible • Can be noticed through "leaking" emotions!	• True emotions never shown subconsciously! • Can only be revealed by deep reasoning!
What we have!	What we want!	Considered unrealistic!

We defined two scenarios for evaluation. The first scenario features a woman encountering a slightly aggressive man. The man asks for change claiming that he has lost his wallet. This scenario will show if spectators can spot suppressed emotional expressions without prior anticipation and how much leakage is necessary for this to happen. The second scenario shows a graffiti-sprayer nearly getting caught in action. The culprit has good reason to hide his guilt resulting in an obvious case of deception. As a consequence spectators will have clearer anticipations about the characters future behavior. Evaluation is looking for the spectator's emotional engagement, compared to using a "child's face"-approach. We also will evaluate the change in perceived naturalism of the displayed behaviour asking spectators to reason about the expressive behaviour displayed by the character.

3 Proposed Model

The basis of the Partial Poker-Face is the concept of a closed body-mind loop similar to [12] (see also Fig. 1). Being able to reason about own affective expressions allows characters to react to their own subconscious emotions. Further intrinsic events (Fig. 1) allows for perceiving upcoming affective expressions much earlier.

We will adapt simulation based ToM as defined in [13] for our model. Meaningful decision to hide emotions requires the character to have expectations about how the hidden emotion would affect perception of self. Also the character should be able to reason about the possible effect the desired expression will have.

The model further generates a dynamic interplay between affective and cognitive computing. Quick and slow thinking, as defined by Kahneman [14], is expected to

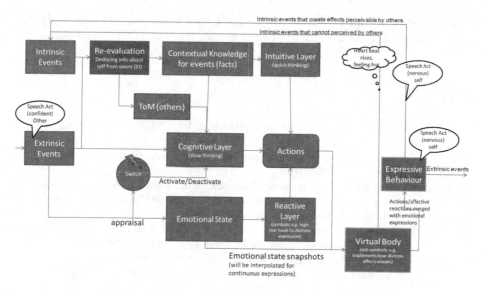

Fig. 1. Proposed model overview

produce more naturalistic behaviour in extreme situations. This introduces two systems of cognitive processes working at different speed and competence. Upon recognising their most intense emotions the characters will thus either use quick thinking (Intuitive Layer in Fig. 1) or slow thinking (Cognitive Layer in Fig. 1), when revealing their true emotions is not an option.

Quick thinking will be modelled as a rule based approach using contextual facts (variables) and common sense (semantic rules). *Quick thinking* only triggers a priori defined intuitive reactions encouraged by certain situations. The rules are created by generalisation and might lead to incomplete conclusions. Applicable situations are

- High cognitive pressure situations (time)
- High emotional arousal situation
- Unclear situation (confusion)

In a less demanding situation the character can try to switch to *slow thinking*. In this mode the character can use their full Cognitive Layer to seek for more appropriate reactions. ToM allows predicting how the altered perception of self changes the emotions of others - assuming everyone will appraise the selected expression the same way as oneself. In EI this skill is called "regulating emotions of others" [10].

Whether the character can utilize only quick thinking or also slow thinking is determined by a switch (Fig. 1). If the character's most intense emotions exceed a threshold, set by its level of emotional awareness, the Cognitive Layer (see Fig. 1) will be deactivated till the emotional arousal has again decayed below the threshold.

To visualize: In the moment our Sprayer is caught he feels both intense surprise and fear. Both emotions will foster quick thinking with their intensity crossing the threshold. Fear makes him show signs of nervousness (both intrinsic and extrinsic events). Intuitively he tries to mitigate the situation by hiding his fear (e.g. look friendly) waiting for the emotional arousal going back below the threshold. Only then he finally can use ToM in order to figure a smooth way out of the situation.

References

1. Breazeal, C.: Emotion and sociable humanoid robots. Int. J. Hum. Comput. Stud. **59**, 119–155 (2003)
2. Paiva, A., et al.: Learning by feeling: evoking empathy with synthetic characters. Appl. Artif. Intell. **19**(3), 235–266 (2005)
3. de Melo, C.M., Gratch, J.: Expression of emotions using wrinkles, blushing, sweating and tears. In: Ruttkay, Z., Kipp, M., Nijholt, A., Vilhjálmsson, H.H. (eds.) IVA 2009. LNCS, vol. 5773, pp. 188–200. Springer, Heidelberg (2009)
4. Lance, B., Marsella, S.: Glances, glares, and glowering: how should a virtual human express emotion through gaze? Auton. Agent. Multi-Agent Syst. **20**(1), 50–69 (2010)
5. Becker-Asano, C., Wachsmuth, I.: Affective computing with primary and secondary emotions in a virtual human. Auton. Agent. Multi-Agent Syst. **20**(1), 32–49 (2010)
6. Poggi, I., Niewiadomski, R., Pelachaud, C.: Facial deception in humans and ecas. In: Wachsmuth, I., Knoblich, G. (eds.) ZiF Research Group International Workshop. LNCS (LNAI), vol. 4930, pp. 198–221. Springer, Heidelberg (2008)
7. Rehm, M., André, E.: Catch me if you can: exploring lying agents in social settings. In: Proceedings of the Fourth International Joint Conference on Autonomous Agents and Multiagent Systems, pp. 937–944. ACM (2005)
8. Hasada, R.: Some aspects of Japanese cultural ethos embedded in nonverbal communicative behaviour. In: Poyatos, F. (ed.) New Perspectives And Challenges In Literature, Interpretation And The Media, vol. 17, p. 83. John Benjamins, Amsterdam (1997)
9. Van Kleef, G.A.: Emotion in conflict and negotiation: introducing the emotions as social information (EASI) model. In: IACM 2007 Meetings Paper (2007)
10. Salovey, P., Mayer, J.D.: Emotional intelligence. Imagin. Cognit. Pers. **9**(3), 185–211 (1989)
11. Goldberg, L.R.: an alternative description of personality: the big-five factor structure. J. Pers. Soc. Psychol. **59**(6), 1216 (1990)
12. Ribeiro, T., Vala, M., Paiva, A.: Thalamus: closing the mind-body loop in interactive embodied characters. In: Nakano, Y., Neff, M., Paiva, A., Walker, M. (eds.) IVA 2012. LNCS, vol. 7502, pp. 189–195. Springer, Heidelberg (2012)
13. Dias, J., Aylett, R., Paiva, A., Reis, H.: The great deceivers: virtual agents and believable lies. In: Proceedings of CogSci2013, pp. 2189–2194 (2013)
14. Shleifer, A.: Psychologists at the gate: a review of daniel kahneman's thinking, fast and slow. J. Econ. Lit. **50**(4), 1–12 (2012)

Emotionally Augmented Storytelling Agent

The Effects of Dimensional Emotion Modeling for Agent Behavior Control

Sangyoon Lee[1]([⊠]), Andrew E. Johnson[2], Jason Leigh[2],
Luc Renambot[2], Steve Jones[3], and Barbara Di Eugenio[2]

[1] Connecticut College, New London, CT, USA
james.lee@conncoll.edu
[2] College of Engineering, University of Illinois at Chicago, Chicago, IL, USA
{ajohnson, spiff, renambot, bdieugen}@uic.edu
[3] College of Liberal Arts and Sciences, University of Illinois at Chicago,
Chicago, IL, USA
sjones@uic.edu

Abstract. The study presented in this paper focuses on a dimensional theory to augment agent nonverbal behavior including emotional facial expression and head gestures to evaluate subtle differences in fine-grained conditions in the context of emotional storytelling. The result of a user study in which participants rated perceived naturalness for seven different conditions showed significantly higher preference for the augmented facial expression whereas the head gesture model received mixed ratings: significant preference in high arousal cases (happy) but not significant in low arousal cases (sad).

Keywords: Virtual humans · Intelligent agents · Dimensional theory · PAD

1 Introduction

Recently, many research efforts toward natural and affective virtual agent capabilities have been undertaken [1]. Several studies have shown that a naturally behaving agent capable of interaction becomes more effective. For example Burgoon and Hoobler pointed out that more than 50 % of social meaning in our communication is carried via nonverbal cues [2]. Although positive effects of emotional agent behavior have been established, it is still challenging to design a computational model for such behaviors.

Dimensional theories of emotion have motivated many prior studies to build a computational model to assess an agent's emotional state and provide a framework to map human emotion in one or more dimensions. To this end the Pleasure-Arousal-Dominance (PAD) model [3] provides well-formed computational foundations. The significance of the PAD model is that continuous changes in emotional state can support a smooth transition between discrete emotion eliciting stimuli. In particular, we investigate the capability of a dimensional model to control agent behavior in the context of storytelling. Given our interests, we have limited our exploration to evaluate the agent's ability to augment emotional behavior for stories

© Springer International Publishing Switzerland 2015
W.-P. Brinkman et al. (Eds.): IVA 2015, LNAI 9238, pp. 483–487, 2015.
DOI: 10.1007/978-3-319-21996-7_53

that dominantly elicit two categorical emotions, happy and sad. The presented model is compared to our previous system that shows a fixed intensity of facial expression and head gesture.

2 Approach: System Model

The nonverbal behavior processor (NVBP) in the system is composed of three components: the Affect Analyzer, the Emotion Processor, and the Gesture Processor.

The Affect Analyzer takes an utterance and executes part-of-speech tagging, affect extraction for words based on WordNet-Affect, and structural analysis to revise word level affect. The gesture predictor uses basic rules adapted from McClave [4] and a data-driven model trained with the SEMAINE video corpus to generate head gesture events. The NVB events are encoded for each word, fed to the speech synthesizer, and the synthesizer then synchronizes NVB events as an agent speaks.

The Emotion Processor takes an affect type event, then processes affect to update the agent's mood with the PAD model; finally, it computes the intensity of an emotional facial expression. PAD vector values are adapted from prior work [5], and the layered model is revised based on Gebhard and Kipp [6]. This final step is an augmentation that may increase or decrease the intensity of facial expression. The computational equations are shown below:

$$E_{evaluated} = e + c_t \times \|e\| \times T + c_a \sum E_{active} \tag{1}$$

$$M_{updated} = T + E_{evaluated} + \sum E_{active} \tag{2}$$

$$E_{intensity} = e_{intensity} \times \frac{\|E_{evaluated}\|}{\|e\|} + R(e) \tag{3}$$

Equation (1) describes how an initial PAD vector, e, is evaluated. c_t and c_a are constant factors toward trait and active emotion. The length of e is denoted by $\|e\|$. Trait vector T and currently active emotions E_{active}, and mood M, are applied to skew the initial vector. Equation (2) shows how the mood is updated based on newly added affect. It is a sum of trait, evaluated new emotion, and all active emotions in PAD. Equation (3) presents augmentation of new emotion to be sent to the facial expression synthesizer. The auxiliary effect, $R(e)$, accounts for repetition of the similar emotion.

When a gesture type event arrives from the speech synthesizer, the Gesture Processor refers to the arousal value of the current mood to compute the intensity of head gesture. For example, when one feels very depressed (low arousal), one may not show much head movement, whereas one may show intense gestures when the arousal value is high. The augmentation ranges from 25 % to 200 % of the baseline intensity.

3   Evaluation

To evaluate whether the presented model can increase the perceived naturalness of emotional facial expressions and head gestures, we designed seven conditions (Table 1). The intensity of facial expression and head gesture ranges from 0.0 to 1.0 as a weight value in our system to map it from no expression/gesture to the strongest expression/gesture. We chose a half intensity for control conditions to avoid extreme cases: intensity 0.0 or 1.0. We assume this as a moderate level of behavior for the system that does not have a computational model to reflect an agent's emotional state dynamically on agent's emotional behavior. A 10 % fixed intensity of a head gesture condition is added to compare very subtle head gesture with the presented model.

The study included three stories from psychological literature and blogs. Each story is a personal experience in the past [7, 8]. The system detected 14 emotion-eliciting words/phrases, 12 happy and 2 sad, and parsed 32 head gestures, 10 nods and 22 shakes in the first story (happy story). For the second story (sad story) a total of 12 emotion-eliciting words/phrases including 10 sad, 1 fear, and 1 surprise and a total of 44 head gestures, 23 nods and 21 shakes were processed. The results were fed to the system to create videos of an agent. The audio track was excluded to avoid the bias caused by audio cues. Instead, subtitles were embedded in the videos.

A total of 24 participants (18 male, mean age 32.61 with SD 11.15) were recruited in this study. The study was composed of three sessions: one training session and two test sessions. During each session, participants (1) read one of the written stories, (2) selected a primary emotion among the six basic emotions that they might feel if they were telling the story, (3) drew a graph depicting the intensity of the primary emotion, and (4) reviewed a video showing the seven conditions and rated them (Fig. 1). The rating was measured as a number of check marks that a participant gave to each condition when one or more agents seemed more realistic than others.

Rating Results. We performed the Wilcoxon signed-rank test to compare ratings between variables: combined cross-variable analysis for model vs. control group in both facial expression and head gesture. The model combined condition in story I for both facial expression ($C1$, $C2$, and $C3$) and head gesture ($C1$ and $C4$) was most preferred; its differences were significant ($p < .05$) except in the comparison with Control IV($C3$ and $C6$) case for head gesture. The model combined condition in story II for facial expression ($C1$, $C2$, and $C3$) was significantly higher than control groups ($p < .05$), whereas the head gesture case ($C1$ and $C4$) was not significant.

Table 1. Combinational behavior model conditions used in the study

Facial expression	Head gesture		
	Model (varied intensity)	Control III (fixed half intensity)	Control IV (fixed 10 % intensity)
Model (varied intensity)	C1	C2	C3
Control I (fixed half intensity)	C4	C5	C6
Control II (Control I w/abrupt transition)	n/a	C7	n/a

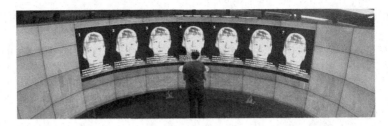

Fig. 1. A participant is reviewing virtual agents video on a large display system. Seven identical agents are telling the same story in sync with different conditions.

In summary, the presented model that can emotionally augment nonverbal behavior received significantly higher preference than the control conditions for facial expression. However, the head gesture model showed mixed results.

4   Conclusions

We designed a PAD space model to compute a virtual agent's emotional state to drive its behavior including facial expressions and head gestures. The presented model uses a shallow parsing of a surface text to extract emotion-eliciting stimuli and generates augmented behavior according to the agent's mood. The result of a user study confirmed that the facial expression model received a significantly higher rating than all control conditions that use fixed intensity of facial expression. However, our head gesture model showed mixed results. We found significant preference for the head gesture model in high arousal cases whereas we obtained meaningful but not significant ratings in low arousal cases. The difficulty of recognizing subtle gestures in low arousal cases may have contributed to the inconsistent rating as some participants noted naturalness of lessened head gesture in a sad/depressed mood. However, more focused future study is required to verify this interpretation.

References

1. Lee, J., Marsella, S.C.: Predicting speaker head nods and the effects of affective information. IEEE Trans. Multimedia **12**(6), 552–562 (2010)
2. Burgoon, J.K., Hoobler, G.D.: Nonverbal Signals. In: Knapp, M.L., Daly, J.A. (eds.) Handbook of interpersonal communication, pp. 240–299. SAGE Publications, Inc., Thousand Oaks (2002)
3. Mehrabian, A.: Pleasure-arousal-dominance: a general framework for describing and measuring individual differences in Temperament. Curr. Psychol. **14**, 261–292 (1996)
4. McClave, E.Z.: Linguistic functions of head movements in the context of speech. J. Pragmat. **32**(7), 855–878 (2000)
5. Zhang, S., Wu, Z., Meng, H.M., Cai, L.: Facial expression synthesis based on emotion dimensions for affective talking avatar. In: Nishida, T., Jain, L.C., Faucher, C. (eds.) Modeling Machine Emotions for Realizing Intelligence. SIST, vol. 1, pp. 109–132. Springer, Heidelberg (2010)

6. Gebhard, P., Kipp, K.H.: Are computer-generated emotions and moods plausible to humans? In: Gratch, J., Young, M., Aylett, R.S., Ballin, D., Olivier, P. (eds.) IVA 2006. LNCS (LNAI), vol. 4133, pp. 343–356. Springer, Heidelberg (2006)
7. DiMarco, L.: My minxy mouse encounter: Disney World. http://www.lolastravels.com/my-3-favorite-travel-memories
8. Ossorio, P.G.: Clinical topics: A seminar in Descriptive Psychology. Linguistic Research Institute, Whittier (1976)

Effect of a Virtual Agent's Contingent Smile Response on Perceived Social Status

Maryam Saberi[✉], Ulysses Bernardet, and Steve DiPaola

Simon Fraser University, Vancouver, Canada
{msaberi,ubernard,sdipaola}@sfu.ca

Abstract. We are investigating if an agent's contingent smile during an interaction with a human participant affects the impression of the virtual character's social status. Psychological studies show lower status individuals are more likely to show contingent feedback [4]. A "Rock-Paper-Scissors" game is used as the scenario to provide an infrastructure for an interaction between a 3D agent and a human participant. During the interaction we are using electromyographic measurements to determine when the human participant is smiling. Immediately after a detected smiling the virtual character mimics the smile. More specifically, we are expecting that participants form the impression that the character has a low social status when the agent shows contingent smiling behavior. We are currently performing the experiment and a next step is to evaluate the system by analyzing the results.

Keywords: IVA · Social status · Contingent smile · Nonverbal behavior

1 Introduction

Intelligent virtual agents (IVA) are more believable if their social behavior are convincing. One of the aspects of social behaviors is the way realistic style 3D character agents communicates social dominance. Behavior such as mimicking the facial expression of addressee in the interaction leads to the impression of submissiveness (lower social status) [4]. Successfully communicating the impression of social status through behaviors such as mimicking smile can reduce the frustration of participants interacting with the agent [2]. Our study, designs a scenario for the interaction between human and a 3D virtual character that provides appropriate context for evaluating the social status of the agent. We use electromyography (EMG) to measure the smile of the human participants in real-time without interference by the researches during the experiment [7]. The question of this study is if contingency of smile in 3D character agents has effect when it comes to creating feelings of low social status? We investigate if having the 3D agent mimicking smile of participants generates an impression of lower social status in comparison to a 3D agent which smiles with the same frequency but not synced with what the participant is doing. Our hypothesis is that IVA which shows contingent smile behavior creates an impression of low social status while interacting with a human participant. On the down side, since human behavior is complex, might not be easy to demonstrate the link between smile mimicry behavior and social status. The competitive nature of the game can affect the results. For

© Springer International Publishing Switzerland 2015
W.-P. Brinkman et al. (Eds.): IVA 2015, LNAI 9238, pp. 488–491, 2015.
DOI: 10.1007/978-3-319-21996-7_54

instance, participants infer IVA's smile after winning the game as a competitive behavior [5]. In future, we assess the effect of smile mimicry in impression of social status in a different scenario to measure the effect of the context. This research is a part of affective virtual humanoid character's model [8]. The model is designed to generate impression of different personality types through nonverbal behaviors of the agent. Thus, generating impression of social status is addressing the social aspect of the personality traits.

2 Computational Background on Expressing Social Status Through Nonverbal Behavior

Prior psychological experiments indicate that facial expressions such as "smile", "eye gaze" and "head tilt" are used to express social status. Following are some of the studies done so far on how nonverbal behavior (specifically mimicking smile of the addressee in an interaction) communicates social status. Lance & Marsella found that a virtual character with a raised head and fast movements is interpreted as more dominant while a bowed head was correlated with impression of submissiveness [6]. As mentioned before, Gratch et al. define contingent feedback as nonverbal movements (e.g., nods or posture shifts) that are tightly coupled to what the speaker is doing in the moment and non-contingent feedback as listener movements that share the same frequency and characteristics of contingent feedback but is not synced with what the speaker is doing [1]. Gratch et al. showed the effect of contingent behavior on harmony and flow is felt engaging in a good conversation [1]. Burleson and Picard used an agent showing sensor-driven non-verbal mirroring with one showing pre-recorded non-verbal interactions to investigate the effect of elements of an affective learning companion's emotional intelligence on participants [2]. There is a lack of work on investigating the effect of contingent smile on impression of social status for IVA. Additionally, most of studies in this area are concentrated on evaluating static images of IVAs while we designed a scenario for human and IVA interaction (specifically 3D realistically rendered and animated real-time IVA). This scenario gives us an infrastructure to experiment the effect of mimicking smile in impression of social status in a social setting.

3 Approach

3.1 Implementation and Scenario

The game of Rock-Paper-Scissors is designed as the interaction scenario. Participants play the game in three sessions: Face-to-face, Responsive and Non-contingent. In face-to-face session, participants play with a confederate face to face. The confederate mimics the smile of the participants. In Responsive and Non-contingent sessions, participants play with the IVA which they see in a monitor in front of them as a full body IVA. IVA's hand gestures (rock, paper or scissors) in each phase are generated randomly. In the Responsive session, the IVA mimics the smile of the human

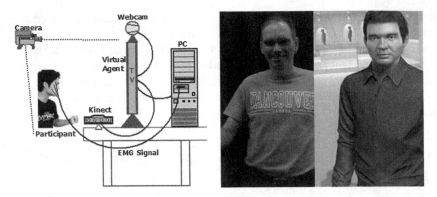

Fig. 1. A participant plays with IVA (right) [9] which behaves based on commands in receives from a Matlab application. A video camera records the interaction of both sides.

participants. In the Non-contingent session, the agent provides smiles with the same frequency but unsynchronized with the human participant's smile. In the Responsive session, an electromyographic (EMG) sensor is used to capture the smile of the participants [7]. In both the Responsive and Non-contingent conditions, data glove sensors are used to capture the hand gesture of the human participant. Matlab simulates the game and sends commands to animate the 3D virtual character and updates the GUI (Fig. 1). Smartbody (Thiebaux et al., 2008) an academic real-time 3D character animation toolkit developed at the University of Southern California's ITC lab is used as our 3D rendering system [9].

3.2   Experimental Procedure and Questionnaires

At the end of each session (Responsive, Face-to-face and Non-contingent), the participant evaluates the social status of the other player using a social status questionnaire. Six adjective pairs from Mehrabian and Russell's Semantic Differential Scale for dominance are used to evaluate the social status [3]. Additionally, we add a question asking how friendly participants thought IVA was to measure the effect of smile mimicry in the impression of friendliness. Participants will go through the three sessions with different order to avoid the order effect. In each of these sessions, the 10 rounds of Rock-Paper-Scissor game are played. In both Responsive and Non-contingent sessions, EMG sensors are attached to the face. Only in the Responsive session are the EMG values are actually used. In the Responsive and Non-contingent sessions, participants see an IVA displayed on a TV monitor derived by our 3D model. The social status scale is presented to participants after each session. A manipulation check will be conducted with an independent sample of 10 students to make sure EMG sensors correctly detect the smile, virtual agent correspondingly mimics the smile, and it is recognizable by participants. Participants will check the plausibility of IVA's smile behavior using a designed GUI while the participants' face and IVA's face are video recorded and experimenters will check the accuracy of mimic behavior after the sessions.

4 Summery and Conclusion

In this study, we expect that the IVA's contingent smile during interaction with human participants, affects the impression participants have of the virtual character's social status. We believe participants get an impression that the IVA has a low social status when the agent shows contingent smile behavior. Successfully communicating the impression of social status through behaviors such as mimicking smile can reduce the frustration of participants interacting with the agent [2]. We are currently performing the designed experiment and a next step is to evaluate the system by analyzing the results. In future, we aim to address generating the impression of social status through gestures, e.g. head and gaze movement and facial expressions, to get a more believable and persuasive behavior.

References

1. Gratch, J., Wang, N., Gerten, J., Fast, E., Duffy, R.: Creating rapport with virtual agents. In: Pelachaud, C., Martin, J.-C., André, E., Chollet, G., Karpouzis, K., Pelé, D. (eds.) IVA 2007. LNCS (LNAI), vol. 4722, pp. 125–138. Springer, Heidelberg (2007)
2. Burleson, W., Picard, R.W.: Evidence for gender specific approaches to the development of emotionally intelligent learning companions. In: IEEE Intelligent Systems, Special Issue on Intelligent Educational Systems, July/August 2007
3. Mehrabian, A., Russell, J.A.: An Approach to Environmental Psychology. MIT, Cambridge (1974)
4. Tiedens, L.Z., Fragale, A.R.: Power moves: complementarity in dominant and submissive nonverbal behavior. J. Pers. Soc. Psychol. 84(3), 558 (2003)
5. Lanzetta, J.T., Englis, B.G.: Expectations of cooperation and competition and their effects on observers' vicarious emotional responses. J. Pers. Soc. Psychol. 56(4), 543 (1989)
6. Lance, B., Marsella, S.C.: The relation between gaze behavior and the attribution of emotion: an empirical study. In: Prendinger, H., Lester, J.C., Ishizuka, M. (eds.) IVA 2008. LNCS (LNAI), vol. 5208, pp. 1–14. Springer, Heidelberg (2008)
7. Blumenthal, T.D., Cuthbert, B.N., Filion, D.L., Hackley, S., Lipp, O.V., Van Boxtel, A.: Committee report: guidelines for human startle eyeblink electromyographic studies. Psychophysiology 42(1), 1–15 (2005)
8. Saberi, M., Bernardet, U., DiPaola, S.: An architecture for personality-based, nonverbal behavior in affective virtual humanoid character. Procedia Comput. Sci. 41, 204–211 (2014)
9. Thiebaux, M., Marsella, S., Marshall, A.N., Kallmann, M.: Smartbody: behavior realization for embodied conversational agents. In: Proceedings of the 7th International Joint Conference on Autonomous Agents and Multiagent Systems, vol. 1, pp. 151–158. International Foundation for Autonomous Agents and Multiagent Systems, May 2008

Author Index

Printed in the United States
By Bookmasters